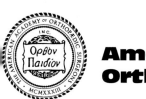

American Academy of Orthopaedic Surgeons

M. Prince, M.D.

OKU

Orthopaedic Knowledge Update

Foot and Ankle 2

American Academy of Orthopaedic Surgeons

OKU

Orthopaedic Knowledge Update

Edited by

Mark S. Mizel, MD
Associate Professor
Boston Medical Center
Boston University
Boston, Massachusetts

Richard A. Miller, MD
Associate Professor
Chief, Foot and Ankle Service
Department of Orthopaedics
University of New Mexico
Albuquerque, New Mexico

Mark W. Scioli, MD
Associate Clinical Professor
Texas Tech Health Sciences Center
Center for Orthopaedic Surgery
Lubbock, Texas

American Orthopaedic
Foot and Ankle Society

Foot and Ankle 2

Developed by the American Orthopaedic Foot and Ankle Society

Published 1998
by the American Academy of Orthopaedic Surgeons™
6300 North River Road
Rosemont, Illinois 60018
1-800-626-6726

Second Edition

Library of Congress Cataloging-in-Publication Data

Orthopaedic knowledge update. Foot and ankle/edited by Mark S. Mizel; developed by the American Orthopaedic Foot and Ankle Society.–2nd ed.

p. cm.

Includes bibliographical references and index.

ISBN 0-89203-178-6

1. Foot–Diseases. 2. Ankle–Diseases. I. Mizel, Mark S. II. American Orthopaedic Foot and Ankle Society.

[DNLM: 1. Foot Diseases. 2. Foot Injuries. 3. Foot Deformities. 4. Ankle Injuries. 5. Orthopedics–methods. WE 880077 1998]

RD781.027 1998
617.5'85–dc21
DNLM/DLC   98-38633
for Library of Congress   CIP

v

Acknowledgments

Orthopaedic Knowledge Update Foot and Ankle 2 Editorial Board

Mark S. Mizel, MD

Richard A. Miller, MD

Mark W. Scioli, MD

American Orthopaedic Foot and Ankle Society Board of Directors, 1998-1999

Ronald W. Smith, MD
President

Thomas O. Clanton, MD
President-Elect

Michael J. Shereff, MD
Vice President

Glenn B. Pfeffer, MD
Secretary

E. Greer Richardson, MD
Treasurer

James A. Nunley, MD
G. James Sammarco, MD
Donald E. Baxter, MD
Past Presidents

Robert B. Anderson, MD
Judith Smith, MD
Members at large

American Academy of Orthopaedic Surgeons Board of Directors, 1998

James D. Heckman, MD
President

Robert D. D'Ambrosia, MD
First Vice President

S. Terry Canale, MD
Second Vice President

William J. Robb III, MD
Secretary

Stuart A. Hirsch, MD
Treasurer

John A. Bergfeld, MD
Alvin H. Crawford, MD
Kenneth E. DeHaven, MD
Douglas W. Jackson, MD
Aaron G. Rosenberg, MD
Thomas P. Schmalzried, MD
Scott B. Scutchfield, MD
William A. Sims, MD
Vernon T. Tolo, MD
John R. Tongue, MD
Edward A. Toriello, MD
William W. Tipton, Jr., MD, (Ex Officio)

Staff

Marilyn L. Fox, PhD
Director, Department of Publications

Bruce Davis, Senior Editor

Joan Abern, Senior Editor

Lisa Moore, Associate Senior Editor

Loraine Edwalds, Production Manager

Sophie Tosta, Assistant Production Manager

Pamela Hutton Erickson, Graphic Design Coordinator

Jana Ronayne, Production Assistant

Geraldine Dubberke, Production Assistant

Alice Levine, Editorial Assistant

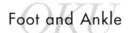
Contributors

David W. Alford, MD
Southern Bone and Joint Specialists
Dothan, Alabama

Richard G. Alvarez, MD
Director, Southern Orthopaedic
  Foot and Ankle Center
University of Tennessee
Department of Orthopaedic Surgery
Chattanooga, Tennessee

Douglas N. Beaman, MD
Director, Foot and Ankle Service
Portland Orthopedic Clinic
Portland, Oregon

Avrill Roy Berkman, MD
Assistant Clinical Professor
  of Orthopaedic Surgery
University of Medicine and Dentistry
  of New Jersey
Newark, New Jersey

James L. Beskin, MD
Assistant Clinical Professor
  of Orthopaedics
Tulane University
Peachtree Orthopedic Clinic
Atlanta, Georgia

Jeffrey T. Brodie, MD
Towson Orthopaedic Associates
Baltimore, Maryland

Loretta B. Chou, MD
Assistant Professor
Division of Orthopaedic Surgery
Stanford University
Stanford, California

Michael J. Coughlin, MD
Clinical Professor of Surgery
Division of Orthopaedics
Oregon Health Science University
Portland, Oregon

Gail P. Dalton, MD
Peachtree Orthopaedic Clinic
Piedmont Hospital
Atlanta, Georgia

Norman L. Donati, Jr, MD
Orthopaedic Surgeon
Upson Orthopaedic Clinic
Thomaston, Georgia

Keith C. Donatto, MD
Assistant Professor of Orthopaedic Surgery
Chief, Foot and Ankle Division
Department of Orthopaedic Surgery
Louisiana State University Medical Center
New Orleans, Louisiana

John E. Femino, MD
Clinical Assistant Professor
Department of Surgery
Section of Orthopaedic Surgery
University of Michigan
Ann Arbor, Michigan

Mark J. Geppert, MD
Orthopaedic Surgeon
Orthopaedic and Trauma Specialists
Somersworth, New Hampshire

Stanley C. Graves, MD
Institute for Bone and Joint Disorders
Phoenix, Arizona

Paul J. Hecht, MD
Assistant Professor, Orthopaedic Surgery
Allegheny University of the Health Sciences
Philadelphia, Pennsylvania

Greg A. Horton, MD
Assistant Professor
Director, Adult Foot and Ankle Service
Section of Orthopaedic Surgery
Kansas University Medical Center
Kansas City, Kansas

David A. Katcherian, MD
Senior Staff Physician
Department of Orthopaedic Surgery
Henry Ford Hospital
Detroit, Michigan

Todd A. Kile, MD
Assistant Professor of Orthopaedics
Mayo Medical School
Consultant, Department of Orthopaedic Surgery
Chair, Division of Foot and Ankle Surgery
Mayo Clinic Scottsdale
Scottsdale, Arizona

Thomas H. Lee, MD
Department of Orthopedics
Ohio Orthopedic Institute
  at Grant Medical Center
Columbus, Ohio

Janet E. Lewis, MD
Foot and Ankle Fellow
Department of Orthopaedics
Baylor College of Medicine
Houston, Texas

Sheldon S. Lin, MD
Assistant Professor of Orthopedic Surgery
Department of Orthopedic Surgery
University of Medicine and Dentistry
  of New Jersey
Newark, New Jersey

James P. Little, MD, MBA
Chairman and Medical Director
Siskin Hospital for Physical Rehabilitation
Department of Physical Medicine and
  Rehabilitation
University of Tennessee College of Medicine
Chattanooga, Tennessee

Jeffrey A. Mann, MD
Orthopaedic Surgery
Oakland, California

Roger A. Mann, MD
Director, Foot Fellowship Program
Oakland, California

Thomas P. Martin, MD
Assistant Professor of Radiology
Department of Radiology
University of New Mexico
Albuquerque, New Mexico

John V. Marymont, MD
Assistant Professor
Team Physician
University of Houston NCAAI
Orthopaedic Consultant
Houston Astros Major League Baseball
Baylor College of Medicine
Houston, Texas

James D. Michelson, MD
Associate Professor
Department of Orthopaedic Surgery
Johns Hopkins
Baltimore, Maryland

Richard A. Miller, MD
Associate Professor
Chief, Foot and Ankle Service
Department of Orthopaedics
University of New Mexico
Albuquerque, New Mexico

Mark S. Mizel, MD
Associate Professor
Boston Medical Center
Boston University
Boston, Massachusetts

David Prieskorn, DO
Assistant Clinical Professor
Michigan State University
College of Osteopathic Medicine
Farmington Hills, Michigan

John F. Ritterbusch, MD
Associate Medical Director
Associate Professor, Orthopaedics
 and Pediatrics
University of New Mexico
 Health Services Center
Carrie Tingley Hospital
Albuquerque, New Mexico

Charles L. Saltzman, MD
Associate Professor
Orthopaedic Surgery
University of Iowa
Iowa City, Iowa

Mark W. Scioli, MD
Associate Clinical Professor
Texas Tech Health Sciences Center and
 Center for Orthopaedic Surgery
Lubbock, Texas

Sean P. Scully, MD, PhD
Associate Professor
 of Orthopaedic Surgery and Cell Biology
Department of Surgery
Division of Orthopaedic Surgery
Duke University Medical Center
Durham, North Carolina

H. Thomas Temple, MD
Associate Clinical Professor
 of Orthopaedic Surgery
Department of Orthopaedic Surgery
 and Rehabilitation
University of Miami
Miami, Florida

David B. Thordarson, MD
Associate Professor
Chief, Foot and Ankle Trauma
 and Reconstructive Surgery
USC Department of Orthopaedics
USC School of Medicine
Los Angeles, California

Keith L. Wapner, MD
Professor and Director
Division of Foot and Ankle Surgery
Orthopaedic Surgery
Allegheny University of the Health Sciences
Philadelphia, Pennsylvania

Marilyn L. Yodlowski, MD, PhD
Section Chief, Foot and Ankle Orthopedics
Boston Foot and Ankle Center
New England Baptist Hospital
Boston, Massachusetts

Table of Contents

OKU Orthopaedic Knowledge Update

Foot and Ankle 2

Preface

The cycle of specialty-oriented Orthopaedic Knowledge Update volumes was completed with the publication of *Orthopaedic Knowledge Update: Shoulder and Elbow.* This volume, the new and updated edition of *Orthopaedic Knowledge Update: Foot and Ankle,* replaces the original, published in 1994. Like the preceding foot and ankle OKU, this book offers the readers a carefully chosen selection of the most up-to-date information, designed to be of use to orthopaedic surgeons who must treat various foot and ankle problems in patients ranging in age from infancy to old age.

We would especially like to thank our individual contributors for the energy and devotion they have shown in sharing their special knowledge with our readers. Also to be thanked for their conscientious efforts in editing and producing this text are the Academy's staff: Bruce Davis, who edited the manuscripts; Sophie Tosta, who coordinated the manuscript review and permissions process; Loraine Edwalds, who supervised the production efforts; and Pamela Erickson, who created the design. We are also deeply grateful to Marilyn Bartlett and Yolanda Lopez from our offices.

As with the previous book, we hope that you, the reader, will find this to be a rich source of information as you seek to update your knowledge of the foot and ankle.

Mark S. Mizel, MD

Richard A. Miller, MD

Mark W. Scioli, MD

Chapter 1
Foot and Ankle Biomechanics

Introduction

Understanding the biomechanics of the foot and ankle is the key to the clinical ability to diagnose and treat problems of this region. As will be demonstrated, a fundamental understanding of the normal and abnormal motions of the various joints and the interrelations between the structures of the foot and ankle allows one to efficiently deduce the underlying etiology of the clinical syndromes that frequently present to the orthopaedic surgeon. This chapter will first endeavor to present the basic terminology, kinematics, and biomechanics of the individual structures of the foot and ankle and for gait overall. These basic principles will then be illustrated via clinical examples.

Kinematics

Kinematics refers to the motion of the joints. In discussing kinematics of joints, 2 basic concepts arise. The first is that any joint can have motions in several planes at the same time. As such, these joints are considered to have a primary plane of motion (such as plantarflexion/dorsiflexion for the ankle) and associated coupled motions in the other plane (such as internal/external rotation in the transaxial plane and varus/valgus in the coronal plane). Implicit in this understanding is the second basic concept, which is that all these motions can be described in terms of 3 perpendicular planes.

These planes are the sagittal, transaxial, and coronal (or frontal) planes. For the ankle, the motions described in these planes are referred to as plantarflexion/dorsiflexion (sagittal plane), internal rotation/external rotation (axial plane), and varus/valgus (coronal plane). The literature is somewhat confusing regarding the description of motions of the hindfoot, midfoot, and forefoot. Much of the ambiguity can be eliminated, however, by using the same reference planes as for the ankle. Therefore, the midfoot and forefoot can be described as having plantarflexion and dorsiflexion in the sagittal plane, abduction and adduction in the axial plane, and supination and pronation in the coronal plane (Table 1). Relating these motions, particularly supination and pronation, to a coordinate reference system eliminates many of the arguments about the differentiation of pronation and supination from inversion and eversion. Because the kinematics of the midfoot and hindfoot joints are understood only in the grossest sense, arguments about such things as the relationship between inversion and supination are somewhat pointless. By referring to an invariant coordinate system of reference planes, the language of communication is rendered unambiguous.

The function of various joints can be gleaned from the plane of their primary motions. For the ankle this is plantarflexion and dorsiflexion, with small contributions of internal-external rotation and varus-valgus through the entire range of motion in the sagittal plane (Fig. 1). For the subtalar joint (Fig. 2), the plane of motion is a modified coronal plane that is externally rotated (on average 67°) and plantar

Table 1
Terminology for motions of the foot and ankle*

	Coronal	Axial	Sagittal
Ankle	Varus/valgus	Internal/external rotation	Plantarflexion/dorsiflexion
Hindfoot	Inversion/eversion	Internal/external rotation	Plantarflexion/dorsiflexion
Midfoot/Forefoot	Supination/pronation, varus/valgus	Adduction/abduction	Plantarflexion/dorsiflexion

* Previous texts have described pronation/supination as an undefined combination of varus/valgus and adduction/abduction. In order to reduce ambiguity in descriptions, this table defines supination/pronation as occurring in the coronal motion plane. Supination/pronation can therefore be defined independent of motions in the other two planes (axial and sagittal). Alternatively, the terms supination and pronation can be complertely discarded in favor of varus and valgus, respectively

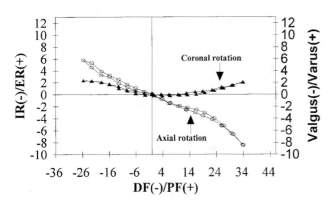

Figure 1

Coupled coronal and axial plane motion that occurs with sagittal ankle motion (plantarflexion-dorsiflexion). As the ankle plantarflexes, the talus internally rotates and goes into slight varus. In dorsiflexion, the talus externally rotates and, again, moves into slight varus.

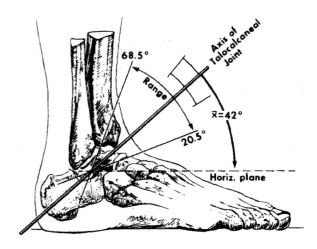

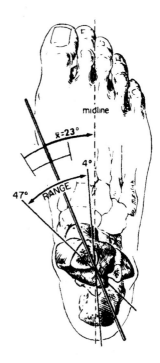

Figure 2

Axis of subtalar joint motion. The axis of motion is perpendicular to the plane of motion, as described in the text. (Adapted with permission from Inman T (ed): *The Joints of the Ankle.* Baltimore, MD, Williams & Wilkins, 1976, p 37.)

flexed (average of 48° from the vertical). There are, in addition, small contributions of plantarflexion/dorsiflexion as well as varus and valgus that occur at the three articulations of the subtalar joint. At Chopart's joint (the transverse tarsal joint consisting of the talonavicular and calcaneocuboid joints) the primary plane of motion is abduction and adduction, with a substantial amount of plantarflexion/dorsiflexion and varus/valgus also occurring. At the transverse tarsometatarsal (Lisfranc) joint, the primary plane of motion is plantarflexion/dorsiflexion, with a very small amount of varus/valgus occurring, and almost no abduction-adduction.

There are many interactions that occur between the primary and coupled motions of each joint as well as between the various joints of the hindfoot. The ankle provides a good example of the first instance. Here, it is well recognized that overtightening a syndesmosis screw will limit dorsiflexion. Although this is typically viewed as a simple sagittal plane obstruction, in reality what is occurring is that the overtightened syndesmosis is limiting external rotation of the talus. External rotation is a normal coupled motion of dorsiflexion of the ankle. Therefore, disruption of the coupled motion will prevent the primary motion from occurring. An example of the second instance is the relationship between Chopart's joint and the subtalar joint. Here, it has been demonstrated that limiting pronation and supination of Chopart's joint by fusing the talonavicular joint will substantially reduce similar motion at the subtalar joint. On the other hand, in situ fusion of the calcaneocuboid joint, which does not similarly inhibit Chopart pronation and supination, has relatively little effect on the resultant motion at the subtalar joint.

Gait

The teleologic reason for the existence of the foot and ankle is to provide a connection between the lower limb and the ground during gait. The mechanical characteristics of the linkage provided by the foot and ankle between the leg and the ground varies according to the needs particular to each phase of gait. The gait cycle is classically broken into 4 distinct segments: heel strike, foot flat, toe-off, and swing. The first 3 comprise the period of limb support, or stance phase, and account for roughly 60% of the entire gait cycle for each limb (Fig. 3). There are 2 elements to the characterization of each phase of the gait cycle. The first is the delineation of the dynamic muscular control of the foot and ankle, which is well demonstrated by electromyographic (EMG) activity of the motor tendon units that control the ankle and foot. The end result of the muscular control is the second element, that being the changing mechanical characteristics of the foot and ankle as it progresses through each cycle.

The EMG data (Fig. 4) can be summarized as follows: During heel strike, the anterior muscle groups of the leg are active to control the progression from heel strike to foot flat. This also serves to absorb energy during heel strike as eccentric lengthening of the extensor motor tendon units occurs during this transition. As the foot moves into the foot flat phase, the anterior muscle groups stop firing and are replaced by activity primarily in the tibialis posterior, which acts to stabilize the foot to prevent overpronation. The peroneal muscle group is recruited at this time to provide varus stability to the hindfoot as the ankle dorsiflexes. The action of the tibialis posterior also initiates push-off at the end of the foot flat stage as the gastrocnemius-soleus complex is also activated and heel rise initiated to progress to toe-off. During the toe-off phase, the calf muscles are firing maximally. Once swing phase is initiated, the gastrocnemius-

Phasic Activity of Muscles During Gait

Muscle Group	0% Heel Strike	7% Foot Flat	30% Heel Rise	60% Toe Off	100% Heel Strike
Tibialis Anterior	███			████	████
Ext. Digitorum Longus	███			████	████
Ext. Hallucis Longus	████			████	████
Gastro-soleus		████	████		
Tibialis Posterior		████	████		
Flex. Digitorum Longus		████	████		
Flex. Hallucis Longus			████		
Peroneus Longus			████	██	
Peroneus Brevis			████	██	
Flex. Hallucis Brevis		████	████		
Ext. Digitorum Brevis		████	████		

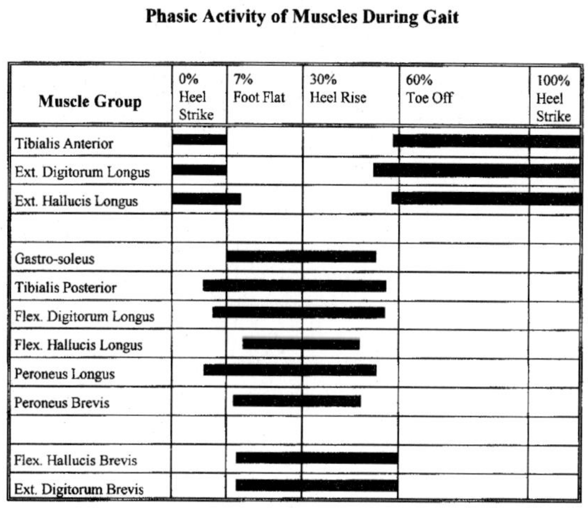

Figure 4

Electromyographic activity of lower leg muscles during gait. The dark line denotes the period of activity for each muscle. (Adapted with permission from Sarrafian SK (ed): *Anatomy of the Foot and Ankle.* New York, NY, JB Lippincott, 1983, p 423.)

soleus complex and other plantarflexors cease firing, and the tibialis anterior and long toe extensors activate to bring the foot out of plantarflexion into dorsiflexion in preparation for the next heel strike.

Complementary to the muscular activity participating in the gait cycle are the changing structural characteristics of the foot and ankle through the phases of stance. During heel strike, the foot is pronated, which serves to unlock Chopart's joint. The flexible midfoot structure that results is optimal for the energy absorption required during the load acceptance phase of gait. The foot is put into a pronation mode by the internal rotation of the leg, which acts through the subtalar joint to cause hindfoot valgus (Fig. 5). This also means that the initial weightbearing region is medial to the midline axis of the foot. As gait progresses to the foot flat stage, the leg rotates externally, which causes midfoot supination via torque conversion at the subtalar joint. This locking mechanism provides a stable platform on which the weight of the body can be supported. This is a critical transition, because failure to establish a rigid midfoot structure will markedly compromise the ability of the foot to bear weight. The weightbearing axis at this time moves laterally on the foot, which is a result of both the external rotation of the leg and the supination of the foot.

As the leg progresses from foot flat to toe-off, the supination of the foot is accentuated by continuing external rotation of the leg, and by the introduction of a new mechanism, the windlass mechanism, which is the name given to the interaction between dorsiflexion of the great toe and

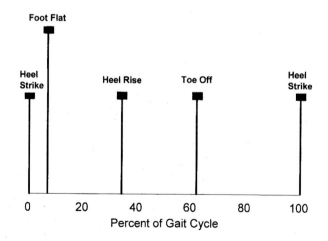

Figure 3

Important landmarks of the gait cycle for a single foot. Between heel strike and toe-off, the foot is in the stance phase. Between toe-off and the second heel strike, the leg is in the swing phase.

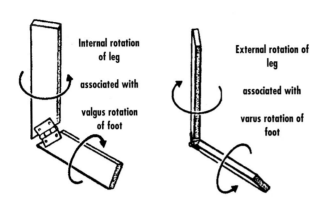

Figure 5
Proposed coupling of leg rotation and foot position through the ankle/subtalar joint complex. (Adapted with permission from Inman TV: *The Joints of the Ankle.* Baltimore, MD, Williams & Wilkins, 1976, p 77.)

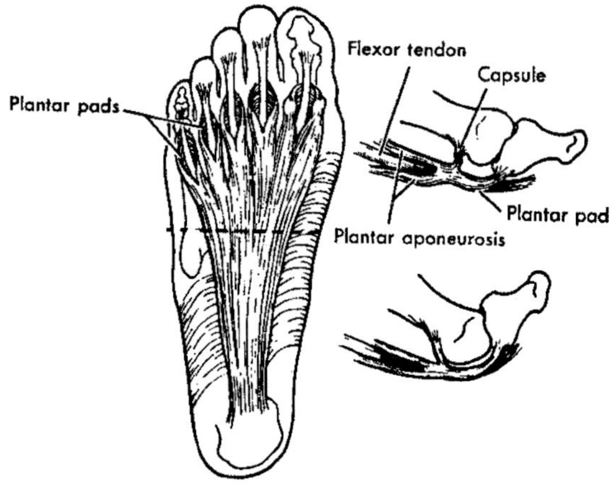

Figure 6
Anatomy of the windlass mechanism. The anterior insertion of the plantar fascia into the flexor mechanism of the hallux is depicted on the left. Progression of the hallux from neutral to dorsiflexion (from upper right to lower right) tightens the plantar fascia, thereby decreasing arch length, thereby increasing arch height. (Adapted with permission from Mann RA, Coughlin MJ (eds): *Surgery of the Foot and Ankle,* ed 6. St. Louis, MO, CV Mosby, 1993, p 26.)

increased tension placed on the plantar fascia (Fig. 6). The plantar fascia originates at the anterior ridge of the inferior calcaneus and runs in the subcutaneous layer anteriorly to end in a broad insertion consisting of the planar plate of the first metatarsophalangeal joint as well as the lesser metatarsophalangeal joints. The orientation of this insertion is such that dorsiflexion of the first metatarsophalangeal joint pulls on the plantar fascia, which results in an increase in midfoot arch height. Consequently, the individual articulations of the Chopart joint become even more nonparallel, further stabilizing the midfoot.

Categorization of Clinical Problems Using Biomechanical Principles

Excepting cosmetic issues, the reasons that patients are seen by orthopaedic surgeons for foot and ankle problems can be characterized as a combination of pain and instability. This can include pain without symptoms of instability (ie, ankle arthritis), pain with instability (ie, lateral ligament incompetence of the ankle), or instability without pain (ie, peroneal motor weakness in Charcot-Marie-Tooth disease). It is critical to distinguish between these various entities, because each of them is emblematic of a different kind of biomechanical malfunction. What follows is a generalized algorithm to

guide the diagnosis and treatment of these problems, accompanied by specific clinical examples. It is assumed that nonmechanical causes of pain, such as infection or obvious unstable fractures, have also been appropriately evaluated and ruled out.

The most common presenting complaint is that of pain. In the absence of such causes as trauma or fracture, joint pain with weightbearing can be traced to 1 of 2 mechanical etiologies. Pain can result from a joint with normal articular surfaces, which is moving in an abnormal way. Although, strictly speaking, this implies some lack of stability, overt instability may be difficult to demonstrate. An example of this would be midfoot pain following an injury to the Lisfranc ligament, which permits abnormally large motion to occur at that joint during the foot flat and toe-off phases of gait. A similar, nontraumatic condition can exist at the Chopart joint, where increased motion occurs as a consequence of an ankle fusion. Under these circumstances, there is a gradual increase in Chopart joint plantarflexion and dorsiflexion in an attempt to compensate for the loss of such motion at the fused ankle joint. Once the biomechanical etiology of pain has been identified, the treatment becomes self-evident, in that it is aimed at reducing or eliminating these abnormal motions. This explains the efficacy of adding a steel shank and rocker bottom sole to the shoe, both of which act to decrease midfoot sagittal motion.

A joint that is subject to normal motion and external forces can also be painful if the joint itself is abnormal at the articulating surfaces. This is probably the most common source of pain, as exemplified by an arthritic degenerated joint. At times, a single joint may cause pain as a result of abnormal motion as well as intrinsic intra-articular pathology. An example of this would be hallux rigidus, in which pain results from both the underlying arthritis and the limitation of dorsiflexion imposed by the secondary dorsal metatarsal osteophyte (Fig. 7). Clinically it may be impossible to distinguish between these sources of pain, but it is important to recognize both etiologies when planning the treatment and explaining the expected outcomes to the patient.

The other biomechanical category of clinical symptoms is instability, which can be either dynamic or static. Static instability includes joint malalignment, such as that seen in a distal tibiofibular fracture that has healed in varus. Alternatively, significant loss of passive restraints of a joint can also lead to static instability. An example of this is the hindfoot valgus that results from chronic posterior tibial tendon insufficiency with secondary loss of ligamentous restraints at the ankle and hindfoot (Fig. 8). What is interesting about these problems is that the patient may be able to overcome these static instabilities by invoking the use of dynamic stabilizers, such as tendons, during normal activities. This can mask the extent of the true instability. An excellent example of this is the patient with chronic lateral ankle ligament laxity who is

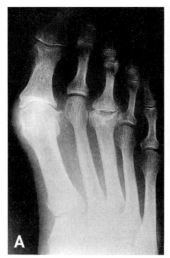
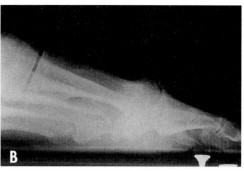

Figure 7

Radiographs of hallux rigidus. The metatarsophalangeal joint is a source of pain due the intra-articular degeneration and the limitation of normal physiologic motion by the dorsal osteophyte. **A,** Anteroposterior radiograph. **B,** Lateral radiograph.

able to function quite well once peroneal strengthening and proprioceptive physical therapy is undertaken.

Dynamic instability, on the other hand, represents the inability of a joint to function normally when under physiologic loads and conditions. It can result from pure weakness of the controlling motor tendon units or from a combination of loss of passive restraint with secondary inability of the dynamic and strengths of motion to control a joint adequately. The physical examination is critical in distinguishing between these 2 possibilities. For instance, a claw toe deformity may be secondary to intrinsic muscle weakness of the foot, which compromises active plantarflexion at the metatarsophalangeal joint (Fig. 9). Because there are no other plantarflexors acting at this joint, it goes into hyperextension, which leads to relative lengthening of the extensor tendons

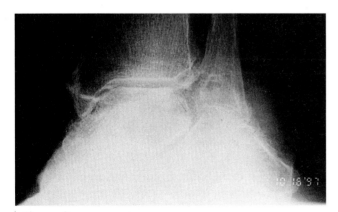

Figure 8

Subluxation of the subtalar joint consequent to posterior tibial tendon rupture. The mortise view of the ankle demonstrates the lateral calcaneal shift relative to the talus, which comprises part of the instability pattern that is seen clinically as pes planus.

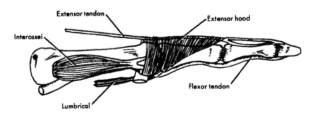

Figure 9

Extensor mechanism of the lesser toes. The plantarflexors of the proximal phalanx are the lumbrical, which inserts onto the extensor hood, and the interossei, which inserts into the side of the base of the proximal phalanx. With extension of the joint, the line of pull of these tendons moves dorsal to the axis of joint rotation, making these tendons become extensors of the proximal phalanx. (Adapted with permission from Sarrafian SK: *Anatomy of the Foot and Ankle.* Philadelphia, PA, JB Lippincott, 1983, p 347.)

6   Foot and Ankle Biomechanics

and relative shortening of the flexor tendons. The change in balance between the extensor and flexor tendons leads directly to the proximal interphalangeal flexion attitude. By comparison, loss of plantar plate integrity at the metatarsophalangeal joint, which can occur in traumatic or inflammatory conditions, will lead to an identical toe position. The distinction between these 2 etiologic entities relies on the physical examination, in which the latter is characterized by a positive anterior drawer sign (known as a Lachman's test or Thompson test) indicative of the plantar plate incompetence. Distinguishing between these 2 etiologies is important clinically because the surgical approaches may be quite different and are specific to the underlying biomechanical cause of deformity.

Biomechanics of Tendon-Joint Interaction

The motions of joints are controlled by passive constraints, such as articular congruity and ligament attachment. Within the extremes of motion permitted by such passive structures, the tendons act to control joint motion. The nature of this control depends on 3 properties of each tendon: the distance of the tendon from the center of motion of the joint, the strength of pull transmitted from the proximal muscle, and the excursion of the tendon through the full range of motion. Of these 3, the tendon excursion is the most important in limiting the range of motion. Muscle strength is hard to gauge because many of the muscles are multipennate and, consequently, the force that they generate is not uniformly related to the square of their cross-sectional area. The easiest parameter to assess in the functional analysis of tendons is their position relative to the joint motion center. Figure 10 schematically shows the position of tendons around the ankle. By breaking the cross section through the ankle into quadrants based on the approximate axis of rotation, one can quickly and easily ascertain the relative contributions of each tendon to sagittal or coronal motion about the ankle and hindfoot. All of the tendons in the anterolateral and posterolateral quadrants contribute to hindfoot eversion, with their proportional contribution based primarily on their distance from the anteroposterior axis line. Therefore, the common extensor tendons anteriorly are relatively weak invertors of the hindfoot, compared to the peroneal tendons posteriorly, because the latter have a greater moment arm (distance from the tendon to the anteroposterior axis of rotation). On the medial side of this axis, the tibialis anterior and tibialis posterior are both substantial originators of hindfoot inversion compared to the flexor hallucis longus

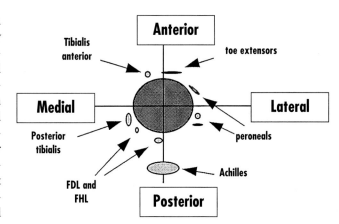

Figure 10

Schematic diagram of the tendons around the ankle (axial section). The action of each tendon can be deduced from its position relative to the axis of joint rotation (see text).

and flexor digitorum longus, again as a consequence of the formers' greater effective moment arm. A more dramatic example is the relative contributions to plantarflexion of the Achilles tendon versus all of the other tendons in the posterolateral and posteromedial quadrants.

The relationship between the actions of the posterior tibial tendon and the Achilles tendon are instructive in demonstrating the effect of changing foot position. At foot flat, the posterior tibial tendon is in the posterior medial quadrant and acts as a primary inverter and secondary plantarflexor. The Achilles tendon is lateral to the axis of inversion and therefore acts as the primary plantarflexor and a secondary everter. As plantarflexion proceeds, the hindfoot is inverted by the action of the posterior tibial tendon. The Achilles tendon now lies in the posteromedial quadrant, where it becomes a strong inverter of the hindfoot. The posterior tibial tendon therefore can be seen as the initiating inverter of the hindfoot, which locks the midfoot into supination and provides a stable foot to proceed into the toe-off phase. The Achilles tendon further contributes to this once it, too, has become an inverter. The Achilles inversion moment actually increases with further plantarflexion as increasing hindfoot inversion occurs. The critical aspect of the relationship between the posterior tibial tendon and the Achilles tendon is that, in the absence of the initiating inversion from the posterior tibial tendon, the hindfoot is never inverted, the midfoot does not become stabilized in supination, and the Achilles tendon is never brought into the posteromedial quadrant where it can act as an inverter. This is why patients with posterior tibial tendon dysfunction are unable to perform a single legged heel rise even though the Achilles tendon is completely normal.

Tendons that cross 2 or more joints have less effect on the middle joints than corresponding tendons that cross a single joint. This occurs because the force developed by tendons spanning several joints is dissipated among the several joints, whereas single joint tendons exert their entire force and excursion across that joint. This explains why the toe extensors are only secondary extensors of the ankle, whereas the tibialis anterior is the primary dorsiflexor.

Similar principles apply at the level of the metatarsophalangeal joint. If one looks at the joint in coronal cross section (Fig. 11), the primary dorsiflexor is the long extensor tendon, which inserts on the extensor hood and around the metatarsophalangeal (MTP) joint. The remaining extensor longus and the entire extensor brevis comprise the secondary dorsiflexors. Balancing these tendons are the primary plantarflexors, which are the lumbricals that insert on the extensor hood and the interossei that insert on the base of the proximal phalanx plantar to the sagittal axis of rotation. The long and short toe flexors act as secondary plantarflexors, because they have no insertions on the proximal phalanx. A significant change in tendon function occurs when the joint is significantly dorsiflexed. In this position, the line of force exerted by the interossei and lumbricals then moves dorsal to the center of rotation, converting these muscles from plantarflexors to dorsiflexors of the proximal phalanx. In this position, there is no remaining active plantarflexor of the MTP joint. This leads to an inherently unstable situation that favors the perpetuation of a fixed dorsiflexed position. This is the etiology of claw toes that occur from wearing high heel shoes that force and hold the MTP joints in a hyperextended position for a prolonged period of time. Conversely, if intrinsic foot weakness is present, such as in neuropathy, the same imbalance across the MTP joint exists,

resulting in a similar claw toe deformity. Recognition of the fundamental biomechanical underpinning of the deformity also explains why some surgeries are more successful at correcting the deformity than others. Simple extensor tendon releases do not consistently restore the motor balance across the joint because no attempt is made to restore a direct plantarflexor to the proximal phalanx. In contrast, the flexor to extensor tendon transfer creates a primary flexor of the proximal phalanx, which does address the motor imbalance across the MTP joint, and thus has a higher rate of success.

Biomechanics of Surgical and Nonsurgical Treatment

The principles of biomechanics of the foot and ankle apply to the selection and underlying rationale of both surgical and nonsurgical treatment modalities. If one understands the biomechanical causes of the clinical syndrome, the formulation of a treatment plan derives directly from biomechanical principles. The simplistic expression of this is in the use of casts and braces to limit the stresses applied to joints, ligaments, and tendons when they are damaged. A less obvious extension of this would be the use of a stiff-soled shoe in the treatment of instability of the MTP joint or plantar fasciitis. In both instances, dorsiflexion of the MTP joints exacerbates the biomechanical problem. In the first instance, this is the dorsiflexion instability of the affected MTP joint. In the second case, the dorsiflexion of the first MTP joint invokes the windlass mechanism, which places tension on the plantar fascia, thereby exacerbating the pain of plantar fasciitis.

The design of surgical treatment is perhaps more obviously related to the underlying biomechanical disorder. Instances of this include the use of arthrodesis to stabilize arthritic joints that cause pain with motion or are grossly unstable (such as triple arthrodesis for posterior tibial tendon insufficiency). Successful fusions, however, require an understanding of the functional position of the foot and ankle, as a solid arthrodesis in a poor biomechanical position can cause more problems than it solves. An example of this would be an ankle fusion placed in plantarflexion, thereby leading to increased dorsiflexion stresses on the midfoot joints, predisposing to premature degeneration.

Fracture treatment, similarly, should be based on an understanding of the underly-

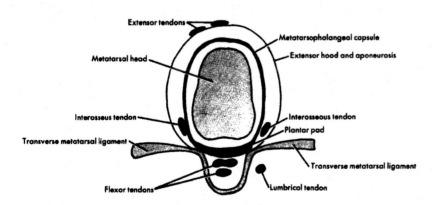

Figure 11

Coronal section of the lesser metatarsophalangeal joint showing the active and passive restraints to motion. (Adapted with permission from Sarrafian SK: *Anatomy of the Foot and Ankle.* Philadelphia, PA, JB Lippincott, 1983, p 347.)

ing biomechanics. Isolated lateral malleolar fractures of the ankle do not require surgical treatment, because the stability of the ankle depends on the medial structures. By extension, bimalleolar ankle fractures are most stable if treated surgically, with restoration of medial malleolar stability. An appreciation for the consequences of nonanatomic surgical reduction are completely related to the effect that such imperfections have on the biomechanical behavior of the relevant joints. For instance, although there is some tolerance for displacement of fractures of the fifth metatarsus because of its relative mobility, such cannot be said of talar neck fractures. The fact that small displacements of 1 mm to 2 mm substantially disrupt the normal motions of the subtalar joint has a profound influence on the decision to pursue surgical treatment as well as the necessity for precision in surgical technique.

Without a detailed understanding of the functional role of specific tendons, tendon transfers and releases cannot be undertaken in any rational way. The use of the extensor hallucis longus (EHL) to substitute for the tibialis anterior is based on both its position relative to the axis of motion in the sagittal plane and the fact that it is active during the same phase of gait as the tibialis anterior. A similar rationale underlies the use of the flexor digitorum longus to reconstruct posterior tibial tendon function. Biomechanics also underlies many of the reasons for failure of various tendon transfers. An EHL-to-tibialis anterior transfer performed for rupture of the tibialis anterior has a much different long-term outcome than a similar surgery done to compensate for tibialis anterior weakness in Charcot-Marie-Tooth disease. In the former, the relative strength of the transferred tendon is not expected to diminish substantially over time. In the latter case, it would be anticipated that the transfer tendon would gradually have less function because of progressive neuropathy and secondary motor weakness. The clinical significance of these differences is profound and should influence the choice and nature of any surgeries offered.

The recognition of the need for tendon lengthening is based completely on the physical examination and appreciation for how tendons influence motion. By simply understanding the basic anatomy of the foot and ankle, one can deduce the site and etiology of tendon pathology. A contracture affecting the flexor digitorum longus is manifest by the development of flexion contractures of the interphalangeal joints of the toes. The contracture can be caused by scarring at the hindfoot (plantaris quadratus) or in the distal leg. Even if neither condition has presented itself, the 2 possibilities could quite easily be distinguished by seeing how the contractures changed with changing the position of the ankle. Because the long flexors originate proximal to the ankle, contractures of these will be accentuated if the ankle is dorsiflexed, because this

increases the distance that these tendons need to traverse. In contrast, when long flexor tendons are contracted because of scarring of the intrinsics or quadratus planti, the position of the ankle does not alter the degree of flexion of the toes. Therefore, assessing the degree of toe flexion contracture in different positions of the ankle will make it easy to distinguish between the 2 sources of pathology.

Annotated Bibliography

Cavanagh PR, Morag E, Boulton AJ, Young MJ, Deffner KT, Pammer SE: The relationship of static foot structure to dynamic foot function. J Biomech 1997;30:243–250.

This prospective study used radiographs to compare various static parameters of the foot (such as calcaneal height, metatarsal inclination, and plantar soft-tissue thickness) to the dynamic function of the same feet using a pedobarograph. By regression analysis, it was found that heel pressure was a function of calcaneal height and first and fifth metatarsal inclination, while first metatarsal pressure was a function of relative first and second metatarsal lengths, plantar skin thickness, and first metatarsal and calcaneal inclination. However, the radiographic parameters could explain a maximum of 38% of the dynamic variation seen between subjects. Consequently, other parameters (such as shoe wear, speed of walking, etc) need to be included in future attempts to predict dynamic function from static data.

Hintermann B, Nigg BM, Sommer C: Foot movement and tendon excursion: An in vitro study. Foot Ankle Int 1994;15:386–395.

This excellent study examines the effective moment arms of tendons, and their excursions, when the foot is in various positions. The total excursions for the tibialis anterior, Achilles tendon, tibialis posterior, peroneus longus, and flexor hallucis longus were found to be 38 mm, 44 mm, 21 mm, 30 mm, and 27 mm, respectively. The effective inversion moment arms for these tendons were 0.59, 0.24, 1.0, -0.82, and 0.62, respectively. The combination of excursion and moment arm provides a guide to potential tendon reconstruction options. They also demonstrate how the Achilles tendon starts out as a weak everter of the foot at neutral, and doesn't become an inverter until the foot has been inverted by other tendons.

Michelsen JD, Ahn UM, Helgemo SL: Motion of the ankle in a simulated supination-external rotation fracture model. J Bone Joint Surg 1996;78A:1024–1031.

In a cadaveric study of 13 specimens, the biomechanical effect of common ankle fracture patterns was investigated. The investigators found that isolated lateral malleolar fractures did not result in any abnormal motion of the ankle when it was moved through a complete range of motion while under axial load. In contrast, ankle injuries that involved both the medial and lateral structures resulted in significantly deranged ankle motion. They also demonstrated that the ankle was not a simple hinge joint but, rather, exhibited coupled rotations consisting of internal/external rotation, and varus/valgus as it was plantarflexed. This study provides a mechanical basis for the surgery of ankle fractures that result in medial injury, while indicating that isolated lateral fractures would not be expected to require surgery.

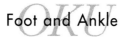

Mizel MS, Marymont JV, Trepman E: Treatment of plantar fasciitis with a night splint and shoe modification consisting of a steel shank and anterior rocker bottom. *Foot Ankle Int* 1996; 17:732–735.

In this study of 57 patients with plantar fasciitis, the authors instituted the use of night splints and the addition of a steel shank and rocker bottom to the shoe sole. The hypothesis was that limiting the tension on the plantar fascia by preventing toe dorsiflexion in the modified shoe, and maintaining it at a physiologically stretched position, would effectively rest the plantar fascia, thereby giving it a chance to heal. The treatment was curative in 59% and resulted in improvement in another 18% at an average follow-up of 16 months. This study demonstrates how basic biomechanical concepts (eg, the relationship of the plantar fascia to toe motion) can be incorporated to develop clinically useful treatment modalities.

Pierrynowski MR, Smith SB: Rear foot inversion/eversion during gait relative to the subtalar joint neutral position. *Foot Ankle Int* 1996;17:406–412.

Many papers in the literature, as well as fabricators of orthotics, refer to the subtalar neutral position (STNP) in describing foot position. Although STNP has been assumed to be the subtalar position when the foot is in a standing neutral position, this study shows that such is not the case. If the STNP is used as a reference, the foot never is inverted during the stance phase of gait in most people. The subtalar position at standing neutral was found to be 5.2° everted with respect to STNP. Furthermore, a single determination of STNP could vary by up to 6.6° from the mean. Consequently, using the STNP for the fabrication of orthotics can lead to unintended clinical results.

Saltzman CL, Aper RL, Brown TD: Anatomic determinants of first metatarsophalangeal flexion moments in hallux valgus. *Clin Orthop* 1997;339:261–269.

This excellent study measured the change in flexor hallucis longus force exerted on the hallux that occurs with hallux valgus. At a hallux valgus angle of 40°, the plantarflexion force on the hallux decreases to 22% of normal. When combined with a 30° pronation deformity, the plantarflexion force is only 5% of normal. In both instances, the laterally directed force on the hallux is increased by an order of magnitude. This study elucidates the mechanism of progressive deformity once hallux valgus has started. It also points out the importance of correcting the flexor hallucis longus position relative to the metatarsal head in hallux valgus surgery, and the results of this study indicate that failure to do so would be expected to be associated with a high recurrence rate.

Steffensmeier SJ, Saltzman CL, Berbaum KS, Brown TD: Effects of medial and lateral displacement calcaneal osteotomies on tibiotalar joint contact stresses. *J Orthop Res* 1996;14:980–985.

The effect of 1 cm medial and lateral calcaneal slide osteotomies on the contact pressures of the ankle were studied in eight cadaver specimens. A medial shift resulted in the center of pressure in the ankle moving medially 1.1 mm, whereas a lateral shift moved the pressure center 1.6 mm laterally on the talus. Although neither shift caused a significant change in total contact area, the lateral shift did lead to a significant increase of lateral talar contact area and pressure. Although there are limitations to the study (static loading with the ankle in neutral, no measurement of medial or lateral gutter pressures), it does point out the potential consequences of displacement osteotomies that should be contemplated.

Thordarson DB, Schmotzer H, Chon J, Peters J: Dynamic support of the human longitudinal arch: A biomechanical evaluation. *Clin Orthop* 1995;316:165–172.

This cadaveric study examined the dynamic contributions to maintenance of the arch when the foot is under 350 N and 700 N of axial load. The Achilles tendon was the main depressor of the arch, decreasing the talar-first metatarsal angle 3.3° and 3.7°, respectively. The posterior tibial tendon was the main tendinous arch elevator, increasing the talar-first metatarsal angle 0.7° and 0.9°, respectively. The primary active arch elevator, however, was the plantar fascia, which was put under stretch by dorsiflexion of the toes. This resulted in an increase of 3.6° and 2.3°, respectively, in the talar-first metatarsal angle. Clinically, this suggests that caution should be used in contemplating plantar fascia release, given the profound effect it would have on arch support.

Yamaguchi K, Martin CH, Boden SD, Labropoulos PA: Operative treatment of syndesmotic disruptions without use of a syndesmotic screw: A prospective clinical study. *Foot Ankle Int* 1994;15:407–414.

The authors conducted a prospective study to validate the biomechanically derived indications for syndesmotic fixation in ankle fractures. Of 21 patients with Weber C fibular fractures, 13 had bimalleolar fractures, and 8 had accompanying deltoid tears proven at the time of surgery. Of the latter, 5 had fibular fractures less than 4.5 cm above the joint, and the remaining 3 had fractures more than 4.5 cm above the joint. Of all these patients, only those in the last group underwent syndesmotic fixation, although all had satisfactory syndesmotic reduction following lateral malleolar fixation. At 1 to 3 years follow-up, no patients demonstrated significant syndesmotic widening. Consequently, syndesmotic fixation appears to be necessary only in those patients with persistent medial injury and a fibular fracture greater than 4.5 cm above the ankle. It should be emphasized that if the syndesmosis remains widened following lateral malleolar fixation, stabilization of the syndesmosis in a reduced position is required.

10   Foot and Ankle Biomechanics

Classic Bibliography

Beaudoin AJ, Fiore SM, Krause WR, Adelaar RS: Effect of isolated talocalcaneal fusion on contact in the ankle and talonavicular joints. *Foot Ankle* 1991;12:19–25.

Engsberg JR, Andrews JG: Kinematic analysis of the talocalcaneal/talocrural joint during running support. *Med Sci Sports Exerc* 1987;19:275–284.

Huang CK, Kitaoka HB, An KN, Chao EY: Biomechanical evaluation of longitudinal arch stability. *Foot Ankle* 1993; 14:353–357.

Jones DC: Foot orthoses, in Heckman JD (ed): *Instructional Course Lectures 42*. Rosemont, IL, American Academy of Orthopaedic Surgeons, 1993, pp 219–224.

Chapter 2
Tumors

Introduction

Tumors of the foot and ankle are relatively common. The differential diagnosis is based on patient age, gender, tumor location, and plain radiographs. Although symptoms may appear early, they are often mistaken for trauma and overuse injuries so that diagnosis is often delayed, sometimes compromising function and more important, oncologic outcome. The histologic type and frequency of tumors of the foot and ankle reflect the quantity and embryologic origin of the tissue from which they arise. It is not surprising that, given the numerous articulations in the foot, cartilage tumors are common.

Foot and ankle tumors, like tumors in other regions of the body, can be separated into bone and soft tissue, benign and malignant, multiple or solitary, and by the underlying tissue from which they arise. The same principles of tumor diagnosis and management, then, apply to lesions that arise in the foot and ankle, specifically, staging, local tumor control, systemic therapy for high grade tumors, metastatic disease, and preservation of function when possible.

Staging

The process of staging fundamentally defines the type and extent of disease. It includes a thorough history and physical examination, followed by appropriate and directed laboratory investigation and radiologic imaging, and culminating in biopsy and pathologic interpretation. It is an organized and methodical approach culminating in definitive diagnosis, so that reasoned and appropriate treatment can be undertaken to control both locally and potentially systemic disease.

History is the most important aspect of staging and directs the physical examination and the adjunct studies that follow. Most patients with benign aggressive and malignant tumors present with pain and discomfort for weeks and sometimes months or even years. Because the foot is cycled thousands of times a day, these symptoms occur early in the disease course but the true etiology is recognized late. Because many common foot and ankle problems are related to injury or overuse, tumors and tumor-related conditions are often not considered in the differential diagnosis at the onset, and delays in

treatment occur. In addition to pain, patients may also complain of swelling or notice a mass. The combination of pain, especially night or rest pain, and a noticeable mass should arouse the suspicion of an underlying neoplasm. Constitutional symptoms are unusual and may signify advanced disease or, more likely, an infection. Some benign and malignant tumors, such as eosinophilic granuloma and Ewing's sarcoma, can also present with signs and symptoms of sepsis, but in the foot and ankle, these tumors are extraordinarily rare. In summary, the onset of symptoms, both type and duration, history of trauma, and a survey of the patient's past medical history are critical in the initial evaluation.

Physical examination must involve both feet, and ideally the entire body, and encompass the basic tenets of examination, including inspection, palpation, occasionally auscultation for suspected vascular malformations, and evaluation of joint, range of joint, and neurovascular assessment. It is important to inspect the nails, web spaces, and the plantar aspects of the feet for skin discoloration, pigmentation, and ulceration. Melanotic lesions can be difficult to detect in subungual locations or in between toes, especially in patients with dark skin. Café au lait spots may be present in patients with neurofibromatosis or McCune-Albright syndrome with associated polyostotic fibrous dysplasia. A bluish hue under the skin suggests a vascular tumor, and, in high flow lesions, pulsations can be seen. Skin ulceration can result from a fungating deep mass or a superficial lesion, such as a melanoma or squamous cell carcinoma. Generally, deep-seated masses will present as a fullness rather than a discrete nodule, whereas more subcutaneous tumors and skin lesions will appear more circumscribed. Disuse and atrophic changes can be seen in patients with long-standing tumors or in conjunction with reflex sympathetic dystrophy, either at initial diagnosis, following treatment, or with recurrent disease. Percussion of soft-tissue masses resulting in paresthesias is suggestive of nerve sheath tumors, which occur about the ankle, or Morton's neuromas, which are peculiar to the web spaces, particularly the third. Pathologic fractures can occur in patients with both benign and malignant tumors and result in pain and deformity. Pathologic fractures are most often seen in the forefoot and may be confused with more common conditions like metatarsal stress fractures or the so-called "march fracture" frequently seen in military recruits.

Palpation should begin away from the suspected lesion and then progress toward the tumor. Size, mobility, and texture of the mass should be noted, as well as the presence or absence of a thrill. A deeply fixed mass or a tumor that is adherent to the dermis will have functional and cosmetic implications following surgical extirpation. When a tumor is suspected, regional nodes in the popliteal fossa as well as the inguinal region should be palpated. In patients with plantar fibromatosis, the hands should be examined because up to 20% of patients with Dupuytren's disease have plantar fibromatosis as well. To complete the foot evaluation, reflex testing, motor and sensory examination, and vascular assessment should be performed. It is important to remember that many disease processes that arise proximally may present as unexplained foot pain, especially lumbar disk disease as well as spinal tumors, infections, and primary neurologic diseases.

Laboratory

Laboratory studies are nonspecific and rarely help in the differential diagnosis of foot and ankle tumors. In general, a complete blood count, erythrocyte sedimentation rate, and routine serum chemistries are adequate. Serum immune electrophoresis and prostate specific antigen are specific tumor markers, but the incidence of metastatic disease or myeloma in the foot and ankle represents only 0.01% of metastatic tumors overall.

Imaging

Plain Radiographs
Every patient with a suspected tumor of the foot or ankle, whether bone or soft tissue, should have plain radiographs in orthogonal planes. The diagnosis is apparent on the radiograph in up to 90% of patients with primary bone tumors.

In evaluating a bone lesion, attention should be directed to the interface between tumor and normal bone. The more narrowly defined the transition from normal to abnormal, the less biologically aggressive the lesion, thus allowing host bone to reinforce itself and contain the tumor. More aggressive lesions are infiltrative, and the surrounding bone is unable to encapsulate the tumor, which creates the illusion of a wider zone of transition. Malignant tumors as well as acute infections can destroy bone in a permeative or moth-eaten pattern with no obvious boundary between normal bone and tumor.

The presence or absence of tumor matrix should be noted and is a valuable clue as to the origin of the lesion. For ex-

ample, osseous tumors make bone and have a "cloud-like" appearance, whereas cartilage tumors produce matrix that resembles "stippled calcifications," "arcs and rings," or "flocculations," or a combination of these 3 patterns. Biologically, matrix represents ongoing endochondral ossification within lobules of cartilage. The plain film is used to assess the degree of endosteal scalloping in cartilaginous lesions; deeper endosteal scallops and cortical erosions imply a more aggressive and potentially malignant disease process. Finally, fibrous lesions have a "ground glass" appearance due to the presence of woven bone intermixed with dense fibrous stroma.

Periosteal reactions can be seen in both benign and malignant disease processes but usually imply a more aggressive tumor. A periosteal response reinforces bone weakened by tumor and, depending on its appearance, can provide information on the lesion's biologic activity. For example, a solid periosteal reaction is seen in patients with less aggressive, usually benign, tumors like osteoid osteoma. An "onion-skin" or "starburst" type reaction is associated with more aggressive, usually malignant, processes like osteosarcoma. In addition to information on margin, matrix and periosteal reaction, pathologic fractures are best seen on plain radiographs.

For soft-tissue tumors, plain radiographs demonstrate soft-tissue shadows, osseous erosions, and mineral densities within the soft-tissue mass which are helpful in establishing a differential diagnosis. Hemangiomata, common benign soft-tissue tumors of the foot, are associated with pheboliths that can be seen on plain radiographs and represent mineralization of organized thrombus within vascular channels. Up to 30% of synoviosarcomas, the most common deep-seated sarcoma of the foot, will mineralize. Injection granulomata, myositis ossificans, soft-tissue chondromas, chondrosarcomas, angioleiomyomas and occasional giant cell tumors of tendon sheath can mineralize and are apparent on plain radiographs.

Computed Tomography
Computed tomography (CT) is the best imaging modality to accurately assess endosteal scalloping and cortical destruction. Tumor matrix is well visualized and, if the CT is formatted correctly, it can detect subtle pathologic fractures. The relationship of soft-tissue tumor extension to normal structures and the intraosseous extent of disease is better demonstrated on MRI. For patients with known malignant tumors, CT of the chest is the most sensitive study to identify early lung metastases, the most common site of distant spread of sarcomas. Finally, fine cut CT and saggital reconstructions can precisely delineate subtle abnormalities like osteoid osteoma in complex bones in the hindfoot, for example.

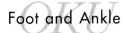

Nuclear Medicine Scans

Radionucleotide scans are rarely helpful in the differential diagnosis of tumors, but they are useful in detecting other sites of tumor in patients with multifocal diseases, like polyostotic fibrous dysplasia, or in patients with multiple skeletal metastases or skip metastases in long bones. The intensity and extent of scintigraphic uptake seen on the early phases of technetium-99 pyrophosphate scans is proportional to the amount of blood flow. For soft-tissue masses, the presence of increased uptake on the early, or blood flow phase, is thought to correlate with malignancy. Radionucleotide uptake on delayed images suggests active bone turnover and offers no information on whether a lesion is benign or malignant. Bone scintigraphy can also be useful in assessing tumor response to chemotherapeutic intervention by comparing the intensity of uptake before and after treatment. More recently, thallium scans have been reported to detect response to neoadjuvant therapy in osteosarcoma. Positron emission tomography (PET) scanning has been used to examine the metabolic activity in both bone and soft-tissue sarcomas before and after neoadjuvant therapy. Unfortunately, changes in metabolic activity do not correlate with tumor necrosis, suggesting that the mesenchymal tissue response associated with the necrosis had metabolic activity similar to that of the tumor. The design and use of more specific markers of tumor cell activity in the future may overcome these initial disappointing results.

Angiography

Angiography provides a road map for resection of lesions near vessels or tumors composed primarily of vessels, particularly high flow arteriovenous malformations and malignant vascular tumors. It also defines the normal vascular anatomy of the lower extremity prior to free flap coverage of soft-tissue defects following tumor resection. In addition, the study can be used for therapeutic embolization in anticipation of or in lieu of surgical resection of some vascular tumors. The therapeutic utility of embolization in the foot, particularly the distal foot, is limited by vessel lumen size and the ability to place a catheter safely to embolize feeding vessels without compromising the viability of the foot. Angiograms, too, have been used to assess the efficacy of chemotherapeutic intervention in patients with malignant tumors. A significant diminution of flow was noted in responsive tumors. Angiography is also a vehicle for delivering chemotherapeutic agents locally, although the results in osteosarcoma are equivalent to those of systemic therapy and the complication rate is higher.

Magnetic Resonance Imaging

Aside from the plain radiographs, this is probably the most informative study to assess intraosseous as well as extraosseous tumor extension and the tumor's relationship to normal tissue. It can be formatted in multiple planes, thus providing excellent spatial orientation in anticipation of surgical excision. Gadolinium administration defines the degree of tumor vascularity as well as the pattern of uptake (diffuse, peripheral, or septal) but adds little to diagnostic specificity. In assessing soft tissue extension, the presence of edema, particularly on T2-weighted pulse sequences, can obscure the relationship between tumor and normal tissue. For this reason, Tl and Tl gadolinium enhanced images may be better in determining whether the neurovascular bundle or an adjacent joint is affected by the tumor.

Biopsy

Once the location and local and distant extent of disease has been established and a reasonable differential diagnosis has been formulated, the biopsy is the final step in the staging process prior to definitive treatment. The approach to the biopsy should involve multiple disciplines, including surgery, radiology, and pathology, in an effort to obtain "diagnostic tissue" for analysis. The pitfalls of biopsy were reported over 15 years ago, and, unfortunately, despite significant educational efforts by the Musculoskeletal Tumor Society, a repeat study 14 years later found the same alarming frequency of errors and complications. These include failure to obtain diagnostic tissue (8.4%), errors in diagnosis (17.8%) and alteration in treatment (19.3%). The recommendations were, and continue to be, that the biopsy be performed in an institution that has expertise in treating patients with musculoskeletal neoplasms and that will provide the definitive treatment. The biopsy should be carried out by an experienced surgeon, recognizing that it must be planned so that future resection and oncologic outcome is not compromised.

A biopsy can be incisional or excisional. Incisional biopsies can be done as an open surgical procedure, by fine needle aspiration or by core needle biopsy, depending on the experience and bias of the institution. Incisional biopsies are generally reserved for tumors exceeding 3 cm in anticipation of adjuvant treatment and definitive surgical treatment for bone and soft-tissue lesions. Excisional biopsies are performed for small lesions (< 3 cm), or in tumors that are thought to be benign based on the staging work-up. The biopsy should be performed through only one anatomic compartment and should avoid neurovascular structures, joints, and reactive areas (periosteal reactions and radiated fields). Excellent hemostasis must be achieved intraoperatively, and drains should be used liberally and brought out through separate sites in line with the biopsy incision. The application of compressive dressings can also be used as an adjunct to control blood extravasation into soft tissue.

Classification

Benign bone and soft-tissue tumors are described as either inactive or latent (stage 1), active (stage 2), or aggressive (stage 3) depending on their radiographic appearance and biologic behavior. Inactive or latent lesions develop a stable relationship with normal bone and have limited capacity for further growth and osseous destruction. An example would be a unicameral bone cyst in the calcaneus or a nonossifying fibroma in the distal tibia. An active lesion has the potential for further growth, albeit slowly, such as an aneurysmal bone cyst. An aggressive lesion can evolve over a short period of time resulting in significant destruction or infiltration of normal tissues. In bone, giant cell tumors, osteoblastomas and chondroblastomas can take on active or aggressive features. In soft tissue, fibromatosis is an aggressive benign tumor with the capacity to grow rapidly and to infiltrate normal tissue. Rarely, so-called benign tumors, such as giant cell tumors and chondroblastomas, can metastasize to lung, creating difficult diagnostic dilemmas and therapeutic options.

The most common classification for malignant tumors is the Enneking staging system, which has been adopted by the Musculoskeletal Tumor Society. Tumors are assigned to 1 of 3 categories based on grade, location within or outside a compartment, and the presence or absence of metastatic disease (Table 1). If the tumor is low grade it is designated I; high grade tumors are designated II. If the tumor has metastasized it is designated III, independent of tumor grade or location within a compartment. Metastases occur distantly in the lungs or skeleton, or regionally in the lymph nodes. If the lesion is confined within the anatomic compartment of origin, it is designated A. Extracompartmental lesions or lesions that have escaped the compartment of origin are labeled B. In the foot, anatomic compartments exist plantarly but are not particularly effective barriers because of the compactness of the muscles and potential communication between muscle layers. Lesions on the dorsum of the foot are considered extracompartmental, and soft-tissue masses in the region of the ankle are also extracompartmental because of the continuity with the dorsum of the foot and lack of identifiable fascial boundaries. Bone itself is a separate compartment, and when tumor breaks out of bone into soft tissue, the tumor is

Table 1

Musculoskeletal Tumor Society Staging System

Stage	Histologic Grade	Compartment	Metastatic
IA	Low	Within	No
IB	Low	Outside	No
IIA	High	Within	No
IIB	High	Outside	No
III	Any	Any	Yes

considered extracompartmental. This classification system is also applicable for soft-tissue tumors.

An alternate classification system is the American Joint Committee Staging Protocol or the TMN classification where T denotes tumor grade, of which there are 4 categories based on cellularity, mitotic activity, and nuclear and cellular pleomorphism. In addition, tumor size and the presence or absence of distant metastases M and lymph node involvement N is considered. An alternative and simpler method is the Hadju classification, which divides malignant soft-tissue tumors by size (< 5cm and > 5cm), grade (high versus low) and depth of involvement (subcutaneous or deep).

Bone tumors

Benign tumors are far more common than malignant lesions in the foot and ankle. In fact, malignant tumors in the foot in particular, are quite rare and most commonly are chondrosarcomas, either primary or secondary (arising in preexisting enchondroma). Relatively common benign tumors include osteoid osteoma, enchondroma, and unicameral bone cyst. In the ankle, fibroxanthoma and osteochondroma, especially in patients with the multiple hereditary form of disease, are not infrequent. Giant cell tumor is a rare lesion in the foot and ankle. Metastatic disease is also exceedingly rare, but should be considered in patients with renal cell carcinoma or gastrointestinal malignancies.

Subungual Exostosis
This is a benign osteochondral excrescence arising from the dorsomedial aspect of the distal phalanx beneath the nail. It is associated with exquisite tenderness and nail deformity.

The etiology of this abnormality is unclear, but it may result from repetitive trauma. Histologically, subungual exostosis resembles osteochondroma, with a fibrous cap with underlying hyaline cartilage and a cancellous base. Subungual exostoses can be hypercellular and exhibit moderate atypia, raising the suspicion of a malignancy. For this reason, clinical, radiologic, and pathologic correlation is essential. Occasionally, skin ulceration can occur with secondary infection. Treatment consists of complete excision, and the rate of local recurrence is low.

Chondroblastoma

Chondroblastoma is probably more common in the foot and ankle than previously thought because up to 50% of them are cystic and often confused with unicameral or aneurysmal bone cysts. The vast majority of unicameral bone cysts in the foot occur in one location, the anterior aspect of the calcaneus just inferior to the angle of Gissane. Alternately, chondroblastomas always occur juxtaposed to articular and apophyseal surfaces, are lytic, slightly expansile, and infrequently demonstrate subtle matrix. Pathologic subchondral fractures have been observed and may be an additional source of pain and discomfort (Fig. 1). These lesions are usually painful, unlike unicameral bone cysts which, being asymptomatic, are usually found incidentally. The majority of chondroblastomas are found in the hindfoot, in the subchondral bone of the talus at the talocrural articulation, and posteriorly in the calcaneal apophysis. Chondroblastoma can be aggressive and although reports of metastases are rare, local recurrence is common. Grossly, the cavity is filled with dark red fluid with sparse solid tissue in the cyst walls. Unless the cavity is thoroughly curetted and burred, the lesion will likely recur. Bone graft is often necessary for large defects that efface subchondral bone. It is important to avoid joint contamination, as chondroblastoma can recur within the joint, particularly the aggressive form of this disease. Overall, local recurrence has been reported to be 25% in one large series despite curetting.

Osteoblastoma

Although quite rare, representing about 1% of all benign tumors of bone, the foot represents the third most common site for this tumor. Most occur in the hindfoot and up to one third occur in the talar neck (Fig. 2). The majority of osteoblastomas are lytic with internal matrix production. Some can be very destructive, particularly the aggressive form of this disease. Malignant transformation to osteosarcoma is possible but rare. Most cases may be osteosarcoma from the onset rather than malignant transformation of benign disease. Osteoblastoma is also seen in the metatarsals

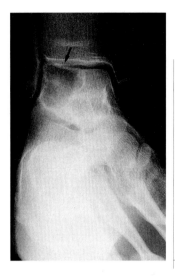

Figure 1

Cystic chondroblastoma arising in the talus. Because chondroblastoma is often cystic in the hindfoot and thus fluid filled, it is often misdiagnosed as unicameral bone cyst. Note that this tumor always effaces a joint surface as in this case, or an apophysis. Pathologic fracture is not infrequent as demonstrated by the arrow. (Reproduced with permission from Fink BR, Temple HT, Chiracosta F, Mizel MS, Murphey MD: Chondroblastoma of the foot. *Foot Ankle Int* 1997;18: 236–242.)

and is always near a growth center. For this reason, it is seen distally in the great toe and the proximal aspect of the lesser metatarsals. In one series, pathologic fracture occurred in 7% of patients and all were in the forefoot. Diffuse osteopenia may be seen locally in patients with osteoblastoma and, rarely, generalized osteomalacia may occur. Radiologically, osteoblastomas tend to be larger than osteoid osteomas but have less sclerosis, are mildly expansile when endosteally based, and often have a soft-tissue mass when subperiosteal in location. Aggressive osteoblastoma can cause extensive osseous destruction, infiltrate soft tissue and evoke aggressive periosteal reactions reminiscent of osteosarcoma. Histologically, osteoblastoma is difficult to distinguish from

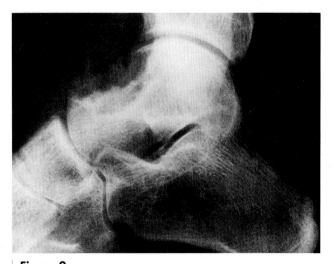

Figure 2

Destructive cavitary lesion in the dorsal aspect of the talus; the most common site for osteoblastoma.

osteoid osteoma, but there is slightly less osteoid than osteoid osteoma and the stromal features are more prominent. The stroma is fibrovascular, with interspersed giant cells and occasional areas of hemorrhage and cyst formation. The trabeculae coalesce centrally and tend to be less organized peripherally than osteoid osteoma. Treatment is enbloc resection, if possible, with or without bone graft depending on the size and location of the defect. Disease recurrence should be monitored closely, as osteoblastoma can recur many years after primary resection.

Osteoid Osteoma

Unlike osteoblastoma, which is progressive, osteoid osteoma is self-limited and usually occurs in the second decade of life. Males are more commonly affected than females. Osteoid osteoma is not uncommon in the foot and ankle representing 6% to 15.6% of reported cases. Patients typically present with pain that is nocturnal and relieved by salicylates. Reactive changes around the lesion are generally more pronounced than in osteoblastoma. Radiographically, there is a radiolucent nidus surrounded by thick sclerosis except in patients with medullary based or periarticular lesions, in whom reactive changes are minimal. Subtle radiographic findings in patients with juxta-articular lesions may lead to long delays in diagnosis and treatment. Enbloc resection has been recommended in the past, but, more recently, nonsurgical treatment with nonsteroidal anti-inflammatory drugs and observation has been endorsed. If surgical intervention is necessary, intralesional curetting and burring is a less aggressive and effective alternative to en bloc resection. Recurrence is common, unless the nidus is completely removed. Radioablation, using a heat probe that is fluoroscopically or CT-directed into the nidus, has been reported with good results. A shortcoming of this approach is the lack of a histologic diagnosis.

Enchondroma

Enchondroma is more common in the collective bones of the hand than in the foot; in one series of 776 cases of enchondroma, only 4.6% of cases occurred in the foot. It is an abnormality of development in which physeal cartilage is trapped or sequestered in growing bone. This anachronistic tissue may remain active in later life and cause symptoms following growth, but, in general, enchondromas are asymptomatic unless pathologic fracture or, rarely, transformation to chondrosarcoma occurs. Radiographically and histologically, enchondroma appears more active in skeletally immature patients and in the small tubular bones of the hand and foot. There is usually mild to moderate endosteal scalloping, sometimes involving two thirds of the endosteal cortex or

more, but no cortical break through or soft-tissue extension should be observed in benign lesions. Expansile changes and cortical disruption are characteristic of malignant transformation. Radionucleotide uptake is usually mild to moderate, but it may be intense when pathologic fracture or malignant transformation occurs. Pathologic fractures are treated by immobilization and observation. In the event of re-fracture, surgery is delayed for approximately 6 weeks or until the fracture is healed, and then curetting, with or without bone graft, is performed. The addition of a chemical adjunct like phenol has been attempted, but there are no studies comparing the risk of local recurrence with or without adjunctive treatment. When curetted material is sent to the pathologist for analysis, one must be certain to include a history of trauma or previous fracture, size, location, and a representative radiograph. Histologically, small regular chondrocytes organized into lobules of varying sizes characterize this disease. Enchondromas of the hands and feet in young patients will appear more worrisome to the pathologist, especially in patients with multiple hereditary enchondromas or Ollier's disease. The association of hemangiomata in conjunction with multiple enchondromas is known as Maffucci's disease. The risk of malignant transformation to chondrosarcoma from enchondroma in patients with multiple enchondromas is 25%. Patients with Maffucci's disease are also at risk for other malignant tumors, including gastrointestinal adenocarcinomas and gliomas, and this risk approaches 100% by the age of 35 years. The degree of cellularity differs with age, location, and degree of cellular activity.

Unicameral Bone Cyst

Typically, unicameral bone cyst is an abnormality of growth plate physiology in young patients whereby cystification supersedes ossification. With time the cyst migrates from the growth plate and eventually consolidates. Pathophysiologically, unicameral bone cyst in the foot is fundamentally different than that in long bones. Almost all unicameral bone cysts in the foot occur in the anterior and inferior aspect of the calcaneus and are usually asymptomatic and discovered incidentally (Fig. 3). This is the location where red marrow converts to white marrow or fat, and, in the place of white marrow, cyst formation occurs. The mechanism by which this happens is unclear. This abnormality occurs in the later part of the second decade and is more common in males than females. In one study the mean age was less than 20 years in 85% of patients. Interestingly, a third of patients presented with a pathologic fracture, albeit subtle in most cases. Because unicameral bone cysts are asymptomatic in most patients and reinforced superiorly by dense osseous trabeculae, initial treatment is observation. For those patients with pain and a

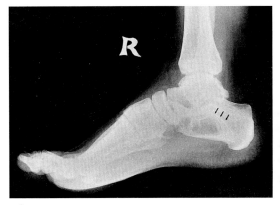

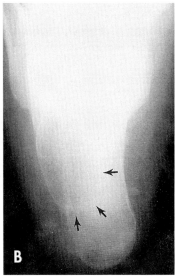

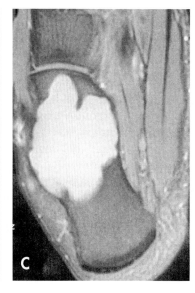

Figure 3

A, A lateral radiograph of the foot and ankle showing a unicameral bone cyst in the anterior calcaneus with reinforced trabeculae (arrows) superiorly. This 20-year-old male presented with heel pain. **B,** Harris view demonstrates this laterally based, slightly expansile radiolucent abnormality with well delineated and sclerotic borders and no matrix production. **C,** An axial T2 pulsed weighted MR sequence shows a homogeneous bright signal abnormality occupying the majority of the anterior calcaneus that is consistent with fluid. There are no fluid-fluid levels to suggest the presence of blood and the cortices are intact circumferentially.

history of pathologic fracture, curetting and bone grafting is preferred. The use of injectable steroids is of unproved benefit in patients with unicameral bone cysts of the calcaneus. It is important to distinguish this tumor from chondroblastoma, which is often cystic and radiographically similar to unicameral bone cyst. Unlike unicameral bone cyst, chondroblastoma is always adjacent to a joint or apophyseal surface and is commonly seen in the talus, generally in patients in their mid 20s.

Intraosseous Lipoma

This is a rare tumor, usually located around the hip in patients in the third and fourth decades and later. In the foot it is found in the calcaneus in the same location as unicameral bone cyst. The mean age of these patients is 36.8 years, compared to younger patients with unicameral cyst. For this reason, there is speculation that the two entities are related and perhaps represent different stages of the same disease. It is difficult to reason why a cyst would evolve into fat, as the natural progression is usually from fat to cyst formation. Of the 9 cases reported in one study, 2 patients had bilateral disease. The treatment for this tumor is curetting, with or without bone grafting, with the expectation of a low rate of recurrence. There is a slight risk of malignant transformation, but none have been reported in the foot.

Epidermal Inclusion Cyst

This is primarily a soft-tissue lesion but can involve bone secondarily, in which case it is described as an epidermal bone cyst. They usually involve the distal phalanx and radiographically appear lytic and slightly expansile with a well-defined sclerotic margin. Pathologic fracture is not uncommon and may be a source of pain and discomfort. They are frequently confused with enchondroma. Treatment is simple curetting, and recurrence is rare.

Fibroxanthoma

Variously known as fibrous cortical defect, fibrous metaphyseal defect, and nonossifying fibroma, this lesion is common in the distal tibia and is usually asymptomatic unless there is an associated pathologic fracture. Radiographically it is an eccentric radiolucent lesion with a "soap-bubble" appearance and a densely sclerotic margin. When the tumor involves greater than 50% of the shaft of the bone and/or exceeds 33 mm in longitudinal extent, it is felt to be at greater risk for pathologic fracture and may be best treated prophylactically with curetting and bone graft. Smaller lesions should be observed, as the natural history of this tumor is to spontaneously regress after many months, or even years. This is probably the most common tumor of long bones in the developing skeleton and is believed to be present in up to

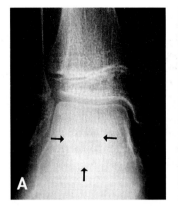
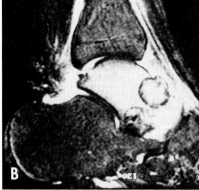
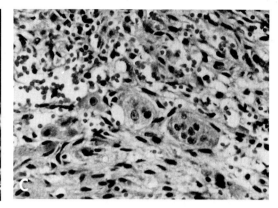

Figure 4

A, AP radiograph of a skeletally immature patient with a radiolucent abnormality with a sclerotic border in the talus that was proven to be giant-cell reparative granuloma histologically. **B,** Sagittal, fast spin echo, T2 weighted pulse sequence demonstrating a hyperintense abnormality in the anterior and dorsal aspect of the talus with surrounding bright signal in the bone and soft tissue representing edema and underscoring the intense inflammatory component of giant-cell reparative granuloma. **C,** Hematoxylin and eosin stain of a giant cell reparative granuloma showing multinucleated giant cells and proliferative spindled fibrous stroma.

30% of individuals. They may be multiple in as many as 8% of patients and when seen multiply, should raise the suspicion of neurofibromatosis or Jaffe-Campanacci syndrome when associated with café au lait spots. Although relatively common in the ankle in both the distal tibia and fibula, this tumor is rare in the foot.

Giant Cell Tumor

This common primary benign bone tumor occurs infrequently in the foot and ankle, accounting for 2% to 5% of cases in several large series. Although there is a wide age range, peak incidence is usually between the second and fourth decades of life, and this tumor is more common in women than men. Multifocal cases have been described and there is a low incidence, less than 1%, of distant metastases. There is an entity, giant cell reparative granuloma, in the small bones of the hands and feet with which giant cell tumor is often confused (Fig. 4). Treatment is curetting and burring, followed by adjuvant therapy, such as phenol or liquid nitrogen, and bone grafting or polymethyl methacrylate packing to provide structural support. The recurrence rate for this tumor is around 25%.

Chondrosarcoma

This is the most common malignant tumor of the foot and may be primary or secondary to pre-existing enchondromas or osteochondromas. The majority of chondrosarcomas are low to intermediate grade tumors, however, high grade tumors can occur, most commonly in the hindfoot. Radiographically there are deep endosteal scallops, cortical destruction with an associated soft-tissue mass, and cartilage matrix production. Radionucleotide uptake is generally intense and often heterogeneous, unlike benign enchondroma where the uptake is usually mild to moderate and homogeneous. MRI usually appears very bright on T2 pulsed sequences, reflecting the high water content within the tumor, while gadolinium enhancement often, but not invariably, has a septal enhancement pattern reflecting the tumor's lobular growth. Histologically, there is great variability, but, in general, there is a relatively high degree of cellularity, myxoid tumor matrix, occasional mitotic activity, and, most important, the presence of tumor surrounding or invading bone. High grade tumors are hypercellular and demonstrate higher degrees of nuclear and cellular pleomorphism and mitotic activity. Occasionally, "dedifferentiation" can occur, with areas of high grade anaplastic spindle cells that, apart from adjacent areas of cartilage tumor, would be unrecognizable as a cartilage neoplasm. Dedifferentiated chondrosarcomas metastasize early and frequently. For this reason, the 5-year survival rate is around 5%. For low and intermediate grade tumors, wide local resection alone is sufficient. For lesions of the foot, this usually involves a ray resection or partial foot amputation. Lesions in the hindfoot, especially higher grade tumors, are best treated by below knee amputation. For patients with high grade and "dedifferentiated" chondrosarcomas, chemotherapy is often given.

Soft-Tissue Tumors

Ganglion Cyst

Ganglia arise from myxoid degeneration of collagen fibers of a joint capsule or tendon sheath, resulting in weakening of the

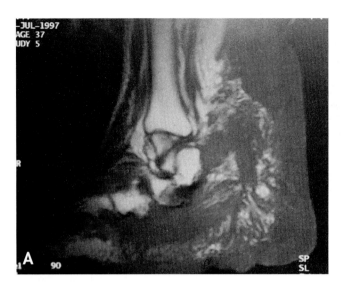 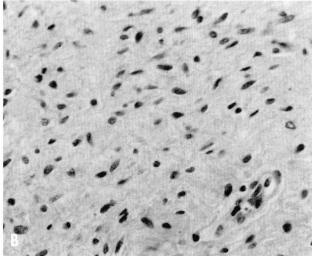

Figure 5

A, T1-weighted sagittal MR image of the ankle showing a large mass that is heterogeneous and predominately hypointense reflecting the underlying tumor with scattered hyperintense areas that represent fat. This is the typical infiltrating appearance of a neurofibroma. **B,** Hematoxylin and eosin stained section revealing a hypocellular spindled proliferation of cells with predominately loose myxoid stroma in a patient with a large neurofibroma.

collagen fibers and cyst formation. The cyst can insinuate around tendons and neurovascular structures and cause mechanical pain or nerve compression. MRI is the best study to delineate the origin and extent of tumor. Aspiration is productive of yellow viscous fluid that has the same constituents as synovial fluid. Treatment is aspiration and injection of a steroid preparation initially, followed by excision for recurrent or persistent tumor. It is important to excise the lesion completely down to and including a portion of the joint capsule.

Neurofibroma

Plexiform neurofibromas occur singularly in 90% of cases, however, multiple lesions are associated with neurofibromatosis of Von Recklinghausen's disease. The latter arises from a genetic mutation and is transmitted in an autosomal dominant fashion. The disease demonstrates a high rate of spontaneous mutation (50%) and a significant rate of malignant degeneration (2% to 29%). Neurofibromas generally present as firm, painless, mobile masses. They are found frequently along peripheral nerves and, when distinct from major nerves, are thought to arise from small sensory fibers. Generally, neurofibromas are not well circumscribed and are interdigitated with surrounding nerve fibers. Surgical excision is frequently not possible without sacrifice of the involved nerve. Neurofibromas in the foot and ankle can reach alarming size and interfere with shoe wear and ambulation (Fig. 5). While debulking of the lesion(s) can provide

some improvement, there are instances when amputation is a better option in spite of the fact that this is a benign process.

Pigmented Villonodular Synovitis (PVNS)

The etiology of PVNS is unclear, but pathophysiologically, it involves synovial proliferation, histiocytic and chronic inflammatory infiltration, and hemorrhage. This results in boggy chronic synovitis with persistent bloody effusions and joint pain. In long-standing disease, joint stiffness and arthritis are present. Radiographically, a soft-tissue mass can be seen on plain radiographs along with subchondral erosions on both sides of the joint in long standing cases (Fig. 6).

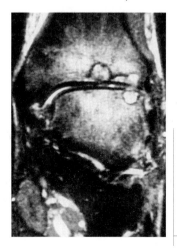

Figure 6

Patients with diffuse pigmented villonodular synovitis can develop subchondral bone erosions on both sides of the joint, as seen in this T2-weighted coronal MRI in a 60-year-old male with long-standing ankle pain and swelling.

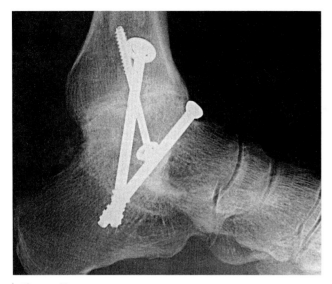

Figure 7

Due to diffuse and multiple joint involvement and persistent disease after several open synovectomies, tibiotalar and subtalar joint fusion was undertaken, resulting in reasonable function and excellent pain relief.

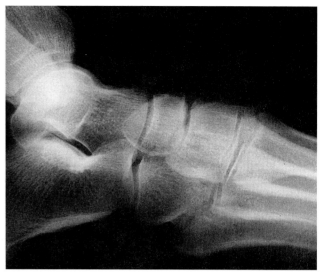

Figure 8

Subtle joint erosions are seen in this patient with giant-cell tumor of tendon sheath or nodular pigmented villonodular synovitis in the navicular and cuneiform bones arising from the dorsal joint capsule.

Magnetic resonance imaging is best at defining the extent of disease and usually appears dark on both T1 and T2 pulsed sequences due to the high hemosiderin content. In the foot and ankle, involvement is usually diffuse, extending from the tibiotalar joint into the subtalar joint and, occasionally, into the transtarsal joints as well. Initial treatment is synovectomy, usually open, but arthroscopic for more limited disease. Because synovectomy is almost always incomplete and involvement is extensive, multiple recurrences are the rule. The use of chemical or radionucleotide synovectomy in the foot and ankle is often impossible due to diffuse involvement, but it may be considered following arthroscopic or open synovectomy for limited disease, either prophylactically or to treat early disease recurrence. The efficacy of these adjuvant therapies in unknown. Low dose external beam radiation has been used for patients with destructive disease in and around joints. In one study, 13 of 14 patients had a complete response following moderate dose radiotherapy (35Gy) with a mean follow-up of 69 months. When pain and arthritic change are functionally limiting, fusion is the only salvage and should include all involved joints (Fig. 7). Fusion eliminates the painful recurrent swelling and, ultimately, improves function.

Giant Cell Tumor of Tendon Sheath

This is a localized or extra-articular form of PVNS and is common in the foot, particularly the forefoot, between the web spaces along the flexor and extensor tendons. The mass itself is relatively painless and can become prodigious before

mechanical symptoms supervene. Usually, patients complain of mild pain and difficulty with foot wear. The mass is usually fixed to a tendon or joint capsule and, in long standing cases, can cause erosions in the underlying bone (Fig. 8). Radiographically, they rarely mineralize and are best seen on MRI as dark signal abnormalities on both T1 and T2 because of hemosiderin deposition (Fig. 9). Few recurrences follow marginal excision.

Hemangioma

Hemangioma, or arteriovenous malformation, is not a neoplasm per se but, rather, a hamartoma, normal tissue in an abnormal location. It is common in the foot and may be capillary or cavernous, high or low flow, and unpredictably symptomatic. When symptoms are present, they are usually mechanical and caused by overuse. Occasionally, in high flow lesions, a "steal" phenomenon can occur, with increased flow to the tumor and decreased flow to normal tissue, which results in a sensation of fatigue or pain similar to that experienced by patients with vascular insufficiency. A bluish discoloration of the skin can be observed in some cases. In general, mechanical symptoms can be managed by modifying activity and the judicious use of nonsteroidal anti-inflammatory medicines. Resection of an arteriovenous malformation must be meticulous and should be proceeded by arteriography and embolization, if possible. Often, the disease is extensive, with involvement of muscle, normal vessels and nerves. Resection in these cases is unsatisfying, and nonsurgical treatment, such

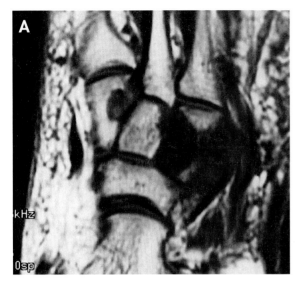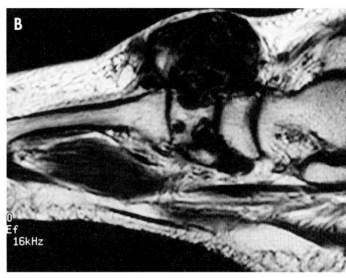

Figure 9

A, The disease process also involves the intercuneiform joint as well and appears dark on T2 pulsed weighted sequences due to hemosiderin deposition. **B,** This tumor can become quite prodigious prior to presentation. This sagittal spin echo T2-weighted pulse sequence reveals a large soft tissue mass arising from the mid-tarsal joint capsule.

as shoe and activity modifications and selective embolization, is more realistic.

Fibromatosis

Also known as Ledderhose's disease, this process is histologically identical to Dupuytren's disease in the hand. It commonly occurs in young individuals and is usually asymptomatic. This disease is a benign proliferation of fibroblasts. The responsible cell is the myofibroblast and the course and extent of disease are variable. Toe contractures, although possible, are not a prominent part of this disease, unlike digital contractures in the hand, but with increased growth of the lesions, shoe wear can be difficult. Bilateral disease has been reported in as many as 50% of patients in some series. Aggressive fibromatosis can be very extensive and insinuate around tendons, nerves, and vessels, making surgical resection impossible. Radiographically, this disease is usually seen in the mid-plantar foot, arising from the plantar fascia medially. It is usually low signal on T1 and intermediate signal intensity on T2 pulse weighted sequences, reflecting the relatively high amount of collagen and low cellularity. This disease is best managed by accommodative shoe wear, padded inserts, and occasional nonsteroidal medicines for symptoms. The value of perilesional corticosteroid injection is questionable. If nonsurgical modalities fail, surgery involves resecting most of the plantar fascia from its origin on the calcaneus to, and sometimes including, the aponeurotic slips along the flexor tendons in

the toes. Resection should be done through an incision that avoids the major weightbearing portion of the medial longitudinal arch. Surgery however, should not be done until all nonsurgical options have been exhausted because of the high rate of local recurrence, skin complications, and loss of the normal windlass effect of the plantar fascia. The addition of radiation, alone or in conjunction with surgical resection, results in good local disease control and may be useful in treating recurrent or inoperable lesions in this location. Fibrosis, stiffness, and, rarely, secondary sarcoma formation in the radiated bed are potential complications. Methotrexate administration and surgery have been used together with satisfactory results in a limited number of patients.

Granuloma Annulare

Granuloma annulare is an uncommon benign reactive or inflammatory dermatosis that manifests clinically as a mass with dermal papules that form rings. These masses can grow rapidly and are generally painless. Reported in multiple locations in up to 60% of patients in one series, they account for about 2% of all benign soft-tissue masses and are more common in children. On MRI, this tumor is hyperintense with muscle on T2 pulsed sequences and isointense on T1 (Fig. 10). These lesions are limited to the subcutaneous tissue, with extension, in some cases, down to fascia. Although unusual in the foot and ankle, they are a cause for concern because of their rapid growth and poten-

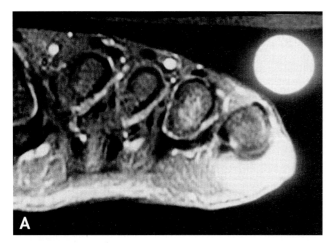
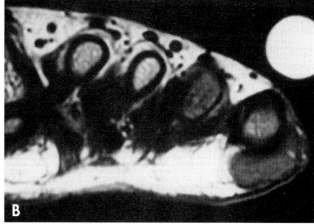

Figure 10
Granuloma annulare is an uncommon but frequently misdiagnosed mass in the foot. It can be deep seated and confused with a more sinister disease process in young patients. They appear uniformly hyperintense to muscle on T1 and enhance markedly with gadolinium administration.

tial confusion with a sarcoma, specifically, synoviosarcoma. Treatment is simple excision, with minimal risk of tumor recurrence.

Melanoma

Melanoma of the foot constitutes approximately 25% of lesions found on the lower extremity and is the most common malignant tumor of the foot. In one study of patients with melanoma of the foot, 65% presented with tumor extending through the dermis and 22% had metastases at initial presentation. Plantar and subungual lesions had a poorer prognosis than dorsal lesions or tumors in other anatomic regions of the body. The poor prognosis was not related to local disease control but to advanced histologic and clinical stage of disease at the time of presentation. Melanomas can be particularly difficult to recognize in a subungual location, particularly in patients with dark skin, and they are often mistaken for subungual hematoma. Wide resection with a 2-cm cuff of normal tissue is the preferred treatment. Such a resection may require split-thickness skin grafting, local advancement flaps, or vascularized soft-tissue transfer.

Clear Cell Sarcoma

This is a relatively rare and highly malignant tumor of soft parts, however, 50% of clear cell sarcomas, also known as amelanotic melanomas, occur in the foot. This mass is generally deep seated and may be present for months or years before it becomes symptomatic. It can involve the underlying bones of the foot secondarily. Melanin deposition causes this tumor to appear dark on both pulse sequences on MRI. It is highly vascular and enhances intensely and diffusely with

gadolinium administration. Clear cell sarcoma is best treated by wide local excision and radiation therapy. There is no role for chemotherapy in small nonmetastatic tumors, and its efficacy in patients with metastatic disease is generally disappointing. Patients should be monitored for many years as recurrences and distal metastases have been reported several years after long disease-free intervals.

Synoviosarcoma

The most common deep-seated sarcoma in the foot, synoviosarcoma, is highly malignant and can be asymptomatic for many months or years before diagnosis. This disease affects adolescents and young adults and is slightly more common in males than females. Radiographically, about 30% of synoviosarcomas will mineralize (Fig. 11), in which case

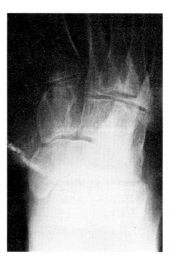

Figure 11
Mineralization in a biphasic synoviosarcoma arising in plantar foot of a 16-year-old girl.

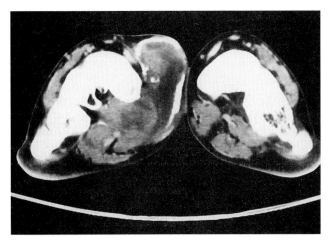

Figure 12
In the mineralization pattern primarily in the periphery of the mass, note the high degree of tumor heterogeneity.

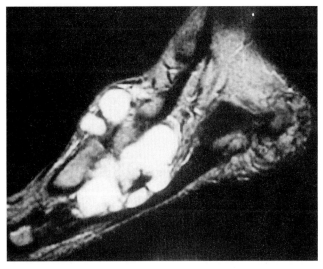

Figure 13
The mass arises from the plantar surface of the foot and wraps around the medial aspect of the foot. Multiple compartments are involved, making limb salvage impossible. This patient underwent above-knee amputation for local disease control.

they are better seen on CT imaging (Fig. 12). Patients with tumors exhibiting extensive mineralization have improved survival compared to patients without mineralization. The tumor is characteristically heterogeneous on T2 due to variable cellularity within the lesion, hemorrhage and hemosiderin deposition, collagen formation, and necrosis. Untreated synoviosarcoma can become quite large, fungate through skin, and track along fascial planes and neurovascular structures (Fig. 13). Histologically, there are two charac-

teristic patterns. The monophasic pattern is primarily spindled with short intersecting fascicles; the biphasic pattern demonstrates both the spindled pattern and a pseudoglandular or "epithelioid" appearance. The former has been reported to have a worse prognosis. Treatment consists of wide local surgical resection and radiation or, in many cases, amputation to achieve local disease control. In spite of adequate local disease control, metastases occur in as many as half of the cases. The role of chemotherapy for nonmetastatic lesions is unclear, and chemotherapy instituted after metastases occur is minimally effective. Because local lymph node spread can occur in 30% of patients, careful examination and imaging are required.

Tumor Resection

Resection is tailored to the biology of the tumor and can be intralesional, through the lesion; marginal, outside the lesion itself but through the reactive zone; wide local, outside the reactive zone of the tumor; or radical, removing the tumor and the entire compartment containing it. For benign bone tumors, intralesional resection is generally acceptable with or without chemical or cryotherapeutic adjuncts, depending on the local activity of the tumor. Marginal resections are appropriate for benign soft-tissue tumors, like giant cell tumors of tendon sheath or hemangiomata, where the risk of recurrent tumor is small. Wide local resection with or without radiation is the treatment of choice for benign aggressive lesions and low-grade malignancies, such as fibromatosis and dermatofibrosarcoma protruberans, as well as some high-grade malignancies, such as soft-tissue sarcomas of the foot and ankle. A radical resection would be appropriate for a large high-grade sarcoma involving multiple compartments or involving the neurovascular bundle. However, local disease control doesn't guarantee a good oncologic result because of the high risk of metastases. Preservation of a plantigrade sensate foot, in full or in part, following wide local resection is preferable to below-knee amputation, as long as local disease is controlled. Metastases occur in a large percentage of patients with malignant soft-tissue tumors of the foot, usually within 2 years of initial treatment, but, in some cases, many years thereafter. Below-knee amputation will achieve local disease control in most patients, but should be reserved for large tumors that involve multiple compartments of the foot, lesions effacing or circumferentally involving neurovascular structures, fungating tumors, and tumors of bone that involve the hindfoot with soft-tissue extension. In the ankle, specifically the distal tibia, low-grade and benign aggressive tumors of bone and occasional high-grade sarcomas with small extraosseous components can be resected en bloc and reconstructed with an allograft, vascularized free fibula or bone transport techniques. For similar lesions of the distal fibula, excision, followed by ankle arthrodesis, produces reproducible and good functional results.

Radiation can be used either before or after surgery for high-grade sarcomas of the foot. The advantage of preoperative radiation is that a lower dose of radiation is used over a smaller field in a well-oxygenated tissue bed. Furthermore, the risk of implanting a tumor in adjacent normal tissue is diminished with preoperative radiation. The disadvantage is that about one third of patients have a higher rate of wound complications.

Summary

Some tumors of the foot and ankle, like plantar fibromatosis and giant-cell tumors of tendon sheath, are relatively common. However, most bone and soft-tissue sarcomas are rare. The same principles of staging and biopsy apply to the foot and ankle as in any other body site. If a malignant disease process is suspected, the biopsy should be done in an institution familiar with musculoskeletal tumors, and all biopsies in the foot and ankle should be longitudinal with excellent hemostasis. Local disease control is one of the few goals that the orthopaedist can predictably achieve for tumors in the foot and ankle. Every attempt should be made to optimize function, whether this involves wide local excision, free-tissue transfer, and adjuvant radiation, or amputation. If foot-preserving treatment is possible, then the goal should be to maintain a foot, in full or in part, that is plantigrade and sensate. Above all, adequate tumor surgery should take precedence. The role of chemotherapy in patients with soft-tissue sarcomas without distant spread of disease is controversial. Malignant tumors of bone in the foot and ankle should be treated like malignant tumors in other sites. In general, these patients will have a better prognosis than patients with larger, more proximal appendicular or axial tumors. The role of gene therapy and biologic modifiers is on the horizon and will almost certainly become part of the overall treatment strategy in treating patients with sarcomas of bone and soft tissue. Until then, early recognition, organized staging, and appropriate local disease control is the standard of orthopaedic care for these patients.

Annotated Bibliography

Staging

Enneking WF, Spanier SS, Goodman MA: A system for the surgical staging of musculoskeletal sarcoma. *Clin Orthop* 1980; 153:106–120.

Classification of musculoskeletal tumors of bone and soft parts based on grade, compartments and presence or absence of metastases.

Mankin HJ, Mankin CJ, Simon MA: The hazards of the biopsy, revisited: Members of the Musculoskeletal Tumor Society. *J Bone Joint Surg* 1996;78A:656–663.

Twenty-five surgeons from 21 institutions submitted 597 cases. This is a follow-up study to the original multi-institutional study in 1982 to determine if the rates of complications, errors, and adverse effects related to the biopsy of musculoskeletal tumors had changed. The data supported the conclusion that no significant change in the number of complications and errors in diagnosis had occurred as a result of the biopsy procedure. Again, errors, complications, and changes in clinical outcomes were 2 to 12 times greater when the biopsy was performed in the referring institution instead of the treating center. This underscores the importance of early referral of all patients with musculoskeletal tumors to centers dedicated to treating these diseases.

Bone Tumors

Arata MA, Peterson HA, Dahlin DC: Pathological fractures through non-ossifying fibromas: Review of the Mayo Clinic Experience. *J Bone Joint Surg* 1981;63:980–988.

Twenty-three fractures were in the lower extremity, and the most commonly involved bone was the distal tibia (10 fractures). In all fractures, the lesions exceeded 50% of the involved bone in both the anteroposterior and lateral planes. The vertical length of the tumor was the greatest dimension and exceeded 33 mm in all cases. Recommended treatment was immobilization and subsequent biopsy, curetting, and bone grafting, or segmental resection for lesions in the fibula.

Casadei R, Ruggieri P, Moscato M, Ferraro A, Picci P: Aneurysmal bone cyst and giant cell tumor of the foot. *Foot Ankle Int* 1996;17:487–495.

In a series of 257 benign foot tumors, the authors identified 24 aneurysmal bone cysts and 21 giant cell tumors. In general, patients with aneurysmal bone cyst (ABC) were younger than patients with giant cell tumor (15 and 27 years, respectively). Although ABCs were rare in the tarsal bones, 19% of giant cell tumors localized to this area. Aggressive radiologic patterns were more commonly seen in patients with giant cell tumor and included cortical destruction and pathologic fracture. ABCs tended to expand bone; giant cell tumors eroded bone. Fluid levels were more commonly seen in patients with ABC. Local treatment of these tumors should consist of curetting, burring, and the use of an adjunct, such as phenol, because of the high rate of local recurrence with curetting only.

Chou LB, Malawer MM: Analysis of surgical treatment of 33 foot and ankle tumors. *Foot Ankle Int* 1994;15:175–181.

In an analysis of 33 patients treated at one cancer center over a 14-year period, there were twice as many benign tumors as malignant lesions. No local recurrences were reported after a period of follow-up ranging from 1 to 13 years (mean 7.2 years). Functional results were considered good to excellent in 82% of patients.

de Palma L, Gigante A, Specchia N: Subungual exostosis of the foot. *Foot Ankle Int* 1996;17:758–763.

This article analyzes 11 cases of subungual exostosis. In 5 cases, 3 separate layers were identified: a fibrous cap, a middle zone consisting of hyaline cartilage, and a deep zone of cancellous bone. In three other cases, the histologic pattern was pleomorphic and disorganized. Based on light microscopy and immunohistochemistry, the authors concluded that subungual exostoses had many features reminiscent of osteochondroma. Complete excision resulted in pain relief and no recurrent tumors.

Fink BR, Temple HT, Chiracosta F, Mizel MS, Murphey MD: Chondroblastoma of the foot. *Foot Ankle Int* 1997;18:236–242.

A review of 42 cases of chondroblastoma of the foot. The majority of patients were male (81%) and the mean age was 25.5 years, which is older than patients with chondroblastoma at other sites (17.3 years). The lesion was most frequently located in subchondral bone of the talus and calcaneus as well as the calcaneal apophysis. The lesion effaced subchondral bone or an apophysis in all cases and was radiolucent, with scant to no matrix production in most cases. Cystic changes were associated with 57% of lesions and were often confused with umicameral bone cysts. Recommended treatment was thorough curetting and bone grafting.

Jackson RP, Reckling FW, Mants FA: Osteoid osteoma and osteoblastoma: Similar histologic lesions with different natural histories. *Clin Orthop* 1977;128:303–313.

Compares and contrasts the clinical, radiographic and pathologic similarities between osteoid osteoma and osteoblastoma. This article highlights the importance of correlating the clinical, radiographic, and pathologic information in distinguishing between these 2 diseases.

O'Keefe RJ, O'Donnell RJ, Temple HT, Scully SP, Mankin HJ: Giant cell tumor of bone in the foot and ankle. *Foot Ankle Int* 1995;16:617–623.

In a series of 308 giant-cell tumors, 12 cases were identified in the foot and ankle. Nine were located in the ankle, the other 3 were located in the hindfoot. The rate of local recurrence was 25%. Of those tumors that recurred locally, all were treated with local measures consisting of curetting or resection; there were no amputations.

Milgram JW: Intraosseous lipomas: A clinicopathologic study of 66 cases. *Clin Orthop* 1988;231:277–302.

Five of 66 cases were in the foot; all in the calcaneus. The mean age was 37 years (range 14 to 75 years). One patient had bilateral disease. There were no recurrences after simple curetting. Because most patients were asymptomatic, observation was felt to be the initial treatment of choice.

Moser RP Jr, Sweet DE, Haseman DB, Modewell JE: Multiple skeletal fibroxanthomas: Radiologic-pathologic correlation of 72 cases. *Skeletal Radiol* 1987;16:353–359.

Of the 900 cases of fibroxanthoma studied in this archival series, 8% were multiple and only 5% with multiple lesions had a history of neurofibromatosis. It was concluded that multiple lesions were probably more common than previously thought.

Murari TM, Callaghan JJ, Berrey BH Jr, Sweet DE: Primary benign and malignant osseous neoplasms of the foot. *Foot Ankle Int* 1989;10:68–80.

In this study, 255 primary benign and malignant tumors of the foot were studied at the Archives of the Armed Forces Institute of Pathology. There were 213 benign and 42 malignant tumors. The most common benign tumor was the giant-cell tumor; chondrosarcoma was the most frequently reported malignant neoplasm. The metatarsals were the most frequently involved bones, followed by the os calcis.

Smith RW, Smith CF: Solitary unicameral bone cyst of the calcaneus: A review of twenty cases. *J Bone Joint Surg* 1974; 56A:49–56.

Of the 20 patients in this series, 11 were treated surgically, with no recurrences at follow-up. Most lesions were asymptomatic, and no changes were observed over time in the 9 patients observed. The authors concluded that unicameral bone cysts of the calcaneus should be treated nonsurgically.

Springfield DS, Capanna R, Gherlinzoni F, Picci P, Campanacci M: Chondroblastoma: A review of seventy cases. *J Bone Joint Surg* 1985;67A:748–755.

Seventy patients with chondroblastoma were reviewed retrospectively. Ten percent of patients had disease in the foot and ankle. The rate of local recurrence was 10%. The preferred method of treatment was curetting, and functional results were good or excellent in 80% of patients.

Surgery

Hain SJ, Koekstra HJ, Eisma WH, et al: The feasibility of hind foot amputation in selected sarcomas of the foot. *J Surg Oncol* 1992;50:37–42.

For high-grade sarcomas of the forefoot that cannot be reconstructed following resection, hindfoot amputation provides adequate margins in most cases as well as good functional results. Specifically, Chopart, Pirogoff, and Syme amputations are reviewed.

Soft-Tissue Tumors

Aluisio FV, Mair SD, Hall RL: Plantar fibromatosis: Treatment of primary and recurrent lesions and factors associated with recurrence. *Foot Ankle Int* 1996;17:672–678.

Risk factors for recurrent disease were multiple nodules, bilateral lesions, and a positive family history of plantar fibromatosis. The authors found that subtotal fasciectomy was most successful in preventing further recurrences of tumor.

Fortin PT, Freiberg AA, Rees R, Sondak VK, Johnson TM: Malignant melanoma of the foot. *J Bone Joint Surg* 199577A: 1396–1403.

In a retrospective clinical review of 60 patients with malignant melanoma of the foot and ankle, overall survival was 63% and overall 10-year survival was 51%. Survival for patients with plantar or subungual lesions was significantly shorter. Lesions in these sites were also found to be more frequently misdiagnosed. Poorer survival in patients with melanoma of the foot and ankle was due to advanced stage of disease and greater depth of invasion, both related to delays in diagnosis.

Lee TH, Wapner KL, Hecht PJ: Plantar fibromatosis. *J Bone Joint Surg* 1993;75A:1080–1084.

An excellent and concise review of this topic.

O'Sullivan B, Cummings B, Catton C, et al: Outcome following radiation treatment for high-risk pigmented villonodular synovitis. *Int J Radiat Oncol Biol Phys* 1995;32:777–786.

Over a 20-year period, the authors treated 21 cases of PVNS. They identified 14 cases that received moderate dose (35 Gy in 15 fractions) and noted excellent disease control in 13 of 14 patients with 69-month follow-up. They recommended subtotal synovectomy followed by radiation in patients in whom subsequent recurrence would significantly compromise function.

Selch MT, Kopald KH, Ferreiro GA, Mirra JM, Parker RG, Eilber FR: Limb salvage therapy for soft tissue sarcomas of the foot. *Int J Radiat Oncol Biol Phys* 1990;19:41–48.

Twenty patients underwent combined radiation and limb salvage surgery for high-grade sarcomas of the foot. Actuarial survival and disease-free survival at 3 years was 83% and 63% respectively. Both early and late complications were reported, but no amputations were performed as a result of complications.

Talbert ML, Zagars GK, Sherman NE, Romsdahl MM: Conservative surgery and radiation therapy for soft tissue sarcoma of the wrist, hand, ankle, and foot. *Cancer* 1990; 66:2482–2491.

Seventy-eight patients treated with limited surgery and radiation with a mean follow-up of 7.9 years had actuarial 5- and 10-year survivals of 80% and 69% respectively. Disease-free rates were 80% and 74% at 5 and 10 years, respectively. Although 15 patients had local recurrence (19%), 12 were salvaged. The authors concluded that "conservative" surgery combined with radiation therapy is oncologically and functionally acceptable.

Varela-Duran J, Enzinger FM: Calcifying synovial sarcoma. *Cancer* 1982;50:345–352.

The authors analyzed the clinicopathologic features of synovial sarcoma in 32 patients with extensively calcified tumors. They noted a focal biphasic histologic pattern in all patients with radiologic and microscopic evidence of extensive mineralization and/or osseous metaplasia. Survival was significantly better (82.5%) in this group compared to other series of patients with synovial sarcoma (25-51%).

Wright PH, Sim FH, Soule EH, Taylor WF: Synovial sarcoma. *J Bone Joint Surg* 1982;64A:112–122.

This study analyzed 185 patients with synovial sarcoma treated at a large cancer center. Overall, 5-year survival was only 38%, with decreased survival seen in patients with tumors greater than 5 cm. Fifteen percent of all cases were located in the foot.

Zindrick MR, Young MP, Daley RJ, Light TR: Metastatic tumors of the foot: Case report and literature review. *Clin Orthop* 1982; 170:219–225.

Seventy-two cases were identified in an extensive literature search. Most lesions were in the tarsal bones (50%). The rest were in the metatarsals (23%), phalanges (17%), and unspecified areas (10%). Genitourinary and gastrointestinal carcinomas were the most common primaries to metastasize to feet. The authors stated that metastatic disease should be considered in the differential diagnosis in any elderly patient with a painful swollen foot and an underlying destructive lesion. Surgery was recommended for local disease control and palliation.

Imaging

Madewell JE, Ragsdale BD, Sweet DE: Radiologic and pathologic analysis of solitary bone lesions: Part I. Internal margins. *Radiol Clin North Am* 1985;19:715–748.

A useful guide to understanding how to analyze bone tumors from plain radiographs in the context of margins, periosteal reaction, and matrix production.

Chapter 3
Skin and Nail Disorders

Introduction

The toenail is an appendage of the skin, and its function is to protect the distal phalanx. Diseases of the toenail pose cosmetic problems, and can be a source of pain and disability as well. The nail is like the horny zone of thick skin (Fig. 1) and consists of flattened, closely apposed squamous cells arranged in lamellae. Three layers of the nail plate are seen on a lateral view by electron microscopy: dorsal, intermediate (the main part of the nail), and ventral layers. The ventral surface is attached to the nail bed. The nail is compact and made up of keratins with a high sulfur matrix component that is not present in the outer layer of the epidermis, which is called the stratum corneum. The fat and water content of the nail is much less than that of the skin; therefore delivery of drugs to the nail is different than that to the skin.

The cuticle is the overlying epidermis on the nail plate. The eponychium is the thin cuticular fold that lies over the lunula and is composed of epidermis. The skin attaching to the undersurface of the nail at the free border is called the hyponychium. The root of the nail lies in a groove in the skin, the body (or nail plate) is the exposed portion, and the free edge is the most distal part. The nail matrix is under the body and root and produces the nail plate. The lunula is white because the papillae are smaller and less vascular than the rest of the nail bed. The germinal matrix is the part beneath the root of the nail and the lunula, and it is the area of growth of the nail. The sterile matrix is the remainder of the nail bed and gives a surface for the nail to glide, but does not participate in growth of the nail.

The 2 digital arteries end in the distal pulp space and give a rich supply of blood to the nail matrix and nail bed. Peripheral vascular disease is one of the common causes of nail deformities.

Toenails grow one fourth the rate of fingernails, at about 1.1 mm per month. It takes about 5½ months to replace a fingernail from the matrix to the free edge, and 12 to 18 months to replace a toenail. Nails grow faster in the summer than in the winter, and the growth rate may increase when there is inflammation around the nail. The growth rate may decrease with systemic illnesses or diseases of the skin.

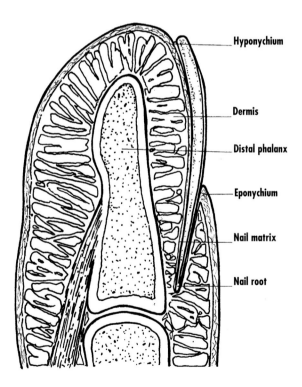

Figure 1

Anatomy of the toenail.

Hyponychium

Dermis

Distal phalanx

Eponychium

Nail matrix

Nail root

Malignant Melanoma

Carcinoma of the melanocytes has increased dramatically in recent times as sun exposure has been increased, with 32,000 new cases and 6,700 deaths in the United States per year. There are 4 types of melanoma: lentigo maligna, acral lentiginous, superficial spreading, and nodular. All have two biologic phases, horizontal and vertical growth phase. The vertical growth phase involves vascularity and is important in the metastatic process.

Whereas superficial spreading melanoma is the most common type in Caucasians (Fig. 2), acral lentiginous melanoma is most common in Asians, Latin-Americans,

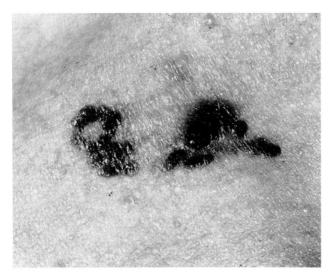

Figure 2

Malignant melanoma. A superficial spreading melanoma shows irregular borders and is black.

disease as stages I and II; stage III has lymph-node and in-transit metastases; and stage IV has distant metastases. The thickness of the tumor is the most important factor that determines prognosis, treatment, and follow-up. There are 5 Clark's levels: level I is limited to the epidermis, level II involves the papillary dermis, level III involves the junction of the papillary and reticular dermis, level IV involves the reticular dermis, and level V involves the subcutaneous fat. Breslow's thickness uses the measurement from the top of the granular cell layer of the epidermis to the deepest aspect of the tumor. A thin lesion measures less than 1.00 mm, intermediate 1.01 to 4.00 mm, and thick greater than 4.00 mm. Microscopic measurement of the deepest levels of melanoma involvement in the skin is a good indicator of prognosis. The prognosis is good for lesions less than 0.76 mm, because these rarely metastasize. The prognosis is poor, however, for lesions greater than 4 to 5 mm. Other factors for prognosis include level of invasion, ulceration, regression, host lymphocytic inflammatory response, mitotic index, angiolymphatic invasion, microsatellitosis, and growth phase (radial or vertical).

In a retrospective study of 60 patients who had a malignant melanoma of the foot or ankle, the most common site of involvement was the plantar aspect of the foot (Fig. 4), followed by the ankle, dorsum of the foot, dorsum of the toe or web, and the subungual area. The overall 5-year survival rate is 80% for all lesions, but 63% for the foot and ankle because of the delay in diagnosis or misdiagnosis. Lesions of the toe and at subungual sites were associated with a higher prevalence of misdiagnosis as compared to those lesions on the ankle or the dorsum of the foot. These lesions have been misdiagnosed as benign nevus, subungual or traumatic hematoma, blister, chronic paronychia, verrucae vulgaris, pyogenic granuloma, eccrine poroma,

and African-Americans. Acral lentiginous melanoma involves the foot or hand. The lesions can be linear or have the appearance of a fungal infection or wart. In the vertical growth phase, massive invasion can occur. In the foot, melanoma usually occurs on the sole, near the toenails and in the webs. With a lesion on the sole of greater than 9 mm and age greater than 50 years, the diagnosis of melanoma must be considered. If the lesion involves the toenail, it may have the appearance of a hematoma, but the adjacent soft tissue will have pigmentation. Also, melanoma may begin in a benign lesion such as a mole, called a dysplastic nevus (Fig. 3).

The American Joint Commission on Cancer classifies local

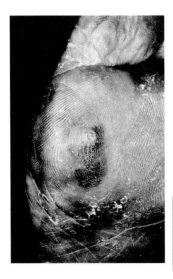

Figure 3

Dysplastic nevus. This benign lesion on the plantar aspect of the foot must be distinguished from a melanoma.

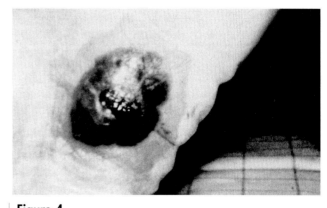

Figure 4

Malignant melanoma. The most common site of foot involvement is on the plantar surface of the foot.

dermatofibroma, and cysts. The prognosis for patients with a subungual melanoma has been poor, with a 5-year survival rate of 16% to 60%.

The treatment is wide excision with a surgical margin of 1 to 3 cm, depending on the thickness of the tumor. Soft-tissue coverage of the plantar aspect can be completed with a split-thickness skin graft for nonweightbearing areas, and large defects at the heel or forefoot may require a free flap or local transpositional flap. Amputation of the toe is indicated for lesions localized to the toe, including subungual lesions. The level of amputation depends on the depth of invasion.

Infectious Diseases

Kaposi's Sarcoma and Acquired Immune Deficiency Syndrome

Kaposi's sarcoma usually is seen on the plantar surfaces of the foot, but can arise on other areas. They are multiple, small, red or purple nodules (Fig. 5). There are 4 types of this disease: classic, African, in immunosuppressed kidney transplant patients, and in patients with human immunodeficiency virus (HIV). The latter form is systemic and can involve the lymph nodes, gastrointestinal tract, lung, brain, pancreas, aorta, and testis. About 15% of HIV-infected homosexual men present with Kaposi's sarcoma. Obstructive lymphedema may be associated with Kaposi's sarcoma, although the mechanism is unclear. The lymphedema may manifest initially, prior to the lesions, which makes the diagnosis difficult.

Current treatment is chemotherapy or radiation. Vincristine, bleomycin, and doxorubicin have response rates as high as 88%. Chemotherapy, however, has limited response, potential toxicity, and progression of the disease once the treatment is discontinued. Liposome-encapsulated doxorubicin shows a high response rate and good patient tolerance, up to 92%, but the development of side effects, such as hand-foot syndrome, may limit its use. This syndrome is seen with continuously administered chemotherapy, and manifests on the palms and soles with swelling, erythema, paresthesias, and, sometimes, cracking of the skin. The pain and swelling can interfere with shoe wear and weightbearing. Resolution occurs following discontinuation of the chemotherapy.

Patients with HIV are prone to chronic fungal infections because of their impaired T-lymphocyte function. Oral candidiasis is the most common fungal infection in these patients, and tinea pedis is the third most common cutaneous fungal infection in HIV patients. *Candida* dermatophytosis is uncommon except in the interdigital and groin areas. It can manifest in nail disease. Treatment with oral ketoconazole is generally successful, but the infection may recur.

Psoriatic disease is uncommon in HIV-infected patients. When present, the disease is often severe and treatment is difficult. A topical immunosuppressive medication can be initiated. A Norwegian form of scabies in which psoriasis-type lesions affect the fingers and toes is most often seen in immunosuppressed patients.

Plantar Warts

The human papilloma virus is the cause of the plantar wart, also called verruca plantaris (Fig. 6). It is a relatively common infection, with a peak incidence in the second decade; about 10% of teenagers are estimated to have warts. It is more commonly seen in athletes, and there is a greater risk of infection with the use of public showers. The virus infects by direct inoculation through a break in the skin. A plantar wart may be difficult to distinguish from a callus because of their similar appearance. Both can be painful with applied pressure, have a thick layer of hypertrophied epithelium, and occur in areas of friction or pressure. The lesion can be trimmed with a scalpel, and the wart will exhibit seeds (punctate hemor-

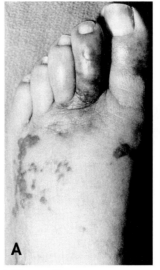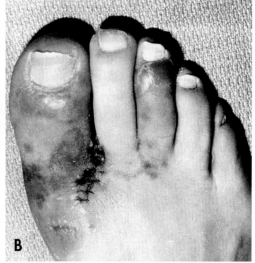

A   **B**

Figure 5

Kaposi's sarcoma. Although these lesions are usually found on the plantar aspect of the foot, they can also involve the dorsum. **A,** These have the typical appearance of multiple small red lesions. **B,** These lesions are purplish, flat, and more diffuse than those seen on the left.

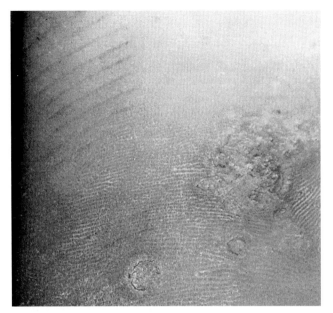

Figure 6

Plantar wart. This lesion on the weightbearing surface is painful. It is composed of multiple lesions.

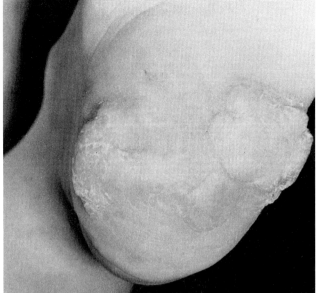

Figure 7

Verruca plantaris. This patient has chronic, multiple, and large warts that cause pain and difficulty with shoe wear.

rhages) and may bleed.

The appearance of a verruca plantaris can be varied. It generally has a hyperkeratotic surface, and may contain multiple capillaries, necrotic tissue, or even pus. The differential diagnosis includes callus, stress fractures, foreign body, and even a neoplasm. If there is suspicion of the latter, a biopsy should be done by the treating physician. The histologic picture of a verruca lesion is thickened epithelium; clumping of keratohyalin granules in the epidermis and viral inclusions can be seen. The infection can manifest as a solitary or multiple lesions (Fig. 7).

Simple trimming of the lesions and placement of chemically treated dressings, such as a 40% salicylic acid transdermal patch, will help decrease symptoms. This can be performed initially by the physician and then by the patient every 48 hours until resolution of the symptoms. Maximal effectiveness requires trimming of the wart prior to placement of the acid patch to allow for increased penetration of the acid into the wart.

Office procedures, such as cryotherapy with liquid nitrogen or cauterization, require local anesthesia. The wart should be trimmed to the level of the seeds before application of the liquid nitrogen, which is delivered with a swab or spray until the area is frozen. Repeated treatments are usually required every 2 to 3 weeks. Surgical excision is generally not recommended, especially on a weightbearing surface,

because a painful scar may result.

Superficial Mycoses

Tinea pedis affects 30% to 70% of the adult population, and is usually caused by *Trichophyton rubrum*. Less common organisms are *T mentagrophytes* and *Epidermidis floccosum*. These mycotic infections present as interdigital, moccasin, and vesicobullous types. The intertriginous or interdigital type is common and usually affects the fourth interspace

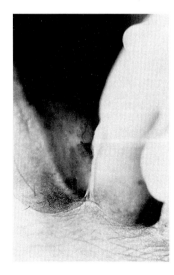

Figure 8

Tinea pedis. The intertriginous type most commonly affects the fourth interspace.

(Fig. 8). The skin appears macerated with erosions. There may be pruritus and a foul odor. The vesicobullous form manifests with vesicles and pustules, and it can extend to the sole or dorsum of the foot (Fig. 9). The moccasin type appears brawny with silvery white flakes on a red thickened base involving the sole, heel, and sides of the feet (Fig. 10).

Patients with immune deficiency have an increased incidence of infection. Diabetes and HIV, for example, have impaired cell-mediated immunity. Environmental factors add to the risk. Shoes, especially plastic ones, are occlusive and increase the risk. Tinea pedis does not occur in the unshod population.

One complication is the development of a secondary bacterial infection. *Pseudomonas* or *Proteus* are the most common organisms, and they can cause lesions that are painful and eroded, with an exudate or odor. Treatment is with antibiotics aimed at the organism identified by culture.

The diagnosis of mycosis is made by microscopic examination with 10% to 20% potassium hydroxide, and the appearance of septate branching hyphae at 10 to 40 power. Treatment involves foot care with topical or even oral antifungal medications in severe cases. The main goal of treatment is to produce a dry environment and avoid closed shoe wear. Frequently changed all-cotton socks, shoe alternation,

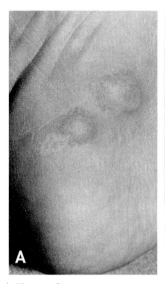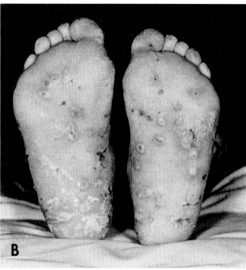

Figure 9

Tinea pedis. **A,** This patient has Hodgkin's lymphoma, and has multiple vesicles on the plantar aspect of the foot. **B,** Vesicobullous type. This form can involve the sole or dorsum, and this patient has diffuse pustules of the sole.

and antifungal powder should be initiated. Topical antifungal agents can be used as well as antibacterial soaps. More involved cases, such as with a secondary infection, may require an oral antibiotic. Oral antifungal agents are used for severe and chronic diseases. Griseofulvin, the most commonly used medication, acts on the cell nucleus. There are multiple side effects associated with use of this medication, including hepatotoxicity, gastrointestinal symptoms, headaches, and impotence. Recently, itraconazole and fluconazole have been used with good results and fewer side effects. These 2 new oral antifungal agents are discussed in the section of diseases of the toenails.

Allergic Diseases

Atopic Dermatitis

Atopic dermatitis is related to hay fever, allergy, asthma, and atopic eczema. In addition to a strong genetic component, there is xerosis of the skin, low itch threshold, and chronic relapsing eczema. Patients with atopic dermatitis lose the normal skin barrier, mostly because of scratching. Their skin has increased transepidermal water loss and loses the ability to bind water. These patients are therefore more susceptible to irritants, resulting in irritant contact dermatitis. There is controversy, however, as to whether patients with atopic dermatitis are more susceptible to allergens. Because there is a defect in T-cell function, they may not be capable of mount-

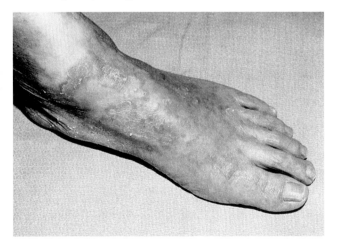

Figure 10

Moccasin type. This form can affect the sole and sides of the foot. This patient was treated successfully with a topical antifungal agent.

ing an allergic response. On the other hand, because the normal skin barrier is lost, patients are more likely to have allergic contact dermatitis because of increased exposure. In a study of 92 children who underwent patch testing for allergic contact dermatitis, the highest yields of positive patch tests were in atopic dermatitis patients with a history of a precipitating contact factor. The most common allergens were metals, fragrances, and rubber compounds.

A clinical entity called juvenile plantar dermatosis that presents in childhood and the early teens is exacerbated by shoe wear. There is an increased association with atopy.

The signs of atopic dermatitis include erythema, exudation, excoriation, dryness, cracking, and lichenification. The sites involved are arms, hands, legs, feet, head and neck, and trunk. These areas can be affected with mild, moderate, or severe disease. The erythema is caused by an increase of blood to the capillaries. The exudation is serous from the inflammation or even scratching. Scratching causes direct skin injury, seen as excoriation. Dryness is seen in the skin, and cracking is a break of the epidermis. Lichenification is the thickening and hyperkeratosis of the skin.

The mainstay of treatment for atopic dermatitis is topical glucocorticosteroids. The steroid usually is combined with an antibiotic, because *Staphylococcus aureus* is often present in eczematous skin of these patients. Severe cases can be treated with systemic prednisolone. Other treatment modalities include phototherapy with high-dose psoralen plus ultraviolet light of the A wave length (PUVA), cyclosporine, and interferon.

Contact Dermatitis

The appearance of contact dermatitis is an eczema, that is, an inflammation of the skin with edema and erythema of the epidermis. Vesicles, papules, weeping, scaling, and hyperkeratosis can be seen. There are 2 separate types of contact dermatitis, irritant and allergic, but their clinical appearance is identical. The irritant type, which accounts for 80% of occurrences, is caused by direct toxic effect of a chemical substance on the skin. An inflammatory reaction is initiated, and the degree of the response depends on the nature of the irritant.

Allergic contact dermatitis makes up the remaining 20% of reactions and is a classic delayed hypersensitivity reaction. It has 2 phases, an initial sensitization phase followed by an elicitation phase. In the initial phase, the allergen sensitizes the lymphocytes, and on reexposure of the skin, an inflammatory reaction occurs by activation of the T cells programmed to recognize it.

The most common cause of contact dermatitis of the foot is an allergic reaction to the shoe. The skin may appear to have an eczematous reaction usually on the dorsum; the sole is less frequently involved. Components of the shoe responsible for the allergic reaction include rubber additives, glue, dyes, and chromate. Other diseases, such as eczema, hyperhidrosis, psoriasis, and dyshidrosis, may be seen with contact dermatitis. Other allergens are poison ivy, poison oak, skin care products (soaps, lotions, and fragrances), and topical medications. Common over-the-counter topical medications, such as neomycin and bacitracin, can cause skin eruptions.

The diagnosis of allergic contact dermatitis is made from patch testing, thus allowing for exact allergen identification. The allergen is placed on a patch on the skin for 48 hours. The reaction of the skin is observed at 48 hours, 72 hours, and 1 week.

Irritant contact dermatitis is diagnosed by history and physical examination. The onset of pain, burning, and itching is within minutes or hours of exposure. Elimination of the irritant will result in predictable healing. There is no patch test available for this disorder. The treatment is avoidance of the inciting irritant. A barrier may be used, such as ointments, barrier creams, or topical corticosteroids.

The treatment of allergic contact dermatitis is avoidance of the allergen. Shoe dermatitis can be treated with foot powder to decrease sweating, which allows for elution of allergens from the shoes. Topical corticosteriods will decrease the inflammation and skin eruptions. Oral antihistamine medication is helpful for sedation and decreasing the itching. Occasionally, a secondary bacterial infection develops, usually a *Staphylococcus* or *Streptococcus* species, and treatment involves a second generation cephalosporin.

Psoriasis

Psoriasis is one of the most common diseases of the skin (Fig. 11). The etiology is activation of T-cell mediated immune responses in the skin, resulting in a chronic, scaly inflammatory dermatosis. There can be epidermal hyperplasia, pustules, and plaque formation, with both acute and chronic inflammation. In severe cases, systemic symptoms, such as fever, arthralgias, and malaise, may accompany the skin manifestations.

There are currently many treatment modalities for psoriasis. Glucocorticoids, phototherapy, and methotrexate have an immunosuppressive effect. The most effective therapy thus far is cyclosporin; however, its use is limited by its side effects, which include hypertension and nephrotoxicity. The topical form is ineffective because of poor absorption by the skin.

Psoriasis is the most common cause of nail deformity; the nail is affected in 50% of patients with this disease, with fingernails involved more than toenails. Nail pitting is a common

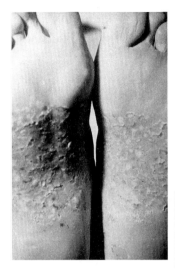

Figure 11

Psoriasis. These plaques have the typical scaly, erythematous, and thickened appearance.

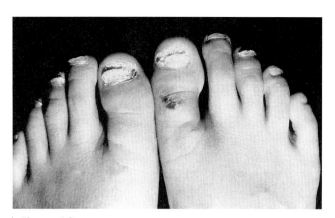

Figure 12

Psoriasis. Nail involvement can occur with or without skin lesions. This patient exhibits abnormality of the nail plate with severe thickening.

manifestation of nail psoriasis. Other causes of pitting are dermatitis, fungal infection, chronic paronychia, and alopecia areata. The pits may be a few to multiple, and may be small (less than 1 mm) or larger. Other associated nail deformities include onycholysis (separation of the nail from the nail bed), abnormality of the nail plate, and thickening (Fig. 12).

There are many types of treatment for psoriasis of the nails, including steroid injections, topical steroids, radiation therapy, phototherapy, and oral retinoids. The disease may recur with cessation of treatment. Also, remission may occur spontaneously with or without resolution of skin lesions.

Diseases of the Toenails

Fungal Infections

Onychomycosis means fungal infection of the nail. The fingernail can be affected, but the toenail is affected 4 times more. It is usually a cosmetic problem, but at times can become painful and interfere with shoe wear (Fig. 13).

Dermatophytes are the most common cause, with *T rubrum* and *T mentagrophytes* as the organisms in 99% of infections. It is a difficult problem to treat, and the prevalence rates have tripled to quadrupled in the last 2 decades. It occurs in about half the population over the age of 70 years. The greater prevalence in the elderly may be due to longer exposure to the fungus, a decrease in immune function, impaired circulation, and previous trauma to the nails.

The keratin of the hyponychium is infected initially by the dermatophyte, which then can involve the nail bed and the nail plate. The fungus first invades the ventral layer, which arises from the nail bed. The intermediate layer can become involved because it has soft keratin, like the ventral layer, but the dorsal layer is rarely involved because it is farther from living cells and is the hardest part of the nail. *T mentagrophytes* destroys the toenail more than *T rubrum* by way of a mechanical or enzymatic process.

The diagnosis is made definitively with microscopic examination of nail scrapings and potassium hydroxide slide preparation and even culture studies. The treatment involves debridement, removal of part or the entire nail, and topical or oral medication. Drugs must target both the matrix and the nail bed for proper treatment of nail involvement. Topical agents have been less effective than oral agents, and they are indicated in the treatment of mild onychomycosis. Once the matrix and nail bed are involved, with moderate to severe disease, the response will be limited because these topical medications are unable to reach the minimum inhibitory concentration for the infecting organism. Topical medication can be used in conjunction with surgery and oral medication.

Oral antifungal agents, such as griseofulvin and ketoconazole, were the most commonly prescribed for the treatment of onychomycosis. The results have been less than satisfactory because the duration of treatment is long (up to 1 year), laboratory monitoring is needed, and there is a high rate of relapse with cessation of treatment.

Recent oral medications such as terbinafine (Lamasil®, Sandoz Pharmaceuticals Corporation, East Hanover, NJ) and itraconazole (Sporanox®, Janssen Pharmaceutica Inc, Titusville, NJ) have been more effective, and treatment time is much less. Itraconazole was approved in September 1995 by the US Food and Drug Administration (FDA) for the treatment of dermatophyte onychomycosis, and it has been marketed to the general population with advertisements and a toll-free telephone number for information. It is a synthetic triazole, and its mechanism of action is at the catalytic

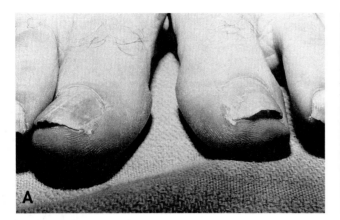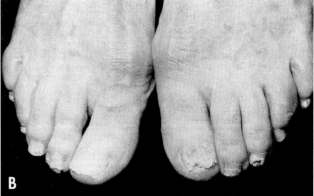

Figure 13

Onychomycosis. **A,** In the early form of the fungal infection, the hyponychium is affected followed by the nail bed and plate. **B,** All three layers of the nail plate are infected. Treatment is difficult and would require an oral antifungal agent to eradicate the infection.

heme iron atom of cytochrome P450 site where it competes for oxygen. It has a higher affinity for fungal cytochrome P450 enzymes than for mammalian ones. The result is a defective cell membrane with altered permeability and function. Terbinafine was approved by the FDA in May 1996. It is a synthetic allylamine derivative, and it inhibits squalene epoxidase, a key enzyme in sterol biosynthesis in fungus.

Itraconazole and terbinafine are taken up both by the nail matrix and the nail bed. They begin to work at 12 to 24 weeks after initiation of treatment, which seems to be less time than that for griseofulvin. Preliminary studies have shown these drugs have a wider range of effectiveness than griseofulvin, and the two have similar efficacies. The spectrum is broad, including *Trichophyton, Microsporum,* and *Epidermophyton.* The drugs remain in the nail for at least 6 months after cessation of the medication. The dosage of itraconazole is 200 mg per day, and can be given continuously or as a pulse dose (200 mg twice daily for 1 week per month for 3 consecutive months). Thus far 88% of patients have marked improvement and 64% mycologic cure at 12 months of follow-up after start of therapy. The treatment is relatively costly; the wholesale price is $336 for a continuous 1 month's supply.

With these oral medications, hepatic enzyme test values should be monitored, especially if there is a history of hepatic dysfunction. Rare cases of hepatobiliary dysfunction have been reported. Also, there have been reports of serious skin reactions, such as toxic epidermal necrolysis, with terbinafine.

Fungal Infection of the Cuticle

While *Staphylococcus aureus* is the most common cause of infection of the nail fold, called paronychia, fungus can be the infecting organism. In the acute process, there can be pain,

erythema, edema, and purulent drainage. *Candida albicans* can be the cause of a chronic paronychia, although less frequently than bacteria. A fungal infection can coexist with a bacterial one, such as *Proteus, Staphylococcus aureus, Streptococcus faecalis,* and *Pseudomonas aeruginosa.* There can be swelling, redness, some tenderness, and irregularity of the nail (ridges, pits, onycholysis, and subungual hyperkeratosis). The nail fold can become thickened with prolonged disease, leading to further damage and loss of the cuticle. Associated diseases, such as eczema or psoriasis, or repeated irritation from occupational exposure may be the inciting event leading to infection. With loss of the cuticle, the risk for nail injury increases, because organisms can access beyond the nail fold.

The diagnosis is made from bacterial and fungal cultures. The treatment can then be determined. If a fungal infection is present, a topical antifungal lotion can be applied. Topical agents are effective in this area. An oral antifungal agent is added if there is nail plate involvement. Topical agents such as imidazole or polyene antifungal lotion are used on a regular basis until complete healing occurs. Other treatment principles should be instituted: keep the affected limb clean and dry, avoid manipulation of the cuticle, avoid irritants, and treat associated skin diseases. A topical steroid can be added to the treatment regimen to decrease inflammation and allow the cuticle to heal. If the condition does not resolve, the diseased cuticle can be excised, which would allow healing and reformation of the cuticle.

Mechanical Problems and Bacterial Infection

Ingrown toenail, also called onychocryptosis, is a common disorder. There are 3 stages of the disease. Stage 1 consists of erythema, edema, and tenderness of the lateral nail fold. Stage 2 has these signs and symptoms of infection and purulent drainage. Stage 3 has worsening of stages 1 and 2 with chronic changes, such as granulation tissue and hypertrophy of the lateral wall (lateral means the affected side of the nail, and not the opposite of medial). The granulation tissue may become quite extensive, involving the entire lateral nail groove.

The cause is usually improper nail trimming. An ill-fitting shoe is an important factor, because it can add external pressure to the affected nail fold. Other causes include diabetes, hyperhidrosis, deformity of the foot and ankle, and trauma.

Treatment is conservative and symptomatic. For stage 1 disease, proper nail trimming, use of open-toed shoes, antibiotics, soaks, and placement of a cotton wick in the lateral groove corners will be successful in most cases. Stage 2 disease may require partial nail avulsion. This can be completed with a digital block, and then cutting the lateral one fourth to one third of the nail with a pair of scissors, taking care to protect the nail bed and matrix. Complete nail avulsion is usually unnecessary and results in a painful exposed nail bed.

A matricectomy procedure may be required to prevent recurrence of the disease, and may be indicated in stage 3 disease. There are several methods of matricectomy, including electrocautery, phenolization, application of sodium hydroxide, laser ablation, or surgical excision (Winograd or Zadik procedures).

The surgical method of lateral matrix removal generally provides a good result. The lateral nail is removed and the proximal nail fold is incised obliquely and lifted to expose the lateral matrix, which is then excised.

With chronic cases of ingrown toenails, the lateral nail fold may become hypertrophied. The disorder can be effectively treated by excising an elliptical wedge of tissue at the distal aspect of the lateral nail fold. The remaining skin is sutured, the lateral nail fold is debulked of soft tissue, and there is less pressure at that site.

Nail Disorders

Trauma is a common cause of toenail abnormality. Repetitive trauma against the end of the shoe with sports activities such as running, tennis, and so forth, or even the use of high heeled shoewear, can cause subungual hemorrhage. The nail may develop ridges, cracking, and onycholysis (separation of the nail plate from the underlying nail bed) (Fig. 14). The treatment is simply avoiding the injury, proper shoe wear, and allowing the toenail to grow out. A subungual hematoma should be distinguished from a malignant melanoma.

Onychogryphosis is a severely deformed nail. It is thick and may have a spiral configuration. These generally do not present with pain, but patients have difficulty with shoe wear. Concurrent diseases such as diabetes mellitus and peripheral vascular disease may increase the risk of infection. These thick hard nails are difficult to trim. Often a burr or drill must be used.

A permanent treatment for this type of deformity is destruction of the nail matrix. Phenol matricectomy is one option. The solution is applied to the germinative cells for 2 minutes. The patient then has daily foot baths with an antibacterial soap until the wound is healed, usually 6 weeks. The prolonged time for healing and drainage from the chemical burn may not be acceptable to some patients.

Alternatively, surgical ablation can be performed. A terminal

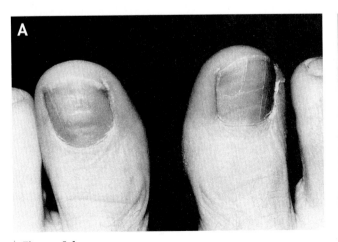 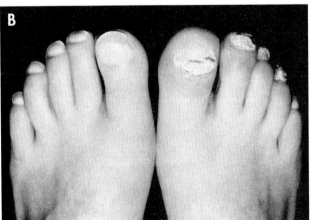

Figure 14
Nail dystrophy. **A,** Multiple ridges can be seen in this mild deformity. **B,** The entire nail plate can be abnormal with thickening and onycholysis.

Syme amputation yields the most reliable results; it involves excision of the entire nail bed and matrix as well as the distal portion of the distal phalanx. The distal plantar pulp is then sutured to the proximal nail fold. The toe will be shortened by this procedure.

Diseases of Sweating

There are 3,000 eccrine glands per square inch in the plantar skin. An increase in sweating can occur with thermoregulatory disturbance, hyperthyroidism, hypoadrenalism, and the intake of fluids or salicylates. Also, emotional hyperhidrosis, an autosomal dominant disorder, can be associated with this disorder. Essential hyperhidrosis is an abnormality of the sympathetic nervous system and is poorly understood. Affected are the hands (hyperhidrosis palmaris) (Fig. 15, A), axillae (hyperhidrosis axillaris), and soles (hyperhidrosis plantaris) (Fig. 15, B). Increased sweating can be associated with plantar bromhidrosis, which is the foot odor caused by bacterial digestion of breakdown products of the stratum corneum. Isovaleric acid is the end product and is the source of foot odor.

The treatment should be directed at reducing sweating and decreasing the growth of bacteria. With bathing, use of foot powders, and changing into clean dry socks and shoes, the symptoms should decrease. The treatment of choice is the use of a 20% aluminum chloride in anhydrous ethanol (Drysol®) at night for 2 nights and then every 3 to 7 nights as needed to decrease sweating. Other treatments include the use of topical antibiotics or iontophoresis. None of the aforementioned modalities give permanent results. Severe cases can affect the patient's psychological, social, and professional well being. Lumbar sympathectomy is the only known permanent treatment to stop all sweating of the foot.

Acknowledgment

Stanford University Department of Dermatology case slide file provided illustrations.

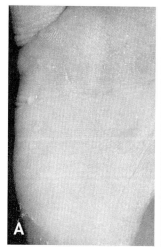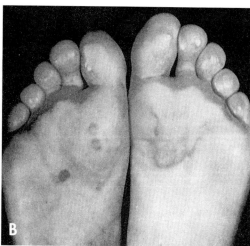

Figure 15

Hyperhidrosis. **A,** An abnormality of the sympathetic nervous system called hyperhidrosis palmaris can affect the hands. **B,** Excessive sweating of the foot can lead to plantar bromhidrosis, which is foot odor. Creating a clean and dry environment is the first step in treatment.

Annotated Bibliography

Malignant Melanoma

Fortin PT, Freiberg AA, Rees R, Sondak VK, Johnson TM: Malignant melanoma of the foot and ankle. *J Bone Joint Surg* 1995;77A:1396–1403.

This is a retrospective review of 60 patients who had a malignant melanoma of the foot or ankle. The most common site was the plantar aspect of the foot. Lesions at the plantar and subungual sites were associated with misdiagnosis.

Su WP: Malignant melanoma: Basic approach to clinicopathologic correlation. *Mayo Clin Proc* 1997;72:267–272.

This is an overview of the clinicopathologic correlation of the 4 different types of malignant melanoma. Microstaging is used for prognostic evaluation of the disease.

Kaposi's Sarcoma and AIDS

Allen PJ, Gillespie DL, Redfield, RR, Gomez ER: Lower extremity lymphedema caused by acquired immune deficiency syndrome-related Kaposi's sarcoma: Case report and review of the literature. *J Vasc Surg* 1995;22:178–181.

The diagnosis and treatment of Kaposi's sarcoma and its associated obstructive lymphedema are discussed.

Gordon KB, Tajuddin A, Guitart J, Kuzel TM, Eramo LR, VonRoenn J: Hand-foot syndrome associated with liposome-encapsulated doxorubicin therapy. *Cancer* 1995;75:2169–2173.

Hand-foot syndrome may be a limiting factor in the use of liposome-encapsulated doxorubicin therapy for the treatment of AIDS-related

Kaposi's sarcoma. This treatment option otherwise seems to have a high response rate and good patient tolerance.

Plantar Warts

Esterowitz D, Greer KE, Cooper PH, Edlich RF: Plantar warts in the athlete. *Am J Emerg Med* 1995;13:441–443.

A case report is presented followed by a complete discussion of the virus, incidence, prevention, treatment, and future use of immunotherapy.

Omura EF, Rye B: Dermatologic disorders of the foot. *Clin Sports Med* 1994;13:825–841.

This is a good survey of foot dermatologic problems, including plantar wart, corns and calluses, toenail disorders, tinea pedis, hyperkeratosis and fissures, contact dermatitis, and neoplasms.

Superficial Mycoses

Masri-Fridling GD: Dermatophytosis of the feet. *Dermatol Clin* 1996;14:33–40.

This author provides a complete review of this type of infection of the foot, detailing etiology, diagnosis, treatment, and complications. Chronic infections can be treated with topical agents, and more severe cases with new oral agents such as itraconazole.

Atopic Dermatitis

Berth-Jones J: Six area, six sign atopic dermatitis (SASSAD) severity score: A simple system for monitoring disease activity in atopic dermatitis. *Br J Dermatol* 1996;135(suppl 48):25–30.

This scoring system was developed to monitor atopic dermatitis, and includes the sites of arms, hands, legs, feet, head and neck, and trunk.

Stables GI, Forsyth A, Lever RS: Patch testing in children. *Contact Dermatitis* 1996;34:341–344.

In 92 children, 45 had atopic dermatitis and had the highest number of positive patch tests. The most common allergens were metals, fragrances, and rubber compounds.

Thestrup-Pedersen K: Atopic dermatitis, in Bos JD: *Skin Immune System (SIS)*, ed 2. Boca Raton, FL, CRC Press, 1997, pp 497–507.

The authors give a detailed description of atopic dermatitis, emphasizing the immunologic aspects.

Contact Dermatitis

Marks JG Jr, DeLeo VA (eds): *Contact and Occupational Dermatology*, ed 2. St. Louis, MO, Mosby, 1997.

This thorough guide to evaluation and treatment of contact and occupational dermatoses lists allergens, and discusses patch testing and occupations commonly associated with contact dermatitis.

McAlvany JP, Sherertz EF: Contact dermatitis in infants, children, and adolescents. *Adv Dermatol* 1994;9:205–223.

Contact dermatitis is the cause of about 20% of all cases of dermatitis, and is divided into two types, irritant and allergic. Allergens are found in plants, clothing, and shoes. Included is a good update on allergens in topical medications and skin care products.

Diseases of the Toenails

Gupta AK, Scher RK, De Doncker P: Current management of onychomycosis: An overview. *Dermatol Clin* 1997;15:121–135.

This is a complete review of current topical and oral antifungal agents for the treatment of onychomycosis. Complete drug information is provided for itraconazole, which has been shown to be more effective than griseofulvin.

Phillips P: New drugs for the nail fungus prevalent in elderly. *JAMA* 1996;276:12–13.

The author discusses why fungal disease is increasingly prevalent in the elderly. Itraconazole and terbinafine have been shown to be effective with a short course of treatment.

Rashid A, Scott E, Richardson MD: Early events in the invasion of the human nail plate by Trichophyton mentagrophytes. *Br J Dermatol* 1995;133:932–940.

An in vitro model was used to determine that fungi invade the nail by a combination of mechanical and chemical factors, thus allowing for further investigation with antifungal agents.

Mechanical Problems and Bacterial Infection

Zuber TJ, Pfenninger JL: Management of ingrown toenails. *Am Fam Physician* 1995;52:181–190.

The 3 stages of ingrown toenails are described, and the appropriate conservative treatment of each type is carefully outlined.

Diseases of Sweating

Noppen M, Vincken W, Dhaese J, Herregodts P, D'haens J: Thoracoscopic sympathicolysis for essential hyperhidrosis: Immediate and one year follow-up results in 35 patients and review of the literature. *Acta Clin Belg* 1996;51:244–253.

Bilateral sympathicolysis was performed on 35 patients with essential hyperhidrosis refractory to nonsurgical treatment. Complete resolution occurred in 52% and patient satisfaction was high. The disease, its incidence, natural history, and other treatment options, are described.

Pedowitz WJ: The malodorous foot. *Foot Ankle Int* 1996;17:54–55.

The author defines different types of smells. He details treatment that is aimed at reducing sweating and inhibiting the growth of bacteria. The current treatment of choice is using a solution of aluminum chloride in anhydrous ethanol.

38 Skin and Nail Disorders

Classic Bibliography

Baran R, Dawber RPR (eds): *Diseases of the Nails and their Management,* ed. 2. Oxford, England, Blackwell Scientific Publications, 1994.

De Berker DAR, Baran R, Dawber RPR (eds): Infections involving the nail unit, in *Handbook of Diseases of the Nails and Their Management.* Oxford, England, Blackwell Science, 1995, pp 53–63.

Hay RJ: Infections affecting the nails, in Samman PD, Fenton DA (eds): *Samman's: The Nails in Disease,* ed. 5. Oxford, England, Butterworth-Heinemann, 1994, pp 32–55.

Samman PD, Fenton DA: Psoriasis, in Samman PD, Fenton DA (eds): *Samman's: The Nails in Disease,* ed. 5. Oxford, England, Butterworth-Heinemann, 1994, pp 56–71.

Tagami H, Aiba S: Psoriasis, in Bos JD: *Skin Immune System (SIS),* ed 2. Boca Raton, FL, CRC Press, 1997, pp 523–530.

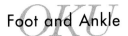

Chapter 4
Ankle Arthroscopy and Sports-Related Injuries

Introduction

Ankle arthroscopy is an innovative and useful addition to the armamentarium of orthopaedic surgeons. It allows direct visualization of intra-articular anatomy without the morbidity of an arthrotomy or malleolar osteotomy. With the advances in arthroscopic instrumentation, indications for ankle arthroscopy have been expanded to include (1) anterior and posterior soft-tissue impingement, (2) syndesmotic impingement, (3) bony impingement, (4) osteochondral lesions of the talus, (5) loose bodies, (6) arthrosis, (7) chronic ankle fractures, (8) ankle arthrodesis, (9) ligament stabilization, and (10) acute ankle fractures. Performing these procedures arthroscopically diminishes disruption of the soft tissues, which allows a more rapid postoperative recovery and an earlier return of function.

Topographic and deep anatomy of the ankle joint, patient positioning, portal placement, arthroscopic instrumentation, and the arthroscopic examination have all been reviewed in the previous foot and ankle update. The focus in this chapter is on specific therapeutic indications and new developments.

Anterior Soft-Tissue Impingement

Single or recurrent inversion injury to the ankle joint can result in anterior soft-tissue impingement or anterolateral impingement. The hypertrophied anterolateral synovial tissue and the injured, redundant anterior talofibular ligament (ATFL) are thought to be responsible for the joint irritation. Impingement occurs primarily in the superior portion of the ATFL, with possible corresponding chondral lesions in the talus and/or fibula. Patients complain of chronic lateral pain and swelling (with or without instability) despite rehabilitation. Radiographic examination is usually normal, but the use of magnetic resonance imaging (MRI) to aid in diagnosis has been proposed. In one study, MRI revealed synovial thickening in the anterolateral gutter in 40% of patients, but a recent investigation concluded that MRI examination is neither beneficial nor cost-effective in the diagnosis of anterolateral ankle impingement. Twenty-two patients with arthroscopic evaluations and preoperative MRIs were reviewed. Anterolateral ankle impingement was confirmed by the arthroscopic examination in 18 patients (82%). Clinical examination was 94% sensitive and 75% specific for impingement; compared with a MRI sensitivity and specificity of 39% and 50%, respectively.

Arthroscopic debridement should be considered following 5 months of failed conservative treatment. A motorized shaver and basket forceps are used to debride the hypertrophic synovium and ligamentous tissues. Use precaution with extensive anterolateral debridement to avoid detachment of the functional ATFL. Distraction is usually not necessary to address anterior pathology. Eighty-seven percent good/excellent results occurred in 55 ankle arthroscopes performed for anterolateral impingement, with 84% returning to sporting activities in one investigation. Similar results were shown in a recent study, with good or excellent results in 84% of anterolateral impingement lesions. Sixty-six percent of these patients reported a subjective feeling of increased range of motion, although objectively only 20% displayed greater than or equal to 5° increase in dorsiflexion at a 2-year follow-up period.

Posterior Soft-Tissue Impingement

Posterior impingement is associated with hypertrophy or tearing of the posterior inferior talofibular ligament (PITFL), transverse tibiofibular ligament, tibial slip, or a tear of the posterior tibial labrum. Diffuse synovitis and fibrosis are viewed arthroscopically in the posterolateral corner of the ankle joint.

The tibial slip, a structure that runs between the PITFL and the transverse ligament, has been noted to hypertrophy and fibrose following ankle trauma. The tibial labrum is analogous to that of the shoulder and can likewise cause impingement.

Distraction and a posterolateral portal are needed for successful posterior debridement. This lesion can be concurrent with anterolateral impingement.

Syndesmotic Impingement

Athletes have an increased incidence of distal tibiofibular injury, with associated prolonged pain and disability. The mechanism of injury is forced external rotation of the foot on the tibia or hyperdorsiflexion of the ankle joint. Physical findings include positive external rotation and fibular squeeze tests, as well as tenderness with palpation over the syndesmotic region.

The syndesmosis is comprised of 3 ligaments: (1) the anterior inferior tibiofibular ligament (AITFL), (2) the PITFL, and (3) the interosseous membrane. Reports vary as to the primary structures involved with impingement. One author states that the AITFL is the predominant ligament involved, with subsequent laxity and talar dome extrusion upon dorsiflexion. Another described a triad of pathologic features—interosseous ligament rupture, chondral fracture of the posterolateral portion of the tibial plafond, and PITFL disruption. This triad was reported in 19 patients who underwent arthroscopy for persistent symptoms of syndesmotic disruption. Of 17 patients available for follow-up, 14 returned to their previous sporting activities after arthroscopic resection of the torn interosseous ligament and debridement of the chondral pathology. Up to 20% of the syndesmotic ligament is intra-articular, and it can be debrided without causing residual instability.

Anterior Bony Impingement

Osteophytes occurring along the anterior lip of the distal tibia and the dorsal talar neck have been associated with athletic activity. A repetitive forced flexion traction on the anterior joint capsule and/or forced dorsiflexion of the ankle joint are the mechanisms of injury. Incidence rates of 45% in football players and 59% in dancers have been reported.

Patients complain of decreased dorsiflexion, swelling, pain, and catching. Radiographic examination (lateral weightbearing and maximal dorsiflexion ankle films) reveal osteophytes on the distal tibia and talar neck. A tibiotalar angle on the lateral view that is not greater than or equal to 60° is consistent with bony impingement. A radiographic classification for anterior ankle osteophytes exists, based on both spur size and amount of arthrosis present. With a type I lesion, spur formation is less than 3 mm. A type II lesion has spur formation greater than 3 mm and associated osteochondral reaction exostosis. Type III impingement exhibits significant bony exostosis with spur formation on the dorsal talar neck. In type IV lesions, there is diffuse pantalar arthritic destruction. Type IV lesions are best treated with arthrotomy.

Arthroscopic debridement is performed through anterior portals with a small burr and fluoroscopy to determine adequate resection. Excessive distraction should be avoided because it can result in tenting of the anterior capsule over the osteophytes, which increases the risk of anterior neurovascular injury. Maintaining visibility and avoiding turning the blade dorsally further protects the neurovascular bundle. Postoperative focus is on early range of motion and activity. One study described 17 patients who underwent arthroscopic resection for anterior impingement, with 16 athletes returning to sporting activities. Mean dorsiflexion increased from 3° to 12° postoperatively, with an average follow-up of 39 months.

Osteochondral Lesions of the Talus

Osteochondral injuries of the talus account for 4% of all osteochondral lesions in joints. The etiology is primarily trauma (acute or repetitive microtrauma), but idiopathic osteonecrosis has also been cited. Medial lesions are more common than lateral lesions, and they tend to be deeper, cup-shaped, nondisplaced, located more posteriorly, and to occur secondary to osteonecrosis. Lateral lesions are generally more shallow, wafer-shaped, and displaced, and are frequently induced by trauma. It is postulated that lateral lesions are produced when the anterolateral aspect of the talar dome impacts the fibula when an inversion/dorsiflexion stress is applied to the ankle. A posteromedial lesion may occur when a plantarflexed ankle is subjected to an inversion/external rotation moment, which causes the posteromedial talar dome to impact the tibial articular surface.

Symptoms include swelling, pain, catching, decreased range of motion, and stiffness. Objectively, one may elicit medial or lateral joint tenderness, decreased range of motion, and swelling. Radiographs are often normal in appearance or display very subtle changes. Radiographs in varying degrees of plantarflexion and dorsiflexion may bring posteromedial and anterolateral lesions in line with the x-ray beam. If the lesion is visible on plain films, a computed tomography (CT) scan is the best staging study. However, if films are negative despite a strong clinical suspicion, MRI is recommended for its increased sensitivity for overall pathology.

The classic classification system by Berndt and Hardy includes 4 radiographic stages: (I) small area of subchondral compression, (II) partially detached fragment, (III) completely detached fragment that is nondisplaced, and (IV) a completely displaced fragment. Ferkel and Sgaglione have since developed a computed tomography (CT) staging classification: (I) cystic lesion within dome of talus, (IIA) cystic lesion with communication to talar dome surface, (IIB) open artic-

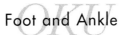
ular surface lesion with overlying nondisplaced fragment, (III) nondisplaced lesion with lucency, and (IV) displaced fragment. Nonsurgical treatment is recommended for stages I and II (of both classification systems) with 6 to 12 weeks of casting. Surgery is advocated for failed conservative treatment and all symptomatic stage III and IV lesions (except for patients with open growth plates). Delaying treatment for up to 12 months to allow a trial of conservative treatment does not compromise the result of subsequent surgery.

Arthroscopic treatment is preferred over arthrotomy because it reduces ankle stiffness, atrophy, and the risk of potential malleolar nonunion associated with a transmalleolar osteotomy. The arthroscopic procedure chosen depends on the location, the extent of osteochondral injury, and the chronicity of the pathology. Standard anteromedial and anterolateral portals are used, with ankle distraction and a 2.7- mm arthroscope. A posterolateral portal may be required for posteromedial and posterolateral lesions. Excision is recommended for lesions that are primarily chondral, with debridement and drilling for larger defects. The base is drilled with a Kirschner wire (K-wire) and an arthroscopic drill guide. The tourniquet should be released to ensure talar bleeding. For lesions smaller than 1 mm, abrasion alone may be adequate. Large osteochondral fragments may be reattached with cannulated Herbert-Whipple screws, absorbable pins, or K-wires.

Most anterolateral lesions are accessible for drilling and/or excision via an anterolateral portal. Posteromedial lesions are often difficult to treat without malleolar osteotomy. Alternatives to osteotomy, however, do exist. Transmalleolar drilling into the medial talus with a 0.062-mm K-wire with a micro vector aiming device at 3.5-mm intervals to a depth of 10 mm is described. Multiple holes are accomplished by plantarflexing and dorsiflexing the ankle. In one investigation, the authors describe a technique that used meniscal repair instrumentation to drill the lesion. The foot is placed in extreme plantarflexion, a partial medial synovectomy is performed, and a curved cannula is inserted through the anteromedial portal into the defect. The lesion is drilled with the 10-in trocar point needle after removing the preattached suture. Lastly, a technique has been presented that avoids violation of intact articular cartilage. A guide pin is placed percutaneously into the sinus tarsi and retrograde drilling into the medial talar lesion is performed over the pin. Calcaneal bone graft is then harvested with a Craig needle, then deposited subchondrally through the talar drill hole.

Bone grafting for osteochondral lesions of the talus has not been well defined. The most appropriate candidate is an adult patient with a detached lesion that still has a congruent articular surface by arthroscopic examination. Arthroscopic techniques consist of retrograde grafting (as described above), transmalleolar grafting (not recommended due to injury to the tibial and talar articular surfaces), and the newer mosaicplasty technique, which inserts an osteochondral plug taken from a nonweightbearing region of the knee into the osteochondral defect. In a preliminary report, the mosaicplasty technique was used in 11 patients with osteochondral lesions 10 mm or greater. All patients returned to full activities with follow-up from 12 to 28 months.

For lesions that were excised and/or abraded, early range-of-motion exercises and weightbearing are begun at 1 week. If the lesion was drilled, bone grafted, or internally fixed, weightbearing is delayed for 4 to 8 weeks, until healing is demonstrated clinically and/or radiographically (to prevent collapse of the articular surface).

In one series, excellent or good results were seen in 88% of patients who underwent arthroscopic debridement and drilling of osteochondral lesions of the talus. Another study of 59 patients, with average follow-up of 40 months, resulted in good to excellent results in 84%. When compared, results of arthroscopic treatment of these lesions are comparable to or better than those of open techniques.

Large osteochondral lesions can progress to tibiotalar arthrosis. A cadaveric study showed a 50% decrease in peak loads in a talus, following a 10° varus/valgus supramalleolar osteotomy. This may be a beneficial adjunctive procedure when large talar lesions exist.

Loose Bodies

These may be of chondral or osteochondral origin secondary to trauma. Patients usually report swelling, catching, and decreased range of motion. Loose bodies will be evident on plain films or CT only if they contain bone. Visualization of chondral defects is possible with MRI with intra-articular contrast. An arthrogram will also reveal the pathology by demonstrating loosened defects on joint surfaces or defect filling caused by the loose body itself.

Preoperative localization of the loose body is critical to facilitate arthroscopic surgical removal. Any chondral/osteochondral defect should be debrided and/or drilled. Excellent and good results after arthroscopic treatment were obtained in 88% of patients with loose body removal.

Degenerative Arthritis

Ankle arthroscopy for degenerative joint disease has been poorly delineated. Candidates are those with loose chondral or osteochondral fragments, osteophytes, limited ankle motion secondary to capsulitis, and a moderate degree of fibroarthrosis. Patients with extensive deformity or advanced degenerative destruction should not be offered arthroscopic intervention.

Although controversy exists concerning this topic, encouraging results have been reported. Twenty-seven patients with degenerative joint disease underwent arthroscopic debridement, loose body removal, and synovectomy. Improvement was documented in two thirds of the patients at an average follow-up of 45 months. Additionally, 10 patients with moderate to severe arthrosis underwent extensive debridement and Achilles tendon lengthening, with subsequent decreased pain and a mean increase in dorsiflexion of 7°.

Arthrofibrosis/Chronic Ankle Fractures

Following osseous union of an ankle fracture, patients often suffer from stiffness, pain, swelling, and activity restriction. Arthroscopy should be considered after several months of unsuccessful rehabilitation. These ankle joints are fibrotic and tight, and viewing can be difficult. Synovitis, fibrosis, adhesions, and loose bodies should be carefully debrided. Any cartilaginous or osteochondral lesions should be identified and treated.

Ankle Arthrodesis

Arthroscopic assisted ankle fusion is indicated in the osteoarthritic joint with minimal deformity. Fusion rates appear faster than with open methods, probably because less distraction and periosteal stripping is required. This procedure is not advised with varus/valgus deformity greater than 15°, malrotation, or anterior-posterior translation of the tibiotalar joint. It should also be avoided in situations of significant bone loss and in neuropathic joints.

The technique involves arthroscopic debridement of all hyaline cartilage and avascular subchondral bone with ring-and-cup curettes, shavers, and burrs. The normal convexity of the talus and concavity of the tibial plafond should be maintained (in opposition to the flattened surface often created in the open technique). Once appropriate positioning is obtained, distraction is released and fixation accomplished percutaneously with transarticular 6.5- or 7.0-mm cannulated screws through the medial and lateral malleoli. A third screw may be necessary in patients with osteoporotic bone. If difficulty is encountered in achieving concentric apposition of the tibial and talar surfaces, fluoroscopy and/or a mini-arthrotomy may be helpful. Lengthening of the Achilles tendon may also aid in neutral reduction of the ankle joint. It is believed that foot biomechanics following ankle fusion are improved with slight posterior talar translation. This is technically impossible with the arthroscopic method (due to the concentric reduction). However, it is not clear whether this is a clinical problem.

Thirty-four ankle arthrodesis were performed arthroscopically. There was a 97% fusion rate, a 9-week average time to fusion, and 86% of patients had good to excellent functional results. There was only 1 malunion. Another investigation reported 16 arthroscopically fused ankles for idiopathic or posttraumatic osteoarthritis and rheumatoid arthritis. A 100% fusion rate was achieved, with a 9.5-week average time to fusion. Fourteen of 16 patients were completely satisfied, and only 1 required shoe modifications. Looking specifically at complications, 42 patients underwent arthroscopic ankle arthrodesis with invasive distraction and demineralized bone matrix-bone slurry. Average follow-up was 27 months. There were 2 fractures, 4 pin infections, 1 deep infection, 4 hardware problems, 4 symptomatic painful subtalar joints, and 3 nonunions. Thirty-one patients had radiographic evidence of fusion; 8 had a fibrous union. Eighty-five percent of patients were satisfied. It is noted that many complications could be avoided by using noninvasive distraction techniques.

Lateral Ankle Instability

Arthroscopic ankle ligament stabilization has limited indications. It is limited to the repair of the anterior talofibular ligament (ATFL). The calcaneofibular ligament (CFL) is extra-articular and requires an open procedure for its reconstruction. The technique for ATFL reconstruction involves abrading a 6- to 8-mm area of the talus 1 cm anterior to the fibula. A suture anchor is used to secure the ATFL to the talus, with the foot held in dorsiflexion and external rotation. A weightbearing cast is worn for 6 weeks, followed by progressive range of motion and strengthening. Further studies will be needed to demonstrate the efficacy of this procedure.

Acute Ankle Fractures

Arthroscopy in association with acute ankle fractures can be used to assess anatomic reduction and to evaluate and treat chondral and osteochondral lesions. After irrigation of the hemarthrosis, fracture reduction can be achieved under arthroscopic visualization, and internal fixation accomplished with cannulated or standard AO screws under fluoroscopic control, using mini-open techniques.

Thirty-three consecutive ankle fractures were arthroscoped to look for intra-articular pathology. Osteochondral lesions were identified in 79% (26 ankles) of the treated ankles. Nine were in the tibia, 16 in the talus, and 1 on the fibula. Fifty-five percent of patients (18 ankles) had loose bodies, and 21% (7 ankles) demonstrated chondromalacia. No randomized prospective studies exist to determine the long-term efficacy.

Complications of Ankle Arthroscopy

As with arthroscopy of any joint, many potential complications can occur. In all series, neurologic complications predominate. One large retrospective review looked at 612 patients who had undergone ankle arthroscopy. The overall complication rate was 9% (55 complications). Twenty-seven of the 55 complications were neurologic (49.1%). The superficial peroneal nerve was injured in 15 cases, the sural nerve in 6, the saphenous nerve in 5, and the deep peroneal nerve in 1 patient. All nerve injuries occurred secondary to direct injury by portal or distractor pin placement. No neurologic injury was caused by tourniquet compression or compartment syndrome. Nerve injury can be decreased by carefully mapping out the nerve distribution, minimizing invasive distraction and minimizing the number of instrument passages.

Other complications consisted of superficial or deep infection, instrument breakage, adhesions, fractures of the tibia and/or calcaneus secondary to invasive distraction, ecchymosis, and reflex sympathetic dystrophy. Superficial wound infections appear to be related to the proximity of portal placement to each other, early mobilization, and the use of tape to close portal sites. Deep wound infections have been correlated with a lack of preoperative intravenous antibiotics.

Distraction Techniques

Visualization in ankle joint arthroscopy may be enhanced by distraction techniques. Invasive distraction techniques use threaded pins inserted into the tibia and calcaneus. Noninvasive techniques require commercially available devices or a gauze roll. Invasive distraction carries the increased risk of pin site infection, fracture, or neurovascular injury; noninvasive distraction minimizes these risks.

A new technique for invasive distraction has been reported that uses a single calcaneal pin and an orthopaedic fracture table. The authors performed more than 100 ankle arthro-scopies with this method, with no complications. This technique allows controlled distraction, does not interfere with portal access, and minimizes the number of osseous pins needed. Most pin related complications occur on the tibial side.

One study, which looked at the relationship between force, magnitude of distraction, and nerve conduction abnormalities using noninvasive ankle distraction, found that distraction with 135 N (30 lbs) of force for 1 hour is associated with reversible nerve conduction changes. The superficial and deep peroneal nerves are affected to a greater extent than the sural nerve.

Subtalar Arthroscopy

Subtalar arthroscopy allows the treatment of osteochondral lesions, loose bodies, degenerative conditions, and assessment of subtalar joint instability. There are 2 commonly used portals, both on the lateral aspect of the hindfoot. The anterior portal is located 2 cm anterior and 1 cm proximal to the tip of the lateral malleolus. The posterior portal is 2 cm posterior and 1 cm distal to the end of the lateral malleolus. The anterior portal is initially used to introduce the camera; the posterior portal serves as an outflow and instrumentation portal. Currently, only the posterior facet can be visualized arthroscopically. A 2.7-mm or a 1.9-mm arthroscope is used, with a 70° camera used to improve visualization. Examination consists of assessment of the synovial lining of the interosseous ligament, followed by assessment of the talar and calcaneal articular surfaces. Posterior advancement of the arthroscope allows visualization of the posterior pouch and its synovial lining. Debridement should be done with a 2.8-mm shaver.

Twenty-nine patients underwent subtalar arthroscopy. The diagnosis at the time of arthroscopy was: (1) synovitis in 7, (2) degenerative joint disease for 5, (3) subtalar dysfunction in 5, (4) chondromalacia in 4, (5) nonunion of the os trigonum in 4, (6) arthrofibrosis in 2, (7) loose bodies for 1, and (8) an osteochondral lesion of the talus in 1 patient. The results were 86% good or excellent following debridement.

A medial portal, recently described, allows better access to posteromedial lesions. It is created from the lateral anterior portal with a trocar directed through the tarsal canal in a posterior direction, angled at 45°. An incision is then made over the tented skin on top of the trocar. This portal was investigated in 6 cadavers. The average distance between the medial portal site and the posterior tibial neurovascular bundle was 1 cm; the closest distance was 0.8 cm. Clinical application has not been assessed.

Soft-Tissue Injuries of the Ankle Joint

Lateral Ligament Injuries

Twenty-three thousand ankle sprains occur in the United States each day. Lateral ankle ligamentous injuries account for approximately 15% of all athletic injuries. They occur in 45% of all basketball injuries, 25% of all volleyball injuries, and 31% of soccer injuries. Following negative radiographs, the "simple" ankle sprain is usually treated with rest from athletic activity, crutches, weightbearing as tolerated, and, in some cases, physical therapy. Up to 20% to 40% of ankle sprains, however, can result in such residual sequela as recurrent sprains and/or chronic instability.

The 3 major structures that comprise the lateral ligamentous complex of the ankle are the anterior talofibular ligament (ATFL), the calcaneofibular ligament (CFL), and the posterior talofibular ligament (PTFL). The ATFL is the most anterior structure with intimate capsular association. The weakest of the 3 ligaments, it is the one most often injured. The CFL is an extracapsular structure that runs deep to the peroneal tendons and spans the subtalar joint. It attaches to the inferior distal surface of the fibula and inserts onto a posterior lateral tubercle on the calcaneal lateral wall. The strongest, and least frequently injured, is the PTFL, which originates from the posterior margin of the lateral malleolus and inserts on the posterior talar surface.

Most ligamentous injuries occur when the ankle is in a plantarflexed, inverted position, without full osseous contact. In this position, the ATFL is usually injured first, followed by the CFL. When the ankle is in a dorsiflexed and inverted position, the CFL is the ligament most likely to be injured. It must be remembered that with severe injury, multiple ligaments may be torn, in conjunction with tendon, bone, and nerve injuries.

On physical examination, it is important to delineate the areas of maximal tenderness and swelling, with complete examination of all surrounding structures. In a systematic manner, one should palpate the ATFL, the CFL, the PTFL, the syndesmosis, calcaneocuboid joint, posterior tibial and peroneal tendons, fifth metatarsal base and shaft, and the medial and lateral malleoli. Specific manual testing maneuvers exist for testing the ATFL and the CFL. The anterior drawer test is performed with the patient sitting, knee flexed to 90°, and the ankle in some plantarflexion. The examiner grasps the heel and applies a forward force, at the same time applying a posterior force to the distal tibia. A positive test results in anterior subluxation of the talus and is indicative of an injured ATFL.

The contralateral ankle should be examined as a reference. The other common manual test is ankle inversion. With the ankle held in dorsiflexion or plantarflexion, the examiner inverts the heel while supporting the medial aspect of the distal tibia with the other hand. A positive test (increased talar excursion) with the ankle in dorsiflexion indicates an injury to the CFL; a positive test with the ankle in plantarflexion indicates damage to the ATFL.

Routine radiographs are often obtained to rule out fracture. It is necessary to have a high index of suspicion for associated fractures of the posterior talar process and lateral talar process, osteochondral fractures of the talus, fractures of the anterior process of the calcaneus, and fractures of the base of the fifth metatarsal (foot radiographs are taken if clinically indicated). Stress radiographs are helpful to help diagnose ankle instability. The anterior drawer stress test and the ankle inversion dorsiflexion and plantarflexion stress tests are performed manually or with the aid of a stress device. It was found that 10 mm of anterior talar subluxation and 9° of talar tilt (or more than 3 mm difference in the contralateral anterior drawer test and/or greater than 3° difference in the contralateral talar tilt) may be indicative of mechanical ankle instability.

Treatment   Multiple prospective studies have shown that functional rehabilitation is the preferred treatment of choice for all grades of acute lateral ligament injury. Functional rehabilitation begins with rest (with crutches, bracing), ice for 15 to 20 minutes (3 times per day for the first several days), compression (with supportive bandages), and elevation to decrease the swelling. Patients are allowed to bear weight as tolerated, and begin range-of-motion exercises as pain decreases. A prospective study looked at early mobilization versus immobilization in the treatment of lateral ankle sprains. Although neither group developed late symptoms and ankle instability, early mobilization allowed earlier return to work and physical activity and greater patient comfort. During this early period of therapy, it is important for athletes to continue upper body training, as well as isometric exercises for the lower extremity.

When ankle pain and swelling diminish, muscle strengthening is instituted. The focus is on strengthening the peroneal and evertor muscles of the ankle in an isometric, concentric, and eccentric manner. A wall will suffice for the isometric stretching and exercises, while rubber tubing can be used for the other exercises. When the patient has near normal range of motion and is virtually painless, he or she may progress to exercises aimed at regaining agility and motor coordination. Proprioception excercises are used to help regain motor coordination. Sports-specific rehabilitation is also begun at this time.

Functional rehabilitation with dynamic bracing has been heralded over immobilization. One study showed earlier and more comprehensive functional recovery in the group of patients who used the dynamic brace, compared to the casted group. The braced patients all had statistically significant better isokinetic performances for peak torque, total work, and average power. Most studies support some mode of functional ankle protection upon return to athletic activity. Many athletes, however, are concerned that the brace will hinder their agility. Twelve high school basketball players wore 3 different ankle braces (Universal, Kallassy, and Air-Stirrup ankle training brace) and performed vertical jumps, standing long jumps, cone runs, and 18.3-meter shuttle run. No brace affected athletic performance in any specific activity, and athletic performance was not decreased by brace wear. Bracing has also been demonstrated to improve ankle joint proprioception, possibly through stimulation of cutaneous mechanoreceptors. The effect of exercise, prewrap, and athletic tape on ankle inversion was studied. Use of ankle tape provided a 10% increase in maximal resistance to inversion moments. This increase, however, was diminished to insignificant levels after 40 minutes of strenuous exercise. Prewrap (underwrap) was found to improve maximal resistance to inversion by greater than 10%.

Most studies evaluating the effectiveness of ankle bracing have measured the restriction of ankle motion at a given torque under static conditions. A recent biomechanical investigation compared the angle-torque relationships with the ankle bare and with the ankle braced under both static and dynamic conditions within the full range of motion. Results showed that the braces aided in stability at 0° of inversion, but did not exhibit velocity-dependent properties. Ankle bracing acted as an additional element in conjunction with the ankle structures. Rather than increase ankle torque, these findings suggest that orthotic devices may help improve ankle stability by preloading and maintaining the tibial-talar joint in anatomic position and by preventing the initiation of inversion in the nonweightbearing ankle during walking, running, or jumping.

Twenty percent of acute ankle sprains will develop into chronic lateral instability. A 20-year study followed 37 patients with a lateral ankle sprain who were treated nonsurgically. Twenty-two patients displayed signs and symptoms of instability. It is in this group of people that surgical stabilization is advocated. Degenerative changes were observed in only 6 of 46 radiographically examined ankles. Acute ligament stabilization in the young athlete with complete lateral tears remains controversial. A retrospective examination was done on 100 patients, 6 to 8 years after acute end-to-end ligamentous repair without reinforcement. Seventy-four patients had good to excellent results. Seventy-five patients showed no sign of instability in their injured

ankles. The overall long-term results were excellent, but no prospective study to date has compared acute repair with functional rehabilitation.

Chronic lateral ankle instability is described as functional (subjective complaints of giving way) and/or mechanical (ankle motion beyond physiologic range of motion). It must be differentiated from sinus tarsi syndrome, subtalar instability, and transverse talar instability. Surgical stabilization is either by anatomic repair or nonanatomic reconstruction. The anatomic Broström repair or a modification of the Broström, advocated by most, does not require sacrifice of any normal tissue, and ankle/subtalar tenodesis is avoided. The most popular nonanatomic reconstructive procedures use the peroneus brevis tendon, in whole or in part.

If reconstruction is mandated, an anatomically oriented reconstruction has been described. Fifteen patients underwent reconstruction with an anatomically oriented split peroneus brevis tendon graft. This reconstruction recreates the ATFL and the CFL without restricting subtalar joint motion. At follow-up (average 42 months), the 12 available patients were functionally improved, there was no mechanical instability, and eversion strength and subtalar motion were maintained.

Deltoid and Syndesmotic Ligament Injuries

Isolated tears of the deltoid ligament are rare injuries. They can be treated closed with 6 weeks of immobilization. Without fracture, these are seen primarily in association with syndesmotic ligament injury.

Syndesmotic ligament injuries are rare, being seen in only 1% to 11% of all ankle sprains. Most commonly seen among professional football players following an external rotation injury, they require a high index of suspicion. Because radiographs may be normal, physical examination is critical. Swelling and tenderness will be seen in the region of the syndesmosis and deltoid ligaments. Specific tests exist to aid in the diagnosis. Pain should be increased with dorsiflexion of the ankle joint, secondary to the wider anterior talus stressing the syndesmosis. There may be a positive Hopkinson squeeze test, in which squeezing the proximal tibia and fibular together produces pain distally. Lastly, pain may be elicited with the Kleiger external rotation test. This test is performed with the patient seated with the knee flexed 90°. The examiner stabilizes the tibia with one hand, while externally rotating the foot. Pain should occur at the level of the syndesmosis.

Plain radiographs of the ankle should be obtained to evaluate for obvious fracture and/or diastasis. The tibiofibular clear space (the clear space between the medial border of the fibula and the lateral border of the posterior tibia as it extends into the incisura fibularis, measured 1 cm proximal to the plafond) should be approximately 6 mm or less on both anteroposterior and mortise views. The tibiofibular overlap (overlap of the fibula and the anterior tibial tubercle) should be greater than 6 mm or 42% of the fibular width on the anteroposterior view and greater than 1 mm on the mortise view. External rotation stress radiographs may elucidate a subtle diastasis. Radionuclide imaging has also been used to detect syndesmotic injury when stress radiographs could not be obtained. Stable injuries are treated conservatively, with functional rehabilitation. It is important for coaches and players to note that recovery time is usually twice that of type III lateral ankle sprains.

Unstable syndesmotic injuries (without fracture) have been classified by Edwards and DeLee. In their study, surgical stabilization involved closed reduction with single screw fixation of the syndesmosis. All patients had tenderness over their deltoid ligament, but only 1 underwent deltoid repair. In situations where syndesmotic injury is associated with a fracture, a previous cadaveric study and a recent prospective clinical study both demonstrate that syndesmotic fixation is not required for rigid bimalleolar fracture fixation or lateral fixation within 4.5 cm of the joint. Following this protocol, no patients exhibited syndesmotic widening at follow-up.

Level of syndesmotic screw placement has been widely debated. A recent biomechanical study of cadaveric specimens found 2.0 cm proximal to the tibiotalar joint to be optimal.

Subtalar Instability

The subtalar joint is extremely complex in both function and shape. There are 2 distinct articulations (anterior and posterior), divided by the tarsal canal and sinus tarsi. The 2 major ligaments are the cervical ligament and the interosseus talocalcaneal ligament. The cervical ligament originates from the distal calcaneus and inserts onto the talar neck. The interosseus talocalcaneal ligament is located deep within the sinus tarsi. It originates from the calcaneus (anteromedial to the posterior facet) and inserts onto the inferior talar body. It is a "Y" shaped structure with anteromedial and posterolateral branches. The lateral talocalcaneal ligament is a small ligament that originates from the lateral process of the talus and inserts onto the calcaneus, anterior and parallel to the CFL.

Ligamentous laxity of the subtalar joint may be associated with an inversion injury of the ankle, with injury to the cervical and lateral talocalcaneal ligaments. Chronic laxity appears in athletes with injury to the interosseous ligament.

Plain radiographs are usually normal, but stress radiographs may be helpful. With the 40° Broden stress view, loss of parallelism of the articular surfaces of the posterior facet is indicative of subtalar instability. Medial displacement of the calcaneus to the talus of more than 3 to 5 mm and/or a talo-calcaneal tilt of greater than 5° are typical indicators. Arthrography may aid in the diagnosis of interosseous ligament injury (and subsequent instability) by demonstrating the disappearance of the normal synovial recess corresponding to the sinus tarsi. MRI can be used to evaluate the structural integrity of the interosseous ligament and cervical ligament.

Treatment Treatment is initially similar to that for acute ankle sprains. Rehabilitation focuses on proprioception and strengthening exercises. It has been suggested that, with acute injuries, it is not important to distinguish between lateral ankle and subtalar instability. However, with chronic symptoms attributed to the subtalar joint, surgical stabilization should be considered. The Chrisman-Snook procedure, described for chronic lateral ankle instability, has been the primary technique used for subtalar instability. In one investigation, 31 of 34 patients who underwent a Chrisman-Snook procedure for isolated subtalar instability (16 ankles) and combined ankle/subtalar instability (18 ankles) had good to excellent results. This technique resulted in a mean supination deficit of 7.2° in 20 patients. Reconstruction of the talocalcaneal interosseous ligament has been done to avoid the tenodesis effect. One author used a split peroneus brevis tendon to recreate the 2 limbs of the interosseous ligament through the sinus tarsi. Thirty-eight of the patients had a minimum follow-up of 2 years. Twenty-nine were satisfied, and 3 showed no improvement. Six patients subsequently underwent a subtalar arthrodesis. Success was based on symptomatic relief, because laxity was difficult to measure objectively.

Soft-Tissue Injuries of the Foot

Midfoot Sprains

Midfoot sprains occur when there is ligamentous injury to the tarsometatarsal joints (the Lisfranc complex). This complex includes 3 columns: (1) the first metatarsal and medial cuneiform medially, (2) the second and third metatarsal and the middle and lateral cuneiform, and (3) the fourth and fifth metatarsal and the cuboid. The keystone to this complex is the second metatarsal, which is recessed between the medial and lateral cuneiforms. The soft-tissue stabilizers include the Lisfranc ligament (from the plantar aspect of the second metatarsal base to the medial cuneiform), the intercuneiform ligaments, and the intermetatarsal ligaments (between metatarsals two through five). It is important to note that there is no intermetatarsal ligament between the bases of the first and second metatarsals. The medial and middle columns stabilize the foot during toe off. This function can be lost with even mild diastasis between the medial and middle columns.

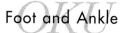

The primary classification system for Lisfranc injury deals with the more obvious fracture/dislocations. It does not address the more subtle Lisfranc longitudinal diastasis seen primarily in athletes. If left untreated, the resultant functional disability can be career limiting and can cause limitations in activities of daily living.

Many athletes give the history of direct injury to their plantarflexed foot. Their foot is driven into the ground by an opposing player falling on their hindfoot, or their plantarflexed foot comes down on another player's leg. A high degree of suspicion is required to diagnose these injuries. With stress applied to the medial, middle, and/or lateral columns, pain should be elicited with minimal dorsiflexion and plantarflexion maneuveurs.

Plain radiographs of the foot should be obtained. Bilateral weightbearing AP radiographs allow enhancement of any diastasis and provide the ability for comparison views. An ankle block may be given to increase the patient's ability to bear weight. In addition to any malalignment between metatarsals and cuneiforms, fractures should be ruled out. A positive fleck sign is commonly seen at the base of the second metatarsal (secondary to avulsion by the Lisfranc ligament), as are compression fractures of the cuboid and/or cuneiforms. The normal amount of space between the first and second metatarsal bases is 1.3 mm; greater than 2 mm is considered abnormal. CT has been shown to be more sensitive than plain radiography in detecting these subtle injuries. As 20% of all Lisfranc injuries are initially incorrectly diagnosed, CT scanning is wise for athletes with midfoot tenderness and normal plain films. Triple-phase bone scanning has also been reported as helpful in diagnosing subtle injury.

Optimal treatment consists of anatomic reduction of the tarsometatarsal joints. The key is to align the lateral border of the medial cuneiform to the second metatarsal to allow healing of the Lisfranc ligament. While greater than 2-mm diastasis is the typical distance accepted between the metatarsal bases, this has been questioned in the athlete. It has been suggested that an anatomic correction be sought in this population. If a patient is diagnosed with a sprain without subluxation, a nonweightbearing cast is used until asymptomatic. Following immobilization, functional rehabilitation is instituted in a brace. If a diastasis exists, open reduction and internal fixation is recommended, with screw fixation. Widening between the base of the second metatarsal and medial cuneiform should be treated with a screw that follows the path of the torn Lisfranc ligament. With frank dislocation, sequential reduction and fixation of the tarsometatarsal joints should be performed.

These injuries can result in prolonged recovery time and residual pain. Identification and correct treatment is manda-tory. A prospective study comparing surgical and nonsurgical treatment of subtle Lisfranc injury is needed.

Tendon Injuries

Peroneal Tendons

The peroneal muscles occupy the lateral compartment of the leg. Distally, the tendons share a common synovial sheath in the fibular retromalleolar space. The peroneal longus contains a sesamoid, the os peroneum, of which 20% is usually bony. The os peroneum lies within the tunnel formed by the long plantar ligament and the groove of the cuboid, approximately 3 cm from the tendon insertion. The primary restraint to subluxation for both peroneals, the superior peroneal retinaculum (SPR), originates from the fibula periosteum and is confluent with the superficial fascia of the leg and the peroneal tendon sheath. The SPR inserts into the Achilles tendon superiorly and the posterior aspect of the lateral calcaneal surface inferiorly. The peroneal brevis is the primary abductor and evertor of the foot and ankle; the peroneal longus functions to plantarflex the first ray and to evert the foot. Both tendons are susceptible to tendinitis, tears, dislocation, and/or rupture.

Peroneus Brevis

The peroneus brevis is susceptible to tendinitis, most commonly seen in athletes who return to activity after a long rest period. Ballet dancers are particularly affected, because of their repetitive stance on the balls of their feet. Symptoms and signs consist of pain, tenderness, and swelling posterior and distal to the lateral malleolus. Initial treatment includes rest, ice, compressive bandages, nonsteroidal anti-inflammatory medication, and range of motion and strengthening as symptoms decrease. Peroneal strengthening exercises are emphasized.

Chronic tendinitis, often indicative of an overuse syndrome, can lead to tendon tearing. Regional tenderness and swelling are evident. MRI may aid in diagnosis by revealing fluid accumulation within the tendon sheath. The integrity of the tendon can also be evaluated, but tears may not always be recognized. A rehabilitation program and nonsteroidal anti-inflammatory drugs are initially emphasized in the treatment; severe cases may require a period of cast immobilization. Stretching, peroneal strengthening, and an ankle brace for athletic activity are stressed. Surgical debridement with tenosynovectomy is performed for recalcitrant cases.

Peroneus brevis tendon tears often occur secondary to the overuse syndromes seen in dancers, runners, and competitive walkers. The position of the brevis in the fibular groove, compressed between bone and the peroneus longus, predisposes it to stress and tearing. The vascularity in the retrofibular region is decreased, which contributes to local injury. Other factors that may be associated with a brevis tear are tendon subluxation, calcaneal and/or fibular fracture (with impingement), degenerative arthritis, and direct trauma. The tear usually occurs distal to the lateral malleolus on its medial aspect and is 2 to 5 cm in length.

Diagnosis of a peroneus brevis tendon tear can be difficult. Radiographs may delineate bony fragments that are causing tendon impingement. MRI allows visualization of fluid within the tendon sheath, as well as intratendinous lesions. Peroneal tenography may confirm peroneal pathology, with pain relief after injection.

Treatment The treatment of peroneus brevis tendon tears depends on the patient's symptoms. For minimal discomfort, treatment consists of anti-inflammatory drugs, physical therapy, and an ankle stirrup brace to prevent inversion. With severe or persistent pain despite nonsurgical treatment, surgical correction consists of tendon debridement and direct repair with a running nonabsorbable suture. In addition to repairing the longitudinal rent in the tendon, some authors suggest tubularization of the tendon to recreate its original shape. Underlying predisposing conditions, such as tendon dislocation and ankle ligament instability should be addressed as well.

With acute complete rupture, direct repair is advised. A chronic rupture may have a proximal stump that is either mobile and advanceable or fixed and contracted. If the tendon is mobile and advanceable, a plantaris graft may be used to bridge the gap between tendon ends and allow continuity of the tendon. If the proximal end is fixed, it may be sutured to the lateral calcaneus. This would only allow minimal tendon excursion, but a varus foot deformity may be avoided. In addition, a fixed proximal stump may also be tenodesed to the peroneus longus.

Anomalous peroneus brevis muscles consist of twin muscle bellies or a muscle belly that extends distally around the lateral malleolus. These muscles are often visible by MRI. With hypertrophy of this muscle in athletes, performance is diminished secondary to pain, particularly during pushoff. Excision of symptomatic anomalous muscles is the treatment of choice. In addition, a peroneus quartus muscle may exist within the retrofibular space. This muscle may also be excised to decompress the retrofibular space.

Peroneus Longus

The spectrum of peroneus longus pathology, described as the painful os peroneum syndrome, includes tendinitis, attritional changes, longitudinal tears, and/or acute and chronic ruptures. With tendinitis of the peroneus longus, patients complain of lateral heel pain particularly with running, cutting, and turning. These symptoms are often seen in the athlete who returns to vigorous play following a period of inactivity. On examination, there is tenderness directly over the tendon, beginning at the lateral calcaneal border. Initial treatment is with anti-inflammatory drugs, physical therapy, and an orthotic device to prevent excessive pronation of the foot. Surgical tenosynovectomy may be required if conservative treatment fails.

Chronic longitudinal tears are attritional and are most common in the middle-aged athlete. Patients complain of chronic lateral heel and foot pain. Tenderness is present directly over the tendon, and swelling may be evident. Treatment with immobilization and therapy may resolve symptoms, but surgical debridement and repair may be necessary.

Both weekend athletes and professional athletes are susceptible to acute ruptures of the peroneus longus tendon, which often occur as an avulsion fracture of the os peroneum. If the injury is missed initially, sequential radiographs may help by revealing positional changes of the os peroneum, as it migrates proximally. If the patient lacks a bony component to the os peroneum, MRI may be required for diagnosis. Minimally symptomatic patients may be treated conservatively with a rehabilitation program. If, however, the patient demonstrates a functional disability, a direct repair of the tendon is recommended. Chronic ruptures may be repaired with a tendon graft, using the plantaris or half of the brevis tendon. As with the peroneus brevis, a fixed contracted tendon should be attached to the lateral calcaneus. It will function as an accessory ankle flexor and will prevent heel varus. With the lost attachment to the first metatarsal, dorsal subluxation of the first ray may occur.

Peroneal Tendon Instability

Both the peroneus longus and brevis are at risk for subluxation and/or dislocation from the fibular retromalleolar sulcus. Peroneal instability is frequently associated with athletic activity. Skiing is often reported as a cause of injury. The usual mechanism occurs when the skier digs his or her ski tips into the snow. This sudden deceleration throws the skier forward into forced dorsiflexion, and the violent peroneal contraction results in dislocation. A second mechanism of injury occurs from forced eversion, as the skier everts his foot in order to edge the downhill ski on a turn. Ice skating, soccer, basketball, rugby, and gymnastics have all been implicated as well.

Initially, patients describe intense pain at the moment of injury, with a popping sensation in the posterolateral ankle. A feeling of instability is noted with attempted return to physical activity. Patients describe a painful snap about the lateral malleolus (or frank dislocation) with dorsiflexion and eversion of their ankle.

Physical examination often reveals tenderness and swelling posterior to the lateral malleolus. Symptoms are exacerbated with active and passive eversion of the foot, while the ankle is held in dorsiflexion. With acute injury, subluxation may not be appreciated secondary to swelling, pain, or patient apprehension. The examiner must be aware of and test for associated lateral ankle instability.

Radiographs demonstrate the pathognomonic sign of peroneal dislocation, an avulsion fracture of the lateral rim of the lateral malleolus (due to avulsion of the SPR), in 15% to 50% of cases. This is best visualized on a mortise view of the ankle. MRI and CT scans will demonstrate the avulsion fracture, but are not usually necessary.

The Eckert and Davis classification described three grades of tendon dislocation. In all cases, the SPR is pulled off its attachment to the lateral malleolus; there are no reported cases of actual tears in the SPR substance itself. In grade I injury, the retinaculum and periosteum are elevated from the lateral malleolus, with the tendons lying between the periosteum and the bone. Grade II injury occurs when the fibrocartilaginous ridge of the lateral malleolus is elevated along with the SPR and periosteum. In grade III injury, a thin cortical rim of bone is avulsed from the lateral malleolus. Grade I pathology is seen most frequently, and grade III injuries are the most rare. Associated tenosynovitis and tears of the peroneal tendons are common.

Nonsurgical treatment for acute peroneal dislocation has a 50% success rate. Surgical treatment is favored to prevent reoccurrence, to return athletes to competition, and to avoid peroneal tendon tears associated with chronic instability.

Acute repair involves reattaching the avulsed superior peroneal retinaculum to the lateral malleolus through drill holes. The patient is placed in a short leg cast with the ankle in a relaxed plantarflexion position for approximately 3 to 4 weeks. A walking cast my be used for another 2 to 3 weeks. Most athletes are allowed to return to their sport at 3 to 4 months, when full motion and strength have returned.

Various techniques exist to address chronic peroneal tendon dislocation/subluxation. Five basic categories of repair have been described. No study has established one procedure to be superior to the others, but the cause of the dislocation should be corrected. The 5 categories are: (1) Anatomic reattachment of the retinaculum as described above for acute injury. This technique alone has been sufficient when there are no underlying predisposing factors. (2) Bone block procedures allow a deeper retrofibular groove and, therefore, containment of the peroneal tendons. This requires a rota-

tional osteotomy of the distal fibula with screw fixation. (3) Reinforcement of the SPR with local tissue transfers can be used for peroneal stabilization. The Jones procedure transfers a slip of Achilles tendon over the retinaculum. Although successful in preventing subluxation, overtightening may result in a stenosing or tenodesis effect. (4) Rerouting procedures primarily use the calcaneofibular ligament to restrain the peroneal tendons. The CFL may be incised and resutured over the peroneals, or some authors describe dividing the peroneal tendons, placing them under the CFL and resuturing the tendons. (5) Lastly, groove-deepening procedures involve the creation of a hinged bone flap on the posterior aspect of the posterior distal fibula. Three sides of the bone are sectioned, and the flap is hinged medially. The underlying cancellous bone is removed and the intact cortical flap of bone is inserted into the former cancellous bed, which allows for a deepened retromalleolar bed without removal of the smooth posterior fibular surface.

When approaching a patient with peroneal instability, it is necessary to address the pathology that is present. Retinacular detachment should be reattached to the fibula. If insufficient retinaculum exists, reinforcement with local tissue may be necessary. A narrow fibular sulcus should be corrected with bone block, groove deepening, or CFL rerouting.

Achilles Tendon

The Achilles tendon extends from the junction of the muscle bellies of the triceps surae (gastrocnemius and soleus) to insert on the posterior superior edge of the calcaneus. The thickest, strongest tendon in the body, it is subjected to tensile loads of up to 8 times body weight and can accept up to 7,000 N of force. The Achilles tendon is poorly vascularized (particularly the region 2 to 6 cm above the calcaneal insertion) for its size and is therefore susceptible to injury. There is a large difference between the force that the gastrocnemius and soleus are able to exert, and that which the tendon is able to transmit without intrasubstance damage. Another important anatomic point is the absence of a true synovial sheath about the tendon. It is surrounded by a peritenon that is prone to inflammatory changes.

Achilles tendinitis is a multifactorial disease. Although overtraining (duration, intensity, and frequency) is the primary culprit, other biomechanical factors that have been implicated are tibia varum, calcaneal eversion, hyperpronation, inadequate heel wedge in running shoes, and tight heel cords and hamstrings. Afflictions of the Achilles tendon occur in 6.5% to 18% of runners.

Pathologic changes typically involve the peritenon first, with changes later seen in the tendon itself. Clinical and histologic studies have resulted in a classification of Achilles tendon injury: (1) peritendinitis, (2) peritendinitis with tendinosis, and (3) pure tendinosis. These entities may be further divided into insertional tendinitis and noninsertional tendinitis. Peritendinitis involves inflammatory changes in the peritenon, with thickening and fibrous adhesion to the tendon. Peritendinitis with tendinosis includes the above findings as well as thickening, softening, and yellowing of the tendon itself. Pure tendinosis can entail tendon thickening with mucinoid degeneration, partial tendon tearing, or complete Achilles rupture. With insertional tendinitis, the pathology occurs in the Achilles bursa (between the calcaneus and the Achilles tendon), with attrition noted in the region of tendon attachment. In conjunction, a Haglund's deformity is commonly seen. This has been cited as the most common form of tendinopathy seen in athletes. Noninsertional Achilles tendinitis primarily involves the hypovascular zone, located 2 to 6 cm proximal to its insertion.

Clinically, patients present either with symptoms of pain and stiffness associated with exercise or with acute rupture without a prodomal phase. History taking is critical and should document acitivities performed, miles run, shoe style, and type of running surface encountered. On physical examination, the region of maximal tenderness, swelling, thickening, bony deformity, and/or tendon gaps or nodularity should be noted. The Thompson test is the best indicator of complete rupture of the Achilles tendon. It is performed by squeezing the relaxed calf with the patient in a prone position. No plantarflexion indicates an incomplete tendon. However, with chronic rupture, fibrosis or secondary scarring may make the Thompson test unreliable. Plain radiographs should be obtained to evaluate bony contour, Haglund's deformity, and possible tendon calcification. MRI is a useful adjunctive test to evaluate tendon pathology. Increased signal intensity on T2 localizes fluid within and around the tendon, as well as defining regions of tendon degeneration and tearing. Ultrasound is also able to distinguish between normal and abnormal tendon substance, edema, and thickening and has a documented specificity of 100% and a sensitivity of 94%.

Treatment The treatment of Achilles tendinopathy should be approached initially with nonsurgical management. Limited immobilization, nonsteroidal anti-inflammatory drugs, and physical therapy (whirlpool and Achilles and hamstring stretching) should be implemented. As the patient returns to physical activity, orthoses with the foot in subtalar neutral (avoiding over pronation), appropriate running shoes (heel wedges of 12 to 15 mm are recommended), avoidance of uneven running surfaces, and diligent stretching are all useful suggestions.

Surgical management is advised in recalcitrant cases that show no improvement after 6 months of nonsurgical treatment, and in cases with extensive tendon damage, as evidenced by MRI or ultrasound. For insertional tendinitis, the tendon should be completely inspected with debulking and repair of tears. The calcaneal prominence should be excised and the Achilles bursa should be removed. Debridement for peritendinitis (noninsertional) depends on the degree and extension of adhesions and thickening and involves either removal of the hypertrophic part of the paratenon or removal of the whole of the paratenon from the entire tendon surface. Care must be taken to not leave hard or narrow edges that will limit tendon gliding.

When tendinosis is present, the tendon must be freed from fibrotic adhesions, and degenerated nodules must be removed. The blood supply to the tendon is enhanced by performing longitudinal scarifications along the tendon, parallel to its fascicles. Some investigators suggest placement of local muscle tissue (ie, soleus) within the tendon to help reestablish nutrition.

Postoperatively, for treatment of insertional tendinopathy, a short leg cast is worn for 2 weeks, followed by functional rehabilitation. With peritendinitis alone, active mobilization is begun immediately; physical therapy is started following suture removal. If tendinosis is addressed, 2 weeks of immobilization is suggested prior to rehabilitation.

Results of nonsurgical and surgical treatment of chronic Achilles tendinopathy have been compared. Forty-one patients initially treated with conservative therapy had a 51% recovery rate. Three additional patients recovered following brisement of the tendon/peritenon interspace (injection of 0.5 cc of 25% marcaine between the peritenon and tendon to distend the inflamed sheath). Seventeen patients required tendon and/or peritenon debridement. Patients who responded to nonsurgical treatment were younger, with an average age of 33. Those who required surgery averaged 48 years of age. Most investigators agree that surgery is essential for recovery in cases in which there are irreversible pathologic changes in the tendon and peritenon as evidenced by ineffective rehabilitation greater than 6 months.

Complete ruptures of the Achilles tendon occur primarily in male athletes between 30 and 50 years of age. Approximately 15% experience prodromal symptoms. Rupture is associated with acceleration-deceleration sports, particularly in the poorly conditioned athlete. There have been few reported cases of Achilles rupture in well-conditioned professional athletes.

Controversy exists concerning nonsurgical versus surgical treatment for Achilles rupture. While studies indicate similar healing rates, nonsurgical treatment results in higher rerupture rates, decreased strength and endurance, and diminished functional levels. The nonsurgically treated Achilles tendon rupture gains only 30% of its preinjury strength—compared to near normal strength in surgically treated groups. Rerupture rates for nonsurgically and surgically treated ruptures are 18% and 2%, respectively. Surgical repair has resulted in a greater resumption of athletic performance to preinjury level. Most investigators recommend surgical repair in young athletes, elite athletes, and very active older athletes.

The multiple concerns involved in Achilles tendon repair include suturing a shredded, "mop-end" tendon, achieving physiologic tension and appropriate tendon length, revitalizing an ischemic tendon, obtaining stable fixation for tendons avulsed from the calcaneal tubersity, and repair of chronic tears. Numerous repair techniques have evolved in an attempt to address these issues.

Direct repair with a large absorbable suture, augmention of direct repair with a fascial turndown, fascia lata graft, plantaris weave, use of synthetic material for augmentation, percutaneous repair, and tendon transfers using the peroneus brevis, flexor digitorum longus, or the flexor hallucis longus have all been done. The long-term results of 23 end-to-end surgical repairs of Achilles tendon ruptures were evaluated. Fifty-four percent of ruptures occurred in patients in their 30s, with 90% occurring during accleration-deceleration sports. All patients had direct end-to-end repair, with 15 augmented with the plantaris tendon. Postoperatively, patients wore a nonweightbearing cast in equinus for an average of 4.2 weeks, followed by a short leg walking cast in neutral for an additional 4 weeks. Physical therapy was then begun, with range-of-motion, stretching, and progressive resistance exercises. There were no reruptures, with 1 attenuated repair noted 9 months postoperatively. Ninety-three percent of patients returned to their preinjury functional level. Seventeen patients had Cybex testing using the contralateral limb as a control, which indicated an average of 92% return of strength. Direct repair, with or without local tissue augmentation, is felt to produce consistent, predictable results associated with a low morbidity and near normal functional outcomes.

A new direct repair technique uses a transverse incision and barbed wire hooks across the tear for 4 weeks. Immediate plantarflexion motion is allowed in an articulated orthosis. This procedure was performed on 78 patients with acute ruptures. Follow-up on 71 patients revealed complete tendon healing without wound complications. Two reruptures occurred proximal to the repair site.

With neglected rupture, a tendon diastasis usually exists, making direct repair difficult. This gap may be bridged with a tendon/fascial turndown if small (1 to 3 cm) or with a tendon transfer if large. The peroneus brevis is most accessible, but supplies the least length. The flexor hallucis longus, transferred to the calcaneus either through a drill hole or secured into the calcaneus with a suture anchor, has proven to be an effective in-phase substitution. A new technique for direct repair has been recently reported in 41 neglected Achilles ruptures (between 1 to 3 months) in recreational athletes. They were treated with primary tendon repair with imbrication (no excision) of the collagenous scar and no augmentation. All patients returned to preinjury level of activity without rerupture. This may serve as a useful additon to the orthopaedist's armametarium for chronic Achilles tendon ruptures.

Flexor Hallucis Longus Tendon

Tendinitis in the flexor hallucis longus (FHL) occurs most often in ballet dancers. The turnout position assumed in ballet predisposes to this condition. To turn out, the hips must be significantly externally rotated. When the feet are forced out further than the hips will rotate, the feet collapse into eversion, resulting in stress to the flexor hallucis longus tendon. The FHL is most commonly affected posterior to the medial malleolus, at the point where it changes direction. With severe inflammation, the great toe may begin to trigger secondary to nodule formation on the tendon.

Patients complain of pain and clicking posterior to the medial malleolus, and these symptoms are exacerbated by dancing en pointe (standing on the tips of the toes). Physical examination reveals localized tenderness, possible swelling, and possible triggering. Ultrasound may assist in diagnosis. Nonsteroidal anti-inflammatory drugs, rest, and physical therapy are used successfully in most cases. However, if a nodule has developed, tendon sheath division with tendon debridement and repair may be necessary. A review of 41 procedures for stenosing tenosynovitis of the flexor hallucis longus tendon and/or posterior impingement syndrome was performed. The tendon tunnel was released from the level of the medial malleolus to the sustentaculum tali and the tendon was debrided or repaired as needed. Thirty ankles had a good or excellent result, 6 had a fair result, and 4 had a poor result. Most dancers return to practice in 6 weeks, followed by full activity in 12 weeks.

Annotated Bibliography

Arthroscopy

Bryant DD III, Siegel MG: Osteochondritis dissecans of the talus: A new technique for arthroscopic drilling. *Arthroscopy* 1993; 9:238–241.

The authors describe a technique for arthroscopic drilling using meniscal repair instrumentation that permits accurate arthroscopic localization and drilling of osteochondral lesions.

Conti SF, Taranow WS: Transtalar retrograde drilling of medial osteochondral lesions of the talar dome. *Oper Tech Orthop* 1996;6:226–230.

The authors provide an alternative to transmalleolar drilling. This method avoids violation of intact articular cartilage.

Cooper PS, Murray TF Jr: Arthroscopy of the foot and ankle in the athlete. *Clin Sports Med* 1996;15:805–823.

This is an excellent review article on athletic foot and ankle pathology that can be treated arthroscopically.

Ferkel RD, Heath DD, Guhl JF: Neurological complications of ankle arthroscopy. *Arthroscopy* 1996;12:200–208.

This is a retrospective study of 612 ankle arthroscopies. There was a 9% overall complication rate, with 27 neurologic complications. The superficial peroneal nerve was injured in 15 cases.

Frey C, Bell J, Teresi L, Kerr R, Feder K: A comparison of MRI and clinical examination of acute lateral ankle sprains. *Foot Ankle Int* 1996;17:533–537.

Physical examination was found to be 100% accurate in the diagnosis of grade III ligament injuries, but only 25% accurate in the diagnosis of grade II injuries.

Glick JM, Morgan CD, Myerson MS, Sampson TG, Mann JA: Ankle arthrodesis using an arthroscopic method: Long-term follow-up of 34 cases. *Arthroscopy* 1996;12:428–434.

Arthroscopic ankle arthrodesis was performed on 34 ankles with a 97% fusion rate. The average time to fusion was 9 weeks.

Hangody L, Kish G, Karpati Z, Szerb I, Eberhardt R: Treatment of osteochondritis dissecans of the talus: Use of the mosaicplasty technique. A preliminary report. *Foot Ankle Int* 1997; 18:628–634.

An autogenous osteochondral grafting technique for the treatment of talar dome osteochondral lesions is reported in 11 patients with talar lesion of 10 mm or greater. The grafts were taken from the ipsilateral knee. Mean follow-up was 16 months with all patients returning to full activities.

Kaikkonen A, Hyppanen E, Kannus P, Jarvinen M: Long-term functional outcome after primary repair of the lateral ligaments of the ankle. *Am J Sports Med* 1997;25:150–155.

This is a retrospective review of 100 patients, 6 to 8 years following a primary repair of ruptured lateral ankle ligaments. Seventy-four patients had excellent/good results and 75 patients had no signs of instability.

Karlsson J, Eriksson BI, Bergsten T, Rudholm O, Sward L: Comparison of two anatomic reconstructions for chronic lateral instability of the ankle joint. *Am J Sports Med* 1997;25:48–53.

Both Karlsson's method of lateral ligament reconstruction and Gould's modification of the Broström, restore mechanical stability. However, the duration of surgery time and surgical complications were greater with Gould's procedure.

Liu SH, Nuccion SL, Finerman G: Diagnosis of anterolateral ankle impingement: Comparison between magnetic resonance imaging and clinical examination. *Am J Sports Med* 1997; 25:389–393.

Twenty-two patients with chronic anterolateral ankle pain were debrided arthroscopically after a preoperative MRI. MRI was not found to be beneficial or cost-effective in the diagnosis.

Ogilvie-Harris DJ, Reed SC: Disruption of the ankle syndesmosis: Diagnosis and treatment by arthroscopic surgery. *Arthroscopy* 1994;10:561–568.

Patients with chronic pain secondary to syndesmotic disruption of the ankle benefit from arthroscopic removal of the intraarticular pathology. The common triad of pathologic features was disruption of the posterior inferior tibiofibular ligament, rupture of the interosseous ligament, and a chondral fracture of the posterolateral portion of the tibial plafond.

Stone JW: Osteochondral lesions of the talar dome. *J Am Acad Orthop Surg* 1996;4:63–73.

An excellent review of the diagnosis and treatment of talar osteochondral lesions.

Ankle Sprains/Instability

Colville MR, Grondel RJ: Anatomic reconstruction of the lateral ankle ligaments using a split peroneus brevis tendon graft. *Am J Sports Med* 1995;23:210–213.

This reconstruction utilizes an anatomically oriented graft to reconstruct the anterior talofibular ligament and the calcaneofibular ligament. Of the 12 patients available for follow-up, eversion strength and subtalar joint motion were maintained after surgery.

Eiff MP, Smith AT, Smith GE: Early mobilization versus immobilization in the treatment of lateral ankle sprains. *Am J Sports Med* 1994;22:83–88.

Although both immobilization and early mobilization in first-time lateral ankle sprains prevent late symptoms and instability, early mobilization allows earlier return to work and is more comfortable for the patients.

Hartsell HD, Spaulding SJ: Effectiveness of external orthotic support on passive soft tissue resistance of the chronically unstable ankle. *Foot Ankle Int* 1977;18:144–150.

External orthotic support is shown to provide greater resistance to torque forces and less inversion range than the unbraced condition.

Hennrikuss WL, Lyone PM, Lapoint JM: Outcomes of the Chrisman-Snook and modified-Broström procedures for chronic lateral ankle instability. *Am J Sports Med* 1966;24:400–404.

A prospective, randomized comparison of the outcomes of the modified Broström and Chrisman-Snook procedures in 40 patients revealed good/excellent results in 80% of patients. The modified-Brostsrom procedure, however, resulted in a higher score and less complications.

Liu SH, Baker CL: Comparison of lateral ankle ligamentous reconstruction procedures. *Am J Sports Med* 1994;22:313–317.

A cadaveric study demonstrated that the modified Broström procedure resulted in the least amount of anterior talar displacement and talar tilt at all forces. There were no significant differences between the Watson-Jones and Chrisman-Snook procedures in anterior talar displacement or talar tilt.

Manfroy PP, Ashton-Miller JA, Wojtys EM: The effect of exercise, prewrap, and athletic tape on the maximal active and passive ankle resistance to ankle inversion. *Am J Sports Med* 1997;25:156–163.

The use of ankle tape provided a 10% increase in maximal resistance to inversion, but this increase decreased to insignificant levels after 40 minutes of play. Use of prewrap improved resistance to inversion by more than 10%.

Pienkowski D, McMorrow M, Shapiro R, Caborn DN, Stayton J: The effect of ankle stabilizers on athletic performance: A randomized prospective study. *Am J Sports Med* 1995; 23:757–762.

Twelve high school basketball players performed various athletic activities while wearing 3 different types of ankle stabilizers. The braces did not alter athletic performance, and there were no differences in the 3 brands of braces.

Regis D, Montanari M, Magnan B, Spagnol S, Bragantini A: Dynamic orthopaedic brace in the treatment of ankle sprains. *Foot Ankle Int* 1995;16:422–426.

Thonnard JL, Bragard D, Willems PA, Plaghki L: Stability of the braced ankle: A biomechanical investigation. *Am J Sports Med* 1996;24:356–361.

The authors hypothesize that the primary function of the brace is to preload the ankle and maintain a proper anatomic position with optimal contact between the articular surfaces.

Deltoid/Syndesmotic Injury

McBryde A, Chiasson B, Wilhelm A, Donovan F, Ray T, Bacilla P: Syndesmotic screw placement: A biomechanical analysis. *Foot Ankle Int* 1997;18:262–266.

This cadaveric study demonstrated that less syndesmotic widening occurs when stressing a syndesmosis following screw placement at 2.0 cm above the tibiotalar joint.

Yamaguchi K, Martin CH, Boden SD, Labropoulos PA: Operative treatment of syndesmotic disruptions without use of a syndesmotic screw: A prospective clinical study. *Foot Ankle Int* 1994; 15:407–414.

This prospective study confirms the earlier cadaveric study that suggested that trans-syndesmotic fixation was not required if rigid bimalleolar fracture fixation was achieved, or lateral without medial fixation was obtained when the fibular fracture was within 4.5 cm of the joint.

Subtalar Instability

Pisani G: Chronic laxity of the subtalar joint. *Orthopedics* 1996;19:431–437.

The author describes reconstruction of the interosseous talocalcaneal ligament using a split peroneus brevis tendon.

Midfoot Injury

Lu J, Ebraheim NA, Skie M, Porshinsky B, Yeasting RA: Radiographic and computed tomographic evaluation of Lisfranc dislocation: A cadaver study. *Foot Ankle Int* 1997;18:351–355.

Six cadaveric feet were used for radiologic and computed tomographic (CT) evaluation of the tarsometatarsal joints following sequential 1-mm increment dislocation of the Lisfranc joint. None of the 1-mm and two thirds of the 2-mm dorsolateral Lisfranc dislocations could be seen on plain radiographs, but all were noted on CT scan.

Peroneal Tendons

Kollias SL, Ferkel RD: Fibular grooving for recurrent peroneal tendon subluxation. *Am J Sports Med* 1997;25:329–335.

Twelve ankles underwent fibular grooving for recurrent peroneal tendon dislocations with an average follow-up of 6 years. There were no resubluxations. Ten patients returned to full activity, including sports. Eleven ankles were rated as excellent.

Mizel MS, Michelson JD, Newberg A: Peroneal tendon bupivacaine injection: Utility of concomitant injection of contrast material. *Foot Ankle Int* 1996;17:566–568.

This article discusses the usefulness of the addition of contrast material to peroneal tendon injections.

Sammarco GJ: Peroneal tendon injuries. *Orthop Clin North Am* 1994;25:135–145.

This is a review article defining the diagnosis and treatment of peroneal tendon injury.

Achilles Tendon

Benazzo F, Todesca A, Ceciliana L: Achilles' tendon tendinitis and heel pain. *Oper Tech Sports Med* 1997;5:179–188.

Achilles tendinopathies are one of the most common overuse problems in athletes. Inflammation or pathologic degeneration of the Achilles tendon itself is one of the causes of heel pain. In athletes refractory to nonsurgical treatment, surgical treatment is indicated.

Motta P, Errichiello C, Pontini I: Achilles tendon rupture: A new technique for easy surgical repair and immediate movement of the ankle and foot. *Am J Sports Med* 1997;25:172–176.

Seventy-eight physically active patients with closed Achilles tendon ruptures were treated with 3 specially designed barbed wire hooks and Aldam's cutaneous approach. This repair allows immediate controlled ankle movement with a brace.

Scioli MW: Achilles tendinitis. *Orthop Clin North Am* 1994; 25:177–182.

The author reports on the pathology and treatment of Achilles tendon injury.

Flexor Hallucis Longus

Hamilton WG, Geppert MJ, Thompson FM: Pain in the posterior aspect of the ankle in dancers: Differential diagnosis and operative treatment. *J Bone Joint Surg* 1996;78A:1491–1499.

A retrospective review of the operative treatment of stenosing tenosynovitis of the FHL tendon or posterior impingement syndrome in 37 dancers yielded 30 ankles with good/excellent results, 6 with a fair result, and 4 with a poor result.

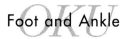
Chapter 5
Shoes and Orthoses

Introduction

External modification of the immediate environment surrounding the foot and ankle can have a major effect on comfort, function, and appearance. This includes not only the particular shoegear worn by a person, but also modifications of the shoe design itself and various types of inserts, braces and accommodative devices that are added to the shoe. Shoes are a major industry, both as a fashion statement, and, as sports and fitness activities have become more popular, so has the specialized shoe as a piece of athletic equipment. However, they also remain a source of potential pathology for the uneducated consumer.

Shoes, their modifications, and the devices that are added to them are an important first line of treatment for many foot and ankle problems. In most cases, before resorting to surgery, these types of nonsurgical treatment modalities should be tried. Symptoms of plantar fasciitis, posterior tibial tendinitis, and many toe deformities can be alleviated by appropriate inserts and devices. Preventive measures in terms of shoe design and insoles can avert the development of more serious problems, such as ulcerations and osteomyelitis, in neuropathic feet. The appropriate selection of athletic footwear can both prevent sports injuries and improve performance.

Shoe modifications refer to internal or external alterations or to additions to the structure of the shoe itself. An orthosis is a brace or body support. Foot orthoses, which are often custom made, are generally referred to as orthotics both by practitioners and by the lay public. The objectives of these devices are to decrease pain, improve function in standing and walking, or enhance athletic performance. The means of accomplishing these goals can be by transferring forces away from sensitive or threatened areas, reducing friction and shear, accommodating or correcting deformities, modifying weight transfer patterns, and limiting motion of painful or unstable joints.

In the past, many of these conservative treatment measures have been ignored by orthopaedic surgeons. There have been relatively few scientifically sound studies on the efficacy of many of the orthotic devices used to treat foot and ankle problems, and, consequently, the medical indications for many of these devices have been unclear. Many orthopaedic surgeons do not have adequate training in the use of orthotics

and shoe modifications for the treatment of foot and ankle problems. Every detailed foot and ankle history and physical examination should include inspection of the patient's shoegear for fit and wear patterns, as well as noting any current or past use of orthotics or other devices. This chapter will cover the basic concepts in shoe construction and design, the rationale for shoe modifications, and the use of various orthotic devices to treat specific foot and ankle problems.

Shoe Design and Construction

Shoes serve to protect the foot, to enhance performance and function of the foot, and, in many cases, to serve a cosmetic function. The style of a shoe refers to the essential design character and particular architecture of the shoe. These are the features that put the shoe into a specific category of footwear. There are 7 basic footwear styles: pump, oxford, sandal, mule, boot, clog, and moccasin. In contrast, fashion is the variation of a particular style, and is determined by the imagination of the designers and the desires of consumers.

The basic anatomy of a shoe is illustrated in Figure 1. Both men's and women's shoes have the same design features, although the proportions tend to be different. These differences may contribute to the increased incidence of foot problems in women. The toe box is the anterior portion of a shoe's upper. It serves to retain the contour of a shoe's toe, and its volume can be altered by changing its height or shape. The space between the floor and the plantar aspect of the tip of the toe is the "toe spring." This can give a rocker effect to the shoe and enhance toe off. A narrow, pointed toe box gives the illusion of a smaller foot, often a fashion desire. However, this type of toe box often compresses the toes from the sides and applies pressure on the dorsum of the toes. The pointed, narrow toe box can push the hallux into valgus, and the lesser toes may be pushed up into a flexed posture, which can lead to hammertoes. As hammering develops, it is further aggravated by the dorsal pressure at the PIP joints, which may lead to painful calluses or ulcerations. In contrast, a wide, high toe box allows ample room for the toes to maintain a natural position without compressing or abrading the skin (Fig. 2).

Just behind the toe box is the vamp, the anterior upper that covers the instep. In a women's fashion pump there is very

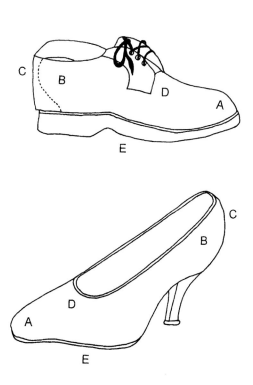

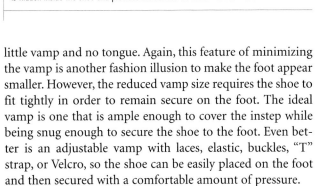

Figure 1

Anatomy of the shoe. **A,** Toe Box; **B,** Quarter; **C,** Counter; **D,** Vamp; **E,** Outsole. The insole is hidden inside the shoe and provides the surface on which the foot rests.

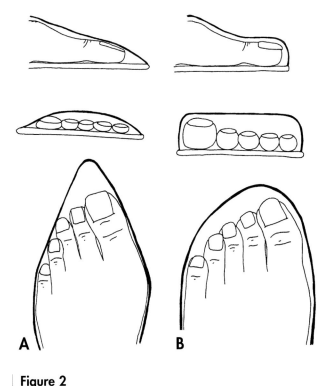

Figure 2

A, A narrow, pointy, receding toe box makes the forefoot look smaller. However, it compresses the toes, pushing the hallux into valgus and applies pressure to the dorsum of the toes. **B,** A wide, high toe box gives ample room for the toes to assume a neutral position. There is no pressure on the dorsum of the toes.

little vamp and no tongue. Again, this feature of minimizing the vamp is another fashion illusion to make the foot appear smaller. However, the reduced vamp size requires the shoe to fit tightly in order to remain secure on the foot. The ideal vamp is one that is ample enough to cover the instep while being snug enough to secure the shoe to the foot. Even better is an adjustable vamp with laces, elastic, buckles, "T" strap, or Velcro, so the shoe can be easily placed on the foot and then secured with a comfortable amount of pressure.

Behind the vamp, the portion of the upper comprising the posterior part of the shoe's upper is called the quarter. This extends to the counter, the area at the rear of the shoe that encases the heel and holds it in position. The counter serves to control the heel and heel fit. Many people who purchase a wide width shoe to accommodate a wide forefoot find that they have difficulty with their heels slipping out of the counter. This is because the manufactures tend to "scale" up all parts of a shoe in the same proportion. However, forefoot width, which can increase from spreading between the metatarsal heads, tends to enlarge more

than the width of the heel, which represents a single bone, the calcaneus.

Inside the shoe is the insole, the hidden component on which the foot rests. This is the area that comes in contact with the plantar aspect of the foot and provides cushioning. The insole also functions in moisture regulation, hygiene and motion control. The bottom portion of the shoe that contacts the ground is the outsole. This is important for friction, insulation, and shock absorption. Again, the fashion desire for a smaller appearing foot leads to soles that are as thin as possible. This often compromises the cushioning effect of the insole and outsole. Many sport-specific shoes have specialized outsole designs based on the degree of traction, shock absorption, and pivoting desired for optimal performance.

Another feature of a shoe is the heel height, although this is generally a fashion consideration. Heel height is measured from the bottom of the outsole where the heel begins, to the plantar surface of the heel. The pitch of the heel is the angle or inclination of the posterior surface of the heel, from the vertical. Generally, the higher the heel the greater the pitch, which reduces the contact of the weightbearing surface with the floor. The advantages of high heels are cosmetic: they give an optical illusion of shortening the foot, slenderizing the ankle and calf, and giving a long-legged look. High heels also change a woman's center of gravity and alter the stride to what is generally considered a more attractive and sensuous appearance. Studies have shown that high heels increase peak pressure under the metatarsal heads. Despite this and other disadvantages of heel height, such as shifting the body weight forward and crowding the toes into the end of the shoe, they have been a popular fashion option. However, a recent study suggests that younger women are wearing high heels to work less often than older ones.

The construction of a shoe is based upon the last, a wooden or plastic model that approximates the size and shape of the weightbearing foot. Most mass produced shoes use a standard last of a medium width. Specialized or functional shoes may have various last shapes such as an extra depth last, or one with a heel narrower than the forefoot of a standard last. Another variation in last is an inflare, in which the forefoot portion has more medial than lateral surface area. An outflare last has more lateral surface than medial surface area anteriorly. Lasts may also be short- or long-toed. Lasting technique is the process whereby the shoe is constructed and attached to the upper sole.

The height of the shoe upper can extend various distances up the ankle, and can contribute to stability of the ankle and hindfoot. A standard oxford upper stops just inferior to the malleoli. A Chukka extends to just above the ankle joint. A high top shoe reaches to 6 inches proximal to the heel. An upper that is 8 or more inches above the heel is defined as a boot.

Shoe Analysis and Fit

When evaluating a patient with a foot or ankle complaint, careful inspection of the shoe is an important part of the physical examination. Wear patterns are generally predictable, with heels worn just slightly to the lateral side (Fig. 3). The inside of the shoe should be examined for pressure points in the forefoot, which contribute to corns, calluses, and toe deformities. Some patients will actually wear a hole in the liner of the shoe or break through the toe box. Treatment of their painful corns can often be accomplished with properly sized and shaped shoes rather than repeated paring, chemical application, or even pads. Removal of the source of the corn, that is, the ill-fitting shoe, will actually alleviate the problem rather than just treat the symptom. In patients with diabetes or other sensory neuropathy, it is essential to avoid

pressure or abrasion from poorly fitting shoes, because this can lead to ulcerations and subsequent infections. Tracing the contour of the patient's weightbearing foot and comparing it to the contour of the shoe will often disclose the source of many foot problems and serves to educate the patient about shoe selection (Fig. 4).

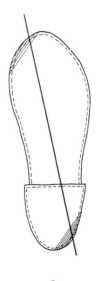

Figure 3

The normal wear pattern on the outsole is slightly medial of center at the toe and just lateral from center at the heel. Abnormalities in this pattern can indicate problems with alignment or gait.

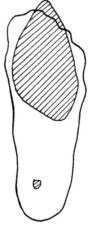

Figure 4

There is often a large mismatch between the contour of a patient's foot (solid line) and the shoe they are wearing (shaded area). Note the compression of the forefoot and the very small contact area of the high heel. Such a tracing can often disclose the cause of a patient's foot pain.

Fit, as well as fashion, can have an impact on the problems caused by shoes. Sizing of shoes dates back to the 14th century. At that time barley corns were used to define length, with 3 barley corns equaling 1 inch. King Edward decreed that 39 barley corns placed end to end would equal the size of the largest foot. This came out to 13 inches, and was designated a size 13, with each smaller size one barley corn, or 1/3 inch, less. Our current system of shoe sizing is still based on this. The most complete measuring device for shoe sizing is the Brannock measuring device generally seen in shoe stores.

Proper measurement of shoe size includes the overall foot length (heel to toe), arch length (heel to arch, or first metatarsal head), and width. A properly sized shoe will have the first metatarsal phalangeal joint at the level of the widest part of the shoe, which is why arch length is important in shoe fitting rather than overall length to the tip of the toes. Historically, shoes in a pair were identical and it wasn't until the 18th century that left and right differences appeared. This symmetry allowed people to get more wear out of their shoes by changing them from one foot to another.

For a shoe to have a proper fit both the size and the shape must be correct. The components of shape include the shape of the sole and the size of the sole, which together are determined by the last. The vamp size and shape contribute to fit as well. For example, pumps or other slip-on type shoes must have a tight vamp in order to stay on the foot. A shoe with laces, however, can provide a secure fit by being tightened after the shoe is put on the foot. If the shoe is the correct shape for the foot, the correct size will allow for 3/8 of an inch between the end of the shoe and the longest toe. In general, as shoes get longer, the manufacturers enlarge all the key internal dimensions in fixed proportions, called scaling. Recent studies have shown that as foot length increases, the forefoot width does increase somewhat, but heel width does not increase significantly. This leads to the common difficulty of having a heel counter that is too loose in a shoe that accommodates the length and forefoot width. Rather than have their feet slip out of the heels, many people buy shoes that are too tight in the forefoot.

Most shoe retailers receive little or no formal training in shoe fitting and it is not surprising that shoes and feet are often poorly matched. The National Shoe Retailers Association has recently begun sponsoring courses across the country to educate retailers on proper shoe fitting techniques, so it is hoped that this situation will improve in the future.

Studies have been done to evaluate the shoes worn by women in an attempt to gain some insight into the effects of shoes on causing foot deformity and pain. The rate of foot problems has been shown to be higher in shoe-wearing societies compared to those where shoes are not worn. Shoes have been implicated as a factor in hallux valgus, bunionettes, calluses, corns, and metatarsalgia. In one study, 80% of women admitted to foot pain, and 76% had some forefoot deformity. In the entire group of women, 88% wore shoes that were smaller than their feet, by an average of 1.2 cm. However, those without foot deformities averaged a discrepancy of only 0.60 cm. Women who did not have foot pain had an average discrepancy of only 0.56 cm. Shoe size also changed with age, increasing as women get older, yet 75% of women had not had their foot measured in more than 5 years.

Educational materials with guidelines for proper shoe selection are available to instruct patients about purchasing new shoes (Fig. 5). Buyers need to be informed on how to select proper fitting shoes, and manufacturers have to have appropriate styles available, with forefoot and heel width proportioned correctly. Most importantly, consumers have to be willing to let foot health, not fashion alone, dictate their shoe selection.

Ten Points of Proper Footwear*

1. Sizes vary among shoe brands and styles. Don't select shoes based on the size marked inside the shoe. Pick the shoe by how it fits your foot.

2. Select a shoe that conforms as nearly as possible to the shape of your forefoot.

3. Have your feet measured regularly. The size of your feet may change as you grow older.

4. Have both feet measured (often one foot is larger than the other). The shoe should be fitted to the larger foot.

5. Have your shoes fitted at the end of the day when your feet are the largest.

6. Stand during the fitting process because the foot lengthens as you are standing. There should be one fingerbreadth (fi in [1.3 cm]) between your longest toe and the end of the shoe.

7. The ball of your foot should fit snugly into the widest part of the shoe, but the shoe should not be too tight.

8. If the shoes don't fit, don't purchase them. Don't expect them to "stretch to fit."

9. Your heel should fit comfortably in the shoe with a minimum amount of pistoning.

10. While you are still in the shoe store, walk to make sure that the fit feels correct.

Figure 5

American Orthopaedic Foot and Ankle Society Ten Points of Shoe Fit. Brochures are available from the American Orthopaedic Foot and Ankle Society, 701 16th Avenue, Seattle, Washington 98122.

Special Types of Shoes and Shoe Modifications

Variations in toe box height, width, and depth can accommodate forefoot deformities such as hammertoes, mallet toes and bunion deformities. A extra depth shoe adds 1/4 to 3/8 of an inch in vertical height. In addition to providing more room for the foot itself, these shoes allow space for a custom insole or other padding, which takes up room in the shoe. An oblique toe is a rounder, mitten-shaped toe box. This conforms to the natural contour of most feet and minimizes compression of the toes. Patients with diabetes or other sensory neuropathy can benefit from therapeutic footwear to minimize skin ulcerations, including soft leather uppers that are easily stretched. Custom-made shoes include a plastizote insole and cloth upper combination that can be made to accommodate a variety of foot deformities. These shoes are primarily for indoor use. For outdoor use, a moldable contour shoe can be fabricated, including Velcro closure straps for patients who have difficulty with laces because of limited hand function.

There are a large number of external shoe modifications that should be in the repertoire of any orthopaedic surgeon who treats patients with foot and ankle problems. These modifications have the advantage of permanent positioning, which eliminates slippage. The disadvantage is that it limits the patient to that particular shoe. Compliance, however, is assured as long as that shoe is worn. External modifications do not affect the shoe volume and therefore do not interfere with fit. However, they are visible and can affect shoe appearance, and they are subject to wear from walking. Shoe modification devices can also be internal, usually attached to the insole. These help to provide conservative measures, which should almost always be tried before resorting to a surgical solution. To optimize the potential results, the orthopaedic surgeon needs to work with the pedorthist, orthotist, or shoemaker by providing the appropriate prescription with information on the patient's diagnosis and desired modifications or at least the goals of the shoe modifications. Any relevant medical conditions (diabetes, peripheral vascular disease) and recent surgery or injuries should also be included on the prescription.

Sole Modifications

The sole of a shoe can be modified with a variety of rocker bottoms. A rocker bar is a piece of stiff material that is beveled at its anterior and posterior edges. The apex of the bar is placed parallel and just posterior to a line from the first to fifth metatarsal heads, and usually extends 0.5 to 1 cm below the level of the sole. This type of bar functions to shift the rollover point posterior to the metatarsal heads. This effectively transfers pressure from under the metatarsal heads to the metatarsal shafts. This rocker bottom can be combined with a steel sole stiffener (Fig. 6). This bar, which is approximately 0.2 cm thick, is inserted between the inner and outer soles of a shoe. The steel bar further limits motion of the sole, but, when combined with the rocker, allows the foot to rollover or flex for a more normal stride. Such modifications can be made to almost any oxford type shoe. The combination of the anterior rocker bottom coupled with a steel sole stiffener can take pressure off the metatarsophalangeal (MTP) joints for patients with MTP pathology, limit dorsiflexion to minimize symptoms of hallux rigidus, and give a more comfortable stride to patients with Lisfranc instability, arthritis, or arthrodeses. Recent studies have also shown that this shoe modification is useful in the treatment of plantar fasciitis because it limits the motion of the windlass mechanism, thereby reducing irritation of the plantar fascia.

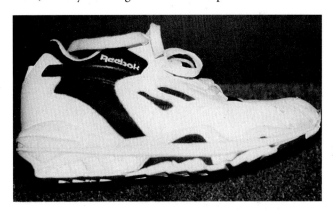

Figure 6

Shoe modified with a steel sole stiffener and anterior rocker bottom. This limits flexion at the MTP and Lisfranc joints and allow the foot to roll off from the contour of the outsole. (Any illustrations of or statements about commercial products are solely the opinion(s) of the author(s) and do not represent an Academy endorsement or evaluation of these products.)

A metatarsal bar also acts to transfer pressure from the metatarsal heads to the shafts. This firm material fixed to the plantar aspect of the shoe, posterior to the metatarsal heads, differs from the rocker bars in that it has a flatter plantar surface, rather than a rounded contour. This gives broader contact with the floor, but less assistance with rollover. Common design names of metatarsal bars are Denver, Mayo, Hauser, and Jones.

The sole of a shoe can be modified with a wedge added to the lateral or medial aspect. A lateral sole wedge will evert or pronate the forefoot, and a medial wedge will do the opposite and invert or supinate a flexible foot (Fig. 7). If there is a fixed

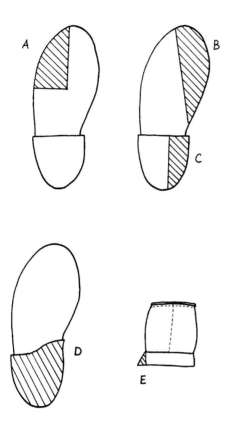

Figure 7

Sole modifications. **A,** Lateral sole wedge shifts the weight from the lateral to medial side of the shoe. **B,** Medial toe wedge in combination with a medial heel wedge. **C,** A Thomas heel **(D)** supports the medial longitudinal arch. **E,** A lateral heel flare resists eversion.

motion and stress at that joint, and also in patients who have had an ankle arthrodesis by providing some "give" with each step at heel strike.

A heel can also be modified with a wedge, which can be inserted in either the medial or lateral side (Fig. 7). The outer border of the wedge is generally 0.2 to .05 cm in thickness. Heel wedges can serve two functions. One is to rotate the foot in eversion or inversion, as would be done by a lateral or medial wedge, respectively. The other function is to accommodate a fixed deformity. One of the side effects of a heel counter on the shoe is that the opposite heel counter will get increased wear from the heel sliding into it, and it must be firm enough to resist any deformity without cutting into the side of the heel and causing skin problems. Application of the wedge to the back of the heel will elevate the whole heel. Such heel elevation is used to accommodate patients with a fixed equinus deformity or leg-length discrepancy. Desired heel elevations greater than 1/4 inch are usually made as external modifications, smaller amounts can be done with pads placed inside the shoe.

A Thomas heel is a 1 cm anterior extension of the heel medial border, and may also include a wedge (Fig. 7, *D*). This type of modification supports the medial longitudinal arch and can be useful for patients with a valgus hindfoot. A reverse Thomas heel has the anterior extension on the lateral edge and provides support to the lateral side of the foot. This modification serves to evert the hindfoot and can be used for patients with a flexible varus.

A heel flare is an outward extension of the medial, lateral, or both sides of the heel along the plantar surface. This gives an increased distance from the border of the flare to the subtalar axis, compared to the normal heel. A lateral flare (Fig. 7, *E*) will resist eversion, and a medial flare will resist inversion. A flare on both sides increases stability of the heel with respect to the subtalar axis.

Foot and Ankle Orthoses

The word "orthotic" is actually an adjective that has been improperly used as a noun by the lay public and medical professional alike. The proper term, "foot orthosis," is a device that serves to brace or support the foot. A patient can obtain such a device from many different venues, including over-the-counter products, often found in pharmacies or sporting good stores, from physical therapists, who may both prescribe and fabricate these devices in some states, or from a physician's prescription.

Many patients come into the office with the idea they "need" an orthotic device, either to accommodate or correct what they perceive as a deformity in their feet, or to improve athletic performance, when in both cases they may have no

forefoot deformity, a sole wedge can balance the plantar contact area closer to neutral. Another type of sole modification is a flare, which provides a broader, enlarged weightbearing surface for the outsole. This can increase stability and help in resisting inversion or eversion of the foot.

There are also a number of heel modifications which can be incorporated in a shoe. The SACH heel is a cushioned heel made by inserting a wedge of spongy material between the outer sole and the bottom of the regular heel. This material acts to absorb impact at heel strike, and will reduce the stress on the heel and ankle. This shock absorption also simulates plantarflexion after heel strike, thereby reducing the range of plantarflexion needed to bring the sole in contact with the floor. The moment of force that tends to flex the knee is also lessened. These effects can be beneficial for patients with ankle arthritis by limiting

pathology in their feet nor any complaint of pain. Other patients may have a congenital or acquired deformity, which can be flexible or fixed, and desire a shoe insert to improve their comfort and function. Still other patients will have feet which appear normal, but will have complaints of either a specific area of discomfort, or generalized, diffuse "sore feet" and look to the orthopaedic surgeon to give them relief with some type of orthotic insert. This has been an area of much confusion with regard to effectiveness because of many anecdotal concepts as well as undocumented biomechanical theories. There have been few scientifically sound studies for many of the indications, yet millions of dollars are spent on orthoses in the United States every year. Recently, as managed care has looked to control costs, the medical necessity of many of these devices has come into question, leading to sharp cuts in coverage by the payers.

An orthopaedic surgeon should be able to evaluate the patient's feet, assess the pathologic process that needs correction or treatment, and write a prescription for the appropriate device. A qualified orthotist or certified pedorthist can then fabricate the device for the patient and work with the orthopaedic surgeon to monitor its effectiveness and make modifications as necessary. There are also many noncustom products, which the orthopaedic surgeon should be familiar with in order to provide guidance to those patients who do not need custom inserts.

The two basic categories of orthotic devices are functional and accommodative. An accommodative orthosis conforms to the contours of the foot to maximize the contact area between the plantar aspect of the foot and the insole. They tend to be soft and resilient in order to decrease contact pressure and shear at bony prominences, thereby preventing ulcerations, skin breakdown, or pain. These inserts are commonly prescribed for the diabetic or rheumatoid foot, or to accommodate a localized deformity like a plantar fibroma. Other types of devices, such as foam athletic insoles or viscoelastic heel cushions, can provide comfort by increasing the cushioning between the foot and the ground. For the patient with a significant deformity or risk of soft-tissue breakdown, a custom-made orthosis may be required. Most of these devices are made of soft materials that may "bottom out" in less than a year. A functional orthotic is one that serves to control or modify the way the foot meets the ground. In some cases, they may be designed to correct a flexible deformity, for example, a valgus hindfoot in a patient with posterior tibial tendon insufficiency. These devices are often rigid, and their stabilizing effect often compromises flexibility and therefore shock absorption. Often, combining materials such as cork and foam will give rigid enough support, yet still provide some cushioning.

Part of the confusion over the use of functional foot orthoses derives from the concept of what constitutes a pathologic condition in the foot requiring treatment. Specifically, arch height and the degree of pronation or supination have been targeted by some as conditions that need treatment, even in asymptomatic patients. Pronation and supination are not single positions of the foot. Rather, they are motions of the foot consisting of components of hindfoot inversion/eversion, forefoot dorsiflexion/plantarflexion, and forefoot abduction/adduction. Pronation and supination are part of the normal motions of the foot during the gait cycle. At the initial phase of gait, the foot contacts the ground in supination. In this position, the midfoot and subtalar joints are rigidly locked. The foot becomes a sturdy platform to accommodate the force of heel strike for the body. As the foot progresses through the gait cycle and the body weight moves forward, the foot begins to pronate. The calcaneus moves laterally, the subtalar joint unlocks, and the forefoot abducts. This makes the foot more flexible so it can adapt to the uneven ground surface.

As the gait cycle continues and toe-off is initiated, the foot again supinates and becomes more rigid to provide an effective lever for push-off. As the foot goes through this cycle, there is a secondary effect on the tibia. As the foot pronates, the tibia rotates internally, and with supination, the tibia rotates externally. This tibial motion, which is based on the mitred-hinge theory, forms the basis for many ideas about pronation and supination of the foot affecting the knee.

Many knee complaints in runners have been attributed to "hyperpronation" of the foot. One study sought to measure the extent of patella deviation with experimental pronation or supination by fitting a valgus or varus wedge in the shoe. Even with a 20° variation in varus/valgus from the inserts, the difference in patellar deviation was only 1.6 mm of motion. Another study placed orthoses in patients' shoes that caused the foot to either pronate or supinate, in an attempt to treat Morton's neuroma symptoms. Not only was there no difference in improvement of symptoms (both groups had 40% improvement), but being placed in forced pronation or supination did not lead to any difference in side effects in terms of knee, hip, or back problems.

Arch height is often equated by the lay public with pronation and supination, which as discussed above, are dynamic events. Normal arches can be low (pes planus) or high (pes cavus), and are not necessarily pathologic conditions that require treatment. There are, however, certain pathologic conditions that are reflected by abnormalities in arch height. For example, an acquired flatfoot can be due to posterior tibial tendon insufficiency, or very high arches can be from neuromuscular disorders like Charcot-Marie-Tooth disease. All children have flexible flat feet and develop arches with maturity. Certainly a child, and even an adult, with an asymptomatic flat foot does not require treatment with expensive, custom-made foot orthoses. If a foot is painful it is more appropriate to determine the specific cause of the pain rather than attribute it to arch height, because most people with both low and high arches are not only asymptomatic, but can function at high-demand athletic levels.

In prescribing foot orthoses, the specific problem needs to be recognized and addressed. It may be something as simple as a foam insole to provide more cushioning, or a custom-made midfoot brace to support the medial arch and prevent valgus deformity in a foot with a nonfunctioning posterior tibial tendon. Foot orthoses can certainly affect measurable parameters such as plantar pressure, ground reaction forces, and subtalar motion. However, there is little scientifically sound evidence to show the clinical and therapeutic efficacy for most conditions. One study has shown that posterior tibial tendonopathy can successfully be treated with UCBL custom orthoses (Fig. 8). Another study has shown that orthoses combined with appropriate shoes are used in the treatment of diabetic neuropathic foot ulcers.

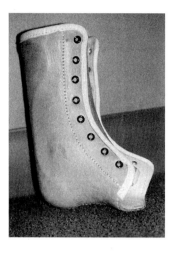

Figure 9

A custom-molded leather ankle brace can treat a variety of problems in the hindfoot and ankle by providing stability and support.

patient may have a vague complaint of "tired feet" or "achy feet," or may just be interested in enhancing athletic performance. The orthopaedic surgeon should be able to provide the patient with information on appropriate shoe selection and terms of style and fit. Prescribing expensive, custom-made orthotic devices should be based on sound principles of treating a defined condition with the specific biomechanical effect of the particular orthosis, as would be done for any other part of the musculoskeletal system.

Annotated Bibliography

Chao W, Wapner KL, Lee TH, Adams J, Hecht PJ: Nonoperative management of posterior tibial tendon dysfunction. *Foot Ankle Int* 1996;17:736–741.

The authors used MAFO splints or UCBL inserts for patients with posterior tibial tendon dysfunction. The authors found that 67% of patients interviewed were pleased with the orthosis and had good to excellent results. These patients tended to be older and have more concurrent medical problems.

Coughlin MJ, Thompson FM: The high price of high-fashion footwear, in Jackson DW (ed): *Instructional Course Lectures 44.* Rosemont, IL, American Academy of Orthopaedic Surgeons, 1995, pp 371–377.

A thorough review of the effects of shoes on development of foot pathology. Common foot problems related to shoewear are discussed, and practical approaches for educating patients and guiding them in shoe selection are provided.

Engle ET, Morton DJ: Notes on foot disorders among natives of the Belgian Congo. *J Bone Joint Surg* 1931;13:311–318.

Feet of natives of the Belgian Congo were examined for pathology. Foot deformities in this group resulted from infection, trauma, or congenital origins. They appeared to be free of the usual forefoot complaints found in the shoe-wearing population.

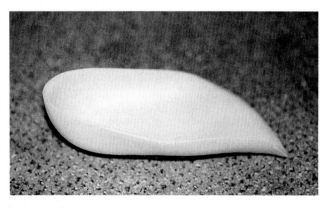

Figure 8

A UCBL (University of California Berkeley Lab) orthosis is an example of a custom-made hindfoot/midfoot brace, which is effective in the treatment of acquired flat foot from posterior tibial tendon insufficiency.

A number of orthoses are aimed at providing stabilization of the ankle (Fig. 9). Treatment of ankle problems is discussed elsewhere in this volume, however, these devices should be included in the armamentarium of every orthopaedic surgeon treating foot and ankle problems. It is important to again emphasize that the pathologic process should be identified in order to provide effective treatment with an orthosis. One of the most difficult problems may be the patient who demands an orthotic, but who does not have any abnormal findings on examination or radiograph. Such a

Frey C, Thompson F, Smith J: Update on women's footwear. *Foot Ankle Int* 1995;16:328–331.

The authors summarize a previously published survey of 255 women between the ages of 20 and 60 years, which compared shoe size with foot measurement. They found that 86% of women evaluated were wearing shoes that were smaller than their measured forefoot width. Those who had foot pain were on average 0.88 cm smaller; those without foot pain had, on average, a 0.58 cm of shoe-foot discrepancy.

Grifka JK: Shoes and insoles for patients with rheumatoid foot disease. *Clin Orthop* 1997;340:18–25.

This review of rheumatoid foot pathology focuses on the physical examination of the rheumatoid foot and nonsurgical treatments such as shoe modifications and custom insoles.

Hayda R, Tremaine MD, Tremaine K, Banco S, Teed K: Effect of metatarsal pads and their positioning: A quantitative assessment. *Foot Ankle Int* 1994;15:561–566.

The authors used 10 normal subjects to measure the effect of 3 different metatarsal pads on plantar pressure beneath the metatarsal heads. They found that a small felt pad reduced pressure at the metatarsal head most consistently (19.15%). In addition, they tested three positions of the pads, normal, 5 mm proximal, and 5 mm distal to the metatarsal heads, and they found that the distal placements gave the lowest pressure readings. It would have been interesting to know if the position and insert with the lowest pressures were also most comfortable.

Janisse DJ: Footwear prescriptions. *Foot Ankle Int* 1997; 18:526–527.

Janisse DJ: Indications and prescriptions for orthoses in sports. *Orthop Clin North Am* 1994;25:95–107.

A short and detailed review of how to write a pedorthic prescription. There are illustrations of various examples of foot orthoses and a discussion of fabrication techniques, as well as applications for their use.

Jones DC: Foot orthoses, in Heckman JD (ed): *Instructional Course Lectures 42.* Rosemont, IL, American Academy of Orthopaedic Surgeons, 1993, pp 219–224.

This is an excellent review of the literature up to 1993, with regard to foot orthoses.

Kaye RA: The extra-depth toe box: A rational approach. *Foot Ankle Int* 1994;15:146–150.

This review of extra-depth shoes includes comparisons of the measured depths of several different models and brands.

Kilmartin TE, Wallace WA: Effect of pronation and supination orthosis on Morton's neuroma and lower extremity function. *Foot Ankle Int* 1994;15:256–262.

Half of a group of patients with Morton's neuroma were fitted with supination felt orthoses, and half with pronation felt orthoses. After a year, there was no statistical difference between the two groups. Interestingly, the authors found no statistical difference between the two groups in new complaints of pain.

Kitaoka HB, Luo ZP, An KN: Analysis of longitudinal arch supports in stabilizing the arch of the foot. *Clin Orthop* 1997;341:250–256.

This study examined the effect of medial arch supports in maintaining arch height and controlling joint rotation in fresh cadaveric specimens. The authors used a magnetic tracking system and found arch position was maintained with significant difference between the two supports and the no support measurements.

Miller CD, Laskowski ER, Suman VJ: Effect of corrective rearfoot orthotic devices on ground reaction forces during ambulation. *Mayo Clin Proc* 1996;71:757–762.

The authors performed a prospective, randomized, single-blinded study to evaluate the effect on ground reaction forces when a semi-rigid custom orthotic insert was placed on asymptomatic flat feet (5° to 10° of calcaneal eversion). They found that vertical and anteroposterior ground reaction forces were reduced to a significant extent with the orthoses, but that medial-lateral differences were not significant.

Mizel MS, Marymont JV, Trepman E: Treatment of plantar fasciitis with a night splint and shoe modification consisting of a steel shank and anterior rocker bottom. *Foot Ankle Int* 1996;17:732–735.

This study employs a molded ankle-foot orthosis (MAFO) night splint and the steel sole stiffener shoe modification for conservative treatment of chronic plantar fasciitis. At 16-month follow up, symptoms were resolved or improved in 77% of the 71 feet studied.

Mizel MS, Michelson JD: Nonsurgical treatment of monarticular nontraumatic synovitis of the second metatarsophalangeal joint. *Foot Ankle Int* 1997;18:424–426.

Conservative treatment of idiopathic second metatarsophalangeal joint synovitis was based on the rocker bottom stiff shoe modification and an intra-articular steroid injection. Symptoms resolved in 70% of patients.

Nyska M, McCabe C, Linge K, Klenerman L: Plantar foot pressures during treadmill walking with high-heel and low-heel shoes. *Foot Ankle Int* 1996;17:662–666.

This study compared plantar pressures as measured in shoes of women wearing low heels and high heels. High heels were seen to cause 40% higher pressures in the medial forefoot. In addition, the force time for the high heel group was 20% higher than for the low heel group.

Shiba N, Kitaoka HB, Cahalan TD, Chao EY: Shock-absorbing effect of shoe insert materials commonly used in management of lower extremity disorders. *Clin Orthop* 1995;310:130–136.

This study used a drop test to evaluate the shock absorption characteristics of three materials. The polymeric foam rubber was found to attenuate force most effectively, while the viscoelastic polymeric material created the highest mean peak force.

64   Shoes and Orthoses

Sim-Fook L, Hodgson AR: A comparison of foot forms among the non-shoe and shoe-wearing Chinese population. *J Bone Joint Surg* 1958;40A:1058–1062.

The incidence of foot deformities was compared between a population in China who wore shoes and another group who did not. Hallux valgus and hammer toe deformities in the shod population occurred at a rate double to that in the unshod group.

Slavens ER, Slavens ML: Therapeutic footwear for neuropathic ulcers. *Foot Ankle Int* 1995;16:663–666.

This article discusses the importance of footwear in treatment plans for patients with neuropathic ulcers. It is presented from a pedorthist's point of view, following 23 patients with neuropathic foot ulcers.

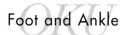

Chapter 6
Pediatric Foot

Introduction

Pediatric foot problems can be classified into those conditions that present in newborns or before age 1, those presenting after age 1, conditions associated with neurologic conditions, and with trauma and infection. Many conditions have a benign natural history, but this natural history needs to be explained to parents so that they understand which conditions require active treatment and which conditions will resolve without treatment.

Conditions Presenting in the Newborn and Before Age 1

Clubfoot

Clubfoot has been classified into 4 groups: congenital, teratologic, part of a syndrome, and positional. Congenital clubfoot is an isolated deformity that is not associated with other musculoskeletal abnormalities. The teratologic form of clubfoot is associated with an identified underlying neuromuscular disorder such as arthrogryposis or myelodysplasia. Clubfoot as part of a syndrome may be autosomal dominant, autosomal recessive, or part of an X-linked recessive disorder. Examples would be clubfoot associated with Larsen syndrome, Pierre Robin syndrome, amniotic band syndrome, and proximal femoral focal deficiency. Positional clubfoot is a normal foot that has been held in a deformed position in utero and should readily correct with casting. Congenital clubfoot is most common, with an overall incidence of 1 per 1,000 live births. Males tend to be more frequently affected and the deformity is bilateral in approximately 5% of cases. Cowell has shown a multifactorial system of inheritance in congenital clubfoot with major influence from a dominant gene. It is important to point out to parents that there is an increased risk to subsequent offspring when the first child has clubfoot.

Although a genetic component has been identified, the etiology of clubfoot is unknown. The talar head and neck deformity is no longer considered to be the primary deformity but is considered secondary to muscle imbalance, soft-tissue contractures, and growth occurring in an abnormal position. Other theories of the cause of clubfoot include muscle fiber disproportion, fibrosis of distal musculature, myofibroblasts in the medial and posterior soft tissues, and arterial abnormalities causing a regional growth disturbance. These current concepts focus on possible neuromuscular causes but further investigations will be necessary to define the precise etiology of clubfoot.

Pathoanatomy The pathoanatomy of clubfoot is complex; however, there is soft-tissue contraction of the triceps surae, tibialis posterior, flexor hallucis longus, and flexor digitorum longus. The long and short plantar ligaments, spring ligament, posterior ankle capsule, subtalar ligament, and lateral ankle ligaments, especially the posterior talofibular and calcaneal fibular ligaments, are also contracted.

Some parts of the bony anatomy are clear-cut. The talus and calcaneus are in equinus. The navicular is medially subluxated on the head of the talus, causing it to abut against the anterior aspect of the medial malleolus. Other aspects of the bony deformity have become more easily understood using 3-dimensional computer modeling of dissected feet and magnetic resonance imaging (MRI) studies. These studies show that there is a posterior deviation of the lateral malleolus, a medial and plantar deviation of the talar neck, and medial rotation and supination of the calcaneus. Often, there is medial subluxation of the cuboid on the head of the calcaneus as well as forefoot cavus. MRI studies on 10 infants with congenital clubfoot revealed that the primary problem is that the deformity of the talar head and neck allows the anterior aspect of the calcaneus to follow the deformed talus, causing a pivot around the interosseous ligament such that the posterior aspect of the calcaneus is forced laterally.

Thometz and Springer in 1990 demonstrated that some treatment failures can be accounted for by unrecognized calcaneal cuboid subluxation. In a study of 100 unoperated feet, 30% had no subluxation, 45% had mild subluxation, and 25% had moderate to severe subluxation. Those feet with moderate and severe subluxation required release and pinning of the calcaneocuboid joint.

Clinical Characteristics Examination of the infant clubfoot reveals hindfoot equinus that can be appreciated by an apparently empty heel pad upon palpation. Hindfoot varus, forefoot adduction, and rigidity are also apparent. Atrophy of the calf and foot may not be obvious in the infant but will become more apparent with age. One of the difficulties in evaluating treatment is that clubfoot varies in severity. In some newborns, the diagnosis is very obvious, with deep medial and posterior creases and approximation of the forefoot to the lower leg. Other cases are mild enough that they are confused with simple metatarsus adductus or positional clubfoot. Only after casting fails is the true diagnosis of clubfoot revealed.

Radiographic Evaluation Radiographs are not helpful in the newborn because of the immaturity of the ossification centers. Radiographs can be helpful when a plateau has been reached in conservative treatment or immediately before surgery. The most common radiographic views used are the weightbearing or simulated weightbearing anteroposterior (AP), and the lateral radiograph with the foot in maximum dorsiflexion. In a normal foot, the lateral view with forced dorsiflexion shows that the os calcis tends to tilt dorsally and the talus maintains its relative position in the ankle mortise. As a result, there is convergence of the anterior talocalcaneal joint on the lateral view. In a clubfoot, the os calcis and talus remain parallel on the lateral view of forced dorsiflexion, with the calcaneus in equinus and almost parallel to the lateral axis of the talus. On an AP radiograph, the kite angle formed by intersection of lines drawn through the axis of the

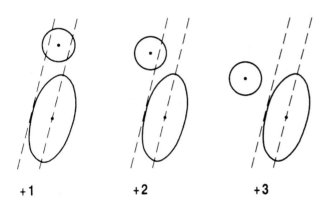

+1   +2   +3

Figure 1

The calcaneal long axis is determined by a line parallel to its lateral border. A parallel medial line passes tangentially to the medial border of the calcaneus. Grade I (normal) demonstrates the midpoint of the cuboid ossification lying between the long axis and the medial line; grade II has the central point of the cuboid ossification lying medial to the medial line; grade III (severe) has the central point of the cuboid ossification moving proximal to the distal end of the calcaneal ossification center. (Reproduced with permission from Thomas GH, Simons GW: Congenital talipes equinovarus (clubfeet) and metatarsus adductus, in Drennan JC (ed): *The Child's Foot and Ankle.* New York, NY, Raven Press, 1992, p 105.)

talus and os calcis normally measures 20° to 40°; an angle less than 20° implies varus, and a true clubfoot always demonstrates a varus kite angle with relative parallelism between the talus and the calcaneus. The navicular, which is known to be medially subluxated on the talus in clubfoot, does not ossify before age 5 or 6 years and therefore is not seen on early radiographs. Some authors have used ultrasound to evaluate the position of the navicular relative to the talus.

The cuboid position can be evaluated on the AP radiograph by noting the relationship of its central point relative to the longitudinal axis of the calcaneus, specifically, a line parallel to the long axis of the calcaneus tangential to the medial border of the calcaneus. If the central point of the cuboid is medial to this line, a grade II calcaneal cuboid subluxation is present. A grade III or more severe subluxation is present if this central point has moved proximal to the distal end of the calcaneal ossification center (Fig. 1). Severe subluxation requires intraoperative reduction and pinning of the joint.

Treatment Treatment will not result in a completely normal foot. Calf atrophy, asymmetry of foot size, limitation of subtalar mobility, metatarsus adductus, or a toe-in gait will probably be present regardless of treatment. The goal of treatment is to produce a near-anatomically normal, pain-free, plantigrade foot that has reasonable mobility and fits into a normal shoe. A cosmetically pleasing appearance is also an important goal.

Treatment should begin as soon as possible after birth and consists of manipulation with serial casting. Taping or malleable splints are alternatives in the hospitalized neonate. The manipulation is directed toward stretching the contracted medial soft tissues, reducing the navicular onto the head of the talus, and then restoring rotational alignment between the calcaneus and the talus. A long leg cast is required because the initial casts will leave the foot in an equinus position, with major attention directed toward reducing the forefoot. A short leg cast would slide off with the foot remaining in the equinus position. Long leg casts also have the theoretic advantage of controlling rotational correction better than below-knee casts. Often, once the equinus has been corrected, short leg casts are used for the family's convenience. Manipulation prior to cast application consists of longitudinal traction followed by forefoot abduction. The thumb can be used to guide the talus back to its normal medial position and to reduce the talonavicular joint. Other authors believe that the talus is locked into the mortise and that the reduction is an attempt to reduce the medially subluxated navicular back onto the head of the talus. Following manipulation the casts are applied and changed at weekly intervals. Complete correction, both clinically and radiographically, should be achieved by 2 to 3 months of age. Failure to achieve clinical and radiographic correction by age 3 months or recurrence following initial correction is an indication for discontinuation of conservative management and proceeding with surgical correction. Further attempts at nonsurgical management may result in a rocker-bottom foot. Results from recent studies suggest that the success rate with conservative treatment is approximately 5%, although Ponseti reported that all feet could be corrected with casting and that the failure or recurrence rate after casting was only 12%. This extensive regime of casting is not frequently used.

Percutaneous heel cord releases are sometimes performed at 3 months of age as part of ongoing treatment. The criteria for percutaneous release as cited by proponents of this approach is persisting radiographic equinus at 3 months of age. After this percutaneous release, serial stretching and casting is continued for an additional 2 months. If adequate correction does not result, surgery is needed. Proponents of this approach have demonstrated that the Achilles tendon reconstitutes itself to its attachment at the calcaneus by the time of surgery at age 1 year. This percutaneous release can be done in the clinic without general anesthesia.

Surgical management is rarely done before the age of 4 months to allow for a trial of cast treatment and for the foot to grow to an adequate size. Those authors who argue for delaying surgery until 12 months of age say that the larger foot size at this age makes surgery easier and less likely to cause iatrogenic damage. In addition, because other diagnoses are uncovered in this first year of life, it is best to delay treatment in order to avoid operating on a clubfoot that is part of a syndrome or a neurologic foot and so that the diagnosis is more clearly established. Advocates of early surgery believe that the amount of pedal growth in the first year of life is considerable, and that early correction permits remodeling of the talus, calcaneus, and navicular. The surgeon should be aware that preterm infants have an increased risk of apnea after anesthesia. Infants with a history of apnea and bradycardia or respiratory distress, intubation, or mechanical ventilation may be at increased risk and should be observed and monitored. Because of these risks, there may be some advantage to delaying surgery in these high-risk infants.

Controversies exist regarding the surgical incisions, the duration of postoperative immobilization, the type and extent of release, and the need for pin fixation. Results are good for feet on which minimal surgery is performed; multiply operated feet have the worst results. It is important to identify all components of the deformity and correct them at the initial surgical setting without doing excessive surgery. Some feet with mild deformities only require posterior or posterior and lateral releases, and these feet would be expected to do well,

both because of the nature of the deformity and because surgical scarring is not extensive. Feet with severe deformity should be corrected in one surgical setting. Techniques for complete soft-tissue releases have been described by Turko, Thompson and associates, McKay, Simons, Carroll and associates, and Goldner. The posterior release typically includes Achilles tendon lengthening, release of the posterior ankle and subtalar joints, including the posterior talofibular ligament, release of the thickened peroneal retinaculum and tendon sheath posterior and inferior to the lateral malleolus, and lengthening of the tendons of the flexor digitorum longus and flexor hallucis longus.

The medial release includes Z-plasty of the tibialis posterior tendon, complete capsulotomy of the talonavicular joint, release of the abductor hallucis tendon, possible release of the medial and plantar surface of the calcaneal cuboid joint, release of the medial aspect of the subtalar joint, and release of part or all of the interosseous ligament.

The lateral release involves the release of the lateral aspect of the subtalar joint and the contracted calcaneofibular ligament, and perhaps release of the calcaneocuboid joint. Sometimes a plantar release is also performed by incising the common origin of the plantar structures from the tuberosity of the os calcis.

Turko first described the posteromedial release more than 15 years ago. McKay expanded the posterior medial release to include the posteromedial lateral release in an effort to address the contracted posterior talofibular and calcaneofibular ligaments, which are believed to cause medial spin and hindfoot varus. Simons proposed a more complete subtalar release that often included the talocalcaneal interosseous ligament, including a release and pinning of the calcaneocuboid joint in more severe deformities. Goldner and others avoid releasing the subtalar joint and obtain correction of hindfoot varus by releasing the deltoid ligaments. Other authors leave the deltoid ligament intact.

Most surgeons place a Kirschner wire (K-wire) across the talonavicular joint; others also use a wire in the subtalar and calcaneocuboid joints. Postoperative plaster is used for 6 to 12 weeks. At the end of casting, orthoses, bivalve casts, or corrective shoes can be used for months to years.

Turko proposed a single posteromedial incision. The Cincinnati incision extends all the way around the heel to the lateral malleolus, or even to the calcaneocuboid joint, to allow a more complete release of structures in that area. Carroll uses a two-incision approach with one medial incision and a second posterolateral longitudinal incision for access to the Achilles tendon and the posterolateral structures.

The incisions do not reflect the surgical release that is employed. Any combination of soft-tissue release can be done through these incisions. The condition of the skin is a concern at wound closure; medial posterior skin is often tight with the foot in the corrected position. One alternative is to leave the wound partially open and allow it to granulate; excellent cosmetic results have been reported with this technique. Another alternative is splinting or casting of the foot in a equinus position, with cast changes in the first week to allow regression of soft-tissue swelling and gradual stretching of the skin into the corrected position. Pins are usually removed after 6 weeks, with casting continuing for another 6 weeks.

Hospitalization is routine for swelling and for pain control. In one study in which a series of clubfoot surgeries using spinal anesthetic were done on an outpatient basis, no cost savings were realized.

Results Because of the variability of involvement of feet before surgery, treatment results are difficult to assess. Recently the results of 3 different approaches to the treatment of clubfoot were studied and found to be clinically similar. Satisfactory long-term results can be anticipated in 70% to 80%. A 35-year follow-up suggests that a sedentary occupation and avoidance of excessive weight gain may improve the overall long-term results. Excessive weakening of the triceps surae may predispose to poor results; therefore, overlengthening of this muscle should be avoided. The outcome could not be predicted from the radiographic result of surgical treatment in this study. The most common residual deformity is dynamic forefoot adduction and supination of the midfoot and hindfoot during ambulation. This is commonly caused by overpull of the tibialis anterior, and correction can be achieved by transferring the entire tendon to the dorsum of the foot into the second or third cuneiform or splitting the tibialis anterior and placing the lateral half into the cuboid.

A fixed cavovarus deformity, which is most commonly caused by a contracted plantar fascia, may represent a recurrence. If the hindfoot remains flexible, the plantar fascia release may benefit the patient, but if a rigid hindfoot varus persists, additional soft-tissue releases, tendon transfers, or bone procedures may be necessary. The bean-shaped foot with residual forefoot adductus may benefit from cuboid decancellation or lengthening of the medial column of the foot with medial cuneiform opening wedge osteotomy combined with closing wedge osteotomy of the cuboid.

Severe pes planus with lateral translation of the calcaneus can be very disabling and can be treated with a calcaneal sliding osteotomy in an effort to place the calcaneus back under the long axis of the tibia. This complication may be related to excessive subtalar and intraosseous release with failure to adequately stabilize the calcaneal talar joint with pins. The surgeon should be aware that after correcting this hindfoot valgus, a supination of the forefoot may become more apparent and a forefoot or midfoot procedure may also be needed in order to regain a plantigrade foot. Recurrence of deformity has been reported in 5% to 20% of patients, repeat surgery is complex because of postoperative scarring, and bony procedures as well as tendon transfers may need to be added.

Calcaneovalgus

Congenital calcaneovalgus foot is the most common deformity of the foot seen at birth. The reported incidence is 30% to 50%, and the condition is secondary to intrauterine molding. The foot is acutely dorsiflexed and the dorsum of the foot is in contact with the anterior shin. The deformity is supple and the foot can be brought into some plantarflexion and supination. This condition resolves without sequelae, and stretching, although frequently recommended, is probably not necessary. This condition needs to be differentiated from posteromedial bowing of the tibia and congenital vertical talus.

Posteromedial Bowing of the Tibia

Congenital posteromedial bowing of the tibia causes a clinical appearance of calcaneal valgus or calcaneus foot deformity at birth and can easily be mistaken for a primary foot deformity. Careful physical examination will reveal the tibial deformity, which corrects spontaneously with growth. Complete angular correction often occurs, with a 2- to 4-cm tibial leg-length discrepancy. Some authors use a short leg cast to help stretch the anterior structures, although this is probably not necessary.

Congenital Vertical Talus

This deformity occurs infrequently and may be idiopathic or inherited. It is associated with arthrogryposis multiplex, neurofibromatosis, nail patella syndrome, and chromosomal abnormalities such as trisomy 13, 15, and 19. It is also associated with myelomeningocele. The differential diagnosis includes calcaneal valgus foot, flexible flatfoot with midfoot sag, and short Achilles tendon or rigid flatfoot associated with tarsal coalition. There are 4 components to true vertical talus: hindfoot equinus, midfoot valgus, forefoot dorsiflexion, and dorsal dislocation of the talonavicular joint.

The dorsiflexed lateral view demonstrates the fixed equinus of the hindfoot with dislocation of the navicular on the talar neck. The plantarflexed lateral view shows that the talonavicular dislocation is not reducible, and that a line drawn through the long axis of the talus and another through the long axis of the metatarsal are not colinear or parallel. The AP view shows midfoot valgus. Older children will develop painful callus over the weightbearing talar head and have degenerative arthritis and pain at the dislocated talonavicular joint.

Treatment Stretching and serial casting can be useful before surgery to help stretch contracted tendons. Surgical treatment is required to reduce the talonavicular dislocation, lengthen the contracted posterior lateral and dorsal musculature, and to release the subtalar joint and talonavicular joints. Some authors have recommended a two-stage procedure to lengthen the long extensor and tibialis tendons with reduction of the talonavicular and calcaneocuboid joints. The forefoot is then reduced and pinned in a markedly plantarflexed position. Six weeks later a second surgical procedure is done, including heel cord lengthening and posterior capsulotomy. Other authors prefer a one-stage open reduction with fixation of the talonavicular joint with a K-wire coupled with posterior capsulectomy. Many series include a planned subtalar arthrodesis at the time of correction and/or a subsequent triple arthrodesis.

Oblique Talus
The lateral plantarflexion radiograph also demonstrates reduction of the navicular onto the talar head. The majority of children with an oblique talus do not require any active form of management.

Metatarsus Adductus
Metatarsus adductus is one of the most common foot deformities in childhood. The terms metatarsus varus, hooked forefoot, skewfoot, serpentine foot, and metatarsus adductovarus have also been used. Skewfoot and metatarsus varus Z foot are distinct diagnoses that will be discussed separately. In true metatarsus adductus the forefoot is adducted and slightly supinated and the lateral border of the foot is convex with an increased prominence of the base of the fifth metatarsus. There is no equinus contracture, and there is normal alignment of the midfoot and hindfoot.

Passive and active mobility have been used to create a three-group classification system. Type I metatarsus adductus is very flexible and the forefoot will correct past neutral into an overcorrected position with two-finger forefoot pressure or with stroking of the lateral border of the foot, causing the peroneals to evert the foot. Type II metatarsus adductus corrects to neutral passively but does not correct to neutral actively. Type III metatarsus adductus is rigid and does not correct to neutral, even with passive stretching.

Treatment Greater than 90% of metatarsus adductus cases resolve without any treatment. Infants with flexible type I and type II deformities can be observed. Infants 6 months of age with type I or type II feet that are not improving may require passive stretching exercises, corrective shoes, or serial casting. Ponseti and Becker observed that only 11% of nearly 400 patients had rigid deformities that required active treatment. In the remaining patients, there was a slight tendency to progression until age 1 or 2 years, and then an improvement over the next 2 years. Passive stretching exercises have been recommended for type II deformities in preambulatory children. The foot is held in the corrected or abducted position for 5 seconds, and 20 repetitions are usually performed with each diaper change. There is no evidence that this treatment alters the natural history of a relatively flexible metatarsus adductus. Corrective shoes may be either straight or reverse last; these are usually hightops with the toes exposed. The shoes are worn 2 to 22 hours a day, and serial casting may be considered when no significant improvement has been achieved after 6 to 8 weeks. The majority of type I and type II deformities will respond satisfactorily to this simple technique.

Pentz and Weiner report the use of reverse last shoes with a straight metal bar. Nearly 800 patients were treated over a 13-year period; there was a 99% likelihood of obtaining a full correction of foot deformity. Their criteria for an excellent result corresponds to a foot that readily reverses to beyond neutral with two-finger pressure without a medial crease. Other authors have criticized the use of the straight bar and shoe orthoses, suggesting that it causes the development of heel valgus. Pentz and Weiner reported no such problems.

Serial casting should be used for type III or rigid metatarsus adductus deformities, and it is better to initiate treatment before 8 months of age. A majority of these feet will correct with 6 to 8 weeks of serial casting. Holding casts for an additional 1 to 2 months or corrective shoes are used after the weekly cast changes.

Surgical management, including release of the abductor hallucis followed by serial casting, release of the metatarsal cuneiform, cuneiform navicular joints, tarsal metatarsal and intermetatarsal releases, and osteotomies of the metatarsals or the medial cuneiform with a closing wedge osteotomy of the cuboid, is almost never needed.

Polydactyly and Syndactyly
Polydactyly occurs in approximately 1.7 per thousand live births. Thirty percent of patients have a positive family history, and this condition may be inherited as an autosomal dominant trait with variable penetrance. Eighty percent of the time there is a postaxial duplication of the fifth digit. Without treatment, at long-term follow-up, 75% of untreated patients experience shoe-fitting problems related to excessive forefoot width, and 20% develop pain.

Preoperative radiographs are important for planning. Duplicated metatarsals should be removed to narrow the forefoot and widened metatarsals should be shaved so that they are not as prominent.

Preaxial duplications may be compounded by hallux varus and have a higher rate of recurrence. Collateral ligament repair is always necessary and in difficult cases, syndactylization of the first and second toes should be considered.

Because syndactyly of the foot does not cause shoe-fitting or functional problems, it usually is not treated. Polysyndactyly may cause painful shoe wear because of disproportionate widening of the forefoot. It is best to remove the duplicated toe without disturbing the syndactyly.

Cock-Up Fifth Toe

The fifth toe is noted at birth to cock up and override the fourth toe. There is a dorsal contracture involving skin, extensor tendon, and capsule of the metatarsophalangeal joint. Taping and stretching will not correct the deformity. A V skin incision centered over the contracted skin allows access to the extensor tendon, which is lengthened, and the capsule of the metatarsophalangeal joint, which is released. A percutaneous 0.045 K-wire stabilizes the fifth toe in the initial postoperative period. The V incision is closed as a Y to relax the skin contracture.

Curly Toe

Curly toe often involves the third or fourth toe and is a flexion deformity of the proximal interphalangeal joint. The toe is often rotated laterally and underrides the adjacent toe. Taping and stretching are ineffectual, and in early childhood a simple open tenotomy of the long and short toe flexors through a longitudinal plantar incision, avoiding the flexor crease, is successful if performed on preschool children. More complex solutions include a flexor-to-extensor transfer, which is not needed in young children.

Congenital Amputations

The majority of congenital foot deformities and partial congenital amputations are sporadic and not inherited. Absent lateral rays may be associated with absence of the fibula associated with a short limb and a malformed foot. Ablation of the foot is recommended between 6 and 18 months of age when it is apparent that the expected limb-length inequality will exceed 10 cm.

Congenital annular constriction bands, also known as Streeter's syndrome, may result in complete or partial amputations of the foot. Toes are often hypoplastic and associated with constriction bands, and clubfoot is frequently associated with this syndrome. Some amputations have incomplete skin closure, and local skin care usually results in secondary healing.

Problems Presenting After Age 1

Flatfoot

All 2-year-olds are flatfooted, whereas the same pattern is seen in only 4% of 10-year-olds. Although many attribute this condition to an arch that is obscured by a fat pad, radiographic studies show actual flattening of the medial arch in toddlers. The flexibility of the foot is more important than the static shape. In flexible flatfoot, there is a longitudinal arch in a nonweightbearing position and in toe standing and with dorsiflexion of the great toe. Treatment is not necessary and the use of arch supports and special shoes will not cause an arch to develop.

Leg aches or growing pains seen in children between 3 and 12 years of age may represent an overuse syndrome that is sometimes relieved by custom arch supports or well-fitted heel cups. The use of expensive orthotics to prevent rapid and uneven shoe wear does not seem to be cost-effective.

The orthopaedist is urged to avoid use of the term pronated as a description of flatfoot. The flexible flatfoot should be distinguished from flexible flatfoot with a short Achilles tendon and peroneal spastic or rigid flatfoot. Stretching exercises should be done to convert the symptomatic flexible flatfoot with a short Achilles tendon to the asymptomatic flexible flatfoot.

Tarsal coalition, a fibrous, cartilaginous, or bony connection between 2 or more tarsal bones that results from a congenital failure of differentiation and segmentation, is a cause of stiff, painful flatfoot. The most common types of tarsal coalitions are calcaneonavicular and talocalcaneal. These occur with equal frequency and account for about 90% of the total number of coalitions. The true incidence of tarsal coalitions is unknown because many asymptomatic individuals are never evaluated. The incidence of bilaterality is also unknown but is likely to be greater than 50%. The onset of symptoms usually correlates with the coalition from cartilage to bone at age 8 to 10 years for calcaneonavicular coalitions, and between 12 and 16 years of age for talocalcaneal coalitions. There may be a progressive valgus deformity of the hindfoot that coincides with ossification of the coalition, with flattening of the longitudinal arch and restriction of subtalar motion. These findings are more severe in feet with talocalcaneal coalitions.

The pain may have its onset with some unusual activity, trauma, or may be insidious. The pain can be in the sinus tarsi region or may be experienced in the ankle region and described as akin to ankle sprains.

Peroneal spasm has been described with tarsal coalitions, and the condition has been called peroneal spastic flatfoot. The spasm may be adaptive shortening; certainly, for some

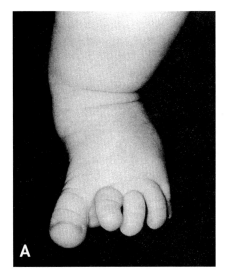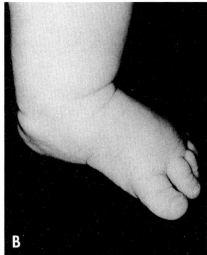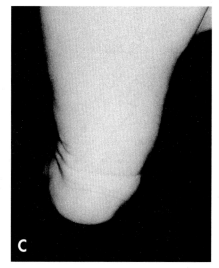

Figure 2

Skewfoot in a 2-month-old boy. **A,** S-shaped foot. Proximal medial convexity with more distal medial concavity. **B,** Medial foot crease. **C,** Heel valgus. (Reproduced with permission from Mosca V: Flexible flatfoot and skewfoot, in Drennan JC (ed): *The Child's Foot and Ankle.* New York, NY, Raven Press, 1992, p 370.)

patients with stress of the subtalar joint there is pain that goes up into the peroneal musculature. Physical examination reveals a rigid flatfoot with the longitudinal arch not recreated with toe standing or by the Jack toe rising test. The severity of pain seems to correlate with the severity of hindfoot valgus deformity. A calcaneonavicular coalition can best be seen on an oblique view of the foot. Talocalcaneal coalitions are best seen on computed tomography images in the coronal plane, that is, perpendicular to the plantar aspect of the foot. Coalitions can be symptomatic while still in the fibrous stage. Conservative measures, such as short leg casting, have been described for this condition and are often unsuccessful. Surgical options of symptomatic tarsal coalition include resection of the coalition, osteotomy, and triple arthrodesis. With excision of calcaneonavicular coalitions and interposition of extensor digitorum brevis, long-term pain relief can be expected in 77% of patients. This procedure is indicated in patients younger than 16 years of age who have no other coalitions present and no degenerative arthroses. Surgical resection of talocalcaneal coalitions has been thought to be less successful than that of calcaneonavicular coalitions. Feet with excessive heel valgus and a coalition of greater than 50% of the area of the posterior facet may have less successful surgical results. A recent paper showed satisfactory results in 8 of 9 cases of middle facet coalitions evaluated more than 10 years after the surgery, regardless of the percentage of middle facet involvement. Degenerative arthritis or persis-

tent pain following resection of a coalition represents an indication for triple arthrodesis.

Skewfoot

This is a rare foot deformity characterized by a forefoot abduction associated with hindfoot valgus (Fig. 2). The condition is not easily diagnosed in the newborn. Clinically, it resembles metatarsus adductus; however, the heel valgus is difficult to appreciate in a chubby newborn and radiographs are difficult to interpret secondary to the limited ossification. With advancing age, the diagnosis becomes more apparent (Fig. 3). The skewfoot adductus is usually rigid, forefoot supination is present, and shortening of the Achilles tendon is noted in the adolescent. Painful skewfoot can be treated with a lengthening of the neck of the calcaneus and lengthening of the Achilles tendon with correction of forefoot adduction by a medial opening wedge osteotomy of the deformed medial cuneiform.

Sever's Disease

Sever's disease is an apophysitis of the skeletally immature calcaneus that may account for heel pain in the adolescent. The condition is characterized by chronic, intermittent pain related to sports activity, with medial and plantar pain located along the calcaneal apophysis. There may be a history of running on hard surfaces with inadequate heel padding. Radiographs are obtained to rule out other abnormalities such as bone cysts or fracture. The radiographic appearance

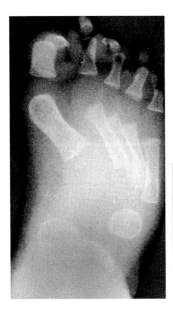

Figure 3

Skewfoot in a 12-month-old child. Note the metatarsus adductus and the lateral displacement of the cuboid relative to the long axis of the calcaneus. (Reproduced with permission from Mosca V: Flexible flatfoot and skewfoot, in Drennan JC (ed): *The Child's Foot and Ankle.* New York, NY, Raven Press, 1992, p 371.)

is one of sclerosis and fragmentation of the calcaneal apophysis. This finding has been observed most often in asymptomatic individuals. Treatment begins with rest, activity modification, and icing. Heel cups or appropriate shoes may be helpful. The problem is self-limited.

Freiberg's Infraction

Freiberg's infraction is an osteochondrosis of the second, or less commonly, third metatarsal head. The condition is typically seen in adolescent females age 10 to 18. They develop pain, swelling, and loss of motion of the involved metatarsophalangeal joint. Radiographs show varying degrees of involvement; in the earliest stages they are normal, although a bone scan may reveal abnormal vascularization. Subchondral fracture can develop later, with joint widening, sclerosis, and flattening of the metatarsal head, and eventual collapse, fragmentation, and osteophyte formation. Degenerative arthritis may ensue. Joint debridement and partial metatarsal head resection may be helpful in cases that do not respond to conservative measures.

Köhler's Disease

Osteochondrosis of the tarsal navicular can be a cause of midfoot pain. Physical examination findings may include tenderness along the medial border of the midfoot and soft-tissue swelling, sometimes accompanied by erythema. The onset is usually between the ages of 3 and 10 with a high male to female predominance. Radiographs are necessary to confirm the diagnosis. The typical radiographic finding is flattening and patchy ossification of the tarsal navicular with preservation of joint surfaces with the talus and cuneiform.

The navicular is the last of the tarsal bones to completely ossify, and delayed ossification can be found in a normal child age 3 to 4 years.

Treatment for Köhler's disease includes immobilization and rest for acute symptoms. Relief of pain and return to activity is reported to occur quicker with a short leg walking cast applied for 6 to 12 weeks followed by an orthotic device supporting the talonavicular joint. The navicular regains its normal radiographic appearance in 8 to 10 months. The clinical results are generally very good, with no long-term problems. Activities can be allowed when symptoms have subsided; some children reportedly have residual symptoms that require use of an orthotic.

Toddler's Fracture of the Calcaneus

One cause of foot pain in children younger than age 3 years is a calcaneal fracture, which has been reported to occur without history of significant injury. In one report, this fracture was not visible on plain radiographs in 5 of the 7 patients studied, and a bone scan was needed to make the diagnosis. Radiographs 2 weeks later revealed an arch of sclerosis across the tuberosity of the calcaneus.

Arthritic Conditions With Foot and Ankle Involvement

Many arthritic conditions present as foot or ankle pain. The pediatric population is affected by rheumatoid arthritis, which can be pauciarticular, polyarticular, or systemic at onset. Other conditions include the seronegative spondyloarthropathies, ankylosing spondylitis, Reiter's syndrome, and psoriatic arthritis as well as arthritis associated with bowel disease. Arthritis should be considered as a cause of foot and ankle pain in a child. Bacterial infections should be considered as well, and will be discussed separately.

Foot Deformities Associated With Neurologic Conditions

Cerebral Palsy

Cerebral palsy is a static encephalopathy that occurs early in brain development, either during the intrauterine period or up until the second year of life. Foot and ankle problems are acquired as a result of muscle imbalance and spasticity.

The typical deformity found in hemiplegia is equinovarus. In spastic diplegia and quadriplegia, equinovalgus is predominant. A reducible malaligned foot can be treated with orthotics, and muscle imbalance in a supple foot can be treated with tendon transfers or lengthenings. Rigid deformities may require bony surgery.

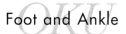

Surgical treatment should be delayed if possible until age 4 to 7 years to allow stabilization of the muscle imbalance and a plateau in gait development. Before this time, nerve blocks, stretching casts, and orthoses are useful in controlling foot deformities.

Conservative measures will work when spasticity in the patient with cerebral palsy is mild. The goals of surgery in the patient with cerebral palsy are to restore muscle balance and to correct fixed deformities. Indications for surgical treatment include increase in rigid deformity despite conservative measures, functional deterioration, or a deformity that presents an obstacle to independent function. For equinus deformity, Achilles tendon lengthening is either done with an open Z-step cut or a two- or three-level sliding lengthening. It is important to avoid overlengthening. Some surgeons prefer lengthening of the aponeurosis of the gastrocnemius, leaving the soleus intact as insurance against overlengthening and a calcaneal deformity. Short leg casts should be worn for 4 to 6 weeks after heel cord lengthening with a plan to resume use of an ankle-foot orthosis thereafter. Calcaneal deformity is most commonly iatrogenic because of excessive lengthening of the gastrocnemius-soleus complex. Treatment of calcaneal deformity remains unrewarding, and prevention is still the best approach. Varus and valgus deformities rarely occur in isolation and are most commonly seen with ankle equinus. Heel varus is usually flexible initially. The tibialis posterior muscle is overactive and can be lengthened, split for posterior transfer to the peroneus brevis, or transferred anteriorly to the dorsum of the foot through the interosseous membrane. Lengthening of the posterior tibia alone is subject to recurrent deformity. If an anterior tibialis tendon transfer is done in conjunction with a posterior tibialis lengthening, a superior result can be expected. An isolated lengthening of the posterior tibialis may have a better chance of success in patients younger than age 6. Lengthening of the intermuscular portion of the posterior tibialis tendon in combination with Achilles tendon lengthening is useful in the 4- to 7-year-old age group. Early ambulation is allowed. When hindfoot varus is fixed, a calcaneal osteotomy, either a closing wedge or slide, is needed in addition to tendon surgery.

Valgus

Hindfoot valgus is common in spastic quadriplegia and diplegia. There is often equinus and there may be peroneal muscle spasticity. Again, surgery is usually delayed until after age 6, if possible. Younger children can be managed with a UCB orthosis with a medial wedge. Peroneal lengthening may be necessary to allow bracing.

Subtalar extra-articular arthrodesis for polio patients was originally introduced by Grice. The current accepted technique uses a cortical screw inserted across the subtalar joint from the talar neck into the calcaneus. Cancellous bone can be used in the sinus tarsi region to achieve an arthrodesis. Frequently the Achilles tendon must be lengthened as equinus becomes evident following realignment of the hindfoot.

Hallux valgus in cerebral palsy can be associated with pes planovalgus or equinovalgus. When there is significant symptomatic crossover of the first and second toes, an arthrodesis of the first metatarsophalangeal joint is indicated. Soft-tissue surgery will not be successful in patients with cerebral palsy.

Myelomeningocele

Almost all children with myelomeningocele will require treatment of their feet. The nonambulatory child requires adequate foot positioning to accept shoewear and to prevent pressure sores. The ambulatory child requires very accurate correction of deformity. Muscle imbalance of the foot is common because the muscles innervated by the sacral roots are abnormal. This muscle imbalance is treated by removing muscle force or by transferring tendons. Because of the decreased sensation and proprioception, Charcot joint changes and skin ulcerations are possible.

Clubfoot is the most common deformity in myelomeningocele. Treatment principles are similar to those used for idiopathic clubfoot, but a more radical operation is necessary in order to obtain sufficient correction. The timing for surgical treatment is chosen so that the child will be ready to stand weightbearing as well as ambulatory orthoses to maintain surgical correction. Contracted tendons in myelomeningocele should be resected rather than lengthened to avoid recurrence of the deformity. If the child has near-normal function, that is, at the sacral level, then the tendons are retained.

Skin coverage and recurrence of the deformity are common problems in myelomeningocele. Forefoot adductus is common and a separate procedure may be necessary when the child is 3 or 4 years old. Usually this consists of closing wedge osteotomy of the cuboid and opening wedge osteotomy of the first cuneiform. Recurrent deformity into equinovarus may be treated by talectomy.

Calcaneal Deformities

Calcaneal deformities in the patient with myelomeningocele are caused by unopposed pull of the anterior tibial, toe extensor, or peroneal muscles. The deformity is usually progressive. Resection of the offending tendons allows the foot to be braced and prevents progressive deformity. In older children, the tibialis anterior tendon can be transferred to the calcaneus with anterior soft-tissue releases. These children may also require osteotomy of the calcaneus with posterior displacement of the os tuberosity.

Valgus Deformity

Valgus deformity can occur in the subtalar joint and in the ankle. The foot should be evaluated with an AP radiograph of the ankle before any treatment is planned. A medial tibial epiphysiodesis can be done with a screw. A calcaneal fibular Achilles tendon tenodesis has been described for valgus associated with a calcaneus deformity. This procedure can lead to progressive improvement of the valgus deformity of the distal tibia. Foot deformity can be treated with a medial displacement calcaneal osteotomy, a subtalar arthrodesis, or a calcaneal neck lengthening. The calcaneal neck lengthening with bone interposition preserves subtalar motion as well as bone growth.

Cavus Deformity

Cavus deformity of the foot is usually accompanied by claw toes and is more commonly encountered in sacral level paraplegia. Children with this condition have sufficient sensation and muscle control for walking, but will frequently develop progressive deformities resulting in ulcerations under the toes and over the metatarsal heads. The cavus is progressive and associated with secondary varus. Ankle-foot orthoses are helpful but many children need surgical treatment. Plantar release, midfoot osteotomies, and calcaneal osteotomies with lateral and backward displacement of the os tuberosity as well as muscle balancing procedures are used for this foot deformity. Muscle imbalance of the toes can be treated with the Jones procedure and transfer of the long extensor tendon to the metatarsal necks with fusion of the interphalangeal joints. This transfer will help elevate the metatarsal heads and prevent recurrent cavus.

Trauma and Infection

Distal Tibial Physeal Injuries

The distal tibial physis is more likely than ankle ligaments to fail with trauma. A variety of mechanisms, including twisting, falls, and direct blows, can cause these injuries, and plain films will confirm the diagnosis in the majority of cases. The Salter-Harris classification is more useful for pediatric patients than mechanistic classification systems. Intra-articular fractures are Salter-Harris types III and IV. Most fractures involve the medial malleolus. If plain films demonstrate gaps of less than 2 mm in the intra-articular surface, these fractures may be immobilized in a cast and followed closely. If the fracture displacement is more than 2 mm or cannot be determined, computed tomography (CT) scanning will be helpful. Indications for open reduction and internal fixation include a gap in the joint surface that is greater than 2 mm, a step-off of the joint surface that is greater than 1 mm, or any misalignment of the physis if significant growth is remaining.

Transitional Fractures

Transitional fractures of the ankle are most often seen in adolescents and occur during the period of transition from fully open distal tibial physis to the closed physis of the adult. The transitional fractures include the juvenile Tillaux and the triplane fractures. These fractures occur when the ankle is forced into external rotation. The distal tibial physeal closure starts peripherally at the anteromedial aspect of the medial malleolus. The anterolateral quadrant of the physis is the last to close, making it most susceptible to separation. It is avulsed by the pull of the anterior tibial fibular ligament as the foot is twist-

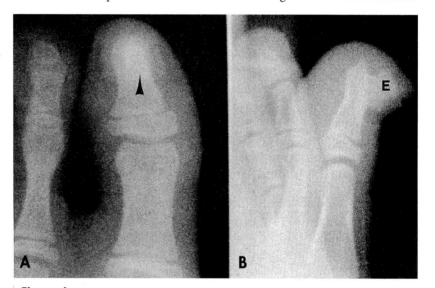

Figure 4

The subungual exostosis clinically mimics ingrown toenail, but does not respond to simple removal of a nail segment. **A,** Only a vague increase in bony density (arrowhead) may be noted on a frontal view, whereas the lateral view **B,** definitively shows the exostosis (E). (Reproduced with permission from Oestreich AE, Crawford AH: *Atlas of Pediatric Radiology*. Stuttgart, Germany, Thieme, 1985.)

ed into external rotation. When this fragment alone is pulled away, a juvenile Tillaux fracture results. The triplane fracture also occurs with external rotation. The fracture line extends into the metaphysis, may involve the physis, and may cross into the epiphysis. There are variable fracture patterns that

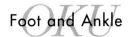

may consist of 2, 3, or 4 parts. In the type I triplane fracture, the metaphyseal fracture line extends down to the physis but does not extend across it. In the type II triplane fracture, the metaphyseal fracture line extends across the physis into the epiphysis and joint. Type II fractures often require surgery. Triplane fractures may also occur in individuals with fully open growth plates. In this situation, the anteromedial portion of the physis is more stable and tends to resist shear. CT scans are indicated for triplane fractures if the diagnosis or extent of displacement is unclear, or surgery is contemplated but the planned exposure will not show the alignment of the physis or joint surface. Treatment may be surgical or nonsurgical, depending on the amount of displacement. Closed treatment is appropriate for fractures that can be reduced to within 2 mm of intra-articular separation.

Subungual Exostosis

A subungual exostosis is a bony lesion that protrudes from the dorsal surface of the distal phalanx, most commonly of the great toe, distorting the overlying nail. It may be misdiagnosed as pyogenic disease or even malignancy. A lateral radiograph demonstrates the osseous portion of the tumor (Fig. 4). The treatment of choice consists of total excision of the lesion in order to prevent recurrence. Adequate exposure requires removal of the overlying nail and longitudinal division of the underlying nail bed. The germinal matrix is preserved so that the nail will grow postoperatively. In excising the exostosis, the soft tissue overlying the exostosis must be removed in order to prevent recurrence. It is difficult to distinguish the nail bed from this overlying soft tissue.

Annotated Bibliography

Clubfoot

Cooper DM, Dietz FR: Treatment of idiopathic clubfoot: A thirty-year follow-up note. *J Bone Joint Surg* 1995;77A:1477–1489.

In patients with idiopathic clubfoot, a sedentary occupation and avoidance of excessive weight gain improves long-term results. Outcome could not be predicted from radiographic results. Excessive weakening of the triceps surae led to poor results.

Downey DJ, Drennan JC, Garcia JF: Magnetic resonance image findings in congenital talipes equinovarus. *J Pediatr Orthop* 1992;12:224–228.

Magnetic resonance imaging scan showed medial angulation of the talar neck and rotation of the calcaneus with the posterior calcaneus forced laterally.

McHale KA, Lenhart MK: Treatment of residual clubfoot deformity: The "bean shaped" foot. By opening wedge medial cuneiform osteotomy and closing wedge cuboid osteotomy: Clinical review and cadaver correlations. *J Pediatr Orthop* 1991;11:374–381.

This procedure improved both forefoot adduction and midfoot supination in older children whose medial cuneiform was ossified.

Ponseti IV: Treatment of congenital club foot. *J Bone Joint Surg* 1992;74A:448–454.

This review reports on a conservative method of treating clubfoot consisting of manipulation and serial casting. Percutaneous Achilles tenotomies were performed during initial casting in 70% of patients. Fifty percent of the patients had a recurrence, requiring repeat casting and often an anterior tibialis tendon transfer. Eighty-nine percent of clubfoot cases could be treated by this method.

Simons GW: Complete subtalar release in club feet: Part I. A preliminary report. *J Bone Joint Surg* 1985;67A:1044–1055.

Simons GW: Complete subtalar release in club feet: Part II. Comparison with less extensive procedures. *J Bone Joint Surg* 1985;67A:1056–1065.

The author describes his techniques for circumferential soft-tissue release of congenital clubfoot and compares this more comprehensive release of the subtalar joint with more limited soft-tissue surgery. The more extensive procedure had better clinical and radiographic results.

Sodre H, Bruschini S, Mestriner LA, et al: Arterial abnormalities in talipes equinovarus as assessed by angiography and the Doppler technique. *J Pediatr Orthop* 1990;10:101–104.

Preoperative angiograms of 30 clubfeet showed that in 28, the posterior tibial artery was the sole blood supply. Doppler studies done postoperatively were not reliable in showing the same findings as the arteriogram.

Thometz JG, Simons GW: Deformity of the calcaneocuboid joint in patients who have talipes equinovarus. *J Bone Joint Surg* 1993;75A:190–195.

In a study of 100 cases of clubfoot, 25% had significant calcaneocuboid joint deformity after surgery. Failure to treat this deformed joint caused residual deformity.

Metatarsus Adductus

Berg EE: A reappraisal of metatarsus adductus and skewfoot. *J Bone Joint Surg* 1986;68A:1185–1196.

This study of 84 patients with 124 involved feet establishes a radiographic classification of metatarsus adduction and skewfoot. All feet classified as simple metatarsus adductus resolved whether treated or not. Feet with more complex deformities required longer periods of casting to achieve correction. The use of the Denis Browne bar to hold the foot in external rotation predisposed patients to a flatfoot deformity.

Farsetti P, Weinstein SL, Ponseti IV: The long-term functional and radiographic outcomes of untreated and non-operatively treated metatarsus adductus. *J Bone Joint Surg* 1994;76A:257–265.

Metatarsus adductus that is passively correctable resolved without treatment. Patients with mild to moderate residual deformity were functional and had pain only after strenuous activities. Surgery is not necessary.

Mosca VS: Calcaneal lengthening for valgus deformity of the hindfoot: Results in children who had severe, symptomatic flatfoot and skewfoot. *J Bone Joint Surg* 1995;77A:500–512.

Severe symptomatic valgus hindfoot deformity can be successfully treated with calcaneal lengthening osteotomy.

Pentz AS, Weiner DS: Management of metatarsus adductovarus. *Foot Ankle* 1993;14:241–246.

In this retrospective review of 795 patients, the incidence of foot deformity was not related to birth weight or birth order. The combination of reverse last shoes and a Denis Browne bar was associated with a 99% incidence of excellent or good results.

Toe Deformities

Hamer AJ, Stanley D, Smith TW: Surgery for curly toe deformity: A double-blind, randomised, prospective trial. *J Bone Joint Surg* 1993;75B:662–663.

The results of flexor tenotomy were compared to those of flexor to extensor transfer in 23 pairs of toes at 4-year follow-up. There was no difference at follow-up, indicating that flexor release was the important part of the surgery and transfer of the flexor to extensor was unnecessary.

Flatfeet

Staheli LT, Chew DE, Corbett M: The longitudinal arch: A survey of eight hundred and eighty-two feet in normal children and adults. *J Bone Joint Surg* 1987;69A:426–428.

Footprints of 441 subjects ranging from age 1 to 80 years were studied. There was a wide normal range of arch height at all ages; low arches are the norm in infants, common in children, and within the normal range in adults. Spontaneous elevation of the arch occurs during the first decade of life.

Wenger DR, Mauldin D, Speck G, Morgan D, Lieber RL: Corrective shoes and inserts as treatment for flexible flatfoot in infants and children. *J Bone Joint Surg* 1989;71A:800–810.

In this prospective controlled clinical and radiographic study, the influence of shoes and orthoses on the development of the longitudinal arch in children was examined. The children were enrolled between 1 and 6 years of age and divided into 3 study groups and 1 control group. At the end of the 3-year study, the height of the arch improved in all groups, including the controls, and there was no significant difference between controls and treated groups.

Tarsal Coalition

Gonzalez P, Kumar SJ: Calcaneonavicular coalition treated by resection and interposition of the extensor digitorum brevis muscle. *J Bone Joint Surg* 1990;72A:71–77.

Seventy-seven percent of 75 feet rated good or excellent results at final follow-up. Talar beaking was not a contraindication to surgery. Best results were seen in patients between 11 and 15 years old at the time of surgery.

Kumar SJ, Guille JT, Lee MS, Couto JC: Osseous and non-osseous coalition of the middle facet of the talocalcaneal joint. *J Bone Joint Surg* 1992;74A:529–535.

In 18 feet treated with resection of the coalition, 16 had excellent or good results.

McCormack TJ, Olney B, Asher M: Talocalcaneal coalition resection: A 10-year follow-up. *J Pediatr Orthop* 1997;17:13–15.

Eight of 9 cases of talocalcaneal coalition resection had a satisfactory result at 10-year follow-up regardless of percent of middle facet involvement.

Painful Problems

Laliotis N, Pennie BH, Carty H, Klenerman L: Toddler's fracture of the calcaneum. *Injury* 1993;24:169–170.

Five of these 7 cases were only diagnosed after scintigraphy. In none was there a history of trauma. The possible presence of this fracture should be considered in limping pre-schoolers.

Schindler A, Mason DE, Allington NJ: Occult fracture of the calcaneus in toddlers. *J Pediatr Orthop* 1996;16:201–205.

Calcaneus fracture can be a cause of limping in toddlers.

Toe Walking

Griffin PP, Wheelhouse WW, Shiavi R, Bass W: Habitual toe-walkers: A clinical and electromyographic gait analysis. *J Bone Joint Surg* 1977;59A:97–101.

Six habitual toe walkers who could walk heel to toe were treated with serial casts. No patient required Achilles tendon lengthening and all patients responded to serial casting. Posttreatment electromyograms demonstrated a return of normal tibialis anterior function.

Katz MM, Mubarak SJ: Hereditary tendon Achilles contractures. *J Pediatr Orthop* 1984;4:711–714.

Eight patients who walked with a toe/toe pattern were treated with serial casting. Toe walking occasionally recurred but Achilles tendon lengthening was not found to be necessary.

Bunions

Groiso JA: Juvenile hallux valgus: A conservative approach to treatment. *J Bone Joint Surg* 1992;74A:1367–1374.

In this study, 56 children with hallux valgus were treated with corrective splinting. Improvement was obtained in 50% and maintained at 2- to 6-year follow-up.

Cerebral Palsy

Barnes MJ, Herring JA: Combined split anterior tibial-tendon transfer and intramuscular lengthening of the posterior tibial tendon: Results in patients who have a varus deformity of the foot due to spastic cerebral palsy. *J Bone Joint Surg* 1991;73A: 734–738.

Combined split anterior tibial tendon transfer and intramuscular lengthening of the posterior tibial tendon, with and without concomitant lengthening of the Achilles tendon, corrected flexible varus in 20 patients with spastic cerebral palsy patients followed for 6 years. Fixed varus or weakness of the anterior tibialis led to the 4 poor results.

Caterini R, Farsetti P, Ippolito E: Long-term followup of physeal injury to the ankle. *Foot Ankle* 1991;11:372–383.

Sixty-eight children with physeal fractures of the distal tibia and fibula were followed for an average of 27 years. All but 6 had been treated conservatively. Sixty of 68 had a satisfactory result. The type of Salter-Harris lesion, the amount of initial displacement, and the quality of reduction were the main factors that affected the end result.

Koman LA, Mooney JF III, Goodman A: Management of valgus hindfoot deformity in pediatric cerebral palsy patients by medial displacement osteotomy. *J Pediatr Orthop* 1993;13:180–183.

Medial displacement osteotomy of the calcaneus gave excellent correction of valgus in 17 of 18 feet followed for an average of 42 months. The distal fragment was displaced 50% or more.

Koman LA, Mooney JF III, Smith BP, Goodman A, Mulvaney T: Management of spasticity in cerebral palsy with botulinum: A toxin. Report of a preliminary, randomized, double-blind trial. *J Pediatr Orthop* 1994;14:299–303.

In order to evaluate local intramuscular injections of botulism toxin in the management of dynamic equinus deformities associated with cerebral palsy, a randomized, double-blind placebo controlled study was done. Five of 6 patients receiving toxin showed improvement versus 2 of 6 receiving placebo. The single patient who did not show improvement in gait had a fixed contracture of the gastrocnemius-soleus complex.

von Laer L: Classification, diagnosis, and treatment of transitional fractures of the distal part of the tibia. *J Bone Joint Surg* 1985;67A:687–698.

Intra-articular fractures with more than a 2-mm gap require open reduction.

Lawnmower Injuries

Dormans JP, Azzoni M, Davidson RS, Drummond DS: Major lower extremity lawn mower injuries in children. *J Pediatr Orthop* 1995;15:78–82.

Two types of lawnmower injuries, a shredding-type injury and a paucilaceration, were identified; the former was seen most often. All patients with a shredding-type injury either ultimately required amputations or had poor results with limb salvage.

Classic Bibliography

Alman BA, Craig CL, Zimbler S: Subtalar arthrodesis for stabilization of valgus hindfoot in patients with cerebral palsy. *J Pediatr Orthop* 1993;13:634–641.

Brage ME, Hansen ST Jr: Traumatic subluxation/dislocation of the peroneal tendons. *Foot Ankle* 1992;13:423–431.

Cowell HR, Wein BK: Genetic aspects of club foot. *J Bone Joint Surg* 1980;62A:1381–1384.

Hensinger RN, Beaty JH (eds): *Operative Management of Lower Extremity Fractures in Children*. Park Ridge, IL, American Academy of Orthopaedic Surgeons, 1992.

Hoffer MM, Barakat G, Koffman M: 10-year follow-up of split anterior tibial tendon transfer in cerebral palsied patients with spastic equinovarus deformity. *J Pediatr Orthop* 1985;5: 432–434.

Howard CB, Benson MK: Clubfoot: Its pathological anatomy. *J Pediatr Orthop* 1993;13:654–659.

Ippolito E, Ricciardi Pollini PT, Falez F: Kohler's disease of the tarsal navicular: Long-term follow-up of 12 cases. *J Pediatr Orthop* 1984;4:416–417.

Laaveg SJ, Ponseti IV: Long-term results of treatment of congenital club foot. *J Bone Joint Surg* 1980;62A:23–31.

Lee EH, Goh JC, Bose K: Value of gait analysis in the assessment of surgery in cerebral palsy. *Arch Phys Med Rehabil* 1992;73:642–646.

McKay DW: New concept of and approach to clubfoot treatment: Section I. Principles and morbid anatomy. *J Pediatr Orthop* 1982;2:347–356.

78 Pediatric Foot

McKay DW: New concept of and approach to clubfoot treatment: Section II. Correction of the clubfoot. *J Pediatr Orthop* 1983;3:10–21.

McKay DW: New concept of and approach to clubfoot treatment: Section III. Evaluation and results. *J Pediatr Orthop* 1983;3:141–148.

McKay DW: Dorsal bunions in children. *J Bone Joint Surg* 1983;65A:975–980.

Peterson HA: Skewfoot (forefoot adduction with heel valgus). *J Pediatr Orthop* 1986;6:24–30.

Peterson HA, Newman SR: Adolescent bunion deformity treated with double osteotomy and longitudinal pin fixation of the first ray. *J Pediatr Orthop* 1993;13:80–84.

Phelps DA, Grogan DP: Polydactyly of the foot. *J Pediatr Orthop* 1985;5:446–451.

Roper BA, Tibrewal SB: Soft tissue surgery in Charcot-Marie-Tooth disease. *J Bone Joint Surg* 1989;71B:17–20.

Saji MJ, Upadhyay SS, Hsu LC, Leong JC: Split tibialis posterior transfer for equinovarus deformity in cerebral palsy: Long-term results of a new surgical procedure. *J Bone Joint Surg* 1993;75B:498–501.

Schlesinger I, Wedge JH: Percutaneous reduction and fixation of displaced juvenile Tillaux fractures: A new surgical technique. *J Pediatr Orthop* 1993;13:389–391.

Seimon LP: Surgical correction of congenital vertical talus under the age of 2 years. *J Pediatr Orthop* 1987;7:405–411.

Walker AP, Ghali NN, Silk FF: Congenital vertical talus: The results of staged operative reduction. *J Bone Joint Surg* 1985;67B:117–121.

Wetmore RS, Drennan JC: Long-term results of triple arthrodesis in Charcot-Marie-Tooth disease. *J Bone Joint Surg* 1989;71A:417–422.

Yadav SS, Thomas S: Congenital posteromedial bowing of the tibia. *Acta Orthop Scand* 1980;51:311–313.

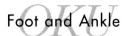

Chapter 7
Neuromuscular Disease

Introduction

Neuromuscular disease, broadly defined, includes all processes that affect the nerves and/or muscles. A more restrictive definition includes only those disease processes that are of a lower motor neuron variety, beginning at the anterior horn cell and extending distally to include the muscle itself. Depending on the specific disease, there may or may not be sensory involvement. Tone may be normal, decreased, or increased.

Although this chapter will focus on management issues related specifically to the foot and ankle, it must be remembered that the focal manifestations of neuromuscular disease are typically the result of a systemic process. Management decisions, therefore, are based on treating the "whole patient." Several issues must be considered related to the disease process itself. Does the disease affect the patient's life span? Is the process limited to the neuromuscular system, or are other organ systems involved? Is the process static, slowly progressive, or rapidly progressive? Will the projected recovery time be altered by the patient's overall health status? Will the patient's postoperative rehabilitation course be altered by the disease itself or by the patient's cardiovascular status? Does the patient have upper extremity involvement that will preclude significant loading of the upper body during the course of rehabilitation? These and other questions need to be considered as one develops an appropriate management scheme. Therefore, discussions related to management of foot and ankle problems resulting from neuromuscular disease must begin with an overview of the various diseases.

Neuromuscular pathology in the foot and ankle, particularly when traumatic and central nervous system origins are included, covers a wide spectrum. Although the focal pathology in the foot may be very similar in a traumatic peripheral nerve injury and anterior horn cell disease, management is very different. Problems related to upper motor neuron pathology require specific attention to spasticity management. Patients with associated sensory involvement are at high risk for tissue breakdown, especially with orthotic inter-

vention. In order to approach the patient from a functional perspective, one must first consider whether or not the patient has upper motor or lower motor neuron problems, and then consider the specific tissue level of involvement, eg, primary muscle disease, peripheral neuropathy, etc. (Table 1).

Upper Motor Neuron Pathology

Patients with upper motor neuron involvement, by definition, have pathology proximal to the anterior horn cell. This results in disinhibition of the motor neurons with secondary increased tone, including spasticity. Depending on the specific level of etiology, patients may additionally have associated sensory loss or even cognitive problems. There is relatively good preservation of the soft tissues as the neurotropic response from the anterior horn cell has been preserved, thus precluding denervation loss of the muscle cells.

Lower Motor Neuron Pathology

Lower motor neuron disease begins at the anterior horn cell and extends distally to include the peripheral nerve, neuromuscular junction, and myofibril. Although some diseases, such as amyotrophic lateral sclerosis, may show mixed upper and lower motor neuron findings, most are characterized by normal to low tone and an absence of upper motor neuron clinical signs. Inasmuch as the nerve supply to the muscle has been interrupted, there will be significant muscle wasting and associated soft-tissue loss, putting the patient at risk for soft-tissue breakdown, particularly at bony prominences. Frequently, the patients have an associated sensory loss, further increasing the risk of skin breakdown as well as adding proprioceptive problems. However, with lower motor neuron etiologies, the physical examination is more straightforward, because these patients do not have spasticity or other central nervous system problems.

Having ruled out central nervous system involvement, it is necessary to consider multiple peripheral etiologies. To simplify the relationship between the history and physical examination and various etiologies, it is perhaps simplest to begin with the most peripheral tissue, the muscle, and then to progress proximally.

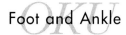
Table 1
Common Neuromuscular Pathologies

	Onset	Prog	Life Span	Mtr	Sns	Sym	Prox	Dist	Hered	UMN	Other Signs	Diagnostic Tests	Treatment
MYOPATHIES													
Muscular Dystrophies													
Dystrophy Duchenne	1-5 yrs	+++	20s	+++	0	+++	+++	+	SLR	0	MR, cardiac	SCK, EMG, Ch X, biopsy degen/regen, fibrosis, bands	Symptomatic, physical rehab, prednisone
Dystrophy Becker	Teens	++	40s	+++	0	+++	+++	+	SLR	0	No MR/ ↓ cardiac	SCK, EMG, Ch X, biopsy degen/regen, fibrosis, bands	Symptomatic, physical rehab, prednisone
Myotonia Congenital (Thompsen Dz)	Birth	+++	Birth to adult	+++	0	+++	++	+++	AD	++	Neonatal hypotonia, early death. If survivers, see below.	Myotonia in parent, amniotic (CTG repeats)	Symp: Quinine, testosterone, calcium blockers
Myotonia Early Childhood	5-10 yrs	++	Adult	++	0	+++	++	+++	AD	++	Endocrine, frontal balding, MR, cardiac	EMG, Ch 19, biopsy, CTG repeats	Symp: Quinine, testosterone, calcium blockers
Myotonia Dystrophy Juv/Adult (Steinert dz)	Teen-Adult	+	Adult	++	0	+++	++	+++	AD	++	Endocrine, frontal balding, MR, cardiac	EMG, Ch 19, Biopsy, CTG repeats	Symp: Quinine testosterone, calcium blockers
Inflammatory													
Polymyositis immune glob, plasma	Teen-Adult	++	50% Remis 15% death	+++	0	+++	+++	++	0	0	Derm precedes myositis, subQ calc., CTD, cancer	EMG, SCK, ESR CTD specific tests Biopsy. Inflam necrosis, phag, fibrosis, perifascic degen	NSAIDs, steroids, mmunosuppress, ie, immune glob, plasma exchange
Dermatomyositis	Child-Adult	++	50% Remis 15% death	+++	0	+++	+++	++	0	0	Derm precedes myositis, subQ calc., CTD, cancer	EMG, SCK, ESR CTD specific tests Biopsy. Inflam necrosis, phag, fibrosis, perifascic degen	NSAIDs, steroids, immunosuppress, ie, immune glob, plasma exchange
NMJ													
Myasthenic gravis	F>20 M>50	+++	Var	+++	0	++	+++	++	0	0	Ptosis, diplopia, dysphagia, thymoma	EMG, Tensilon test ACH receptor antibody, TFTs	Thymectomy, neostigmine, prednisone, immunosup, plasma exchange, immune glob
Myasthenic Syndrome (Lambert-Eaton)	Adult	++	Adult	++	0	++	+++	++	0	0	Cancer (2-3s)	EMG, Tensilon test ACH receptor antibody, TFTs	ACH Inh, guanidine, immunosup
Postpolio Syndrome	20 yr PD	+	NML	+	0	0	Var	Var	0	0	Pain, fatigue	Hx of polio, EMG	Symptomatic, activity limitations

Table 1 (Continued)
Common Neuromuscular Pathologies

	Onset	Prog	Life Span	Mtr	Sns	Sym	Prox	Dist	Hered	UMN	Other Signs	Diagnostic Tests	Treatment
Botulism	Var	Depends on acute phase treatment		+++	0	++	++	++	0	0	Nausea, ileus, resp, dysphagia, diplopia	EMG, Toxin	Antitoxin, guanidine, supportive
Organophosphates (insecticides, nerve gas)	Var	Depends on acute phase treatment		+++	+	+++	+++	++	0	0	Cranial neuropathy, GI, resp failure	EMG	Atropine, supportive
Meds: "Mycins," Curare	Var	Depends on acute phase treatment		++	0	+++	+++	++	0	0	Bulbar, resp failure	EMG	DC drug, symptomatic anti-cholinesterases, calcium

PERIPHERAL NERVE

Acquired Traumatic

	Onset	Prog	Life Span	Mtr	Sns	Sym	Prox	Dist	Hered	UMN	Other Signs	Diagnostic Tests	Treatment
Direct Trauma	Var	Var	Var	++	++	Var	Var	Var	0	0	Fractures, dys-esthesias, RSD	EMG	Symptomatic, seizure meds, antidepressants, surgery
Iatrogenic: Post-operative, injection	Var	Var	Var	++	++	Var	Var	Var	0	0	Dysesthesias, RSD	EMG, GTT	Insulin, symptomatic, (pain meds, antidepres, seizure meds)

Acquired Nontrauma

	Onset	Prog	Life Span	Mtr	Sns	Sym	Prox	Dist	Hered	UMN	Other Signs	Diagnostic Tests	Treatment
Diabetes Mellitus	10 yr PD	+	Var	++	+++	Var	+	+++	MF	0	↑Glu, 3 Ps, PVD vision, dysesthesias	EMG, Glucose	Oral agents, insulin, symptomatic, organ system specific
Vitamin def (B1, B6, B12)	Var	++	Var	++	++	++	+	+++	0	+	Paresthesias, pain tend. Ataxia, mental, anemia	EMG, serum vitamin levels	Vitamin replacement, symptomatic
Heavy metal (lead, arsenic)	Child-Adult	++	Var	+++	+	++	++	+++	0	0	GI, ataxia, anemia, encephalopathy	X-ray: Lead lines. RBC: Stip. Urine: UCP and ALA, Serum: Lead. Hair: Arsenic	Chelation: BAL, EDTA Hydration, DC exposure
SLE	Teens-30s	+	Var	++	++	++	+	++	MF	0	Rash, arthritis, myositis, nephritis, PUD, cardiac, cns	ANA, LE prep, EMG, biopsy	NSAIDs immunosuppressants symptomatic

Hereditary (HMSN)

	Onset	Prog	Life Span	Mtr	Sns	Sym	Prox	Dist	Hered	UMN	Other Signs	Diagnostic Tests	Treatment
CMT I	Teens-Adult	++	NML	++	++	+++	+	+++	AD Ch 17	0	Pes cavus, claw toes	Family hx, EMG, Ch, biopsy	Symptomatic
CMT II	Teens-Adult	++	NML	++	++	+++	+	+++	AD Var	0	Pes cavus, claw toes	Family hx, EMG, Ch, biopsy	Symptomatic
Dejerine-Sottas III	Infant	+	Var	+++	++	+++	++	+++	AD/AR Var	0	Delayed motor milestones	Family hx, EMG Ch, biopsy	Symptomatic

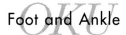
Table 1 (Continued)
Common Neuromuscular Pathologies

	Onset	Prog	Life Span	Mtr	Sns	Sym	Prox	Dist	Hered	UMN	Other Signs	Diagnostic Tests	Treatment
IV - VII	Var	++	Var	++	++	++	++	+++	AD/AR Var	++	CNS-hearing, vision, MR, ataxia cardiac	Family hx, EMG, Ch, biopsy	Symptomatic
INTRASPINAL													
Anterior Horn Cell													
Werdnig-Hoffmann	Birth	++++	< 2 yrs					+++	AR Ch 5	0	Fasciculations, hypotonia	EMG, Biopsy, Ch 5	Supportive, symptomatic
SMA I				+++	0	+++	+++		AR Ch 5	0	Fasciculations, hypotonia	EMG, biopsy, Ch 5	Supportive, symptomatic
SMA II	18 mo.	+++	> 2 yrs					++	AR Ch 5	0	Fasciculations, hypotonia	EMG, biopsy, Ch 5	Supportive, symptomatic
Kugelberg-Welander SMA III	Child	++	Young adult	++	0	+++	++		AR ch 5	0	Fasciculations, hypotonia	EMG, biopsy, chrom 5	Supportive, symptomatic
Adult motor neuron disease Lou Gehrig's Disease (ALS)	Adult	+++	3-5 yrs PD	+++	0	++	++	+++	< 5%	++	Muscle cramps, fasciculations, bulbar dysfunction, resp	EMG, biopsy	Supportive, symptomatic, Riluzole: Min. ↑ survival
Poliomyelitis	Var	0	NML	+++	0	0	++	+++	0	+	Muscle pain, fever, GI sx, bulbar sx	EMG	Supportive, symptomatic,
Congenital													
Overt Meningomyelocele	Birth	0	Var	+++	+++	+	+	++	MF	++	Hydrocephali, Neurogenic B&B	MRI, EMG	Surg closure, symptomatic
Occult Tethered Cord (Traction myelopathy)	Adol	+	NML	+	+	+	+	++	MF	+	Dysesthesias, B&B incontinence	MRI, EMG	Surg decompress, symptomatic

AD = Autosomal dominant	CTG = DNA repeats	Mtr = Motor	Sens = Sensory
Ach = Acetylcholine	DC = Discontinue	NML = Normal	SCK = Serum creatnine
AR = Autosomal recessive	GTT = Gluocose tolerance test	PD = Post diagnosis	SLR = Sex-linked recessive
B&B = Bowel & bladder	Inh = Inhibitors	Prog = Progressiveness	TFT = Thyroid function test
Ch = Chromosome	MF = Multifactorial	PVD = Peripheral vascular disease	Var = Variable
CTD = Connective tissue disease	MR = Mental retardataion	RSD = Reflex sympathetic dystrophy	

Specific Diseases

Muscular Diseases

Myopathic processes include the well-known, X-linked recessive dystrophies (Duchenne and Becker) and inflammatory processes (polymyositis) as well as rare congenital muscle diseases (central core disease and nemaline myopathy) and metabolic muscle diseases (phosphorylase deficiency and acid maltase deficiency, etc). Classic Duchenne muscular dystrophy, frequently suspected due to delayed ambulation, is always evident by school age. Laboratory testing reveals at least a tenfold increase in muscle enzymes, especially serum creatinine phosphokinase (SCK). Muscle biopsy demonstrates an absence of dystrophin, an abnormal variation muscle cell size, and an increase in connective and fat tissue. The inheritance pattern is X-linked recessive, and DNA studies reveal a Duchenne-type mutation within the dystrophin gene. Even with the best of management, these patients require assisted devices by the age of 13 years. They typically lose their ambulation abilities by their late teens and rarely survive beyond their twenties.

A less severe form, Becker muscular dystrophy, has a later onset and progresses more slowly. There is a greater than five-fold increase in SCK, and muscle biopsy shows changes that are similar (although they are less severe) to those seen in Duchenne muscular dystrophy. Patients typically do not become wheelchair dependent until after their teens, and they frequently survive into their fifth and sixth decade.

Muscular dystrophies are characterized by low tone and can usually be managed conservatively. However, in order to lengthen the time of ambulation, these patients occasionally require heel-cord lengthening and other limited surgical procedures. The dystrophies are characterized by low tone, calf hypertrophy, and proximal weakness. The inheritance pattern varies from X-linked recessive (Duchenne and Becker) to autosomal dominant (myotonic). Carrier detection and prenatal diagnosis are accomplished through DNA studies using polymorphic markers. In spite of the limiting anatomic name (muscular dystrophy), these patients frequently have "nonmuscular" problems, including endocrine abnormalities (particularly myotonic), cardiomyopathy, and mental retardation. Additional muscular dystrophies include Emery-Dreyfus muscular dystrophy (EMD), facioscapulohumeral muscular dystrophy, and limb-girdle muscular dystrophy.

Myotonic dystrophy has 3 clinical varieties, depending on the age of onset. The congenital form can be a cause of stillbirth or severe neonatal weakness. Early childhood types begin between the ages of 5 and 10 years and are characterized by myotonia, mental retardation, and generalized weakness. Juvenile/adult form (classical) demonstrates myotonia and weakness of the ocular, pharyngeal, and distal limb muscles. Minimal myotonic dystrophy typically occurs after age 50, with symptoms similar (though milder) to those of the classical disease. The most common inheritance pattern of the various forms of myotonic dystrophy is autosomal dominant.

Inflammatory myopathies are similar to dystrophies in their clinical presentation. Patients have normal to low tone, an absence of upper motor neuron findings, and a symmetrical pattern of weakness that tends to be more pronounced proximally. Patients with inflammatory myopathies often have muscle soreness and tenderness as well as markedly elevated muscle enzymes. There is frequently multisystem involvement, and inflammatory myopathies are believed to be related to connective tissue diseases. Associated disorders include interstitial lung disease, cardiomyopathies with arrhythmias, esophageal dysmotility, and various autoimmune syndromes. The muscle biopsy is characterized by necrosis and phagocytosis of muscle cells, with areas of regeneration and increased connective tissue. Patients with dermatomyositis have an incidence of associated cancer (lung, gynecologic, prostate, and gastrointestinal), which ranges anywhere from 5% to 50%, the greatest incidence occurring in older males. Management of inflammatory myopathies is typically nonsurgical, including the use of pharmacologic agents (prednisone and immunosuppressants) and physical therapy modalities. Myopathic problems can additionally be seen with endocrine abnormalities (particularly thyroid disease), prolonged steroid use, and exposure to ethanol and other toxins.

Neuromuscular Junction Diseases

Before considering peripheral neuropathic processes, one should consider disease processes of the neuromuscular junction. Classically, one initially considers myasthenia gravis or myasthenic syndrome, which affect the neuromuscular junction postsynaptically and presynaptically. Diagnosis of myasthenia gravis is based on a positive Tensilon test and the presence of serum antibodies. Pharmacologic treatment includes anticholinesterase inhibitors and immunosuppressants. Familial neuromuscular junction syndromes exist, but these are relatively rare.

Toxins, including botulinum, nerve gas, and insecticide, affect the neuromuscular junction directly as well. Therapeutic use of botulinum will be discussed later related to the management of spasticity. Interestingly, although poliomyelitis is a disease of the anterior horn cell, postpolio syndrome is believed to be a result of inadequate transmission at the neuromuscular junction itself. Patients with postpolio syndrome who have direct involvement of the foot and ankle are managed similarly to patients with a peripheral neuropathic process, but they do not have an associated sensory loss.

Peripheral Nerve Diseases

Processes directly affecting the peripheral nerve are the major subject of this chapter. Although we will focus specifically on the management of patients with Charcot-Marie-Tooth disease, these management principles can be applied to neuropathic processes from multiple etiologies. Peripheral nerve problems can be focal or systemic, demyelinating or axonal. They can result from multiple inherited or acquired etiologies, including traumatic, metabolic, vascular, and inflammatory processes. Although neuropathies can selectively affect motor, sensory, or autonomic fibers, they more typically affect all peripheral nerves (mixed pattern).

Acquired traumatic peripheral nerve problems that affect the foot are seen in combination with other injuries. For example, patients with acquired brain injuries frequently have extremity fractures and associated peripheral nerve involvement. Proximal incomplete sciatic nerve injuries have significant peripheral manifestations, usually involving the peroneal more than the tibial portion of the nerve. Occasionally, foot and ankle neuropathic manifestations are iatrogenic, including injection neuropathies and postoperative peroneal palsy. Pharmacologic iatrogenic problems (eg, isoniazid [INH] therapy) tend to be self-limited and therefore do not require definitive intervention. Less common traumatic etiologies include compartment syndromes and burns.

Acquired nontraumatic etiologies include metabolic diseases, such as diabetes mellitus and vitamin deficiencies, toxic neuropathies, and inflammatory neuropathies (eg, Guillain-Barré syndrome). These diseases may have demyelinating or axonal components, and frequently have both. Clinical manifestations include weakness, atrophy, and sensory loss. Diabetes mellitus, by far the most common etiology, typically involves all extremities, with the distal lower extremities being involved first. However, although diabetes is a systemic disease, one may occasionally see isolated severe involvement of only a few nerves with relative sparing of other nerves (eg, mononeuropathy multiplex).

Immune polyneuropathies can occur in isolation, eg, Guillain-Barré syndrome, or in combination with known collagen-vascular disease. Pathology can be predominantly demyelinating with secondary axonal involvement (Guillain-Barré syndrome) or mainly axonal (chronic immune polyneuropathies). Associated diseases include rheumatoid arthritis, systemic lupus erythematosus, polyarteritis nodosa, and amyloidosis. Diagnosis, often made based on clinical presentation and electrodiagnosis, frequently requires biopsy of nerve and muscle, particularly for chronic forms. Pharmacologic treatment depends on the specific etiology, but typically includes nonsteroidal anti-inflammatory drugs, prednisone,

and other immunosuppressants. Some patients benefit from plasma exchange.

Charcot-Marie-Tooth disease is an example of a hereditary motor sensory neuropathy (HMSN). HMSN I is hypertrophic and demyelinating, resulting in significantly slowed nerve conduction velocity. HMSN II is predominately axonal with only minimal slowing of nerve conduction velocities, but with significant reduction of evoked potential amplitudes. Clinical manifestations and management of Charcot-Marie-Tooth disease are discussed later in the chapter. HMSN III (Dejerine-Sottas) is an inherited (both dominant and recessive) severe demyelinating nonprogressive neuropathic disease that manifests itself in infancy. Weakness is diffuse and more pronounced distally. Motor milestones are delayed. Four other relatively rare HMSN diseases (HMSN IV to VII) are characterized by varying degrees of central nervous system involvement, including visual and hearing impairment and cognitive deficits.

Some hereditary neuropathies, called hereditary sensory autonomic neuropathies (HSAN), spare the motor neurons and affect only the sensory and autonomic fibers (HSAN I to V). More well known are the hereditary sensory neuropathies that have additional associated pathology. These include Friedreich's ataxia, ataxia telangiectasia, Tangier's disease, and Fabry's disease. In addition to dysesthesias related to sensory neuropathy, these rare familial diseases are characterized by ataxia, long tract signs, cardiovascular disease, and visceral involvement.

Intraspinal Diseases

There are multiple intraspinal sources of neuromuscular pathology. These can be at the cellular level (eg, anterior horn cell diseases), in the intraspinal peripheral nerves (eg, cauda equina syndrome), and in the spinal cord itself. Etiologies include hereditary, mechanical, metabolic, toxic, inflammatory (infectious and noninfectious), neoplastic, and vascular. Depending on the level of involvement, clinical manifestations may be upper motor neuron, lower motor neuron, or a mixed neurologic pattern.

Various disease processes involve the anterior horn cell directly. Some, like spinal muscular atrophy (SMA) type I (Werdnig-Hoffman) and SMA type II, manifest themselves in infancy and in early childhood and result in early death. SMA type III (Kugelberg-Welander) occurs much later in childhood and progresses more slowly, as patients become wheelchair dependent by the fourth decade but have near normal life spans. SMA type IV (adult onset) manifests itself in the third to fifth decades. The disease is slowly progressive and life span is unaffected. Diagnosis, based on clinical presentation, is confirmed by neuropathic elec-

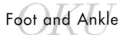
tromyography (EMG) and biopsy. Treatment for SMA is symptomatic.

Adult motor neuron disease has a variety of clinical presentations, inheritance patterns, and ages of onset. The most common and well-known form, amyotrophic lateral sclerosis (Lou Gehrig's disease), is a nonfamilial disease of middle age to later years. Distal extremity weakness, particularly in the hands, is a frequent presenting complaint. The weakness progresses proximally, and patients eventually demonstrate bulbar (cranial nerve) involvement. Muscle fasciculations and atrophy are primary signs. Patients have upper motor neuron findings, including hyperreflexia and other corticospinal abnormalities. Only 5% of the cases are familial. Diagnosis is based on clinical presentation and electrodiagnosis, and biopsy confirms a neuropathic process. Treatment is mainly supportive, although multiple pharmacologic interventions have been attempted. Death in amyotrophic lateral sclerosis typically occurs 3 to 5 years following diagnosis.

Poliomyelitis, a more patchy and nonprogressive form of anterior horn cell disease, presents a special challenge. In addition to the residual weakness, atrophy, and contractures from the original polio, patients frequently present with postpolio syndrome. As stated above, postpolio syndrome is believed to result from the drop out of individual myofibrils secondary to failure at the neuromuscular junction itself. Management of associated foot and ankle problems from remote polio is necessarily affected by superimposed symptoms of muscle pain and easy fatigability related to postpolio syndrome. Limited exercise is tolerated, and patients have minimally progressive weakness in the involved muscles (1% to 2% per year).

Congenital sources of intraspinal neuromuscular problems are varied. Typical dysraphism demonstrates itself as an obvious congenital abnormality, meningomyelocele. Occult dysraphism may appear as a tethered cord with traction myelopathy symptoms in a growing child or teenager. Residual sequelae of postoperative meningomyelocele include leg-length discrepancies, contractures, severe atrophy, sensory deficits, and neurogenic bowel and bladder. These patients frequently have "soft" central neurologic findings related to an associated hydrocephalus. Less commonly, progressive peripheral lower extremity manifestations may be the result of syringomyelia or even an occult tumor.

Common mechanical etiologies include severe arthritis with secondary spinal stenosis and disk disease. Patients with spinal stenosis can show both upper and lower motor neuron findings, including urogenital involvement. Patients with bilateral distal lower extremity sympotoms should be asked specifically about problems with bowel and bladder control.

Pure upper motor neuron spinal cord paralysis is typically the result of trauma. Less common etiologies include inflammatory processes (infectious and noninfectious), tumors (benign and malignant), and vascular events (postoperative aneurysm repair, embolic, etc). Management of foot and ankle problems in patients with significant spasticity will be discussed later.

Intracranial Disease

The most proximal etiology of any neuromuscular problems of the foot and ankle relates to intracranial pathology. The degree of involvement of the distal lower extremities relates to the location of the pathology within the brain itself. Middle cerebral artery distribution lesions tend to involve the distal extremities more severely, with some sparing proximally. By contrast, anterior cerebral lesions typically impair proximal muscle control more than distal muscle control.

By far, the most common intracranial etiology in children is cerebral palsy, with an incidence of approximately 1%. Classic cerebral palsy (spastic diplegia), typically seen in premature infants, results from paraventricular ischemia/hemorrhage. The greater the extension of pathology away from the ventricles, the more severe the lower extremity involvement, with eventual involvement of upper extremities as well.

Acquired intracranial problems include stroke, brain injury, multiple sclerosis, and tumors (malignant and nonmalignant). Specific peripheral manifestations are related to anatomic location and extent of involvement. The most common pattern seen in stroke relates to carotid/middle cerebral artery involvement, with significant lower extremity distal weakness and spasticity. Acquired brain injury, by contrast, does not follow a predictable pattern. Although virtually all brain-injured patients have increased tone, specific motor, sensory, and cognitive deficits are related to trauma-induced focal damage.

History and Physical Examination

History

Management of similar foot and ankle problems may differ based on findings in the history and physical examination. A foot and ankle surgeon is expected to develop an extended differential diagnosis. The surgeon should obtain adequate historical information to detect factors that could affect long-term rehabilitation potential. Behavioral or cognitive problems should be considered in relationship to the patient's ability and/or desire to cooperate during the recovery process. Vision, hearing, and balance problems should be defined. The patient's fitness, endurance, and lifestyle are important. If the patient has a progressive process, one has to establish the rate of progression and the degree of involvement of other organ systems. Unrelated upper extremity problems (such as carpal tunnel syndrome or unresolved rotator cuff symptoms) may be exacerbated by increasing reliance on the upper extremities during the recovery period. The patient should be questioned about associated cervical or lumbar pain or radicular symptoms. All patients should be asked about any changes in bowel or bladder control. Important psychosocial elements of the history, including such habits as smoking and alcohol and drug use, should be elicited, along with details of the social support system.

Physical Examination

General physical examinations should include a brief assessment of the central and peripheral cardiovascular function. Skin should be checked for hair loss, evidence of delayed healing, and general color and status.

A careful neurologic assessment is critical in neuromuscular disease. Deep tendon reflexes should be assessed for symmetry and for upper and lower extremity differences. Passive movement should be evaluated for increased or decreased tone and for clonus. Resistance to passive movement may be rackety (basal ganglia) or smooth (corticospinal). Sensory modalities, including pain and temperature, pressure, vibration, and position sense, may be affected selectively (eg, posterior column disease) or globally (diabetic polyneuropathy). Patterns of sensory loss (dermatomal, stocking, glove, etc) should be noted. Strength testing should include axial and peripheral muscles. Rate of muscle fatigue should be noted, particularly when there is a possibility of neuromuscular junction disease. Distribution of weakness is characteristic for specific etiologies, eg, symmetrical proximal weakness in myopathy and distal weakness in neuropathy (notwithstanding notable exceptions cited earlier). Functional testing should include limited evaluation of balance, coordination, stance, and gait. Gross evaluation of cranial nerves and mental status requires only a couple of additional minutes.

Diagnostic Tests

Laboratory Tests

Simple screening laboratory testing, including complete blood count with erythrocyte sedimentation rate, chemistry screen with creatine phosphokinase, antinuclear antibodies, refractory anemia, and urinalysis, may be in order to rule out inflammatory processes and muscle and connective tissue pathology. Disease-specific laboratory testing is delineated in Table 1.

Electrodiagnostic Studies

Electrodiagnostic studies are extremely helpful in establishing diagnosis and in providing information related to management. These should be considered an extension of the history and physical examination, and therefore the specific nerves and muscles to be tested depend on available clinical information. Characteristic findings are noted for each category of neuromuscular disease.

In myopathic processes, such as muscular dystrophy and polymyositis, electrodiagnostic findings include small polyphasic potentials with a myopathic (early) recruitment pattern. Depending on the severity, one can additionally see significant electrical membrane instability (positive waves and fibrillation potentials) as degenerating myofibrils spontaneously depolarize. In advanced disease, electrically silent areas are noted as electrically active muscle tissue is replaced by connective tissue. Although motor-evoked potential amplitudes can be reduced due to loss of muscle mass, nerve conduction studies (velocities, distal latencies, etc) are normal in myopathies, because the pathologic process involves the myofibril rather than the conducting nervous tissue.

In diseases that affect the neuromuscular junction, electrodiagnostic studies do not typically reveal electrical membrane instability, because the myofibril itself is not directly affected. Similarly, nerve conduction velocities along the course of the nerve are normal. However, repetitive nerve stimulation across the junction itself results in a characteristic progressive decrement in the generated electrical potential, as increasing numbers of neuromuscular junctions demonstrate failed transmission.

A variety of electrodiagnostic abnormalities are found with diseases directly involving the peripheral nerve. Both diabetes mellitus and Charcot-Marie-Tooth disease characteristically demonstrate pathology in the myelin sheath and in the axon. The absence of myelin results in impaired conduction. Therefore, proximal (nerve conduction velocities) and distal (latencies) conductions are slowed. With increasing axonal loss and accompanying denervation, positive waves and fibrillation potentials are noted. The progressive reduction in myofibrils results in a reduced evoked potential amplitude. By the time a patient demonstrates a typical cavus foot, there is near total loss of all residual viable motor units. The myofibril recruitment pattern is severely reduced (neurogenic).

In diseases that affect the anterior horn cell, such as poliomyelitis and amyotrophic lateral sclerosis, one can see varying abnormalities, depending on the rate of progression and degree of severity of the underlying neuropathic process. In amyotrophic lateral sclerosis, initial electrodiagnostic studies reveal enlarged motor units (a denervation/reinnervation pattern as a few anterior horn cells drop out, with

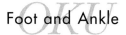

residual neurons sprouting to pick up greater numbers of muscle cells) with a neuropathic recruitment pattern. Early on, there tends to be very little residual denervation. Because only the axon itself is affected (the myelin remains intact), conduction velocities remain normal. As the disease progresses, increasing numbers of anterior horn cells are destroyed, and "denervation potentials" (positive waves and fibrillation potentials) are noted, particularly in the most distal muscles. Inasmuch as the degenerative process results from proximal (anterior horn cell) pathology, electrodiagnostic abnormalities may be found in all muscles, even if the only clinical evidence is distal extremity weakness. If the cause of the neuromuscular process affecting the foot and ankle is above the level of anterior horn cell, no peripheral electrodiagnostic abnormalities will be noted. However, central nervous system conductions, such as somatosensory evoked potentials, will demonstrate abnormalities in both intraspinal and intracranial pathology.

In addition to assisting with making the diagnosis, electrodiagnostic studies can be used to help direct the management of the foot and ankle in neuromuscular disease. Through the use of needle electromyography (EMG), individual muscles can be tested for degree of spasticity at rest and amount of volitional control at both minimum and maximum recruitment. This is particularly helpful if a tendon transfer is considered. Additionally, one can determine the degree of denervation and reinnervation as well as relative numbers of residual viable motor units.

Other Special Testing

In most neuromuscular diseases, the diagnosis can be made through the history and physical examination, limited laboratory testing, imaging, and electrodiagnostic studies. Occasionally, particularly with inflammatory processes, the diagnosis can be confirmed through either muscle (sample intermediately involved rather than severely or mildly involved muscles) or nerve (eg, sural) biopsies. Chromosomal studies are increasingly available for familial forms of neuromuscular disease.

Consultation

It may be helpful to consult with a physical medicine and rehabilitation specialist (physiatrist) or a neurologist for a performance of electrodiagnostic studies and for assistance in the patient's nonsurgical management, particularly in areas such as spasticity management, pain management, and neuromuscular reeducation. With multisystem diseases, consultation will depend on the specific organ systems involved.

Nonsurgical Management

Many patients respond to a conservative program of treatment. Specific management should consider both the focal problem and the generalized process causing that problem. If there are significant upper motor neuron findings, particularly severe spasticity, successful treatment must begin with management of the spasticity. The Ashworth Scale rates spasticity from 0 (normal tone) to 4 (rigid due to tone). Patients with mild spasticity frequently respond to home exercise and stretching with varying degrees of physical therapy assistance. If spasticity remains significant and involves more than 2 or 3 muscle groups (making motor point blocks impractical), one needs to consider oral pharmacologic intervention.

Although this treatment is usually carried out by a physiatrist or neurologist, the treating orthopaedic surgeon should be familiar with the multiple regimens. Baclofen, active at both the spinal and supraspinal level, is considered to be the drug of choice for spasticity resulting from spinal cord injury or multiple sclerosis. Treatment starts with a relatively low dose of 5 mg, 2 or 3 times per day, progressing to a maximum dose of 20 mg 4 times per day. Patients may experience some sedation initially, but this typically resolves. Discontinuation requires a tapering schedule, because abrupt withdrawal can result in hallucinations and/or seizures. Diazepam has been used successfully in spinal cord injuries for many years, but it carries with it the problems of sedation and habituation. In patients whose spasticity is typically controlled on baclofen during the day, but who have problems with spasticity at night, 5 mg or 10 mg of diazepam at bedtime is particularly helpful.

In pediatric patients and adult brain injury patients, dantrolene sodium is considered to be the first-line drug. Patients are typically started on a dose of 25 mg once or twice a day, progressing to a maximum total daily dose of 200 mg. In patients with significant associated weakness, doses must be titrated to reduce spasticity without impairing mobility. Dantrolene sodium is believed to exert a direct effect on the skeletal muscle, presumably by interfering with calcium release. Dantrolene sodium causes some sedation, which can largely be avoided by a gradually increasing dosage schedule. Due to potential liver toxicity, liver enzymes should be monitored on a periodic basis. In view of the direct effect on muscle cells, additional precautions include monitoring for pulmonary and cardiac disease. Tizanidine, a central alpha 2-noradrenergic agonist, (similar to clonidine) has been used in Europe for many years. Patients, started at 4 mg per day, are increased by 2 to 4 mg every 3 to 4 days to an average daily dose of 18 to 24 mg in divided doses. This drug was recently approved in the United States for use in multiple sclerosis and spinal cord injury. The primary mechanism of action is spinal (polysynaptic) and supraspinal. There are fewer complaints of subjective weakness than with other antispastic agents. Side effects are similar to those of baclofen and dantrolene, and liver enzymes must be checked on a periodic basis.

In patients with spasticity that involves only 2 or 3 muscles, nerve or motor point blocks may be considered. Direct nerve blocks are avoided because they result in an associated sensory loss. Electrodiagnostically guided motor point blocks, by contrast, result in significant reduction in tone without an associated sensory impairment. Patients may initially be locally injected with a short-acting anesthetic, such as lidocaine, followed by postinjection evaluation of gait. Postinjection evaluation can be based on simple clinical observation or on a formal evaluation in a gait analysis laboratory. If a temporary block results in significant improvement, treatment can progress to a more permanent block. Traditionally, permanent blocks have been performed with phenol through electrodiagnostically guided injection techniques. More recently, motor point blocks are performed using botulinum toxin (Botox). Regardless of the agent used, the involved muscle typically recovers from the "permanent" block in several months. Hopefully, by that time, through various other interventions, including stretching, serial casting, and splinting, the patient has adequate range and function. If not, a second block can safely be performed.

When spasticity has been adequately controlled, range of motion can be gained using physical therapy modalities and a vigorous stretching program. However, some patients may require a program of static or dynamic splinting. Additional range may be gained through a program of serial casting, altering the cast on a periodic basis to make incremental gains. If serial casting is used, patients (particularly those with an associated sensory loss) must be checked periodically for skin breakdown.

In patients who continue to have significant spasticity, intrathecal baclofen should be considered. More invasive neurosurgical procedures include selected posterior rhizotomy and spinal cord stimulators.

Electrical stimulation has several benefits. Patients who use home units can stimulate the involved denervated muscles several time per day, reducing the degree of atrophy. There is an associated reduction in spasticity in the antagonistic muscle. Additionally, in patients who have good residual sensation, there is a neuromuscular reeducation effect as proprioceptive sensory signals from the moving muscle and tendon are transmitted back to the brain.

Patients who have central nervous system involvement can benefit from neuromuscular reeducation through EMG biofeedback. An electrical monitoring disk is placed over the involved muscle, and a second monitoring disk is placed over the antagonist. Both signals are differentiated as they are sent through auditory and/or visual amplifiers. Through a series of neuromuscular reeducation sessions (2-channel EMG biofeedback units are available as well), the patient is able to demonstrate improving selected control of the involved muscle group with selective inhibition of the antagonists. EMG neuromuscular reeducation is particularly useful following a tendon transfer.

Managing Specific Disease Entities

Diagnostic and management concepts discussed above can be applied in general to varied neuromuscular diseases. As stated in the introduction, management decisions demand consideration of the whole patient, including focal and systemic manifestations of the disease as well as the patient's psychological status. It is beyond the scope of this chapter to delineate specific diagnostic and management considerations for each listed disease. Charcot-Marie-Tooth disease (CMT) offers most of the diagnostic and management challenges seen in typical neuromuscular diseases. Therefore, we have selected this particular disease entity as our prototypic example.

Charcot-Marie-Tooth Disease
Hereditary motor and sensory neuropathies (HMSN) are a group of familial diseases characterized by slowly progressive distal muscular weakness and atrophy with minor deficits in sensation. Life expectancy for most individuals will be normal, and females will be more severely affected than males.

CMT disease is the most common inherited neuropathy, affecting 1 in 2,500 people, or 125,000 individuals in the United States alone. In the 1800s, Charcot and Marie in France and Tooth in England described independently the condition that still bears their names. It is also known as peroneal muscular atrophy and hereditary motor sensory neuropathy. The 2 most common types of hereditary motor sensory neuropathy are types I and II. Type I patients have thickened nerves and abnormal fatty myelin covering the nerves, hence the term hypertrophic CMT disease. Type II patients have deterioration of the axons, hence the name neuronal CMT disease (Table 2).

Classification of CMT Disease
The most useful classification, from Dyck and Lambert, is based on 4 criteria: clinical findings, electrophysiologic data, genetics, and neuropathology.

Table 2
Charcot-Marie-Tooth clinical evaluation

Type	Pattern	Chromosome	Protein	Age O/S	Sex	NCV	Path
IA	Dom	17	PMP 22 (1)	22 to 30	M/F	Slow	"Onion" hypertrophy
IB	Dom	1	PO (2)	20 to 30	M/F	Slow	"Onion" hypertrophy
II	Rec			10 to 15	M/F	NI	Axonatrophy
X-linked	Rec	X	CX 32 (3)	< 10	M		

PMP 22, Peripheral myelin protein; PO, Protein Zero (adhesive); CX 32, Connexin 32 (gaps); The expressivity of Charcot-Marie-Tooth gene can be variable in terms of symptoms. Some individuals may be severely affected while other affected members may have hardly noticeable symptoms

HMSN Type I This is the autosomal dominant form of CMT disease. Electrodiagnostic studies are characterized by dramatic slowing of motor nerve conduction velocity and hypertrophic onion bulb changes of the nerves on biopsy. Two subgroups are identified, type I-A and type I-B. Type I-A is not linked to Duffy blood group focus on chromosome 1 (not associated with slow motor nerve conduction velocity [NCV] and onion bulb changes on nerve biopsy). Type I-B is linked to Duffy blood group on chromosome 1, which has the associated slow motor NCV and onion bulb changes on nerve biopsy. Bird documented that these 2 subgroups represent mutations at separate genetic foci and are not allelic. The large group of HMSN type I includes Roussy-Levy syndrome.

HMSN Type II This is also inherited as a recessive dominant, but is the neuronal form of CMT disease. The motor NCV is slightly decreased or normal. Nerve biopsy lacks the hypertrophy found in type I.

HMSN Type III This is inherited as an autosomal trait, with the motor NCV being very slow and nerve biopsy showing onion bulb formation with sequential demyelination. Type III contains the familiar hypertrophic interstitial neuritis of infancy and childhood called Dejerine-Sottas disease.

HMSN Type IV This is characterized by serum elevation of phytanic acid and represented as Rejsam's disease. Motor nerve conduction is slow and nerve biopsy shows onion bulb formation. Inheritance is an autosomal recessive.

HMSN Type V Characterized by spastic paraplegia, type V is inherited as an autosomal dominant gene.

HMSN Type VI Although similar to type I, type VI additionally demonstrates optic atrophy.

HMSN Type VII Type VII comprises type I patients who have retinitis pigmentosa.

Incidence
Males are affected more frequently, but females are affected more severely. According to Jacobs and Carr, blacks are believed to be exempt from CMT disease.

Pathology
Motor nerve roots and peripheral nerves show degenerative changes, with a loss of myelin and fragmentation of the axon cylinders. HMSN type I nerve biopsies show hypertrophic changes with onion bulb thickening, which is histologic evidence of repetitive demyelination and remyelinization. HMSN type II shows degenerative changes with minimal hypertrophy on nerve biopsy. A secondary loss of anterior horn cells and degeneration of the posterior columns and posterior roots (dying back) occurs in the spinal cord. Muscle biopsy shows the changes of neuronal atrophy with infiltration of fat and changes in fiber-type groupings and blastic proliferation.

Clinical Findings
In type I, onset of symptoms is usually delayed until the third decade of life. Type II onset is typically between 5 and 15 years. Sixty percent will be male and 40% female. Muscle cramps in feet and legs, shoe wear problems, difficulty in running on uneven ground, or pain under the metatarsal head with prolonged walking or standing are among the pre-

senting complaints. Paresthesias in the legs is occasionally reported. The initial deformity, mild cavus and claw toes, gradually increases in severity.

Distal muscular atrophy is symmetrical. Fascicular twitching is often present, but the paralysis is flaccid with atrophic muscle evident. Intrinsic muscles of the feet are affected first, followed by the peroneus brevis. This results in early pes cavus. Atrophy soon spreads to the anterior compartment, affecting the anterior tibialis and toe extensor muscles. Because of a strong posterior compartment and peroneus longus, forefoot and ankle equinus gradually develop. Drop foot is evident with a "marionette" gait. Gastrocnemius and other calf muscles eventually atrophy.

Approximately 94% of CMT disease patients have a foot deformity. Of these, 85% have pes cavus, 40% have claw toes, and 25% have varus of the hindfoot. Bilateral equinovarus and pes cavus with drop foot are common, producing fractures and recurrent ankle sprains of the lower extremities. With decreased proprioception, foot deformities, and distal weakness, the patient is unstable in stance and gait. Knee flexion activates the proprioception sensation of the knee itself and, additionally, lowers the body's center of gravity.

By the time the calves atrophy, the upper limbs become involved. This latter stage begins as symmetrical atrophy of the hand intrinsic and forearm muscles. Intrinsic wasting and clawing of the hand are common. Thumb opposition may not be possible. Fine motor movements become impaired, making writing, button fastening, and turning door knobs difficult. Upper extremity involvement will be less severe in type II than in type I. Pelvic, shoulder, arm, thigh, trunk, and facial muscles are spared. In advanced cases, legs, feet, forearms, and hands are wasted and slender, while the thighs and upper arms remain normal. This contrast of plump thighs and slender legs has been likened to an "inverted champagne bottle" or "ostrich legs." The weakness of the lower extremities is more pronounced in type II than in type I, hence, the classic "stork leg" appearance is more often seen in HMSN type II.

The deep tendon reflexes are decreased to absent, with the most distal reflexes being affected first. The patellar, triceps, and biceps reflexes remain present. Sensory loss in the hands and feet may be present with dysthesias. There may be decreased vibratory and position senses with associated disturbance of gait, but ataxia is not present. Central nervous system, respiratory, and bowel and bladder problems are rare, but chronic fatigue and weakness are common. Intellectual function and life span are unaffected. Patients often remain ambulatory. Many remain free of serious physical impairment until well past the fourth decade. Pregnancy can lead to worsening of CMT disease, but symptoms can subside after

parturition. In a study group with an average age of 22.3 years at the time of delivery, marked worsening of symptoms occurred. In comparison, a group of women with an average age of 34.3 years at the time of delivery had minimal worsening of symptoms. Scoliosis is present in about 40% to 50% of patients. It is usually not severe, and only 10% to 15% of these scoliosis patients require surgical intervention.

Neurotoxic Drugs in Neuromuscular Disease
The CMT Association continually monitors and publishes a list of drugs that can be neurotoxic to patients with CMT and other neuromuscular diseases. These drugs can potentially worsen the symptoms of neuromuscular diseases. It is recommended that they either be avoided or that they be used with caution (Outline 1).

Evaluation
Criteria for diagnosis of CMT disease are not strict. Diagnosis in most cases is established by family history, in conjunction with clinical findings of distal extremity weakness and pes cavus. However, with mutations, spontaneous cases do occur and may present diagnostic problems in individuals with mild cavus or weakness. Nerve conduction studies show slow conduction velocities. A nerve biopsy is seldom necessary.

Clinically, patients with CMT disease will have foot and ankle complaints. The skin of the foot will have plantar calluses and painful corns on the toes. Because the toes rub the top of the toe box, wearing shoes is painful. Weakness, from easy fatigability to frank drop foot, is common. A progressively higher arch is accompanied by increasing symptoms of ankle instability. Anesthesia is rare.

Lower Extremity Examination
Hindfoot varus, cavus deformity, and forefoot valgus are typical of CMT disease. Forefoot valgus is primarily the result of plantarflexion of the first metatarsal. Initially supple, the hindfoot varus will become progressively fixed. The lateral block test of Paulos and Coleman determines the flexibility of the subtalar joint and the contribution of forefoot valgus to the deformity. The heel and lateral forefoot are placed on a wooden fi-inch-thick long block. The first ray is allowed to be off and drop to the floor (Fig. 1). The flexible hindfoot allows the calcaneus to correct to neutral or slight valgus. Therefore, if the plantarflexed first ray is eliminated from the deformity by the block, the hindfoot varus should correct. However, if the hindfoot remains in varus on the block, the deformity is rigid, and surgical dorsiflexion of the first ray alone will not correct the deformity.

Cavus deformity can be midfoot, hindfoot, or forefoot. In hindfoot cavus, the pitch of the calcaneus will be greater than

Outline 1
Drugs potentially toxic to patients with neuromuscular disease

Adriamycin

Alcohol

Amiodarone

Chloramphenicol

Cis-platium

Dapsone

Diphenylhydantoin (Dilantin)

Disulfiram (Anabuse)

Glutethimide (Doriden)

Gold

Hydralazine (Apresoline)

Isoniazid (INH)

Mega Dose of Vitamin A

Mega Dose of Vitamin B6 (pyridoxine)

Mega Dose of Vitamin D

Metronidazole (Flagyl)

Nitrofurantoin (Furadantin, Macrodantin)

Nitrous Oxide (chronic repeated inhalation)

Penicillin (large IV doses only)

Perhexiline (Pexid)

Taxol

Vincristine

Zoloft

Use with caution:
    Lithium
    Misonidazole

apex of deformity at or near the tarsometatarsal joints. The first metatarsal is always involved. Global anterior cavus includes all the metatarsals.

Forefoot valgus is frequently found in CMT. The first ray is flexed downward in relation to the rest of the lesser toe metatarsals. This flexion is measured by placing the calcaneus in a neutral position and visualizing the plantar forefoot, which faces laterally. The toe deformities are fixed or flexible claw toe. The plantar fat pad migrates distally, and calluses can form under the metatarsal heads over the proximal interphalangeal joints of the toes. The great toe also has the same deformity, with calluses under the sesamoids and at the interphalangeal joint.

Neurologic evaluation is very important. Sensory impairment is much less severe than motor deficits and appears late. Vibration, joint position, and 2-point discrimination are affected first. Superficial sensation is affected in only 24% of the cases. Deep tendon reflexes are frequently absent or decreased, but motor examination is variable. In a typical pattern, deep and superficial posterior compartment muscles are of normal strength. The anterior tibialis and peroneus brevis are usually weak, resulting in weak ankle dorsiflexion and subtalar eversion. The peroneus longus retains good power. To compensate for foot drop in swing phase, the pelvis is elevated with moderate hip and knee flexion. The extensor digitorum longus and extensor hallucis longus are recruited as ankle dorsiflexors, giving rise to hyperextension of the metatarsophalangeal joints. Foot contact is toe-heel or foot flat. This pattern of muscle strength and weakness leads to the "marionette" gait typical of CMT. With the gradual decrease of elevation at heel strike and the foot supinated to gradual pronation, normal shock absorption is lost. The hindfoot remains inverted, locking the subtalar and midtarsal joints.

Radiographic Evaluation
Radiographic evaluation starts with the anteroposterior weightbearing and lateral weightbearing radiographs. The anteroposterior view shows forefoot adduction. In patients with forefoot cavus (typical of CMT), the lateral view should demonstrate the plantarflexed first ray. Hindfoot cavus is associated with a calcaneus inclination angle of greater than 30° (Friedreich's ataxia). Because of the external rotation of the tibia resulting from the supinated foot (calcaneus in varus and forefoot in valgus), the fibula will appear almost posterior to the tibia. The Harris view shows the calcaneus in varus.

Cavus: Deforming Forces of Muscles
Forefoot valgus, created by overpull of the peroneus longus, which plantarflexes the first ray, can be noted in the unloaded foot with the hindfoot held in neutral position. In addition,

30°. This vertical position of the calcaneus is documented by measuring the angle formed by the inferior border of the calcaneus and the floor as viewed on the lateral weightbearing radiograph. In midfoot cavus, the apex of deformity falls between the anterior tuberosity of the calcaneus and the medial cuneiform. Anterior cavus (forefoot cavus) has the

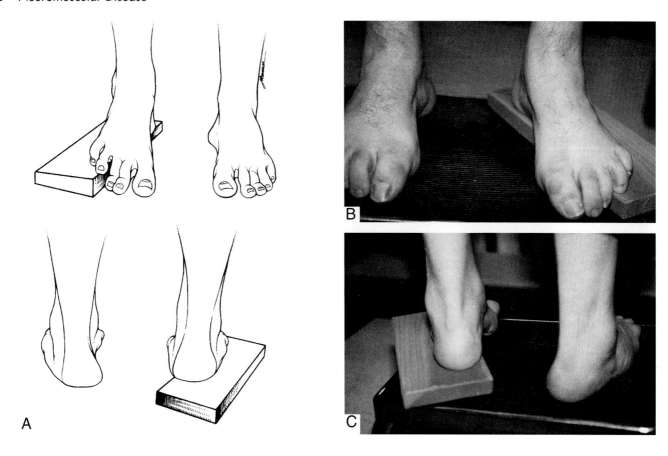

Figure 1

A, Line drawing illustrating lateral block test. (Reproduced with permission from Alexander IJ: Evaluation of frontal plane mechanics, in *The Foot: Examination and Diagnosis*. New York, NY, Churchill Livingstone, 1990, pp 41–54.) **B,** Photograph showing anterior view of lateral block test. **C,** Posterior view photograph of lateral block test demonstrating a flexible hindfoot.

the peroneus brevis is weak, leaving its antagonist, the posterior tibialis, unopposed. The additional force of the unopposed posterior tibialis with the peroneus longus increases the high arch.

Intrinsic muscle atrophy with secondary claw toes contributes to complaints in patients with cavus feet. Limited space for toes in shoes and increased pressure under the metatarsal heads are among the first complaints in these patients. Flexion of all metatarsophalangeal joints is lost, with intrinsic weakness. The flexor digitorum longus flexes the proximal and distal interphalangeal joints, increasing the clawing posture of the toes. As the extensor digitorum longus and extensor hallucis longus work to overcome the weakness of the anterior tibialis, the deformity is accentuated. In skeletally immature patients, prolonged muscle imbalance will cause bony deformity; in adults, untreated soft-tissue contractures will lead to rigid deformity.

Cavus: Evaluation of Frontal Plane Deformities

In the frontal plane, the motion of the foot is described as inversion and eversion. In inversion, the foot tilts so that the plantar aspect of the foot is toward the midline. In eversion, the foot tilts so that the plantar aspect of the foot is away from the midline. If the foot is maintained in the inverted or everted position, it is in a static position. The inverted position is termed varus, and the everted position is termed valgus.

When the position of the foot is rigid and not in normal alignment, secondary abnormalities occur in the position of the uninvolved portion of the foot. Rigid forefoot valgus with flexible hindfoot varus is perhaps the most common pattern, but hindfoot valgus with compensatory forefoot varus also exists. This chapter is concerned with the most common deformity, forefoot valgus with hindfoot varus.

The neutral hindfoot position is determined with the patient lying prone, with the feet dangling over the edge of the table in the "figure-of-4" position. The natural external rotation of the extremity to be examined is eliminated by laying the medial malleolus of the opposite ankle over the popliteal space. This "figure-of-4" position tilts the pelvis internally, rotating the extended leg internally, thus putting the foot and ankle in a neutral position (Fig. 2). A line can then be drawn down the midcalf to the ankle and another line drawn along the sagittal axis of the calcaneus (posterior heel area) (Fig. 3, A). The fifth metatarsal is grasped, and the ankle is placed in neutral as the other hand palpates the medial aspect of the talonavicular joint so that the joint comes into alignment (Fig. 3, B and C). With the talonavicular joint aligned, the calcaneus is by definition in neutral position. From this point of neutral, the normal subtalar motion is two thirds inversion and one third eversion (Fig. 3, D).

To determine the position of the forefoot, the patient's foot is placed in the neutral midfoot position as discussed above. The inverted forefoot, relative to the neutral position of the calcaneus (the sole of the foot pointed inward from the midline), is in varus (Fig. 3, E). The everted foot (the sole of the foot pointed away from the midline) is in valgus. This information, together with the lateral block test, allows assessment of the flexibility of the hindfoot varus and the associated rigid forefoot valgus. The block is placed under the lateral heel and extended under the lateral metatarsals, allowing the first ray to drop to the floor (Fig. 1). A flexible compensatory hindfoot deformity will correct. A rigid hindfoot deformity will remain deviated in varus or the same position as when the patient is standing without the block.

Planning Treatment of a Cavus Foot

Sequential approach to evaluation of a cavus foot is important in planning its nonsurgical management or surgical correction. Japas, Alexander and Johnson, and later Holmes and Hansen addressed several questions to facilitate decision making when planning treatment of cavus foot. The following principles apply to all cavus feet, not just the deformity in Charcot-Marie-Tooth disease. Because of the progressive muscular imbalance, this deformity is most prone to recurrence.

1. Is the deformity bilateral? Unilateral pes cavus is usually secondary to poliomyelitis or trauma such as cauda equina trauma, incomplete spinal cord injuries, deep posterior compartment syndrome, or a crushed foot. Bilateral involvement is mostly frequently from CMT, but consideration must be given to other etiologies, such as diabetic neuropathy, Friedreich's ataxia, spinal cord tumor, spinal dysraphism, diastematomyelia, etc. In a young person, these must be thoroughly investigated.

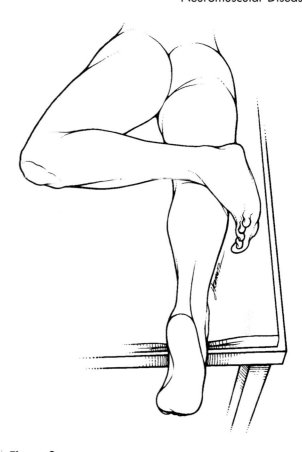

Figure 2

Line drawing illustrating the "figure-of-4" position. (Reproduced with permission from Alexander IJ: Evaluation of frontal plane mechanics, in *The Foot: Examination and Diagnosis.* New York, NY, Churchill Livingstone, 1990, pp 41–54.)

2. Is the cavus deformity primarily hindfoot or forefoot? A calcaneal pitch angle of greater than 30° is hindfoot cavus found in poliomyelitis, cauda equina injury, or incomplete spinal cord injury. This cavus foot is caused by weakness of the gastrocnemius-soleus muscle complex. Calcaneocavus deformity is unlikely in CMT, because weakness occurs in sequence from foot intrinsics to peroneal brevis and anterior tibialis. The gastrocnemius, soleus, and posterior tibialis are last to atrophy, and hindfoot equinus is frequent in CMT, because these muscles are unopposed. In these patients, the cavus deformity is secondary to muscle imbalances of the mid and anterior tarsals and metatarsals and is referred to as anterior cavus. The calcaneal pitch will be less than 30°.

3. Is the forefoot deformity global or primarily first metatarsal? Global deformity implies flaccid paralysis of toe extensors, whereas first ray plantarflexion suggests CMT as the etiology.

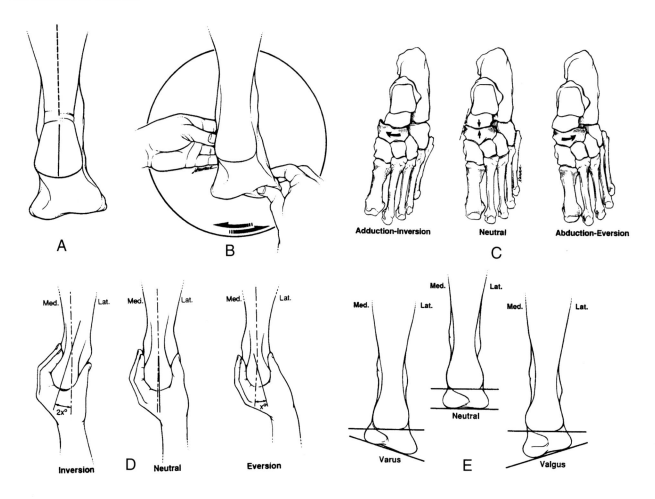

A

B

Adduction-Inversion   Neutral   Abduction-Eversion

C

Med.   Lat.   Med.   Lat.   Med.   Lat.

2x°   x°

Inversion   D   Neutral   Eversion

Med.
Lat.

Med.   Lat.   Med.   Lat.

Neutral

Varus   E   Valgus

Figure 3

Evaluating the frontal plane. A, Line showing the axis of the central calf and heel. B, Defining neutral position based on palpation of the talonavicular joint. C, The talonavicular joint in adduction-inversion, neutral, and abduction-eversion. D, Defining inversion and eversion of the hindfoot. E, Defining forefoot varus and valgus. (Reproduced with permission from Alexander IJ: Evaluation of frontal plane mechanics, in *The Foot: Examination and Diagnosis.* New York, NY, Churchill Livingstone, 1990, pp 41–54.)

4. Are the deformities fixed or flexible? In the forefoot, when passive dorsiflexion of the metatarsals is not possible, tarsometatarsal joint stiffness or soft-tissue contraction produces a fixed deformity. Both bone and soft-tissue procedures may be required in order to obtain a satisfactory correction. In the hindfoot, the "fixed or flexible" question is answered with the lateral block test. Fixed hindfoot deformity may require bony realignment to produce a neutral position of the calcaneus. Unopposed action of the posterior tibialis and long-toe flexors will produce hindfoot varus. Hindfoot varus can also be secondarily produced by forefoot valgus. By identifying the pathologic biomechanics, treatment can be specifically directed.

5. What are the deforming forces? In the forefoot, the peroneus longus plantarflexes the first metatarsal by overpowering the weak anterior tibialis, thus causing forefoot valgus. Claw toes formed by the extensor hallucis longus and extensor digitorum longus acting as ankle dorsiflexors aid the weak anterior tibialis. As they pull against the weak foot intrinsics with normal long toe flexors, claw toes form. The strong posterior tibialis overwhelms the weak peroneus brevis, causing forefoot adduction and hindfoot varus.

6. Are the toe deformities fixed or flexible? Toes that can be corrected passively can be managed by soft-tissue procedures. Fixed contractures may require both bony and soft-tissue correction.

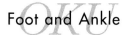
7. Is the ankle unstable? Patients with hindfoot varus may complain of chronic ankle instability. If the symptoms persist after correction of the cavovarus foot, ligamentous instability needs to be addressed.

8. What are the patient's goals? Unrealistic patient expectations can undermine the result of an excellent surgical correction. The need to explain the magnitude of the problem and the anticipated functional ability after surgery cannot be overemphasized. Specific, well-defined goals must be understood and agreed on by the patient and the orthopaedist.

Nonsurgical Management

The goals of nonsurgical management are to maintain function, insure safety, maintain comfort, protect weakened joints, and conserve energy. Because of the nature of the disease, many patients with CMT cease vigorous activity and become increasingly sedentary. Reduced activity results in disuse weakness of normal muscles as well as generalized deconditioning and weight gain. Therefore, function can be improved by establishing a program of generalized strengthening and conditioning exercises. Resistance exercise must be carried out with caution, to avoid the damage of overstraining. Swimming or stationary cycling may be more suitable than walking, and appropriate stretching exercises can minimize deformity.

Superimposing injury on already weakened muscles can further compromise performance. A program of strengthening is directed toward improving the function of weakened muscles and maximizing the strength of uninvolved muscles. Each patient should undergo a complete evaluation by a physical therapist familiar with CMT to establish a level of exercise for each muscle group that will result in strengthening without injury. By increasing the resistance and/or increasing the number of repetitions, exercises are progressed. For the foot and ankle, resistance exercise can progress from lifting the weight of the limb to lifting the limb with a weight attached to it. Using Therabands allows for an escalating program by starting with the least resistive color and progressing to no further than red or blue. Pain and excessive fatigue must be avoided. When the patient is ready to increase the resistance, the number of repetitions is decreased. Gradually, the number of repetitions with the new resistance is increased again.

CMT patients will also benefit from improved conditioning. An inactive lifestyle contributes to deconditioning, and more effort is required to accomplish a task. Conditioning exercises must accommodate the patient's weakness. Swimming or stationary cycling may be more suitable than walking. Benefits of exercise include increased muscle strength and cardiovascular endurance, allowing the patient to be more active in everyday life.

Appropriate stretching exercises can minimize deformity. For example, in CMT disease, dorsiflexor muscles become weak and plantarflexor muscles pull and become contracted. This makes it difficult to stand with the feet flat on the floor. These patients fear falling backward and tend to select shoes with higher heels. Abnormal pressure and pain in the foot puts abnormal stress on other joints. In this case, the stress is a backward pull of the knee predisposing the patient to recurvatum. Avoiding or minimizing these deformities is the focus of the strengthening exercises. Specificity in stretching is important. The specific muscle imbalance must be identified. Stretching of the weaker muscle is to be avoided, because doing so will increase the imbalance. Stretching is taught by the physical therapist, with emphasis on isolating individual muscles for stretching and for strengthening.

Orthotic Devices and Bracing

Orthotic devices and braces support the weakened limbs. They are used to assist walking or to prevent contractures. The molded ankle foot orthosis (AFO) is the most common device used. Worn as a night splint, it helps prevent Achilles contracture and dropfoot. Worn during ambulation, the AFO stabilizes the weakened ankle and clears the foot during the swing phase of the gait cycle. The extremity requires less flexion at the hip and knee as the leg swings forward, which decreases movement and energy expenditure. The plastic molded AFO has the advantage over metal braces because of its lighter weight. Also, its total contact decreases pressure points, and it can be worn inside the shoe and pants, making it cosmetically more acceptable.

Orthoses can also be used to accommodate foot deformities. For example, the plantarflexed first ray can be accommodated by elevating the heel and the lateral forefoot, allowing flexion of the first metatarsal. This allows the unstable hindfoot to correct and makes the ankle feel more stable. It can also be used to decrease pressure areas and to provide comfort and skin protection.

Surgery

Soft-Tissue Procedures

First ray plantarflexion is caused by the imbalance of the strong peroneus longus and the weak anterior tibialis. In conjunction with this, the peroneus brevis is weak in eversion. Transferring the peroneus longus to the peroneus brevis eliminates the first ray strong plantarflexion force and restores the ankle eversion power.

Cavovarus is partially caused by the relatively strong pathologic force of the posterior tibialis against the unopposed peroneus brevis. Two transfers with the posterior tibialis are recognized as valuable methods of eliminating its contribution to the cavus. The 2 are: (1) transfer of the posterior tibialis tendon to the dorsum of the foot through the interosseus membrane, and (2) transfer of the posterior tibialis tendon around the ankle to the cuboid.

In long-standing cavus, the plantar fascia is usually tight and persists as a prominent deforming force. As an important part of treatment of any cavus foot, the plantar fascia release can be partial, or radical, as required for the neurogenic cavus foot. When considering transfer of the anterior tibialis tendon as a split or entire tendon laterally to restore balance dorsiflexion, caution is advised, because the anterior tibialis muscle can be very weak in CMT and in other disease states, causing cavus. As a rule, muscles will loose 1 grade when transferred. Lengthening of the heel cord is a very important

part of managing CMT cavus. The imbalance between strong plantarflexors and weak dorsiflexors leads to forefoot drop and to a contracted Achilles tendon.

Claw toes, the most frequent forefoot deformity, are the result of intrinsic weakness. When flexible claw toes do not resolve spontaneously with surgical correction of the midfoot cavus, transfers of the Girdleston-Taylor type can be effective (Fig. 4). This addresses the extensor digitorum longus (EDL), the weak intrinsics, and the strong long flexors' contribution to the typical claw toe deformity. The EDL acts to aid weak ankle dorsiflexors. This causes hyperextension at the metatarsophalangeal (MTP) joints, which are normally flexed by the pathologically weak intrinsic muscles. To accentuate the deformity, the strong flexor digitorum longus (FDL) acts to flex the toes at the distal interphalangeal (DIP) joint, thus increasing the claw toe deformity. The flexor-to-extensor transfer takes the FDL as a splint tendon and transfers it dorsally to the extensors, thereby flexing the MTP joints. The

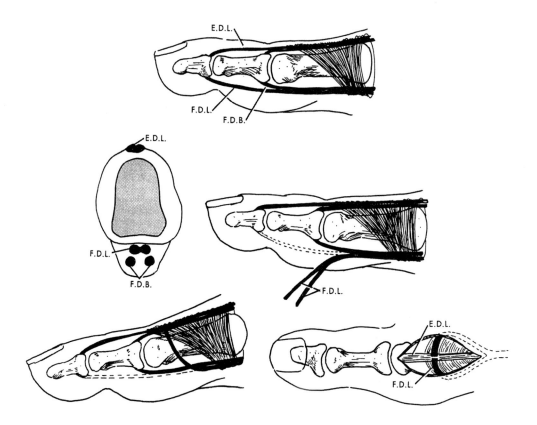

Figure 4

Flexor-to-extensor tendon transfer for correction of flexible hammer toes. EDL = extensor digitorum longus. FDL = flexor digitorum longus. FDB = flexor digitorum brevis. (Reproduced with permission from Coughlin MJ, Mann RA: Lesser toe deformities, in Mann RA (ed): *Surgery of the Foot*, ed 5. St. Louis, MO, CV Mosby, 1986, pp 132–157.)

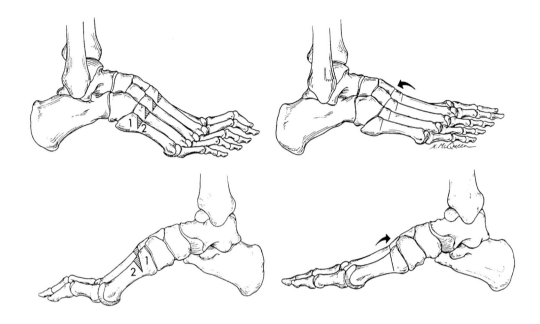

Figure 5

Closing wedge osteotomy for correction of plantarflexed metatarsals. (Reproduced with permission from Richardson EG: Neurogenic disorders, in Crenshaw AH (ed): *Campbell's Operative Orthopaedics*, ed 8. St. Louis, MO, Mosby Year Book, 1992, pp 2777-2834. Redrawn from Gould N: Surgery in advanced Charcot-Marie-Tooth disease. *Foot Ankle* 1984;4:267-273.)

claw hallux is treated successfully by the Jones procedure, an interphalangeal (IP) joint arthrodesis and transfer of the extensor hallucis longus (EHL) to the first metatarsal neck. Other successful transfers in the cavus foot are available. EDL and EHL attachment to the metatarsal necks, bases, or cuneiforms eliminates their influence in claw toes, allowing them to act as dorsiflexors for the ankle.

The surgical goal is to produce a plantigrade foot. With early deformities in which the foot is supple, soft-tissue procedures such as tendon transfers and plantar fascial releases may be all that is necessary. The younger the individual, the higher the probability that several procedures may be necessary during growth. If a specific bony deformity exists in a supple foot and prevents it from becoming plantigrade, an osteotomy to correct the deformity, along with the appropriate soft-tissue procedure to balance the power, will be necessary. It is better to maintain a flexible foot than to carry out an arthrodesis. Even when the foot is fairly rigid, osteotomies are more beneficial than fusions.

Bony Procedures

At the metatarsal level, rigid plantarflexion of the first metatarsal with fixed forefoot valgus can be treated with a dorsal closing wedge osteotomy. In global deformities, multiple dorsal wedge osteotomies (Fig. 5) may be necessary. Prior

to doing the dorsal wedge osteotomies, a plantar fascia release is recommended. Transfer of the peroneus longus to the peroneus brevis eliminates the deforming plantar force and should improve hindfoot varus.

Other methods of correcting at the metatarsal level are

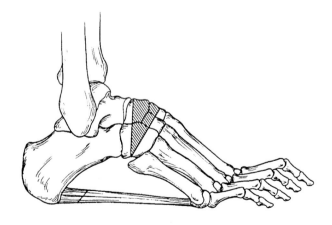

Figure 6

Cole anterior tarsal wedge osteotomy. (Reproduced with permission from Richardson EG: Neurogenic disorders, in Crenshaw AH (ed): *Campbell's Operative Orthopaedics*, ed 8. St. Louis, MO, Mosby Year Book, 1992, pp 2777-2834.)

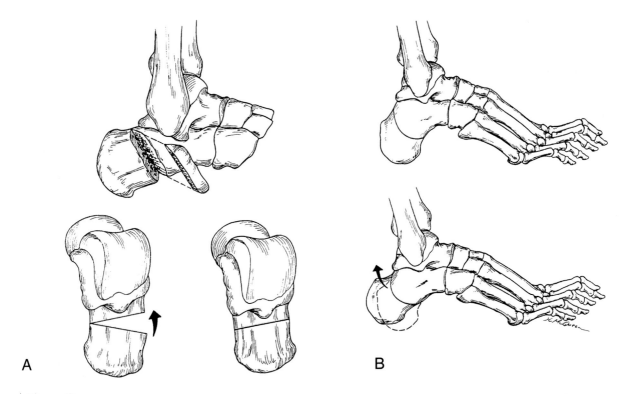

Figure 7

A, Dwyer calcaneal osteotomy. B, Samilson crescentic calcaneal osteotomy. (Reproduced with permission from Richardson EG: Neurogenic disorders, in Crenshaw AH (ed): *Campbell's Operative Orthopaedics*, ed 8. St. Louis, MO, Mosby Year Book, 1992, pp 2777-2834. Part B was redrawn from Bateman JE (ed): *Foot Science*. Philadelphia, PA, WB Saunders, 1976.)

truncated metatarsal osteotomies and arthrodeses with wedge resection of the articular surfaces of Cole (Fig. 6). Interestingly, a pseudarthrosis rate of 30% is reported with the Cole ostectomy. Ideally, correction of the deformity at its apex would achieve the best cosmetic result, but no publication to date has provided a technique to determine the exact apex of cavus.

Hindfoot varus is usually associated with a cavus foot. Flexibility of the hindfoot is determined by the lateral block test (Fig. 1). The hindfoot that fails to correct is considered rigid, and realignment can only be achieved by osteotomy. Lateral wedge osteotomies (Fig. 7, A) and crescentic osteotomies (Fig. 7, B) correct the hindfoot varus and hindfoot cavus. A lateral calcaneal slide osteotomy by itself is usually not enough to correct a moderately severe hindfoot varus.

Although now used less frequently, the triple arthrodesis has been a key procedure in the management of cavus. Currently, its use is restricted to patients with severe rigid cavus deformity with markedly limited subtalar mobility. In the triple, the hindfoot varus is corrected through the talocalcaneal joint resection. The cavus deformity is corrected

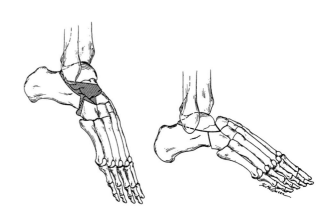

Figure 8

Lambrinudi triple arthrodesis to correct cavus. (Reproduced with permission from Richardson EG: Neurogenic disorders, in Crenshaw AH (ed): *Campbell's Operative Orthopaedics*, ed 8. St. Louis, MO, Mosby Year Book, 1992, pp 2777-2834.)

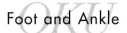
through resection of the transverse tarsal joint. For advanced deformities, the Lambrinudi triple arthrodesis (Fig. 8) gives the greatest correction.

Annotated Bibliography

Alexander IJ: Evaluation of frontal plan mechanics, in *The Foot: Examination and Diagnosis.* New York, NY, Churchill Living stone, 1990, pp 41–54.

An understanding of the biomechanics and correct nomenclature of the normal foot and deformities related to the frontal plane are necessary for successful management of any hindfoot and forefoot problem. This chapter makes it easier to understand the problem of cavus and enables one to communicate what the problem is to colleagues and patients.

Alexander IJ, Johnson KA: Assessment and management of pes cavus in Charcot-Marie-Tooth disease. *Clin Orthop* 1989; 246:273–281.

Offering a sequential approach to evaluating any cavus foot, this article suggests the most appropriate surgical management based on nature of deformity and its rigidity.

Angus PD, Cowell HR: Triple arthrodesis: A critical long-term review. *J Bone Joint Surg* 1986;68B:260–265.

A review of 80 feet followed for an average of 13 years found a high incident of arthritic changes in the ankle and midfoot as well as pseudarthrosis, avascular necrosis of the talus, and residual deformity. Preoperative rigid equinovarus had the majority of poor results causing the authors to suggest that bone resection may not be the best method of correcting severe equinus.

Cochrane S, Bergoffen J, Fairweather ND, et al: X-linked Charcot-Marie-Tooth disease (CMTX1): A study of 15 families with 12 highly informative polymorphisms. *J Med Genet* 1994;31: 193–196.

Bergoffen JI, Scherer SS, Wang S, et al: Connexin mutations in X-linked Charcot-Marie-Tooth disease. *Science* 1993;262 2039–2042.

The authors identified the CMT disease gene found on the X chromosome. he gene's function is to encode fora protein called connexin 32. It forms the gap functions between cells which are two connections between cell interiors that allow diffusion of the small molecules and transmission of electrical signals.

Coleman SS, Chesnut WJ: A simple test for hindfoot flexibility in the cavovarus foot. *Clin Orthop* 1977;123:60–62.

Paulos L, Coleman SS, Samuelson KM: Pes cavovarus: Review of a surgical approach using selective soft-tissue procedures. *J Bone Joint Surg* 1980;62A:942–953.

Both of these articles discuss the treatment of cavus based on a flexible hindfoot evaluated by the lateral block test. This test has become a standard in evaluation of the cavovarus foot.

Gould N: Surgery in advanced Charcot-Marie-Tooth disease. *Foot Ankle* 1984;4:267–273.

This is one of the first articles to emphasize osteotomies instead of triple arthrodeses for treatment of advanced Charcot-Marie-Tooth. The metatarsal ostectomies are at the bases. The first metatarsal cut is in 2 planes to correct the adduction as well as the plantar flexion. A little less bone is taken sequentially from each base as one goes from the first to the fifth metatarsal.

Holmes JR, Hansen ST Jr: Foot and ankle manifestations of Charcot-Marie-Tooth disease. *Foot Ankle Int* 1993;14:476–486.

This article covers strategies of orthopaedic management of CMT disease foot and ankle deformities and is an outstanding review on the subject. It includes algorithms that will help the surgeon who infrequently treats cavus foot problems.

Mann DC, Hsu JD: Triple arthrodesis in the treatment of fixed cavovarus deformity in adolescent patients with Charcot-Marie-Tooth disease. *Foot Ankle Int* 1992;13:1–6.

This article points out that triple arthrodesis offers adolescent patients with Charcot-Marie-Tooth disease a stable plantigrade foot in the face of a progressive disorder. "Post operative pain was related to a non plantigrade foot and not to the presence of pseudoarthrosis." However, they could not determine if the nonplantigrade foot was due to incomplete surgical correction or to progressive muscle imbalance.

Mann RA, Missirian J: Pathophysiology of Charcot-Marie-Tooth disease. *Clin Orthop* 1988;234: 221–228.

In their review of 8 adult patients with a strong family history of Charcot-Marie-Tooth disease, the authors hypothesize that deformity of the foot is caused by weakness of the tibialis anterior, peroneus brevis, and intrinsic muscles which are then overpowered by their strong antagonist, the peroneal longus and tibialis posterior.

Mann RA: Pes cavus, in Mann RA, Coughlin MJ (eds): *Surgery of the Foot and Ankle,* ed 6. St. Louis, MO, Mosby-Year Book, 1993, pp 785–801.

This is an outstanding chapter on the management of cavus. Mann emphasizes correction of deformity but also motor balancing of the corrected foot, while he offers the triple arthrodesis as a last resort.

Oatis C: Physical therapy and rehabilitation of the Charcot-Marie

Tooth disease patient: Conservative management of the functional manifestations of Charcot-Marie Tooth disease, in Reiss A (ed): *Charcot-Marie Tooth Disorders: Pathophysiology, Molecular Genetics, and Therapy.* New York, NY, John Wiley & Sons, 1990.

This article demonstrates that function can be improved dramatically by establishing a generalized program of strengthening and conditioning exercises. Even neurologically involved muscles can be strengthened. Resistance should increase the difficulty of the exercise without causing pain or making it impossible to complete the exercise correctly.

Roa BB, Garcia CA, Sater U, et al: Charcot-Marie-Tooth disease type 1A: Association with a spontaneous point mutation in the PMP22 gene. *N Engl J Med* 1993;329:96–101.

This article studied a patient with a spontaneous mutation in the peripheral gene PMP22, who has the CMT disease phenotype.

Roper BA, Tibrewal SB: Soft tissue surgery in Charcot-Marie-Tooth disease. *J Bone Joint Surg* 1989;71B:17–20.

This review of 10 patients with an average of 14 years follow up resulted in the authors concluding that soft-tissue procedures can postpone the need for triple arthrodesis.

Shapiro F, Bresnan MJ: Orthopaedic management of childhood neuromuscular disease: Part 1. Spinal muscular atrophy. *J Bone Joint Surg* 1982;64A:785–789.

Shapiro F, Bresnan MJ: Orthopaedic management of childhood neuromuscular disease: Part II. Peripheral neuropathies, Friedreich's ataxia, and arthrogryposis multiplex congenita. *J Bone Joint Surg* 1982;64A:949–953.

Part II particularly provides an excellent review of HMSN and their management.

Westmore RS, Drennan JC: Long-term results of triple arthrodesis in Charcot-Marie-Tooth disease. *J Bone Joint Surg* 1989; 71A:417–422.

Sixteen patients with 30 triple arthrodeses with an average follow-up of 21 years had 47% poor results and 30% fair results. Patients with a poor result had severe impairment of function and needed an arthrodesis. Progressive muscle imbalance resulted in a recurrence of cavovarus in 7 patients. They concluded that triple arthrodesis should be limited to those patients with severe rigid deformity.

Wukich DK, Bowen JR: A long-term study of triple arthrodesis for correction of pes cavovarus in Charcot-Marie-Tooth disease. *J Pediatr Orthop* 1989;9:433–437.

A review of 22 patients with a follow-up of 12 years found 88% good and excellent function with 86% satisfaction rate. Talonavicular pseudarthrosis was present in 15% of the feet with only 1 that was asymptomatic. Radiographic evidence of arthritis was evident in 62% of the feet and 24% of the ankles.

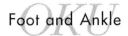

Chapter 8
Nerve Problems of the Foot and Ankle

Applied Surgical Anatomy and Anatomic Variations

Knowledge of the neurological anatomy about the foot and ankle is essential to planning and performing any surgical procedure. Despite a postoperative radiograph showing a perfect fracture reduction or solid arthrodesis, the outcome of the surgical procedure may be compromised if an incisional neuroma or neuropraxia results. Anatomic and surgical texts often show a single course of each nerve that may differ slightly between references. A review of the literature reveals that while some consistent anatomic nerve courses do prevail, there are numerous anatomic variations, particularly of the tibial, superficial peroneal, and sural nerves. An understanding of the applied surgical anatomy and potential anatomic variations is useful in planning incisions for surgical exposure or decompression and avoiding iatrogenic injury.

Superficial Peroneal Nerve
The superficial peroneal nerve provides sensation to the anterior lateral ankle and the dorsum of the foot. Common approaches for fracture fixation and arthroscopic portals place the nerve and its branches at risk. The nerve is typically described as a single branch coursing in the lateral compartment deep to the peroneus longus, then descending between the peroneus longus and brevis muscles, and exiting the crural fascia 12 to 15 cm above the level of the ankle, where it becomes subcutaneous. Two consistent branches arise, the medial and intermediate dorsal cutaneous that subsequently arborize to provide sensation to the dorsal aspect of the foot and toes, save the first web space.

Most commonly, the superficial peroneal nerve branches into the medial and intermediate dorsal cutaneous nerves after exiting the crural fascia approximately 4 to 5 cm above the ankle joint. However, in 25% to 30% of patients, the medial and intermediate dorsal cutaneous nerves arise independently from the superficial peroneal nerve and have unique exit sites from the lateral or even the anterior compartment. In this subset, the primary concern is the intermediate branch of the superficial peroneal nerve, which

penetrates the fascia of the lateral compartment 5 cm above the ankle joint. The nerve may course parallel to the anterior border of the fibula, or it may actually cross the fibula to reach the dorsum of the foot. Although the lateral approach to the fibula is frequently used for fracture fixation, clearly this common approach has the potential for iatrogenic nerve injury in a significant number of cases. These anatomic variations should also be considered when performing fasciotomies of the leg for compartment syndromes.

The dorsomedial cutaneous nerve provides sensation to the dorsomedial aspect of the great toe. A communicating branch to the deep peroneal nerve may also be present. The more lateral terminal branch provides sensation to the dorsolateral aspect of the second toe and the dorsomedial aspect of the third toe. The medial terminal branch originates either lateral or dorsal to the extensor hallucis longus (EHL) tendon and then crosses over the EHL. Distal to the first metatarsocuneiform joint, the nerve is consistently medial to the EHL. This nerve is frequently at risk during procedures about the first metatarsocuneiform and metatarsophalangeal joints.

Deep Peroneal Nerve
The deep peroneal nerve courses in the anterior compartment along with the anterior tibial artery. The position of the nerve is anterior to the vessels, although direct anterior, anteromedial, and anterolateral positions have been reported. The nerve bifurcates into lateral and medial terminal branches. The site of bifurcation has been reported above, at, or below the level of the mortise. Bifurcation just distal to the mortise is most common.

The lateral terminal branch provides motor function to the extensor digitorum brevis muscle. The medial terminal branch courses over the dorsum of the foot and is crossed by the tendon of the extensor hallucis brevis. An anastomosis from the superficial peroneal nerve may be present in approximately 30% of patients. The nerve bifurcates proximally to the first web space to provide sensation to this area.

Anterocentral arthroscopy portal placement has been associated with an unacceptably high incidence of injury to the deep peroneal nerve and the anterior tibial artery. While the plane between the extensor digitorum longus and the EHL

Tibial Nerve

Descending distally between the soleus and the posterior tibial muscle, the tibial nerve passes along the posterior aspect of the medial malleolus deep to the flexor retinaculum, where it divides into the medial and lateral plantar nerves. Proximal bifurcation of up to 14 cm above the medial malleolus has been demonstrated in 13% to 31% of specimens. Cadaveric studies have revealed multiple calcaneal branches that may originate from both the medial and lateral plantar nerves. Up to 70% of the time these calcaneal branches originate proximal to the tarsal tunnel. The so-called first branch of the lateral plantar nerve has received attention as a source of heel pain, with potential for entrapment between the deep fascia of the abductor hallucis muscle and the medial caudal margin of the medial head of the quadratus plantae muscle. Cadaveric dissection has indicated that injury to the medial or lateral plantar nerves could result with placement of intramedullary rods through the heel into the tibia, or with endoscopic plantar fascia release.

Saphenous Nerve

A terminal sensory branch of the femoral nerve, the saphenous nerve is the only nerve to provide sensation to the ankle and foot that is not of sciatic origin. After becoming subcutaneous between the tendons of the sartorius and gracilis muscles at the level of the knee, the nerve courses distally near the greater saphenous vein. Several medial crural cutaneous branches arise during its course. In the lower leg the terminal divisions pass anterior to the medial malleolus to provide sensation to the medial and dorsomedial aspect of the foot. Anteromedial arthroscopy portal placement and incisions about the anterior aspect of the medial malleolus place the saphenous nerve at risk.

Sural Nerve

While the origin of the sural nerve is fairly consistent, the terminal branching pattern is variable. The sural nerve originates 10 to 20 cm proximal to the tip of the lateral malleolus. The medial sural nerve originates from the tibial nerve, which courses between the heads of the gastrocnemius muscle to become subcutaneous in the distal third of the leg. It is joined at this level by the lateral sural nerve, which is a branch of the common peroneal nerve. The nerve runs adjacent to the lesser saphenous vein and is either anterior lateral or anterior medial to the vein. The nerve and vein are less closely associated below the level of the lateral malleolus.

The sural nerve is consistently located adjacent to the peritenon of the Achilles tendon at a distance of 7 to 10 cm above the tip of the malleolus. The sural nerve gives off a variable number of lateral calcaneal branches to provide sensation to the lateral and retrocalcaneal areas. Cadaveric specimens have shown 1 to 5 lateral calcaneal nerve branches. A lateral malleolar branch may form descending anteriorly at the tip of the malleolus. The sural nerve lies 10 to 15 mm below the tip of the fibula and below the sheath of the peroneal tendons, and it consistently crosses superficial to the peroneal tendons. The sural nerve then bifurcates and the lateral branch of the bifurcation bifurcates again about the base of the fifth metatarsal. Because of its small size and anatomic variations, the nerve is susceptible to iatrogenic injury from surgical approaches about the lateral aspect of the foot and ankle. Procedures about the Achilles tendon, the peroneal tendons, lateral ankle ligaments, sinus tarsi, and the fifth metatarsal all place the sural nerve at risk for problematic incisional neuromas.

Incisional Neuromas

Despite admonitions to avoid nerve injury, incisional neuromas are not infrequent. Most nerve injuries give rise to sensory disturbances or dysesthesia. Symptoms may range from negligible sensory loss to severe dysesthesia, possibly resulting in causalgia. Differential injections with local anesthetic are useful to determine which nerve is involved, and to possibly eliminate other sources of pain. A report on treatment of incisional neuroma on the dorsum of the foot described satisfactory results in 12 of 14 patients. Severed nerves resulting in stump neuromas were treated with proximal nerve resection. So called spindle neuromas, in which the nerve is enveloped in fibrous cicatrix, were treated with neurolysis. The sural nerve is most amenable to proximal resection, because the sensory loss is usually well tolerated and the nerve stump can be buried in the surrounding peroneal musculature. More proximal resection of the deep peroneal nerve will cause a motor deficit of the extensor digitorum brevis.

A recent report has advocated the use of a centrocentral anastomosis with autologous nerve graft for treatment of foot and ankle neuromas. This technique involves simple epineural repair of two cut nerve endings. An additional nerve transection and subsequent neurorrhaphy is made 5 to 10 mm proximal to the epineural repair. This in effect creates a loop, with axonal regeneration from both ends into the

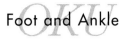
nerve graft. The concept is to prevent chaotic axonal sprouting, as regenerated axons grow into the graft but do not cross the contralateral suture line. Four of 5 patients showed definitive subjective and objective improvement with this technique. A patient with persistent symptoms following Morton's neuroma excision had the least improvement.

Peripheral Anesthesia for Foot and Ankle Surgery

Many surgical procedures about the foot and ankle can be performed using regional anesthetic techniques with or without the use of intravenous analgesia and amnesia. There are many potential advantages in the ambulatory setting; lower cost and increased patient satisfaction have been documented. Even when general anesthesia is used, placement of a peripheral nerve block is useful for postoperative pain relief. The agents administered for regional anesthesia typically include a combination of lidocaine and bupivacaine hydrochloride. The maximum safe dose of lidocaine without epinephrine should not exceed 4.5 mg/kg or a maximum total dose of 300 mg. The maximum safe dose of bupivacaine without epinephrine should not exceed 2.5 mg/kg. In a 70 kg adult, this amounts to a maximum dose of 35 ml of 0.5% bupivacaine and approximately 30 ml of 1% lidocaine. Because the toxic effects of these agents are additive, proportionate uses of these two compounds should not exceed the proportionate maximum safe dosages.

Digital Block
The technique of digital toe blockade is useful for procedures isolated to the digit, such as nail procedures, hammertoe repair, or fracture reduction. Injection of local anesthetic at the level of the web space on both sides of the toe blocks the common digital nerves to the toe. A portion of the injection is placed in the more dorsal and central soft tissues at the base of the toe to anesthetize the dorsal cutaneous nerves. Epinephrine should be used with caution, as the vasospasm produced may be associated with vascular embarrassment. Less than 5 cc of solution is usually sufficient to achieve a satisfactory block.

Ankle Block
Nearly all forefoot procedures and many mid- and hindfoot procedures can be performed using an ankle block. The published results of ankle blocks performed by orthopaedic surgeons have shown this to be an effective surgical anesthetic technique with minimal complications. Two series with a combined total of 1,650 patients reported frank fail-

ure of the block in only 5 cases. The combination of ankle block anesthetic and an ankle tourniquet has been reported to have a similar success rate. The technique involves blocking the major nerves at the level of the ankle. It may be possible to block only those nerves expected to innervate the operative field, however, a complete ankle block is preferred, particularly if an ankle tourniquet is used. The branches of the superficial peroneal nerve and the saphenous nerve lie in the subcutaneous tissue and can easily be anesthetized by a generous ring type of block about the anterior ankle. The sural nerve also lies in the subcutaneous tissue and is blocked several centimeters above the ankle. A subcutaneous injection between the anterior border of the Achilles tendon and the posterior border of the fibula is used. The deep peroneal nerve lies just lateral to the palpable dorsalis pedis pulse and is injected over the dorsum of the foot. The success of an ankle block is usually dependent on satisfactorily anesthetizing the tibial nerve. Because the nerve lies deep to the flexor retinaculum, a subcutaneous injection is of little value. The course of the nerve may be estimated by palpating the posterior tibial pulse behind the medial malleolus and injecting immediately behind this. Alternatively, one can inject from a more posterior direction several millimeters medial to the Achilles tendon. The needle is advanced until the tibia is reached, is slightly withdrawn, and then the injection is performed. Aspiration should be performed in this area prior to injection to make certain that an intravascular injection is avoided.

Popliteal Block
The use of sciatic nerve blockade in the popliteal area has been shown to be a very successful mode of regional anesthesia. This may be used as a primary anesthetic or administered perioperatively for postoperative pain management. Potential advantages of a more proximal block include increased volume of injection about the nerve and the ability to add epinephrine to prolong the block. The technique involves the use of a nerve stimulator and an insulated stimulating needle to isolate the nerve 7 to 8 cm above the popliteal crease. An injection of 30 ml of 0.5% bupivacaine with 1:200,000 epinephrine is injected in this area, where the sciatic nerve bifurcates into the common peroneal and tibial branches. The saphenous nerve may also be injected subcutaneously at the knee or ankle to ensure complete sensory block. The results of popliteal sciatic nerve block for postoperative anesthesia revealed a very high patient satisfaction rate and low use of postoperative narcotics. The average duration of the block has been shown to be 20 hours, with over 80% of patients experiencing relief between 12 and 28 hours.

Entrapment Neuropathies

Tarsal Tunnel Syndrome

Tarsal tunnel syndrome is a term used to describe the symptom complex associated with entrapment neuropathy of the tibial nerve or one of its terminal branches. While analogy to carpal tunnel syndrome in the upper extremity has been suggested, the only thing that is truly analogous is the similarity of the name. Carpal tunnel syndrome is common, easily diagnosed by clinical and electrodiagnostic means, and very responsive to release of the transverse carpal ligament. Tarsal tunnel syndrome is less common and lacks definite diagnostic criterion. The results of release have unfortunately not paralleled the results of carpal tunnel release.

The tarsal tunnel is a fibro-osseous tunnel bordered anteriorly by the tibia and laterally by the posterior process of the talus and the calcaneus. The flexor retinaculum courses over the contents of the tarsal tunnel, which include the tibial nerve, the posterior tibial artery and vein, and the tendons of the posterior tibialis, flexor hallucis longus, and flexor digitorum longus. The flexor retinaculum has attachments to the sheaths of each of these tendons. The proximal extent of the retinaculum may be up to 10 cm above the medial malleolus. The vascular supply to the nerves in the tarsal tunnel has recently been investigated. The tibial nerve and its lateral and medial plantar branches receive an abundant vascular supply and are unlikely to be susceptible to ischemia brought about by regional compression. However, in some cases, the vascular supply to a portion of the lateral plantar nerve may potentially be compromised or subject to compression. This may help to explain the relative greater frequency of lateral plantar nerve symptoms in tarsal tunnel syndrome.

Numerous causes of tarsal tunnel syndrome have been reported. Space-occupying lesions such as a ganglion, lipomas, or neurilemoma may result in increased pressure within the fibro-osseous tunnel. Varicosities or proliferative synovitis may also cause nerve compression. The anterolateral bony borders of the tunnel may also contribute to nerve compression. Tarsal tunnel syndrome has been associated with bony pathology, including talocalcaneal coalition, enlarged or displaced os trigonum, and nonunion of the sustentaculum tali following calcaneus fracture.

The clinical symptoms of tarsal tunnel syndrome are frequently diffuse and poorly localized. Patients may describe paresthesias, and they frequently complain of pain that is burning in nature. While some patients complain of pain over the posterior medial aspect of the ankle, it is common for them to complain of global pain in the foot. Symptoms are typically exacerbated by activity, however, some patients may complain of pain at night. Percussion over the nerve may result in recreation of symptoms or radiating paresthesias. Radiation may be present either into the plantar aspect of the foot or up the lower aspect of the leg. Gross sensory examination is typically normal. While longstanding dysfunction of the tibial nerve may lead to intrinsic weakness or atrophy, this is an unusual finding.

Because the symptoms are frequently poorly defined, electrodiagnostic testing has been used in an attempt to provide an objective measure of the problem. Recent literature has reported that electrodiagnostic studies are nearly 90% accurate in identifying tibial nerve entrapment. There has also been electrodiagnostic support for distal lateral plantar nerve entrapment in heel pain syndrome. Unfortunately, electrodiagnostic testing for tarsal tunnel syndrome has not been shown to correlate with intraoperative findings or ultimate clinical outcome. It should also be noted that a negative test does not preclude the clinical diagnosis of tarsal tunnel syndrome. Although the value of electrodiagnostic tests as a predictor of surgical outcome is unproved, they are potentially useful for identifying other sources of pain, such as radiculopathy or neuropathy. Plain film radiographs are useful to identify potential bony sources as a cause of symptoms. If a strong suspicion exists for a space-occupying lesion, a magnetic resonance imaging (MRI) scan can be useful. One study found that 88% of 40 feet with tarsal tunnel syndrome had identifiable MRI abnormalities.

For patients without evidence of a space-occupying lesion, conservative treatment should be tried initially. Nonsteroidal anti-inflammatory medication and local steroid injections may be used. If a pathologic postural abnormality is felt to be contributing to the symptom complex, an orthotic device can be used. A period of immobilization may be beneficial. For patients with a space-occupying lesion, surgery is typically recommended if the symptoms are severe. It is clear that the most favorable outcomes from release of the tarsal tunnel are in cases in which a space-occupying lesion exists. Symptomatic resolution or considerable improvement in symptoms should be expected if a source of increased volume, such as a ganglion, lipoma, or neurilemoma, is removed. One reported cause of tarsal tunnel syndrome is an anomalous muscle located deep to the flexor retinaculum. The results of posterior tibial nerve neurolysis and resection of the anomalous muscle have been less favorable than resection of other space-occupying lesions. In one series, pain reduction and patient satisfaction were reported in 4 of 6 patients, but only one patient was symptom free at follow up.

Release of the tarsal tunnel should include incision of the flexor retinaculum overlying the nerve. There is no established role for internal neurolysis, and avoiding significant dissection about the nerve has been suggested to protect its vascularity and minimize scarring. The extent of distal release has been debated, and an inadequate distal release of either the medial or lateral terminal nerve branches has been suggested as one reason for surgical failure. If a space-occupying lesion is present beneath the flexor retinaculum, it is unlikely that a distal release of either the medial or lateral plantar nerves is necessary. Medial tibial nerve entrapment may occur along the medial aspect of the foot at the fibromuscular tunnel formed by the tarsal navicular and the abductor hallucis muscle. Entrapment at the level of the knot of Henry has also been recognized. Entrapment of the lateral plantar nerve may occur as the nerve courses beneath the foot. Entrapment of the first branch of the lateral plantar nerve has been recognized as a potential source of heel pain. This nerve may be entrapped beneath the deep fascia of the abductor hallucis muscle in its course to innervate the abductor digiti quinti. If this is an isolated phenomenon, a local nerve release may be indicated. As the best chance for an optimal result is usually the index procedure, an extensile release of the posterior tibial nerve from the proximal aspect of the flexor retinaculum to the level beneath the abductor hallucis is recommended. If supported by preoperative clinical symptoms, further plantar dissection of the medial plantar nerve through the knot of Henry or the lateral plantar nerve beneath the plantar fascia may be considered.

From a review of the literature, satisfactory results are expected in 75% to 90% of patients who do not have a space-occupying mass. The results of a composite review of 24 articles comprising 122 patients who underwent tarsal tunnel release revealed that 69% of patients had complete resolution of symptoms, and another 22% had substantial improvement. However, the results of a recent study reviewing the clinical results after tarsal tunnel decompression were much less favorable. Only 14 of 32 feet (44%) had a good or excellent result. Nineteen percent had some continued pain and disability while 38% were clearly dissatisfied with the result, with no long-term pain relief. Of the 5 patients who were completely satisfied, 3 had some sort of space-occupying lesion. Despite the fact that 82% of patients with preoperative electromyograms (EMGs) demonstrated abnormalities consistent with the diagnosis of tarsal tunnel syndrome, there was no correlation between the clinical outcome and the EMG findings.

Failure following tarsal tunnel release may be secondary to an inadequate release or secondary to cicatrix formation about the nerve. Of course, it is possible that the pain may be from another source altogether. Patients with an additional, more proximal nerve lesion in the same lower extremity with coexistent tarsal tunnel syndrome have been shown to respond poorly to tibial nerve release. The clinical course fol-

lowing the initial operation may provide insight into the reason for persistence or recurrence of symptoms. An inadequate release may be indicated by the length and location of the incision as well as the patient's symptoms. The area of inadequate release is typically distal and may include the medial or lateral plantar nerves. For patients who initially do well, but who later develop recurrence of symptoms, scarring about the nerve may be the cause. This is a most difficult problem to treat, because simple removal of the scar and repeat neurolysis will likely have the same ultimate outcome. Preliminary investigation of nerve wrapping with autogenous vein grafts, or peripheral nerve stimulation may have potential merit, but the outcome of these modalities is unknown at this point.

The clinical results following revision tarsal tunnel release have provided insight into the difficult problem of persistent symptoms following tarsal tunnel surgery. In a report involving 13 revision tibial nerve releases, three distinct groups of patients were identified based on preoperative and intraoperative findings. The first group, consisting of 4 patients, had evidence of extensive scarring about the nerve, but an adequate distal release from the initial surgery. All patients in this group did poorly, with 1 patient ultimately having a below knee amputation secondary to chronic infection and intractable pain. A second group, of 5, had intraoperative evidence of significant nerve scarring, but also had an inadequate distal release requiring further decompression. The results of this group were somewhat mixed, but overall they were improved. The third group of 4 patients did not have significant scarring, but had evidence of inadequate distal release. All patients in this group did well. The authors summarized that revision tibial nerve epineurolysis is not recommended if the previous surgical procedure adequately released the tibial nerve and its distal branches. They cautioned that revision release in the face of abundant scarring has less predictable results.

The use of a radial forearm free flap has been reported in two patients who had recurrent tarsal tunnel syndrome as a result of scarring of the tibial nerve. It is hypothesized that the pliable vascular tissue over the nerve may provide a suitable bed which may limit scar formation. While both patients were reported to be pain free at follow up, a larger study group is needed before this can be universally recommended.

Anterior Tarsal Tunnel Syndrome
The term anterior tarsal tunnel has been used to describe the relatively rare entrapment neuropathy of the deep peroneal nerve. The nerve may be compressed anywhere along its course by both intrinsic and extrinsic sources. Potential sites of entrapment include the inferomedial band or super-

omedial band of the extensor retinaculum, or the tendon of the extensor hallucis brevis muscle. Mechanical irritation can also occur from ganglia, degenerative osteophytes, or from an os intermetatarseum, and can be exacerbated by extrinsic forces, such as tight-fitting or lace-up shoe wear, or ski boots. Crush injuries to the dorsum of the foot frequently lead to irritability of the deep peroneal nerve. This may be from neuropraxia as the result of the crush as well as swelling or constriction of the surrounding anatomy in the perineural region.

Symptoms of entrapment vary depending on whether the deep peroneal nerve proper, the lateral terminal branch, or the medial terminal branch is involved. The entrapment may be purely sensory if only the medial terminal branch is involved, but more proximal entrapment can affect the motor branch to the extensor digitorum brevis muscle and cause weakness of the short toe extensors or pain referred to the sinus tarsi region. It should be noted that while weakness, atrophy, or EMG findings consistent with extensor digitorum brevis dysfunction may be noted, a terminal branch of the superficial peroneal nerve has been demonstrated to innervate this muscle in 22% of patients.

Patients may complain of neuritic pain along the course of the nerve, and these may be subtle sensory changes in the first web space. Evaluation should include plain radiographs to rule out bony pathology as a contributing factor. Electrodiagnostic testing may be helpful in determining the level of entrapment by examining the extensor digitorum brevis muscle. This may also identify other sources of nerve dysfunction, such as radiculopathy or peripheral neuropathy. Sensory nerve conduction velocities can be compared to the contralateral foot and may be useful in establishing a diagnosis.

Local anesthetic injection combined with corticosteroid may be of both diagnostic and therapeutic value. Temporary improvement or relief of symptoms should be expected from the local anesthetic. If no relief is obtained, the diagnosis should be questioned. Patients should be counseled to avoid constrictive shoe wear, which can cause extrinsic pressure on the nerve. For patients refractory to conservative measures, decompression of the nerve may be warranted. If the source of entrapment is at the level of the ankle, division of the extensor retinaculum alone or in combination with removal of offending osteophytes has been shown to result in symptomatic relief. The results of release of the nerve over the dorsum of the foot have been described. In addition to neurolysis of the nerve, excision of a section of the extensor hallucis brevis tendon as it crosses over the nerve was advocated. Excellent or good results were obtained in 80% of patients. Of the 4 patients that did not improve, one did not have incision or

excision of the extensor hallucis brevis tendon, one had a surgically identifiable neuroma as the result of a crush injury, and two had painful neuropathy from diabetes. It was recommended that the finding of a true neuroma was an indication for resection rather than simple decompression. Additionally, patients with sensorimotor neuropathy were not considered good candidates for this procedure.

Superficial Peroneal Nerve Entrapment
Neuritis of the superficial peroneal nerve may be associated with direct trauma, ankle sprains and instability, fibular fracture, or ganglia. Entrapment of the superficial peroneal nerve may occur as the nerve becomes subcutaneous, as it pierces the crural fascia 12 cm to 15 cm above the level of the ankle. Superficial peroneal nerve symptoms may accompany exertional compartment syndromes of the anterior and lateral compartments. Muscle herniation through the fascial defect has also been reported to be associated with nerve entrapment. Physical examination typically reveals pain over the nerve exit site, and, in a few patients, a muscle bulge may be palpated. Sensory dysesthesias over the course of the nerve on the dorsum of the foot may be elicited. Local steroid injection and activity modifications may prove useful. For refractory cases, neurolysis with compartment fasciotomy is recommended. Instability of the lateral ankle ligaments may also be addressed if this is felt to be a contributory factor.

Sural Nerve Entrapment
Entrapment of the sural nerve is exceedingly rare and typically occurs as the result of traumatic bony pathology or an associated ganglion. An aponeurotic band of the Achilles tendon causing sural nerve entrapment has also been described. Potential sites of involvement from fracture include the lateral malleolus, calcaneus, an os peroneum, or the fifth metatarsal base. Nonsurgical treatment includes shoe wear modifications and local corticosteroid injection. Surgery may be indicated for decompression of the nerve and to address the underlying bony or soft-tissue pathology. If a traumatic neuroma is found at time of surgery, proximal transection outside of the zone of injury and burying of the proximal segment in muscle is recommended.

Plantar Interdigital Neuroma

Plantar interdigital neuroma, frequently referred to as Morton's neuroma, is generally thought to result from entrapment of the common digital nerve as it passes beneath the transverse metatarsal ligament. With dorsiflexion of the toes, the nerve is thought to compress beneath the distal aspect of the ligament. However, as the incidence is 8 to 10 times greater in females than males, extrinsic sources, such as shoes with a constricting toe box and high heels, obviously play a significant role in the development of pathology. Although previously thought to involve predominantly the third web space, second and third web space involvement has been reported to be similar. This has been supported by both clinical and cadaveric studies. Interdigital neuroma of the first and fourth web space is exceedingly rare.

That this is an entrapment neuropathy is supported by studies, which demonstrate that the histology of the nerve proximal to the transverse intermetatarsal ligament is normal and that changes in the nerve are distal to the ligament. Fusiform swelling of the nerve may be present, and it is from this morphologic appearance that the term "neuroma" was derived. Histologic examination of the involved nerve reveals sclerosis and edema of the endoneurium, thickening and hyalinization of the endoneural vessels, perineural thickening and fibrosis, and demyelinization and degeneration of nerve fibers.

Other factors may contribute to or cause symptoms associated with plantar interdigital neuroma. As the common digital nerve to the third web space may receive contributions from both the medial and lateral plantar nerves, it has been speculated that the nerve may have increased thickness or be subject to tethering. However, 1 cadaveric study failed to support an increased incidence of third web space neuroma formation based on a communicating digital nerve branch. A communicating branch was absent in over 73% of the 71 cadaveric feet dissected. Data from that study revealed that the relative space in the metatarsal head/transverse metatarsal ligament region was smaller in web spaces 2 and 3, supporting the notion that mechanical factors are contributory to interdigital neuroma formation. Other factors that may play a role in the development of symptoms include trauma, angular deviation of the toe, or inflammation of the bursa that overlies the transverse intermetatarsal ligament.

The symptom complex in patients with plantar interdigital neuroma typically consists of pain located on the plantar aspect of the foot at or just distal to the level of the metatarsal heads. Patients often describe a neuritic, burning type of pain with radiation into the affected toes, or less often proximally along the plantar aspect of the foot. Symptoms are typically worse with activity and with shoe wear, particularly shoes that are tight across the forefoot, or with heels having heights that require significant toe dorsiflexion. Physical examination should reveal tenderness in the plantar web space area, occasionally with reproduction of the radiating pain out into the toe. The metatarsophalangeal joints should be carefully palpated and ruled out as the source of the symptoms. With

compression of the foot in a medial-lateral direction, recreation of symptoms may occur accompanied by a palpable click (Mulder's sign). A mass, such as a ganglion or synovial cyst, may occasionally be palpated.

While the diagnosis of interdigital neuroma is based on history and careful clinical examination, the use of soft-tissue imaging techniques to make or confirm the diagnosis has been advocated by some authors. Electrodiagnostic sensory action potentials have not proven to be useful in the diagnosis of plantar interdigital neuroma. Ultrasonography has been shown by one group to have a very high predictive value, accurately predicting the presence, size, and location in 98% of 55 neuromas without any false positives. Another smaller study presented similar results in 8 patients with clinically diagnosed interdigital neuromas unresponsive to conservative measures. Sonography revealed a round or oval echogenic mass that was confirmed at surgery in all cases with no false positives. Normal digital nerves and the transverse metatarsal ligament are not identified in normal subjects using a 7.5 MHz transducer. The exact role of more expensive imaging such as MRI is unclear at this point. While useful for soft-tissue imaging, one study reported a high incidence of false negatives using both ultrasound and MRI. It should be noted that the MRI resolution used in this study was relatively low, and not comparable to high resolution scanners. The optimal sequence for MRI evaluation continues to be debated in the radiology literature, as conventional images, even with high resolution scanners, may not satisfactorily image the pathology. These imaging techniques assume that symptoms from interdigital neuroma are associated with macroscopic morphological changes in the nerve. Although several studies have shown few false negatives and have advocated MRI to assist in the diagnosis as well as offer alternative diagnoses (ie, stress fracture, ganglion), its routine use cannot be recommended.

Initial treatment of an interdigital neuroma is nonsurgical and may involve relatively simple measures. Patients should be counseled to avoid shoes that constrict the forefoot, or elevated heels that require dorsiflexion of the metatarsophalangeal joints. Metatarsal padding may also be used in an attempt to relieve pressure beneath the metatarsal head area. A prospective randomized study investigated the use of pronation and supination orthoses in patients clinically diagnosed with Morton's neuroma. The hypothesis was that potential restriction of subtalar joint pronation would limit hypermobility of the metatarsals and reduce stresses across the forefoot. The results of this study failed to show any significant effect of the orthoses in the 33 patients enrolled in the study. The authors suggested that some placebo effect may exist, but they questioned the significance of excessive foot pronation as the cause of Morton's neuroma.

Corticosteroid injections have been shown to be of value in the nonsurgical treatment of interdigital neuroma. When combined with local anesthetic, the injection may be of diagnostic value in helping to confirm the diagnosis and determine the degree of pain reduction in the immediate post-injection period. An investigation studied the results of a single webspace injection for treatment of third webspace interdigital neuroma. Eighty percent reported benefit from the injection, and 46% had relief longer than 3 months. Forty-seven percent ultimately required surgical excision, and the majority of those who did not undergo surgery continued to have symptoms. The authors concluded that a single corticosteroid injection may be temporizing but not curative. A successful surgical result was not precluded by the injection. The results of multiple corticosteroid injections (average, 3.8) performed in 1 or more web spaces over a 1- to 3-week period have been reported. Fourteen percent had total relief after 1 injection, and 30% experienced total relief after 4 or more injections. Another 50% experienced significant partial pain relief with multiple injections. Results actually improved over time, and, at 2-year follow-up, 60% of patients had complete relief and 29% had slight residual pain. Potential side effects of corticosteroid injections in this area include the possibility of skin and fat atrophy as well as altered pigmentation at the injection site.

When symptoms become refractory to conservative measures, surgical excision of the neuroma through a dorsal incision is most frequently recommended. The main advantage of the dorsal approach is that it avoids scar formation on the plantar aspect of the foot. It should be noted that the use of a plantar approach does have many advocates, and satisfactory results and high patient satisfaction have been reported. A large series reported on the use of 172 plantar incisions in 137 patients for a variety of problems including excision of interdigital neuromas and stump neuromas. The satisfaction rate with regard to the plantar incision was 96%. Four patients were dissatisfied secondary to incisional tenderness or incisional punctate keratosis. No long-term problems with hypertrophic scarring, wound healing, or severe tenderness were reported. The authors did state that they felt a plantar incision was unwise in patients with hyperkeratotic plantar skin.

Regardless of the choice of approach, the nerve must be transected well proximal to the weightbearing metatarsal heads or painful stump neuroma symptoms may develop, leading to surgical failure. The existence of multiple plantarly directed branches have been observed in cadaveric dissection, and it is hypothesized that these could prevent proximal nerve retraction following transection. An accessory nerve branch may anastomose with the common digital nerve from either a medial or lateral direction. If cut during resection of the common digital nerve, this accessory branch may retract beneath the weightbearing metatarsal head region, potentially resulting in a painful stump neuroma. Suture of this accessory nerve branch to the side of the metatarsal has been recommended to prevent this potential problem.

Unfortunately, the reported rate of surgical failure for resection of plantar interdigital neuroma is in the range of 15%. This may be secondary to inaccurate diagnosis, improper web space selection, or formation of painful stump neuroma. In patients who never really obtain significant relief from their index procedure, it is unlikely that stump neuroma formation is the source of their pain. When the diagnosis indicates painful stump neuroma, it may be addressed by more proximal resection from either a plantar or dorsal approach. The published results of both approaches are similar, resulting in symptomatic improvement in 75% to 80%. The use of a plantar approach has been advocated, as it allows more proximal dissection through a previously unoperated field. Patients should be counseled that, despite the approach used, the published results of re-exploration document continued discomfort in more than 50% of patients.

Recognizing that plantar interdigital neuroma may in fact represent an entrapment neuropathy, some authors have recommended division of the transverse intermetatarsal ligament and simple neurolysis rather than surgical excision. A recently published report indicated a very high patient satisfaction rate (98%) with this procedure. Seventeen of 35 patients demonstrated complete pain relief and 12 of 35 reported minimal discomfort with activity. Preoperative relief of symptoms with local lidocaine injection was found to correlate with postoperative symptom relief. This procedure avoids potential painful stump or recurrent neuroma formation and does not preclude neuroma resection in the future.

The incidence of adjacent or multiple interdigital neuromas in the same foot appears to be quite low. In fact, skepticism has been raised about the existence of such. In patients with Morton's neuroma, the reported incidence of two primary interdigital neuromas ranges from 1.5% to 4%. Some authors have suggested that adjacent web space exploration is unwarranted, and the use of diagnostic web space injections can help to delineate the source of the pathology. The results of simultaneous adjacent interdigital neurectomy have been reported in a series of 19 feet in 15 patients. Eighty-four percent of patients had complete symptom resolution (53%) or minimal residual symptoms (31%). Reported sequelae of the procedure, dense sensory loss of the plantar aspect of the third metatarsal head to the tip of the third toe, was recognized in 9 of 15 patients. Although not encountered, poten-

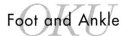

tial vascular embarrassment of the toe could occur if the vascular supply on each side of the toe was injured. In an effort to lessen the dorsal sensory loss, a single curved dorsal incision was found to be preferable to two longitudinal dorsal web space incisions. The overall improvement of 84% in this study is similar to results reported for resection of a single web space neuroma. Although it was not performed in this study, the authors suggested that in cases where adjacent interdigital neuromas occur, resection of the larger neuroma and transverse metatarsal ligament release and neurolysis in the adjacent web space may be considered to avoid desensitization of the toe.

Reflex Sympathetic Dystrophy

The symptom complex that comprises reflex sympathetic dystrophy (RSD) was first reported following peripheral nerve injuries as the result of gunshot wounds in American Civil War soldiers. Causalgia, initially termed "erythromelalgia," was described as chronic burning pain with associated hyperalgesia, allodynia, temperature and trophic changes of the affected extremity. Sudek later described a related condition without associated nerve injury calling it inflammatory bone atrophy secondary to associated patchy osteoporosis. Reflex sympathetic dystrophy syndrome is a term that has been used to include a group of disorders including RSD and causalgia. A multitude of authors have attempted to define the diagnosis, classification, and treatment of this complicated pain phenomenon. Unfortunately, this has resulted in a variety of confusing names for a confusing problem.

In 1986, the International Association for the Study of Pain (IASP) subcommittee on taxonomy attempted to defined RSD and causalgia. While the symptom complex of RSD and causalgia are similar, causalgia is distinguished by a definable associated injury or trauma to a peripheral nerve. In 1993, the IASP coined the term complex regional pain syndrome (CRPS), subdividing it into 2 forms. CRPS type I refers to RSD in describing a complex disorder or group of disorders that may develop as a consequence of trauma without any obvious nerve lesion. CRPS type II refers to causalgia in defining a similar symptom complex. However, a definable nerve injury or trauma differentiates this from CRPS type I. Pain management specialists are a critical part of the multidisciplinary approach to this problem, and it is important to understand the taxonomy used by their profession. Whether or not this distinction has therapeutic or prognostic implications is not known.

RSD is typically thought to have 3 fairly distinct stages. While an overlap of stages may occur in patients with a mixed clinical presentation, determining the stage may be useful in estimating prognosis and treatment options. The first or acute stage occurs following an antecedent injurious stimulus, but onset may be delayed for days to weeks. This stage is typically hyperemic with hyperpathia, allodynia, and pain of a burning nature. Demineralization of bone begins to develop after the first month. The second phase usually occurs 2 to 4 months following onset of symptoms. This phase is dystrophic and ischemic. Hyperpathia and allodynia persist, and swelling may become firm with the early development of contractures. Hyperhidrosis and cyanosis give way to dryness and pallor, which become prominent in this stage. This stage may last for 6 months. The third phase, described as atrophic, is associated with subcutaneous atrophy, muscle atrophy, joint stiffness, and muscle contracture. While hyperpathia may lessen, diffuse burning pain may persist. Blood flow may show normalization, but the skin is often dry and cool with a glossy appearance. In addition to the physiologic changes, psychological changes may also develop. Anxiety, depression, and hopelessness may accompany the chronic pain personality.

The diagnosis of RSD may be suggested in the posttraumatic or postsurgical setting when the magnitude of the subjective complaints seems to be discordant or out of proportion to the objective findings. Swelling, stiffness, and discoloration may accompany and also be out of proportion to that expected with the trauma or disease. The use of 3-phase radionuclide bone scanning has been reported to be extremely sensitive in establishing the diagnosis of RSD of the foot. Patients with RSD have been shown to demonstrate a characteristic delayed bone-scan pattern consisting of diffuse increased tracer throughout the foot, with juxta-articular accentuation of tracer uptake. In evaluating a patient with possible RSD, a dynamic assessment of the lower extremity can be useful to examine the thermoregulatory capacity in a stressed state and confirm the diagnosis. Isolated cold stress testing applies a cold thermal stress to an extremity and uses the skin surface temperature as an index of blood flow. Abnormal thermoregulation is evidenced by asymmetric responses in the extremities to isolated cold stress testing.

Early recognition of the diagnosis and institution of treatment are critical. Presumably with early recognition and treatment, the course of the disease may be altered so that the degree of symptoms is decreased and irreversible trophic changes can be lessened or avoided. A multidisciplinary approach that includes the use of physical therapy, pharmacotherapy, and sympathetic blocks should be instituted. Physical therapy should include desensitization in addition to both active and passive assisted exercises, although excessively painful stimuli should be avoided. Desensitization in the form of massage, contrast baths, whirlpool, and transcutaneous electrical nerve stimulation has been advocated. Patients should also perform manual desensitization of the extremity themselves. Edema control with the use of a compression garment may also be useful. The psychological component of this symptom complex may also benefit from counseling as a component of the comprehensive approach.

A number of pharmacological interventions have been advocated in the treatment of RSD. Nonsteroidal anti-inflammatories, calcium channel blockers, alpha and beta andrenergic blocking drugs, serotonin antagonists, and antidepressants have all been used with varying degrees of success. Because of the risk of tolerance in the face of a chronic pain syndrome, the use of narcotics should be minimized. The use of sympathetic blockade has been shown to be the most effective treatment for RSD. If no relief of symptoms is obtained by interruption of the sympathetic efferent impulses to the affected limb, the diagnosis must be questioned. A series of lumbar sympathetic blocks is used in conjunction with physical therapy. Regional Bier blocks using guanethidine, reserpine, or bretylium have been used in some centers. In chronic recalcitrant cases, implantable peripheral nerve stimulators as well as dorsal column stimulators have been used, but typically are reserved as a last resort.

Annotated Bibliography

Surgical Anatomy and Anatomic Variations

Santi MD, Botte MJ: Nerve injury and repair in the foot and ankle. *Foot Ankle Int* 1996;17:425–439.

A recent comprehensive reference on surgical anatomy and nerve repair with an extensive bibliography.

Incisional Neuromas

Lidor C, Hall RL, Nunley JA: Centrocentral anastomosis with autologous nerve graft treatment of foot and ankle neuromas. *Foot Ankle Int* 1996;17:85–88.

Describes the concepts and technique of this newly applied approach to traumatic neuromas in the foot and ankle.

Peripheral Anesthesia for Foot and Ankle Surgery

Lee TH, Wapner KL, Hecht PJ, Hunt PJ: Regional anesthesia in foot and ankle surgery. *Orthopedics* 1996;19:577–580.

The technique and success of ankle block are outlined in this report.

Rongstad K, Mann RA, Prieskorn D, Nichelson S, Horton G: Popliteal sciatic nerve block for postoperative analgesia. *Foot Ankle Int* 1996;17:378–382.

The technique of popliteal block is described. Lasting postoperative pain relief was reported in this series.

Entrapment Neuropathies

Beskin JL: Nerve entrapment syndromes of the foot and ankle. *J Am Acad Orthop Surg* 1997;5:261–269.

This recent review article discusses nerve compression syndromes and surgical treatment.

Tarsal Tunnel Syndrome

Sammarco GJ, Chalk DE, Feibel JH: Tarsal tunnel syndrome and additional nerve lesions in the same limb. *Foot Ankle* 1993;14:71–77.

Patients with an additional proximal lesion were shown to respond poorly to tarsal tunnel release.

Skalley TC, Schon LC, Hinton RY, Myerson MS: Clinical results following revision tibial nerve release. *Foot Ankle Int* 1994;15:360–367.

Poor results were reported with revision release when a previous complete release of the tibial nerve and its branches was complicated by nerve scarring. Satisfactory results were obtained if the previous release was inadequate, particularly if no significant scarring was present.

Plantar Interdigital Neuroma: Diagnosis and Nonoperative Treatment

Greenfield J, Rea J Jr, Ilfeld FW: Morton's interdigital neuroma: Indications for treatment by local injections versus surgery. *Clin Orthop* 1984;185:142–144.

Corticosteroid injections were shown to have a beneficial effect with 60% of patients reporting no pain and 29% reporting minimal residual symptoms at 2 years.

Rasmussen MR, Kitaoka HB, Patzer GL: Nonoperative treatment of plantar interdigital neuroma with a single corticosteroid injection. *Clin Orthop* 1996;326:188–193.

A single steroid injection was shown to be beneficial but not curative. The injection did not preclude a successful surgical result.

Shapiro PP, Shapiro SL: Sonographic evaluation of interdigital neuromas. *Foot Ankle Int* 1995;16:604–606.

This article supports the use of ultrasound in the evaluation of plantar interdigital neuromas and documents a high correlation with surgical findings.

Plantar Interdigital Neuroma: Surgical Treatment

Alexander IJ, Johnson KA, Parr JW: Morton's neuroma: a review of recent concepts. *Orthopedics* 1987;10:103–106.

A review article which details the pathology, histology, and results of treatment.

Amis JA, Siverhus SW, Liwnicz BH: An anatomic basis for recurrence after Morton's neuroma excision. *Foot Ankle* 1992;13:153–156.

This article highlights plantar branches of the digital nerve which may potentially tether the nerve and cause persistent symptoms following neurectomy.

Beskin JL, Baxter DE: Recurrent pain following interdigital neurectomy: A plantar approach. *Foot Ankle* 1988;9:34–39.

The results of a plantar approach were equivalent to the use of a dorsal approach. Potential benefits include an unoperated surgical field and the ability to trace the nerve proximally. Despite the approach, 50% of patients still have complaints of continued discomfort.

Richardson EG, Brotzman SB, Graves SC: The plantar incision for procedures involving the forefoot: An evaluation of one hundred and fifty incisions in one hundred and fifteen patients. *J Bone Joint Surg* 1993;75A:726–731.

This large series reports successful use of a plantar incision for a number of forefoot problems. Minimal complications were reported.

Flanigan DC, Cassell M, Saltzman CL: Vascular supply of nerves in the tarsal tunnel. *Foot Ankle Int* 1997;18:288–292.

Galardi G, Amadio S, Maderna L, et al: Electrophysiologic studies in tarsal tunnel syndrome: Diagnostic reliability of motor distal latency, mixed nerve and sensory nerve conduction studies. *Am J Phys Med Rehabil* 1994;73:193–198.

Lawrence SJ, Botte MJ: The sural nerve in the foot and ankle: An anatomic study with clinical and surgical implications. *Foot Ankle Int* 1994;15:490–494.

Levitsky KA, Alman BA, Jevsevar DS, Morehead J: Digital nerves of the foot: Anatomic variations and implications regarding the pathogenesis of interdigital neuroma. *Foot Ankle* 1993; 14:208–214.

Seale KS: Reflex sympathetic dystrophy of the lower extremity. *Clin Orthop* 1989;243:80–85.

Stanton-Hicks M: Complex regional pain syndrome: A new name for reflex sympathetic dystrophy and causalgia. *Curr Rev Pain* 1996;1:34–40.

Stanton-Hicks M, Janig W, Hassenbusch S, Haddox JD, Boas R, Wilson P: Reflex sympathetic dystrophy: Changing concepts and taxonomy. *Pain* 1995;63:127–133.

Classic Bibliography

Adkison DP, Bosse MJ, Gaccione DR, Gabriel KR: Anatomical variations in the course of the superficial peroneal nerve. *J Bone Joint Surg* 1991;73A:112–114.

Cimino WR: Tarsal tunnel syndrome: Review of the literature. *Foot Ankle* 1990;11:47–52.

Davis TJ, Schon LC: Branches of the tibial nerve: Anatomic variations. *Foot Ankle Int* 1995;16:21–29.

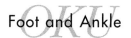

Chapter 9
The Insensate Foot

Introduction

The insensate foot remains a significant challenge to the practicing orthopaedic surgeon. This insensitivity is attributed to a variety of causes, including peripheral neuropathies, leprosy, tabes dorsalis, and diabetes mellitus. Diabetes is the most common cause of peripheral neuropathies in the Western world, and it will be the primary focus of this chapter. Attributes of the pathophysiology, peripheral neuropathy, and angiopathy, as well as new advances in the detection and treatment of the insensate foot, also will be presented. Education, which is the chief cornerstone to the prevention of ulcers and other sequelae of the insensate foot, will also be discussed.

Epidemiology

The American Diabetic Association estimate that in the United States there are 14 million individuals with diabetes; the condition is undiagnosed in approximately 50% of these individuals. It is well recognized that as the age of the general population increases, the incidence of diabetes, particularly type II diabetes, also increases.

The cost of diabetes and the rates of major amputation in the United States remain high, in part because present knowledge regarding the prevention and management of foot disease is not widely applied in clinical practice. The increased cost for home care and social services were a main part of the total cost, averaging between 45% and 57% each year. Recently, a Swedish study noted the annual cost per patient for home care and social services is $17,900 after a minor amputation and $34,700 after a major amputation.

Foot and ankle complications remain the most common diagnosis for which patients with diabetes are admitted to hospitals, and these complications are the leading cause of amputation. The long-term mortality in patients with diabetes who have foot ulcers has been estimated to be increased twofold compared to their sex- and age-matched nondiabetic counterparts. Vascular disease is 30 times more common and the incidence of gangrene is 70 times more common in patients with diabetes than among the general population. The risk of peripheral vascular disease increases with the duration of diabetes. Over 50,000 amputations related to diabetes are performed in the United States each year, representing a significant morbidity and mortality; in patients with diabetes, 30% of amputees lose their contralateral limb within 3 years, and, following the amputation of a leg, nearly two thirds of these patients die within 5 years.

The severity of diabetes-related complications is not related to disease severity. In fact, patients with the milder form of diabetes, noninsulin-dependent (type II), have more complications than patients with insulin-dependent type I diabetes. In another Swedish study, the prevalence of current and prior foot ulcers was 2% in the type I patients and 10% in the type II patients. Age-adjusted risk for lower extremity amputation has been reported to be 15 to 40 times higher in patients with diabetes than in normal patients. In 1990, National Hospital Discharge Data indicated that in 54,000 patients with diabetes, at least 1 extremity had been amputated. The actual number of patients in the United States undergoing at least 1 nontraumatic diabetes-related amputation per year increased 70% from 1979 to 1990.

Demographics

Specific studies have reported elevated risk for amputation among males with diabetes, ranging from 1.4 to 2.7 times greater than their female counterparts. A higher rate of amputation also exists among blacks than in whites, and amputation rates tend to be lower in the western United States and generally higher in the northeast. In 1986, chronic skin ulcers alone accounted for $150 million of the $1.6 million in direct costs related to type II diabetes mellitus.

Atherosclerosis obliterans, as indicated by the presence of intermittent claudication, was reported in the Framingham study to be 3.8 and 6.5 times more common in males and females with diabetes, respectively. Cigarette smoking, lipoprotein abnormalities, and hypertension are major alterable risk factors that have been implicated in the development of atherosclerosis in normal subjects and are assumed to be similarly atherogenic in patients with diabetes. Smoking was a statistically significant risk factor for amputation in an Indianapolis study but these data have been contraindicated in other studies. Lipoprotein abnormalities, including elevated plasma triglyceride levels, may be more prevalent among diabetic individuals.

Many investigators have postulated that the presence of chronic hyperglycemia accelerates the development of the chronic complications of diabetes. Among patients with diabetes and higher blood glucose levels, a twofold increased risk of leg lesions, including gangrene, was noted as compared to patients with lower blood glucose concentrations. Studies demonstrate statistically significant increased amputation risk with elevated plasma glucose levels.

Pathophysiology

Fifteen percent of all patients with diabetes will develop a foot ulcer during their lifetime. Peripheral vascular disease is present and the diagnosis made in 8% of new onset diabetic patients, in 15% after 10 years, and in 42% after 20 years. Thus, peripheral vascular disease is not considered to be the primary cause of foot ulcers.

Peripheral Neuropathy

The most common syndromes that involve the foot are the distal, symmetric, sensory, and motor polyneuropathies. These result in pain, paresthesias, muscle atrophy, loss of sensation, and autonomic neuropathy, with dry, scaly feet, radiculopathy, and entrapment syndrome. Peripheral neuropathy in the patient with diabetes is not always a secondary occurrence, and other causes, such as alcoholism, herniated nucleus pulposus, heavy metals, vitamin deficiencies, and malignancies, should be considered. The incidence of polyneuropathy in the patient with diabetes is estimated to be over 80% in those with foot lesions, regardless of the length of time one has had diabetes.

The etiology of diabetic neuropathy is not clearly understood. Changes within the vasonervorum and the resulting ischemia to the nerve have been seen in autopsy studies. One hypothesis implicates the accumulation of sorbitol within these feeding vessels, which impedes oxygen transport. Another hypothesis implicates intraneural accretion of advanced products of glycosylation. Although attempts have been made to block the biochemical pathways to sorbitol synthesis, the neuropathy has remained an essentially irreversible process. This neuropathic phenomenon includes all three neural systems: sensory, autonomic, and motor.

Sensory Neuropathy

Sensory deficits and symptoms, which generally predominate over motor involvement in diabetic neuropathies, appear first in the most distal portions of the extremities and progress proximally in a "stocking" distribution. Loss of large sensory fibers diminishes light touch and proprioception, whereas involvement of small fibers diminishes pain and temperature perception, leading to repeated injury, especially to the feet. Typical neuropathic paresthesias or dysesthesias may accompany either large or small fiber involvement. Sensations may include burning, stabbing pain, or a deep ache. The sensation of numbness, cold, or "dead feet" is sometimes elicited. Patients may begin to lose deep tendon reflexes and vibratory sense and proprioception. It is important to document the amount of sensory loss qualitatively and quantitatively in order to track the natural history of the deficit. This will be discussed in greater detail.

An active injury, along with a sensory neuropathy, received by a bare foot is required to produce ulceration. The theory of repetitive stress notes that a moderate level of stress, which is acceptable for a few repetitions, may be harmful when continued for a long period of time. When a tissue becomes injured, the inflammatory response with resultant hyperemia develops. If the irritation continues, the tissue is damaged, with subsequent ulceration. Once there is an opening in the skin, infection may occur, with the potential for significant complications.

Dorsal ulcerations are a product of a shoe exerting too much pressure on the dorsum of a foot. Such pressure can produce ulcerations in as little as 1 hour.

Autonomic Neuropathy

The autonomic system is responsible for control of the eccrine and apocrine glands in the extremity. These glands, along with the vascular control at the arterial level, control the limbs' thermoregulation and the normal hyperemic responses needed to fight infection. With the loss of this system, there is loss of normal sweating and skin temperature regulation. The skin becomes dry, scaly, and stiff, and it cracks easily, which opens pores for bacterial invasion.

Motor Neuropathy

Intrinsic muscle atrophy results in a gradual dorsiflexion of the toes with a distal migration of the plantar cushion, thus making the plantar forefoot more susceptible to injury. The metatarsophalangeal joints are hyperextended and the proximal interphalangeal joints are hyperflexed. The flexion contractures at the proximal interphalangeal joints can cause pressure of the dorsal aspect of the toe against the type of toe box of the shoe. Subsequently, this pressure can lead to ulcerations on top of the toes in addition to increased pressure areas on the plantar aspect of the metatarsal head. Motor neuropathy can involve a single proximal nerve, such as the common peroneal nerve, resulting in a unilateral foot drop.

Patient Evaluation

Examination for the insensate foot necessitates removal of shoes, stockings, pantyhose, and trousers so that the examination can extend to the level of the knees. Both feet should be examined in comparison. Patients with insensate feet should have them examined at least 4 times per year by an orthopaedist and 3 times daily in self-examination. Examination of patient data would indicate that the 5.07 Semmes-Weinstein monofilament test demonstrates the appropriate level of protection against neuropathic ulceration (Fig. 1). However, up to 10% of patients who meet this threshold criteria of protection still may experience skin breakdown.

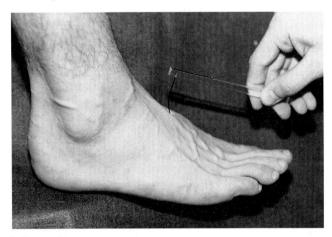

Figure 1

A 5.07 Semmes-Weinstein monofilament is demonstrated. Ten grams of pressure is exerted on the skin when the filament buckles as shown.

Vascular Evaluation

Because would healing depends directly on local blood flow, the adequacy of local circulation is paramount. In addition to evaluation for pulses, the limb should be observed for dependent rubor, varicose veins, shiny atrophic skin, pallor on elevation, and delayed capillary filling time. The femoral, popliteal, dorsalis pedis, and posterior tibial pulses should all be palpated, and auscultation for bruits can sometimes identify the presence of atheromatous plaques. Skin temperature is also noted at the time pulses are palpated. If the pulses are nonpalpable, vascular screening with Doppler ultrasound may be indicated. Doppler data are expressed as both absolute pressure and a ratio of foot and ankle pressures to brachial Doppler arterial pressure. Pressures are measured using pneumatic tourniquets at least 1.5 times the circumference of the limb, and readings are taken with Doppler probes. A ratio of 0.45 or greater is necessary to heal an ulcer in the

diabetic foot. In a nondiabetic patient, the ratio is 0.35. These studies are performed bilaterally and include wave tracings and toe pressures.

Doppler arterial readings are subject to several potential distortions. Rigid arterial calcifications can cause a decrease in arterial wall compliance and commonly result in falsely elevated pressure readings. Arterial brachial indices greater than 1 are one indication of this type of false reading.

Recent studies have indicated that absolute toe pressures, rather than ratios, are more predictive of distal wound healing. Minimum toe pressures of 40 to 50 mm Hg are necessary for healing; if the levels are low, arteriography and arterial reconstruction may be appropriate. Advancements in transcutaneous oxygen measurements, xenon clearance, and fluorescein angiography hold promise as newer predictors of the likelihood of amputation healing. However, to date, no technique is as inexpensive and simple to perform as the Doppler ultrasound.

If a patient complains of painful ulcers or specific pain in the foot, ischemia should be suspected. It should be remembered that ulcers occur as a result of lack of sensation, although the neuropathy can be a source of pain.

Every diabetic foot with serious infection or ischemia requires a vascular evaluation. Aggressive vascular reconstruction with a thorough and complete debridement of infected and necrotic tissue is the key to limb salvage. Limbs that in the past required a below-the-knee amputation can now sometimes be salvaged with a Syme's amputation. The salvage of insensate limbs is important both in maximizing function and in minimizing the amount of energy necessary for ambulation. Oxygen consumption during ambulation increases as the amputation level becomes more proximal, and associated morbidity and mortality are also increased.

Radiographic Evaluation

On the plain radiograph, osteolytic changes in the distal phalanx are typical of the insensate foot. These changes can easily be confused with infection, but a relative absence of osteopenia surrounding these changes suggests typical diabetic findings as found with the Charcot joint. Radiographs should also be closely inspected for any signs of gas, bony deformities, or foreign bodies beneath the skin. Arterial calcification is typical and a "lead pipe" appearance is often noted on radiographs of diabetic patients.

A recent radiographic review of 456 diabetic subjects revealed the presence of arterial calcification in 75% of those with contralateral amputation compared to only 39% of patients without a contralateral amputation. Moderate or severe claw toes, present in 70% of patients with previous amputations, were seen in only 55% of patients with no contralateral amputation. Charcot changes were noted in less than 1% of this diabetic population. This study led to the conclusion that the emphasis Charcot deformities receive in the literature is probably the result of their severity rather than their prevalence.

Nuclear Medicine

Nuclear medicine studies provide important information regarding vascular perfusion of both bone and soft tissue. Technetium 99m (Tc 99m) has been shown to be of limited value when used alone in order to rule out osteomyelitis in patients with peripheral neuropathy. Gallium-67 scanning, either alone or in combination with Tc 99m is of little diagnostic value and gives little additional information. The combination of 3-phase technetium and indium-111 has been shown to have the highest degree of efficacy (100% sensitivity, 80% specificity, and 91% accuracy), followed closely by indium-111 alone (100% sensitivity, 70% specificity, and 96% accuracy).

In the adult patient with diabetes with a clinical suspicion of osteomyelitis with no radiographic findings of the disease, indium alone, is an appropriate nuclear evaluation for ruling out infection. If, however, the indium scan is positive, a technetium scan performed simultaneously is often helpful in making the differentiation between osteomyelitis and infection limited to the soft tissue.

Computed Tomography and Magnetic Resonance Imaging

Computed tomography (CT) has been valuable in localizing pathologic anatomy, including abscesses and abnormal bony changes; however, its ability to differentiate between normal and abnormal soft tissue is limited.

The sensitivity and specificity of magnetic resonance imaging (MRI) for the diagnosis of osteomyelitis were 100% and 81%, respectively, for diabetic patients, with an accuracy of 95% in one study. MRI was deemed positive with T1-weighted marrow images showing areas of decreased signal intensity with corresponding high density areas on both short tau inversion recovery and T2-weighted images. Accurate delineation of the extent of involvement of infection allows for limited surgical resection in selected patients, making an MRI-guided approach clinically useful and cost-effective. The use of gadolinium enhancement and fat suppression further reduces the number of false negatives.

Foot and Ankle Ulcers Foot and ankle ulcers occur as a result of a "loss of awareness" to trauma. They are the single most common complication for which diabetic patients seek medical assistance.

Classification The Wagner's classification grades ulcers in the following manner. Grade 0, ulcers have intact skin (may have bony deformities). In grade I, there is a localized superficial ulcer; in grade II, a deep ulcer to tendon, bone, ligament, joint; in grade III, a deep abscess and osteomyelitis; in grade IV, gangrene of toes or forefoot; and in grade V, gangrene of the whole foot. In this system, the formation of ulcers and gangrene are classified together and assumed to be related along the same continuum. New classification systems, such as a depth ischemia classification, define the grades more precisely and separate the natural history of ulceration (caused by a neuropathy) from the natural history of gangrene (caused by vascular insufficiency). Classification of the ulcer also requires a recognition of the location of the lesion. Forefoot ulcers typically have lower associated mortality rates and higher incidence of limb salvage. More proximal lesions leave fewer salvage options.

Patient Education The most important role of the orthopaedic surgeon is in prevention of ulcers through patient education. Patients are cautioned never to walk barefoot, to inspect their feet every 2 hours, and to change their shoes every 4 hours to relieve pressure. Patients should also be advised not to expose their feet to potential trauma, such as heating pads or hot bath water. The temperature of bath water should always be checked with the hand prior to immersing the feet. The patient should be cautioned never to perform "home surgery." Because of the lack of sensation and poor eyesight, patients often trim calluses too much, resulting in infection. Most importantly, patients should be cautioned to discontinue smoking in order to protect arterial circulation.

The clinician should evaluate the fit of the shoes, and the patient should be advised to wear cushioning socks in order to help decrease pressures. A gradual introduction to new shoes by wearing them for only a short period daily for a week can reduce blister formation. Shoes with extra-depth toe boxes should be prescribed when appropriate. A rigid rocker sole type shoe often is helpful in reducing stresses placed on the forefoot or midfoot. New developments in this area include in-sole pressure measurement devices used to help customize prescriptions.

Nonsurgical Treatment Nonsurgical management must be designed to relieve pressure. It has been noted that having calluses trimmed can reduce localized pressure by 30%. Patients should also be instructed in proper cuticle care and be advised not to bevel the toenails when they trim them.

The most important form of nonsurgical treatment is the use of a total contact cast, the preferred device of many orthopaedic surgeons for protecting neuropathic ulcers during ambulation (Fig. 2). The goal of the total contact cast is to distribute pressures over the entire surface of the foot and leg. Patients with ulcers cannot adequately be treated by shoe modifications alone. The total contact cast can be used in Wagner's grades I and II type ulcers. Once osteomyelitis is apparent, nonsurgical treatment is no longer appropriate. Total contact casts also enclose the toes, thereby reducing the risk of patients bumping their toes while undergoing treatment. The weight of the cast adds inertia to the swing phase of gait and subsequently can actually be injurious unless the toes are adequately protected. Webril should be placed between the toes in order to reduce the maceration that occurs from sweating in this region. Felt should be placed over bony prominences such as the medial and lateral malleoli and the anterior tibial region. Generally, it is believed that plaster can be molded more accurately than fiberglass and, as a result, a better fit and a more uniform pressure distribution can usually be obtained using plaster.

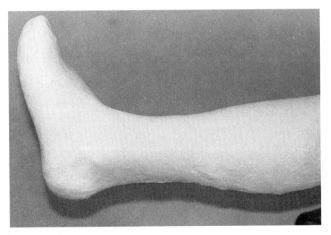

Figure 2
A total contact cast is demonstrated.

It is critical that excess padding not be placed over the foot and leg in the cast. If more than 3 layers of Webril are used, sheer movement can occur between the layers of Webril, resulting in friction within the cast. The first cast must be removed within several days of application, because a significant change in swelling often occurs soon after the cast application. Failure to change the cast during that period of time can result in a dead space within the cast and subsequent movement between the skin and the cast material. The average time for cast wear is 8 to 10 weeks.

When these principles are followed, a total contact cast will limit toe motion and immobilize the joints of the foot. The cast also reduces shear stresses on the skin providing that casts are changed frequently as swelling recedes. Healing rates of 90% have been reported with the use of total contact casts as long as no infection is apparent.

The debridement of necrotic tissue and the application of a sterile dressing along with frequent inspections are necessary for adequate healing. Heat, soaks, and whirlpool therapy can damage tissue and promote infection. In a double-blind randomized trial, topical hyperbaric oxygen was found to be beneficial; however, it is still considered controversial Recently, the use of topical growth factors has been advocated to assist in ulcer healing. This treatment also remains controversial and is not widely accepted. Diabetic patients do not tolerate undrained suppuration, and drainage by needle aspiration is considered inadequate.

Surgical Treatment If diabetic ulcers fail to heal by conservative treatment or if a Wagner's grade III, IV, or V lesion is identified, excessive internal bony pressures must be identified. The purposes of surgery are to relieve any internal area of pressure produced by bony prominences and to debride necrotic or infected tissue. Thorough vascular evaluation is necessary prior to surgery to avoid progression of tissue necrosis. Aminoglycosides should generally be avoided in favor of nonnephrotoxic antibiotics.

Wagner's classification grade IV and grade V ulcers require amputation. Care must be taken in the choice of the appropriate amputation level. Total lymphocyte count and total protein, and albumin levels provide a good indicator of the patient's nutritional state and systemic ability to combat infection and heal postoperatively. Tissue perfusion, measured by Doppler ultrasound, transcutaneous oxygen measurements, or temperature readings, determines wound healing potential locally. Effective healing can be expected in diabetic patients when Doppler indices are greater than 0.5 at the level of the amputation being planned. Arteriography has not been helpful in planning the level of amputation. A Syme's amputation is indicated when forefoot or midfoot infection and ischemia is profound.

The Charcot Joint
In 1868, Charcot first described the bizarre and painless changes that were associated with tabes dorsalis. He attributed the bone and joint changes to an "atrophic effect." The first to describe the neuroarthropathy associated with diabetes was Jordan in 1936. Today, diabetes is the most common cause of Charcot changes within joints, but other causes include syphilis, leprosy, and syringomyelia.

The two most widely held opinions for the cause of this neuroarthropathy are the neurotraumatic theory and the

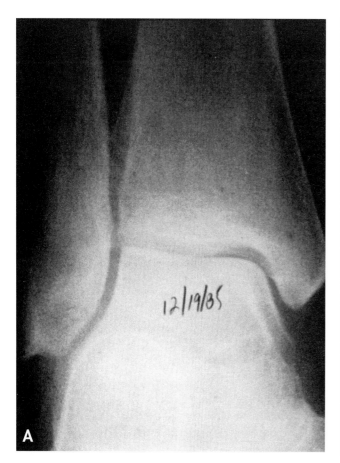
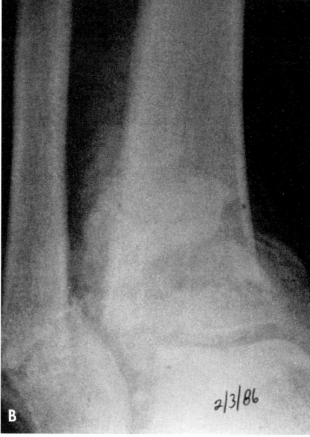

Figure 3

A, The appearance of an Eichenholtz 0 ankle after a recent slip and fall. The initial examiner failed to ask this 82-year-old woman if she was diabetic. She was placed in an Ace wrap and allowed to bear weight. **B,** The appearance of the same ankle 2 months later.

neurovascular theory. The neurotraumatic theory attributes the cause to a decreased protective sensation resulting in cumulative mechanical trauma, which ends in fracture and joint destruction. Not well explained by this theory, however, is the fact that many patients do complain of pain associated with their arthropathy. According to the neurovascular theory, a neurally initiated vascular reflex leads to increased reabsorption by osteoclasts. Glycolization of the supporting structures of the foot is thought to occur secondary to high glucose levels in the blood. This results in increased stiffness and increased collagen cross linkage. As the joints become more brittle, bone dissolution and fragmentation can occur, resulting in a change in foot function.

The diagnosis of a Charcot joint can often be difficult, resulting in a missed or delayed diagnosis in approximately a quarter of presenting cases. Gout, cellulitis, osteomyelitis, and posterior tibial tendinitis can all mimic this disorder. Clues to making a diagnosis, however, come from knowing the history of diabetes or other systemic disorders, constitutional signs of infection, and radiographic assessment of the joints in question. Often, patients recall a trivial injury to which they attribute their complains. Physical examination often reveals intact pulses, warm skin, swelling, and erythema, and can often demonstrate crepitus with motion of the bony architecture.

Early radiographic changes include osteopenia, which is secondary to the loss of subarterial control. The use of a bone scan specifically Tc 99m and indium-111 has shown the highest diagnostic efficacy followed closely by indium-111 alone. When the diagnosis cannot be made by any other means, a biopsy is appropriate to evaluate the bone histologically. In Charcot joint destruction, the pathognomonic change seen is bony particles imbedded within the synovium.

As described by Eichenholtz, the staging of a Charcot foot entails both a clinical and radiographic criteria. In stage I, the patient presents with acute inflammatory process characterized by edema, hyperemia, and erythema. Bone fragmentation is seen radiographically, which causes confusion with osteomyelitis. Stage II involves the body's reparative process. There is noted to be swelling, warmth, and redness, and radiographs show coalescing new bone at the site of the fracture or dislocation. Stage III is a continuum of stage II, with resolution of the clinical inflammation, and bony consolidation radiographically visualized. A stage 0, added to this classification, refers to the diabetic patient with a peripheral neuropathy who has suffered an acute sprain or fracture (Fig. 3). The stage 0 underscores the importance of education for diabetic patients with a foot or ankle injury.

Various patterns of disintegration of the tarsus have been reported. Use of the term disintegration emphasizes the fact that often a bone injury or infection is involved, rather than joint incongruity. In pattern I, a posterior pillar injury, the calcaneus fractures as a result of a heavy step during normal gait. In pattern II, a central (body of the talus) injury occurs, with disintegration of the talus caused by subtalar incongruity. Interestingly, the ankle is rarely damaged in a patient with leprosy but often is involved in patients with tabes dorsalis. In pattern III, an anterior pillar (medial arch) injury occurs when weakening or slackening of the plantar tension of the foot (from intrinsic paralysis or imperfect reflex coordination) results in angulatory forces on the bones and joints, particularly the dorsal edge of the foot (Fig. 4). This pattern is common in diabetic patients. Pattern IV is an anterior pillar (lateral arch) injury, in which the pattern seen is dominated by sepsis. This pattern occurs most often in a foot with varus orientation. Because of poor cushioning, the lateral bony rim of the foot is exposed to concentrated weightbearing. This pattern occurs much more often in leprosy than in tabes dorsalis or diabetes because of the paralysis of the common peroneal nerve seen in leprosy patients. In pattern V, a cuneiform (metatarsal base) injury occurs as a result of walking on a foot with a cracked cuneiform and typically occurs from a twist of the foot or from weights falling on the dorsum of the foot. The crack forms a weak point in the long lever of the foot, which then propagates the fracture across the foot, forming a broad flail pseudoarthrosis.

This anatomic classification has been simplified relative to its effect on the diabetic foot. Type I Charcot changes affect the midfoot area in and about the metatarsal cuneiform and navicular cuneiform joints and are most common, occurring

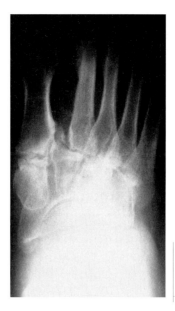

Figure 4

A pattern III Charcot midfoot collapse is demonstrated.

in 60% of Charcot feet. This pattern is characterized by symptomatic medial and plantar bony prominences that can lead to ulcerations. Type II involves the hindfoot, represents 20% of the neuroarthropathic feet, and is characterized by instability requiring long periods of immobilization. Type III A involves the ankle and results in the severest instability, requiring the longest time for healing. Type III B, which involves the os calcis, represents the pathologic fracture of the tuberosity of the calcaneus.

Most surgeons would agree that in the inflammatory stage (Eichenholtz stage I) conservative treatment in the form of casting and nonweightbearing is most appropriate. After the inflammatory stage resolves, however, some authors have advocated surgical intervention if a bony prominence exists or if the foot is unstable. If the foot is stable and has a chronic midfoot deformity, an exostectomy may be all that is required to allow any ulcers present to heal. Traditionally, arthrodeses have been discouraged in neuropathic joints because of the increased risk of nonunion. However, conservative care also has risks, and recently some surgeons have advocated arthrodesis in any foot that is unstable as a result of a mobile joint, in order to remove bony prominences and aid in the healing of ulcers. In one study, 8 consecutive patients with Charcot changes were treated with a triple arthrodesis, and clinical union was achieved. However, in another study, 50% of patients with preoperative ulcers had recurrent ulcers that took 5 months to consolidate, during which time patients were wheelchair-bound. The use of a retrograde intramedullary nail has also been advocated for providing rigid fixation in the neuropathic joint, but nailing has significant potential complications and its final place in the treatment regimen remains to be determined.

Conservative care involves elevation of the foot, restricted or complete nonweightbearing, and total contact casting. If after 8 weeks the acute inflammation has resolved, a custom-made ankle-foot orthotic lined with Plastazote or Pelite may allow normal ambulation.

Annotated Bibliography

Apelqvist J, Ragnarson-Tennvall G, Larsson J, Persson LL: Long-term costs for foot ulcers in diabetic patients in a multidisciplinary setting. *Foot Ankle Int* 1995;16:388–394.

The authors discovered the expected total cost per patient following a minor amputation was in excess of $43,000 and was $63,000 after a major amputation. The authors concluded that the long-term cost in diabetic foot care is considerable, mainly because of the need for increased home care and social service, and also the cost of treatment of recurrent ulcers and amputations.

Birke JA, Franks BD, Foto JG: First ray joint limitation, pressure, and ulceration of the first metatarsal head in diabetes mellitus. *Foot Ankle Int* 1995;16:277–284.

The authors noted that sensory loss, duration of diabetes, and limited range of motion at the hip, ankle, and foot were related to ulcerations at all forefoot locations.

Brand P: The insensitive foot, in Jahss MH (ed): *Disorders of the Foot and Ankle,* ed 2. Philadelphia, PA, WB Saunders, 1991, vol 3, pp 2170–2186.

This chapter is a concise review of the author's research regarding the insensate foot.

Caputo GM, Cavanagh PR, Ulbrecht JS, Gibbons GW, Karchmer AW: Assessment and management of foot disease in patients with diabetes. *N Engl J Med* 1994;331:854–860.

The authors present an excellent review on diabetic foot care, emphasizing early detection and immediate surgical intervention and including revascularization when necessary.

Chang BB, Shah DM, Darling RC III, Leather RP: Treatment of the diabetic foot from a vascular surgeon's viewpoint. *Clin Orthop* 1993;296:27–30.

The authors review the improvements in the identification and treatment of patients in whom correction of arterial occlusive disease is necessary for healing.

Early JS, Hansen ST: Surgical reconstruction of the diabetic foot: A salvage approach for midfoot collapse. *Foot Ankle Int* 1996;17:325–330.

The authors report their experience of 18 patients with 21 feet undergoing surgical reconstruction for diabetic neuropathy. They note aver-age time to union was 5 months; 47% of patients were without any complication throughout their postoperative course, and 70% of the ulcers healed without incident.

Fletcher F, Ain M, Jacobs R: Healing of foot ulcers in immunosuppressed renal transplant patients. *Clin Orthop* 1993;296:37–42.

The authors confirmed the long-held clinical suspicion that a higher failure rate may occur with limb salvage surgery in the immunosuppressed patient.

Johnson JE, Kennedy EJ, Shereff MJ, Patel NC, Collier BD: Prospective study of bone, indium-111-labeled white blood cell, and gallium-67 scanning for the evaluation of osteomyelitis in the diabetic foot. *Foot Ankle Int* 1996;17:10–16.

The authors concluded that for adult diabetic patients with clinical suspicion of osteomyelitis but not radiographic findings of that disease, indium-111 alone is an appropriate nuclear medicine evaluation for ruling out infection if it is negative, however, if an area of indium-111 white blood cell uptake is present, a simultaneous technetium 99m scan is often helpful in providing the anatomic correlation to differentiate osteomyelitis from infection that is limited to soft tissue.

Larsson J, Agardh CD, Apelqvist J, Stenstrom A: Clinical characteristics in relation to final amputation level in diabetic patients with foot ulcers: A prospective study of healing below or above the ankle in 187 patients. *Foot Ankle Int* 1995;16:69–74.

The authors note older age, history of cerebrovascular disease, and low hemoglobin levels were associated with above-ankle amputations in diabetic patients with foot ulcers. However, the authors warn that none of these factors should be taken as a cause to choose a primary amputation above the ankle and the authors recommend more attention should be paid to biologic factors than to chronologic age.

Martin RL, Conti SF: Plantar pressure analysis of diabetic rocker-bottom deformity in total contact casts. *Foot Ankle Int* 1996;17:470–472.

The authors showed the use of short leg casts and total contact casts both significantly reduced the midfoot pressure.

Moore TJ, Prince R, Pochatko D, Smith JW, Fleming S: Retrograde intramedullary nailing for ankle arthrodesis. *Foot Ankle Int* 1995;16:433–436.

Authors note retrograde intramedullary rodding may allow stable fixation in neuropathic ankles with significant collapsed tali.

Myerson MS, Henderson MR, Saxby T, Short KW: Management of midfoot diabetic neuroarthropathy. *Foot Ankle Int* 1994;15:233–241.

The authors present their management protocol for 68 patients with diabetes and neuroarthropathy of the midfoot in which they note it was found to be successful in 82 of 85 feet treated.

Olmos PR, Cataland S, O'Dorisio TM, Casey CA, Smead WL, Simon SR: The Semmes-Weinstein monofilament as a potential predictor of foot ulceration in patients with noninsulin-dependent diabetes. *Am J Med Sci* 1995;309:76–82.

The authors demonstrate Semmes-Weinstein monofilament testing as an important predictor of foot ulceration.

Patel VG, Wieman TJ: Effect of metatarsal head resection for diabetic foot ulcers on the dynamic plantar pressure distribution. *Am J Surg* 1994;167:297–301.

Sixteen diabetic patients with neuropathic plantar ulcers were assessed for a mean of 36 weeks following metatarsal head resection, and their plantar pressure distributions were measured. The authors concluded that reduction of plantar pressure is crucial for plantar ulcer healing and metatarsal head resection leads to reduced peak plantar pressures and expedites ulcer healing.

Perry JE, Ulbrecht JS, Derr JA, Cavanagh PR: The use of running shoes to reduce plantar pressures in patients who have diabetes. *J Bone Joint Surg* 1995;77A:1819–1828.

Inexpensive running shoes relieve plantar pressure in the forefoot and heel by a mean of 31%, with the most relief occurring in feet that had highest pressures when they were unshod. The authors conclude that individuals with insensate feet should be discouraged from wearing leather-soled oxford style shoes, and inexpensive running shoes should be viewed as the least acceptable choice for foot wear for these individuals if they are free from deformity.

Pinzur MS, Stuck R, Sage R: Benchmark analysis on diabetics at high risk for lower extremity amputation. *Foot Ankle Int* 1996;17:695–700.

The authors note patients with long-standing adult onset diabetes, identified as at high risk for foot ulcer development, have a substantially increased risk for lower limb amputation, multiple organ system failure, hospitalization, and institutionalization.

Schon LC, Marks RM: The management of neuroarthropathic fracture-dislocations in the diabetic patient. *Orthop Clin North Am* 1995;26:375–392.

The authors review present classification systems used for grading Charcot joints and their experience with reconstruction of these deformities.

Smith DG, Barnes BC, Sands AK, Boyko EJ, Ahroni JH: Prevalence of radiographic foot abnormalities in patients with diabetes. *Foot Ankle Int* 1997;18:342–346.

This article reviews the radiographic findings of 456 veterans with diabetes who were not necessarily seen for foot and ankle complaints. Charcot changes were seen in 1.4% of patients. Other deformities, such as arterial calcifications and claw toes, are much more common.

Tisdel CL, Marcus RE, Heiple KG: Triple arthrodesis for diabetic peritalar neuroarthropathy. *Foot Ankle Int* 1995;16:332–338.

The authors noted clinical union in all 8 patients of their study following triple arthrodeses in patients with diabetes mellitus with sensory loss. Follow-up was 44 months and included repeat physical examination and radiographs.

Weinstein D, Wang A, Chambers R, Steawart CA, Motz HA: Evaluation of magnetic resonance imaging in the diagnosis of osteomyelitis in diabetic foot infections. *Foot Ankle* 1993; 14:18–22.

Magnetic resonance imaging applications for diabetic feet are reviewed.

Classic Bibliography

Eichenholtz SN: The Charcot Joint. Springfield, IL, CC Thomas, 1966, pp 220–223.

Pinzur MS: Amputation level selection in the diabetic foot. *Clin Orthop* 1993;296:68–70.

Chapter 10
Hallux Valgus Deformity in the Adult

Introduction

The hallux valgus deformity is a lateral deviation of the phalanx, an increased intermetatarsal angle, and an enlarged medial eminence. The degree of deformity however, is extremely variable.

Types of Deformities

The hallux valgus deformity may consist of an enlarged medial eminence with little or no deviation of the proximal phalanx on the metatarsal head. In these patients, it is usually the pain over the medial eminence that brings the patient for consultation. As the hallux drifts in a lateral direction, more severe deformities emerge, including marked lateral deviation of the proximal phalanx on the metatarsal head, a large medial eminence, increased intermetatarsal angle, attenuation of the medial joint capsule, contracture of the lateral joint capsule, and displacement of the metatarsal head off of the sesamoids. Due to the severity of the deformity, the second toe may be involved secondary to crowding caused by the hallux. The changes involved in the second toe may be either overlapping or underlapping of the hallux or possibly subluxation or frank dislocation of the metatarsophalangeal joint (Fig. 1).

Pathologic Anatomy

Congruent Joint

A congruent joint is one in which there is no lateral deviation of the proximal phalanx on the metatarsal head, a "perfect fit." If any surgical alteration is made to the joint, it must be done in such a way that the phalanx is not rotated on the metatarsal head, or the "perfect fit" will be altered and may become painful or arthritic (Fig. 2).

Incongruent Joint

The incongruent joint is one in which there is lateral deviation of the proximal phalanx on the metatarsal head. This may be anywhere from a minimal subluxation of a millimeter up to a

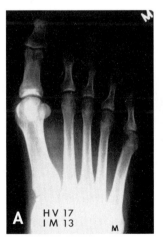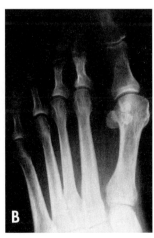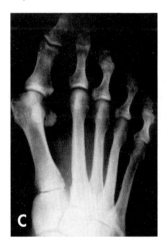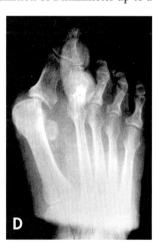

Figure 1

A spectrum of hallux valgus deformities. **A,** Congruent joint with large medial imminence. **B,** Mild subluxation of the metatarsophalangeal joint. **C,** Moderate subluxation of the metatarsophalangeal joint. **D,** Severe subluxation of the metatarsophalangeal joint. Note that as the deformity becomes more severe, the metatarsal head is pushed off of the sesamoid sling. The hallux places increasing stress on the second toe as the severity of the deformity increases.

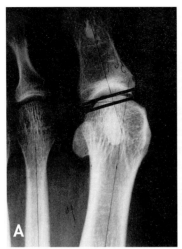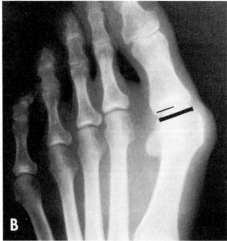

Figure 2

Congruent joint in which there is a "perfect fit" between the proximal phalanx and the metatarsal head. Any attempt to alter this relationship will result in joint surfaces which are no longer congruent and can lead to eventual stiffness or arthrosis or both.

significant subluxation of the joint. In this situation, the imperfect fit is corrected by moving the proximal phalanx back into a congruent position. The incongruent joint is usually present in a more advanced deformity and will continue to deform with time. It represents an instability of the joint, which will increase as the patient gets older (Fig. 3).

The pathologic anatomy of the incongruent joint is one of progressive attenuation of the medial joint capsule caused by

the stretching brought about by the lateral deviation of the proximal phalanx on the metatarsal head, contracture of the lateral joint structures, particularly the joint capsule and adductor hallucis tendon; an increase in the intermetatarsal angle due to pressure of the proximal phalanx against the metatarsal head; and, with time, pronation of the great toe due to the mismatch between the weaker dorsal medial joint capsule and the stronger plantar medial capsule.

The other pathologic change that occurs about the joint is the displacement of the sesamoid sling. The sesamoid sling, which normally is centered beneath the metatarsal head, is anchored laterally by the adductor hallucis tendon and the transverse metatarsal ligament. As the deformity of the great toe increases, the sesamoid sling remains anchored laterally and the metatarsal head is literally pushed off of the sesamoids. As this occurs, because the sesamoids are attached to the base of the proximal phalanx by the sesamoidal phalangeal ligament, rotation of the proximal phalanx is brought about. This results in the pronation of the proximal phalanx in the more severe hallux valgus deformities. At times, it may be so severe that the proximal phalax is rotated almost 90° on its long axis.

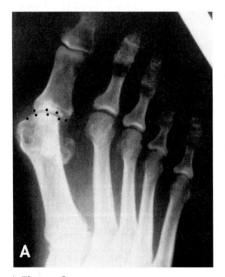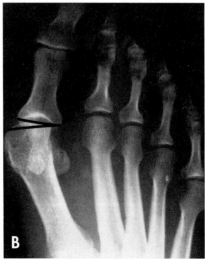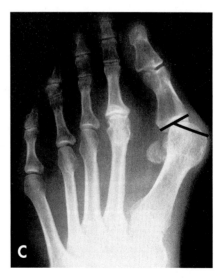

Figure 3

Examples of an incongruent joint. **A,** When the lateral aspect of the proximal phalanx deviates lateral to the lateral aspect of the metatarsal head, the joint is considered incongruent or subluxed. **B,** Moderate subluxation. **C,** Severe subluxation.

Arthrosis of the Metatarsophalangeal Joint

Arthrosis of the metatarsophalangeal joint is carefully looked for when evaluating the patient with hallux valgus deformity. This is important because if a significant degree of arthrosis is present and the joint is realigned, the possibility of the patient developing stiffness and pain following the procedure is very great. This obviously would result in an unsatisfactory result for the patient and may require further surgery (Fig. 4).

Hallux Valgus Interphalangeus

The hallux valgus interphalangeus deformity represents the lateral deviation within the proximal phalanx of the great toe. This is an intrinsic bony deformity that is present in the proximal phalanx. As a rule, this deformity is not significant, although in some cases it is the main deformity, and it can result in a prominence over the interphalangeal joint and occasionally a painful callous along the plantar medial aspect of the hallux (Fig. 5).

Distal Metatarsal Articular Angle (DMAA)

The distal metatarsal articular angle represents the relationship between the articular surface of the metatarsal head and the long axis of the metatarsal. As a rule, up to 10° of lateral deviation is considered normal. In some individuals, however, this angle is significantly greater, resulting in a hallux valgus deformity with a congruent metatarsophalangeal joint. As noted earlier, any alteration of the congruent joint can lead to stiffness or arthrosis. An increased DMAA is noted most frequently in juveniles and in males with hallux valgus deformity (Fig. 6).

Metatarsal-Cuneiform Joint

Stability of the metatarsal-cuneiform is extremely variable. This saddle-shaped joint should always be carefully evaluated along its normal axis, which produces motion in a dorsal-medial and plantar-lateral direction. One school of thought proposes that instability of the metatarsal-cuneiform, per se,

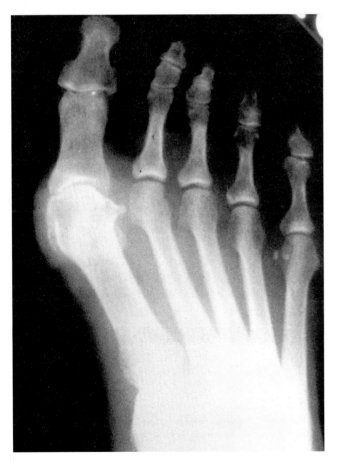

Figure 4

Arthrosis of the first metatarsophalangeal joint.

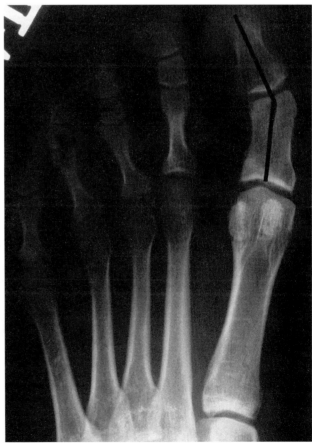

Figure 5

Hallux valgus interphalangeus.

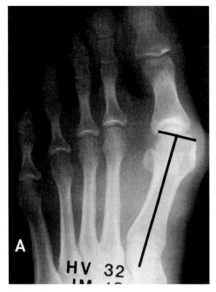
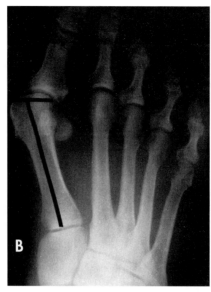
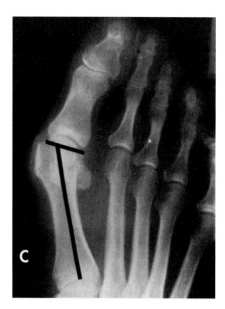

Figure 6

Distal metatarsal articular angle (DMAA). **A,** Normal DMAA. **B,** Increased DMAA. **C,** Increased DMAA with congruent joint.

is responsible for the hallux valgus deformity, but most of the scientific evidence points towards the conclusion that it is rarely the cause of a hallux valgus deformity. In our experience, only 2% to 3% of patients with hallux valgus deformity have significant instability of the metatarsal-cuneiform joint.

Evaluation of the Patient With Hallux Valgus

History

When evaluating the patient with hallux valgus, it is extremely important to obtain a careful history. The chief complaints range from patients who localize pain to a specific area to patients who are dissatisfied with their shoe wear. It is very important for the clinician to appreciate why the patient is seeking attention.

The patient's occupation is carefully considered. It is important to determine how much time patients spend on their feet throughout the work day, and whether they are working at heights. Individuals who work on their feet all day probably should not undergo hallux valgus correction until they are sufficiently disabled to make it difficult for them to carry out their occupation. Patients who do spend all day on their feet may not be able to return to work after their hallux valgus repair, and this can represent a financial disaster. From an occupational standpoint, one must carefully determine

whether the patient is seeking correction of the problem because of inability to wear a stylish shoe or because they truly have a painful deformity.

Recreational activities also require careful consideration. If a patient is participating in running activities at a competitive level, whether it be long-distance running, racquet sports, gymnastics, basketball, or other sports, our philosophy is that correction of a hallux valgus deformity should be carried out only when the patient is no longer able to continue his or her recreational or professional activity. This philosophy recognizes that following hallux valgus surgery, the metatarsophalangeal joint may be painful and patients may not be able to return to their previous level of performance.

Shoewear is another very important factor that must be discussed with the patient. Women often have an unrealistic expectation as to what type of shoe they should be able to wear. Many times a woman with a wide, square foot seeks to wear a stylish shoe that, unfortunately, does not fit her foot. This results in pain over the medial eminence and, as a result, the patient seeks medical attention. In our experience, prior to bunion surgery, two thirds of the patients could not wear the shoes they wished; after surgery, two thirds could. This still leaves one third of the patients who are unable to wear the shoes they desire, usually because of a discrepancy between the size of the foot and the shape of the shoe. It is much better to change a patient's shoe than to carry out a hallux valgus repair.

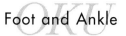
Physical Examination

A careful physical examination is essential in the work-up of the patient with a hallux valgus deformity. With the patient standing, the foot posture is carefully observed in order to evaluate the longitudinal arch, the severity of the deformity of the great toe and any deformities that may be present in the lesser toes. The patient's gait should be observed for evidence of motor weakness or abnormal alignment of the lower extremity. Next the patient is seated and the range of motion of the ankle, subtalar, transverse tarsal and metatarsophalangeal joints of both feet are compared. When observing the range of motion of the metatarsophalangeal joint, note carefully how much dorsiflexion and plantarflexion is present on the involved side versus the uninvolved side. Attempt to correct the hallux valgus deformity while moving the great toe in dorsiflexion and plantarflexion. This maneuver demonstrates approximately how much correction can be obtained at the time of surgery while maintaining satisfactory range of motion.

If dorsiflexion is severely restricted, the patient probably has an increased DMAA, and the hallux valgus cannot be completely corrected without carrying out some type of an osteotomy to realign the distal articular surface. The patient with arthrosis will also demonstrate restricted motion, and crepitation may be noted when the joint is moved.

The size and configuration of the medial eminence and overlying bursa is also noted. At times, the dorsal medial cutaneous nerve may be irritable and a Tinel's sign is present over this region. The plantar aspect of the joint is also palpated looking for pain about the sesamoids, although this is not common in patients with hallux valgus deformity. The degree of pronation of the hallux is observed.

The neurovascular status of the foot is carefully evaluated, and if there is any question as to the blood supply, arterial doppler studies are obtained. From a sensory standpoint, look for the presence of a peripheral neuropathy. As the last part of the physical examination, evaluate the patient's typical shoe wear as well as the shoes the patient is wearing at the time of the examination.

Radiographic Evaluation

Radiographic evaluation of the foot requires a weightbearing radiograph, which will accurately show the severity of any deformity. The following assessments should be made.

The metatarsophalangeal joint is carefully evaluated for arthrosis, which narrows the joint space and is associated with sclerosis and possible subchondral cyst formation. It is important to identify arthrosis preoperatively, because it acts as a prognosticator for the final result. When significant arthrosis is present, most bunion operations, except those that result in obliteration of the joint, are contraindicated. Also, measure the metatarsophalangeal joint congruency.

The hallux valgus angle represents the relationship of the long axis of the proximal phalanx to the long axis of the first metatarsal. Up to approximately 15° of lateral deviation is considered normal.

The intermetatarsal angle is the relationship of the first metatarsal to the second metatarsal. As a general rule, this angle is approximately 9° or less.

Radiographic evaluation of the metatarsal-cuneiform joint is difficult because varying angles of the X-ray tube give varying configurations of the joint surfaces. Significant lateral sloping of the metatarsal-cuneiform joint alerts the clinician to the possibility of instability of that joint and the patient is reevaluated. In juvenile patients, radiographs sometimes demonstrate a deficiency along the medial aspect of the medial cuneiform and a significant increased lateral slope to the cuneiform.

The DMAA is measured by using the best approximation of the articular surface and then drawing a line between the medial and lateral aspect of this. Another line is then drawn down the long axis of the metatarsal. The angle described by the articular line and the metatarsal line defines the distal metatarsal articular angle, which is usually 10° or less of lateral deviation. Increased lateral deviation can be a factor in the choice of the procedure to be carried out, and may be predictive of the possible result in certain cases.

Hallux valgus interphalangeus is measured by drawing a line connecting the condyles at the proximal aspect of the proximal phalanx and then drawing a line through the long axis of the phalanx. In hallux valgus interphalangeus, there is lateral deviation of this line.

The alignment of the sesamoids is carefully noted. They usually sit directly beneath the first metatarsal head, but in hallux valgus associated with an incongruent joint, there is progressive uncovering of the sesamoids. Arthrosis of the sesamoids is looked for, but this finding is quite uncommon and rarely has clinical significance.

Conservative Management

After one has carefully evaluated the patient with a hallux valgus deformity, a decision must be made regarding management. In general, patients can be managed initially with conservative treatment, such as changing the patient's shoes and possibly placing pads or mole skin over the painful areas. Conservative treatment also provides insight as to the compliance of the patient and his or her willingness to work with the physician to resolve the problem. Occasionally, the deformity is so severe and painful that conservative management would not be of significant benefit to the patient. In such cases I believe it is appropriate to proceed directly with surgical intervention.

Conservative management of the patient with a hallux valgus deformity begins with explaining to the patient the nature of their problem, including the basic pathologic anatomy, the cause of pain, and ways of reducing or preventing pain. As a general rule, the most frequent first step in conservative management is to change the patient's shoes. The patient must be made to realize that the shoe size and style they are wearing is not the same as the size and shape of the weightbearing foot. Even patients who desire to wear a pointed toe shoe should be encouraged to get a larger size, made of material that is soft enough to expand, thereby taking the pressure off the medial eminence. If the main problem is metatarsalgia secondary to the loss of stability of the first metatarsophalangeal joint, a soft support in the shoe may be of benefit.

When recommending athletic shoes, encourage the patient to obtain shoes that do not have a seam over the area of the medial eminence. A simple solution for work shoes used in gardening or other such activities is to get an old shoe and cut out a section over the medial eminence, which will relieve the pressure and make the shoe more comfortable. If other toes are involved, such as a cross-over or cross-under toe, some type of padding around the toe (lamb's wool) or a toe sling may help reduce the patient's symptoms. In general, orthotic devices are not useful in treating patients with hallux valgus unless metatarsalgia is present. Elevation of the longitudinal arch, per se, has not been demonstrated to be effective in preventing or decreasing the severity of the hallux valgus deformity.

Decision Making

In treating hallux valgus deformity, the first decision that must be made is whether to treat the patient conservatively or surgically. Conservative management must be presented to the patient, because most patients will prefer to avoid hallux valgus surgery, if possible. As long as the patient is able to function comfortably, I believe hallux valgus surgery can be put off as long as the patient desires. Performing a hallux valgus repair in order to prevent progression of deformity is not indicated.

If the decision is made to carry out surgery, then the patient's chief complaint, occupational exposure, and recreational activities must be correlated in order to define their overall level of activity. The physical findings must be carefully compared with the radiographic findings and a decision

reached as to what type of surgical procedure would best benefit the patient.

Last, but not least, the patient's expectations must be considered. What does the patient expect to gain from the surgical procedure? Do they expect to wear a narrow, pointy, high-heeled shoe or do they simply desire relief from the pain over the medial eminence?

Surgical Procedure

A foot and ankle surgeon must choose from a number of possible procedures the one that will best treat the pathologic anatomy presented. The following algorithm has been developed in order to help the clinician in the decision-making process with regard to surgical management (Fig. 7). The basis of the algorithm is whether the patient has a congruent joint or an incongruent joint. If the patient has a congruent joint, in which the proximal phalanx should not be rotated on the metatarsal head, the surgical procedure must respect this condition. Conversely, if the patient has an incongruent joint, in which the proximal phalanx can be rotated about on the metatarsal head, an entirely different group of surgical procedures are possible. Some similarities exist between the various procedures. If the indication for a given procedure is stretched too far, failure may occur. The procedures presented in the algorithm can usually be relied on to give the best possible result within the limitations of the procedure selected.

Viewing the algorithm, it is noted that the hallux valgus deformity is divided into four groups, those with a congruent joint, those with an incongruent joint, those with instability of the metatarsal-cuneiform joint and those with arthrosis of the first metatarsophalangeal joint. The juvenile hallux valgus patient basically fits into this scheme, but there are certain circumstances surrounding the juvenile hallux valgus that can make their deformities unique. This is covered in the chapter on juvenile hallux valgus.

Congruent Metatarsophalangeal Joint

The congruent metatarsophalangeal joint is one in which there is no lateral deviation or subluxation of the proximal phalanx on the metatarsal head. In the majority of these cases, the main problem is an enlarged medial eminence or a hallux valgus interphalangeus. As pointed out previously, a patient with a congruent joint may have a markedly increased DMAA that can result in a significant hallux valgus deformity. In general, this combination is seen in the juvenile patient, and it is covered in that section. The congruent joint is treated with a periarticular procedure, such as a Chevron procedure, or an Akin procedure with excision of the medial eminence.

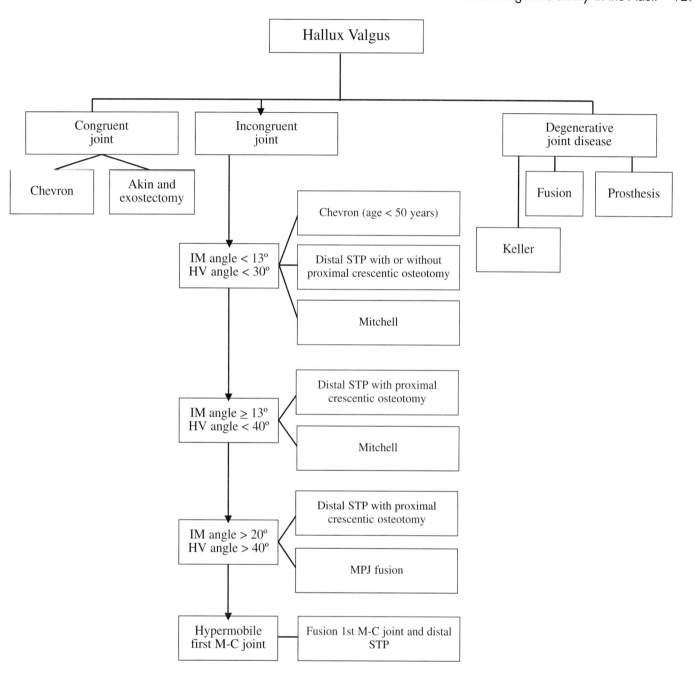

Figure 7
Algorithm for determining treatment for hallux valgus. (Courtesy of The Curtis Center, Philadelphia, PA.)

Incongruent Metatarsophalangeal Joint

Patients with an incongruent joint are divided into 3 groups depending on the severity of the deformity: a mild deformity, in which the hallux valgus is less than 30° and the intermetatarsal angle less than 13°; moderate deformity, in which the hallux valgus angle is between 20° and 40°, and the intermetatarsal angle is between 13° and 20° and a severe deformity, in which the hallux valgus angle is greater than 40° and the intermetatarsal angle is greater than 20°.

As noted in the algorithm, not all procedures are capable of correcting the entire spectrum of deformity. Once the hallux valgus angle is greater than 30° to 35°, a distal metatarsal osteotomy, such as the chevron, is no longer capable of obtaining enough correction. Likewise, a soft-tissue procedure alone usually will not correct this much deformity without the addition of a proximal metatarsal osteotomy.

The incongruent joint with a mild deformity, in which the hallux valgus angle is less than 30° and the intermetatarsal angle less than 13°, may be treated with a distal soft-tissue procedure with or without an osteotomy, a chevron procedure, or a Mitchell procedure.

The incongruent joint with a moderate deformity, in which the hallux valgus angle is less than 40° and the intermetatarsal angle between 13° and 20°, may be treated with the distal soft-tissue procedure with an osteotomy or with the Mitchell procedure. Note that the chevron procedure is not capable on a routine basis of correcting a deformity of this severity.

The incongruent joint with a severe deformity, in which the hallux valgus angle is greater than 40° and the intermetatarsal angle greater than 20°, may be treated with a distal soft-tissue procedure and a proximal metatarsal osteotomy or an arthrodesis, if indicated. Note that the Mitchell procedure cannot be used for deformities of this severity on a routine basis.

In the patient with arthrosis of the metatarsophalangeal joint, an arthrodesis of the metatarsophalangeal joint is the procedure of choice in an active individual; in an older inactive person, one might consider a Keller procedure. As a general rule, the use of a prosthetic replacement for the first metatarsophalangeal joint is not an indicated procedure, especially in young active individuals. Although some surgeons have used this procedure over a long period of time, the results have not stood the test of time, and most people now believe it should be used only under certain special circumstances.

Metatarsal-Cuneiform Instability

In the patient with a hallux valgus deformity and a hypermobile first metatarsal-cuneiform joint (which occurs in about 2% to 3% of patients with hallux valgus deformity), a first metatarsal-cuneiform arthrodesis along with a distal soft-tissue procedure is indicated.

Transfer Lesions

If a callous is present beneath the second metatarsal head in a patient who has an advanced hallux valgus deformity, it is probably the result of the loss of stability of the first metatarsophalangeal joint brought about by the severity of the deformity. In most of these cases, when the hallux valgus deformity is corrected and the normal windlass mechanism functions to depress the first metatarsal head, the callous beneath the second metatarsal head dissipates once it is unloaded. For this reason, unless specific pathology exists in the second metatarsophalangeal joint, such as a subluxation or dislocation, surgical treatment of the callous can generally be avoided.

The following is an outline of the surgical procedures, their postoperative management and most frequent complications for those listed in the algorithm.

Surgical Procedures

Distal Soft-Tissue Procedure

In the distal soft-tissue procedure, the contracted structures on the lateral side of the metatarsophalangeal joint are released through a dorsal web space dissection; these structures consist of the adductor hallucis tendon, the lateral joint capsule, and the transverse metatarsal ligament. The medial eminence is exposed through a medial midline approach, and the exostosis is removed in line with the long axis of the metatarsal shaft followed by plication of the medial capsule. The joint is kept immobilized in a postoperative shoe for 6 to 8 weeks, with weekly dressing changes to maintain alignment.

The most frequent complication associated with this procedure is recurrence of the deformity when it is used in a patient with a fixed intermetatarsal angle that was not corrected by the soft-tissue procedure alone. A second complication is iatrogenic hallux varus, in which the great toe deviates in a medial direction. Possible results are a cocking-up deformity or chaffing against the medial aspect of the patient's shoe.

Distal Soft-Tissue Procedure With Proximal Crescentic Osteotomy

In this procedure, the increased intermetatarsal angle is corrected with a proximal metatarsal osteotomy. We prefer to use the crescentic osteotomy because it is relatively easy to cut and to manage postoperatively. Other types of proximal osteotomies can be used for patients who have a fixed increased metatarsal angle.

The distal soft-tissue procedure is carried out as discussed earlier, and proximal osteotomy is carried out approximately 1 cm distal to the metatarsal-cuneiform joint. The metatarsal shaft is displaced laterally while the proximal fragment is displaced medialward. When using this procedure, it is critical to achieve adequate correction through the osteotomy.

Postoperative care consists of immobilization in a firm gauze bandage and 1/2-inch adhesive dressing, which is changed on a weekly basis for 8 weeks. The patient is permitted to ambulate in a postoperative shoe as tolerated.

The most common complications following this procedure are incomplete correction through the osteotomy or inadequate plication of the medial joint capsule. Hallux varus deformity may also recur as previously described.

Distal Soft-Tissue Procedure and Metatarsal-Cuneiform Joint Fusion

In the patient with a hypermobile metatarsal-cuneiform joint, an arthrodesis of the metatarsal-cuneiform joint is performed at the time of the correction. When the first metatarsal-cuneiform joint is arthrodesed, it is important that it be brought into a plantar-lateral direction, which respects its normal plane of motion, so that the metatarsal does not end up in an elevated position. The arthrodesis is stabilized using one or two interfragmentary screws across the metatarsal-cuneiform joint. The distal soft-tissue procedure that is combined with this procedure is the same as was described previously.

Postoperatively, the patient is placed in a removable cast for 4 weeks. The dressing is changed about the first metatarsophalangeal joint on a weekly basis. A walking shoe is used for the second 4-week period. As a rule, the fusion occurs at approximately 8 to 10 weeks.

The main complication following this procedure is nonunion of the metatarsal cuneiform joint, which even if present may not be symptomatic.

Chevron Procedure

The chevron procedure is a distal metatarsal osteotomy, which is carried out through a medial longitudinal incision. The metatarsal head is exposed from the medial aspect as it is for the distal soft-tissue procedure. After the medial eminence is removed at an oblique angle starting in the sagittal sulcus, a chevron-shaped cut in the transverse plane is produced. The apex of the cut should be no closer than 8 to 10 mm to the articular surface of the first metatarsal head. The osteotomy site is translated laterally approximately 5 to 7 mm, depending on the size of the individual metatarsal shaft. Once it has been displaced, it can be fixed with either a single Kirschner wire or a screw. The medial prominence created by

the lateral displacement is then removed.

Occasionally, a medial closing wedge is added when the patient has an increased DMAA, and rotation of the metatarsal head in a medial direction is required to realign the articular surface with the long axis of the metatarsal. Under these circumstances, usually a 2- to 3-mm wedge of bone is removed.

The main complication is incomplete correction, usually due to the preoperative presence of moderate or severe deformity. Osteonecrosis of the metatarsal head is always possible whenever a distal osteotomy is carried out, but usually can be avoided if stripping of the soft tissues is kept to a minimum.

Akin Procedure

The Akin procedure is carried out through a medial approach, exposing the proximal three fourths of the proximal phalanx and the medial eminence. If it is being carried out only for a hallux valgus interphalangeus, the metatarsal head does not need to be exposed, but if it is being carried out in association with a large medial eminence, then the medial eminence obviously must be exposed. The exposure of the medial eminence is the same as for the distal soft-tissue procedure. The osteotomy at the base of the proximal phalanx is carried out 3 to 4 mm distal to the articular surfaces of the proximal phalanx. It must be kept in mind that the proximal phalanx articular surface is concave and, as such, the osteotomy must be made distal enough so as to not violate the metatarsophalangeal joint. Usually a medially based wedge measuring 3 to 5 mm is removed, after which the osteotomy site is closed. The osteotomy can be stabilized either by suture material or with a small screw. If this is carried out in conjunction with excision of the medial eminence, the medial eminence is exposed as described for the distal soft-tissue procedure, the medial eminence is removed in line with the metatarsal shaft, and the medial capsule plicated.

Postoperative management consists of immobilization in a gauze and adhesive tape dressing and ambulation is allowed in a postoperative shoe. In general, immobilization continues for approximately 6 to 8 weeks until the osteotomy site appears to be healed.

The major complication associated with this procedure occurs when it is used on an incongruent joint, resulting in incomplete correction or recurrence of the deformity. When this procedure alone is carried out on an incongruent joint, the destabilizing forces are not addressed, and the deformity may progress.

Keller Procedure

The Keller procedure is carried out through a medial midline incision. A proximally based flap is created, and the medial eminence is removed. The proximal third of the proximal phalanx is excised. Because excision of the proximal phalanx releases the short flexor tendons, an attempt should be made to reattach these into the proximal phalanx through a drill hole, or the short flexor tendons may be attached to the flexor halucis longus tendon. The medial capsule is plicated and a longitudinal pin is used to stabilize the metatarsophalangeal joint for approximately 3 weeks. After removal of the pin, mobilization of the joint is begun.

The major complication following this procedure is loss of stability of the first metatarsophalangeal joint, resulting in a recurrent deformity. Occasionally, a transfer lesion occurs beneath the second metatarsal head due to loss of stability of the first metatarsophalangeal joint.

Fusion

The metatarsophalangeal joint is approached through a dorsal incision, exposing the articular surfaces. The surfaces can be cut flat, or a ball and socket configuration can be created, using specialized reamers. The ideal position for a fusion is approximately 15° of valgus and 10° of dorsiflexion in relation to the plantar aspect of the foot. Fixation is by an interfragmentary screw and dorsal plate, or in some cases, only two interfragmentary screws. Postoperative management is immobilization in a postoperative shoe for approximately 10 to 12 weeks until union has occurred.

Major complications are a nonunion at the fusion site or malalignment, which results in increased stress of the interphalangeal joint of the hallux.

Annotated Bibliography

Badwey TM, Dutkowsky JP, Graves SC, Richardson EG: An anatomical basis for the degree of displacement of the distal chevron osteotomy in the treatment of hallux valgus. *Foot Ankle Int* 1997;18:213–215.

The study was designed to define the amount of lateral displacement of the ct. The authors concluded that in 97.5% of the cases, the distal fragment can be translated laterally 6 mm in males and 5 mm in females.

Blum JL: The modified Mitchell osteotomy-bunionectomy: Indications and technical considerations. *Foot Ankle Int* 1994; 15:103–106.

A modified Mitchell procedure with 2 to 3 mm of plantar displacement and one third or less lateral displacement of the metatarsal head and pin fixation was used on 204 patients. Average metatarsal shortening was 3.2 mm, with 91% good and excellent results. Of 5 cases of osteonecrosis, only one was symptomatic. The author's criteria for procedure was an intermetatarsal angle less than 17° and a hallux valgus angle less than 30°.

Coughlin MJ, Abdo RV: Arthrodesis of the first metatarsophalangeal joint with Vitallium plate fixation. *Foot Ankle Int* 1994;15:18–28.

In this review of 58 feet fused using a small vitallium plate after creation of congruent joint surfaces with reamers there were 93% good or excellent results with only one nonunion. Postoperative hallux valgus angle was 17.1°, a correction of 18.4°; 1-2 intermetatarsal angle was corrected to 9.5°, a correction of 2.4°. Postoperative dorsiflexion was 22.6°.

Coughlin MJ: Hallux valgus. *J Bone Joint Surg* 1996;78A: 932–966.

This review article covers the entire spectrum of hallux valgus surgery, describing treatment principles, surgical techniques, and causes of failure.

Coughlin MJ: Juvenile hallux valgus: Etiology and treatment. *Foot Ankle Int* 1995;16:682–697.

An 11-year retrospective study of 45 patient's with juvenile hallux valgus treated with a multiprocedural approach resulted in good and excellent results in 92% of cases.

Dreeben S, Mann RA: Advanced hallux valgus deformity: Long-term results utilizing the distal soft tissue procedure and proximal metatarsal osteotomy. *Foot Ankle Int* 1996;17:142–144.

In this retrospective study of 28 cases of hallux valgus deformity with an intermetatarsal angle 14° or greater, followed an average of 5.5 years, loss of correction of the hallux valgus angle was 3.8° and of the intermetatarsal angle 1.4°. The authors concluded that there is sufficient inherent stability of the first metatarsocuneiform joint that it does not require stabilization to obtain a satisfactory long-term result.

Easley ME, Kiebzak GM, Davis WH, Anderson RB: Prospective, randomized comparison of proximal crescentic and proximal chevron osteotomies for correction of hallux valgus deformity. *Foot Ankle Int* 1996;17:307–316.

The prospective study compared the results following a proximal crescentic or chevron osteotomy for correction of moderate to severe hallux valgus deformity. Good results were achieved with both procedures and no statistically significant differences were found with respect to correction of the intermetatarsal angle or functional outcome.

Mann RA, Donatto KC: The chevron osteotomy: A clinical and radiographic analysis. *Foot Ankle Int* 1997;18:255–261.

This retrospecive analysis of 23 feet demonstrated that, depending on the measuring technique, the degree of correction varies considerably. Measurement bisecting the metatarsal shaft and phalanx demonstrated a correction of 5° of the hallux valgus angle and none of the intermetatarsal angle. Using the center of the head method, the intermetatarsal angle corrected 4° and the hallux valgus 11°. There was no sesamoid correction.

Markbreiter LA, Thompson FM: Proximal metatarsal osteotomy in hallux valgus correction: A comparison of crescentic and chevron procedures. *Foot Ankle Int* 1997;18:71–76.

Retrospective study of 50 feet corrected with a proximal osteotomy of either the crescentic or the chevron type. In all parameters there were no statistical differences between the two procedures. Both surgical techniques offer equally excellent and predictable results.

Miller RA, Firoozbakhsh K, Naraghi F, Ferries J: Determination of in vitro metatarsocuneiform pressure before and after surgical modification of the great toe. *Foot Ankle Int* 1995;16:84–87.

Contact pressures measured at the first metatarsocuneiform joint demonstrated a significant decrease in both the maximum pressure and total force following a resection arthroplasty (Keller procedure) versus first metatarsophalangeal arthrodesis. These results demonstrate the loss of weightbearing by the first metatarsal following a resection arthroplasty, which accounts for the lateral metatarsalgia.

Myerson MS, Komenda GA: Results of hallux varus correction using an extensor hallucis brevis tenodesis. *Foot Ankle Int* 1996; 17:21–27.

The authors demonstrated satisfactory correction of a hallux varus deformity using an extensor hallucis brevis transfer. The tendon was detached proximally, passed underneath the transverse metatarsal ligament and placed through a drill hole in the first metatarsal. A loss of dorsiflexion of approximately 10° was noted following the procedure.

Pelto-Vasenius K, Hirvensalo E, Vasenius J, Rokkanen P: Osteolytic changes after polyglycolide pin fixation in chevron osteotomy. *Foot Ankle Int* 1997;18:21–25.

Retrospective study of 94 metatarsal heads following a chevron osteotomy, which initially demonstrated osteolytic changes in 21(22%). At 2.1 years follow-up, 16 of the 21 resolved, 4 partially resolved, and one was still visible. There was one case of osteonecrosis related to the Chevron procedure.

Peterson DA, Zilberfarb JL, Greene MA, Colgrove RC: Avascular necrosis of the first metatarsal head: Incidence in distal osteotomy combined with lateral soft tissue release. *Foot Ankle Int* 1994;15:59–63.

In a study of 58 Chevron procedures with a lateral soft tissue release with follow-up of 2.5 years, there was 1 case of osteonecrosis, which was asymptomatic at 4.2 years follow-up. Authors concluded that a lateral soft-tissue release is safe when combined with a chevron procedure.

Pochatko DJ, Schlehr FJ, Murphey MD, Hamilton JJ: Distal chevron osteotomy with lateral release for treatment of hallux valgus deformity. *Foot Ankle Int* 1994;15:457–461.

The retrospective study of 23 feet following a chevron and lateral capsular release, which included the adductor tendon, demonstrated no evidence of osteonecrosis. Soft-tissue release did not appear to increase the incidence of definite radiographic evidence of osteonecrosis.

Pouliart N, Haentjens P, Opdecam P: Clinical and radiographic evaluation of Wilson osteotomy for hallux valgus. *Foot Ankle Int* 1996;17:388–394.

This retrospective study of 32 Wilson osteotomies for hallux valgus demonstrated a 35% incidence of metatarsalgia with an average shortening of 10.2 mm. Those patients without metatarsalgia demonstrated 7.7 mm of shortening. Patient satisfaction was 90% good and excellent.

Saragas NP, Becker PJ: Comparative radiographic analysis of parameters in feet with and without hallux valgus. *Foot Ankle Int* 1995;16:139–143.

The authors demonstrated in a series of 118 feet, of which 52 had a hallux valgus angle of greater than 15°, that there was no difference between the groups with respect to sesamoid position relative to the second metatarsal, incidence of pes planus, relative length of the first metatarsal, and the first metatarsal-medial cuneiform articulation.

Small HN, Braly WG, Tullos HS: Fixation of the chevron osteotomy utilizing absorbable polydioxanon pins. *Foot Ankle Int* 1995;16:346–350.

Radiographic review of 100 consecutive chevron osteotomies without internal fixation revealed 8% incidence of displacement at the osteotomy site. The study group of 71 feet fixed with two absorbable pins showed no evidence of delayed union. Follow-up averaged 1.3 years and pin tracks remained visible in 100% of cases. Four patients demonstrated lytic areas around one or both pin sites.

Thomas RL, Espinosa FJ, Richardson EG: Radiographic changes in the first metatarsal head after distal chevron osteotomy combined with lateral release through a plantar approach. *Foot Ankle Int* 1994;15:285–292.

Retrospective review of 80 chevron procedures with lateral soft-tissue release through a plantar incision usually associated with a fibular sesamoidectomy. The authors concluded that the bone and soft-tissue procedure did not place the head of the metatarsal at risk for clinically significant avascular changes with persistent bone death, cartilage necrosis, joint space collapse, loss of motion, or articular pain.

Tourné Y, Saragaglia D, Zattara A, et al: Hallux valgus in the elderly: Metatarsophalangeal arthrodesis of the first ray. *Foot Ankle Int* 1997;18:195–198.

This retrospective study of 41 feet with an average age of 67 years reported a pain-free first ray using normal footwear in 90% of cases and normal gait on flat terrain in 95% of cases. Fixation with an interfragmentary screw and 1/4 tubular plate resulted in 4 nonunions.

Trnka HJ, Zembsch A, Wiesauer H, Hungerford M, Salzer M, Ritschl P: Modified Austin procedure for correction of hallux valgus. *Foot Ankle Int* 1997;18:119–127.

In a retrospective study of 94 feet, the authors added to the Austin (chevron) procedure an extensive lateral release, which enabled them to gain increased correction of the intermetatarsal angle, hallux valgus angle, and sesamoid position. They had 3 cases of osteonecrosis, of which one was symptomatic. Hallux varus resulted in 8 cases, 2 of which were symptomatic.

Classic Bibliography

Coughlin MJ: Juvenile bunions, in Mann RA, Coughlin MJ (eds): *Surgery of the Foot and Ankle,* ed 6. St. Louis, MO, Mosby-Year Book, 1993, pp 297–339.

Hattrup SJ, Johnson KA: Chevron osteotomy: Analysis of factors in patients' dissatisfaction. *Foot Ankle* 1985;5:327–332.

Johnson JE, Clanton TO, Baxter DE, Gottlieb MS: Comparison of Chevron osteotomy and modified Mcbride bunionectomy for correction of mild to moderate hallux valgus deformity. *Foot Ankle* 1991;12:61–68.

Mann RA, Coughlin MJ (eds): *Video Textbook of Foot and Ankle Surgery.* St. Louis, MO, Medical Video Productions, 1991, pp 146–184.

Mann RA, Coughlin MJ: Adult hallux valgus, in Mann RA, Coughlin MJ (eds): *Surgery of the Foot and Ankle,* ed 6. St. Louis, MO, Mosby-Year Book, 1993, pp 167–296.Mann RA, Rudicel S, Graves SC: Repair of hallux valgus with a distal soft-tissue procedure and proximal metatarsal osteotomy: A long-term follow-up *J Bone Joint Surg* 1992;74A:124–129.

Mann RA: Decision-making in bunion surgery, in Greene WB (ed): *Instructional Course Lectures XXXIX.* Park Ridge, IL, American Academy of Orthopaedic Surgeons, 1990, pp 3–13.

Myerson M, Allon S, McGarvey W: Metatarsocuneiform arthrodesis for management of hallux valgus and metatarsus primus varus. *Foot Ankle* 1992;13:107–115.

Richardson EG: Keller resection arthroplasty. *Orthopedics* 1990;13:1049–1053.

Sangeorzan BJ, Hansen ST Jr: Modified Lapidus procedure for hallux valgus. *Foot Ankle* 1989;9:262–266.

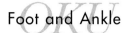

Chapter 11
Juvenile Hallux Valgus and Other
First Ray Problems in Orthopaedics

Introduction

The onset of hallux valgus in children is uncommon. While many bunion deformities become symptomatic in older age groups, the onset may occur as early as 10 years of age or younger. Early onset is often associated with increased severity and with a congruent metatarsophalangeal (MTP) joint. Many reports have stressed the importance of delaying surgery until skeletal maturity has been reached based on an increased rate of recurrence following hallux valgus correction; however, the increased rate of recurrence may indeed be due to the fact that a congruent metatarsophalangeal joint has been surgically corrected with an intra-articular repair.

Juvenile hallux valgus is more common in the female population. Although the mode of inheritance has not been well defined, inheritance from one generation to another has been noted in as high as three quarters of juveniles with hallux valgus. By definition, a juvenile hallux valgus deformity occurs in the pre-teenage and teenage years. Often, although the bunion may have developed at an early age, the patient does not seek treatment until much later in life. Some bunion deformities treated in later years are much more difficult to correct surgically and may indeed have had their onset during adolescence.

A juvenile hallux valgus deformity differs from an adult hallux valgus deformity in several ways. Usually, the hallux valgus angle and intermetatarsal angle are not as severe as in the adult. Rarely is there an enlarged medial eminence. Epiphyseal growth plates at the base of the first metatarsal and proximal phalanx may still be open in the juvenile patient. Hypermobility of the first metatarsocuneiform joint may be present as well.

Etiology

Juvenile hallux valgus has been associated with several anatomic factors. While pes planus and ligamentous laxity have been implicated, it is likely that pronation is no more common in the juvenile with hallux valgus than in the general population. A long first metatarsal in comparison to the second metatarsal is associated with a high rate of MTP joint congruency. High fashion footwear implicated in the progression of hallux valgus deformities in adults does not appear to be a significant factor in a juvenile with a bunion deformity. Metatarsus adductus has a high rate of association with juvenile bunions and may present as a difficult anatomic variant to correct because of its association with a large hallux valgus angle and a relatively small 1-2 intermetatarsal angle. A contracted Achilles tendon may place the foot at risk for a hallux valgus deformity.

Anatomy

First Metatarsophalangeal Joint

The orientation and shape of the articular surface of the distal first metatarsal and proximal phalanx have a significant effect on the predisposition of a hallux valgus deformity. Radiographic analysis of the first MTP joint may demonstrate either a subluxated (non-congruent) or non-subluxated (congruent) MTP joint (Fig. 1). The articular surface of the first metatarsal and proximal phalanx are rarely oriented at a right angle to the longitudinal axis of the respective bones. A slight valgus inclination of the great toe (approximately 6°) is considered to be normal. When the articular orientation of the MTP joint is abnormally high, a static fixed hallux valgus deformity may be present. The distal metatarsal articular angle (DMAA) (Fig. 2A) quantitates the magnitude of the lateral slope of the distal first metatarsal articular surface. While 6° is felt to be normal, it is not uncommon for the DMAA to measure 10° to 15° without any joint subluxation in juvenile hallux valgus. The proximal phalangeal articular angle (PPAA) (Fig. 2B) establishes the orientation of the articular surface of the proximal phalanx in relationship to the axis of the proximal phalanx. Slight valgus inclination may be present, but it rarely exceeds 5°. Where this angle is significantly higher, a hallux valgus interphalangeus deformity occurs. Hallux valgus deformities that are characterized by angulation of the articular surface of either the proximal phalanx or first metatarsal (congruent joint) are felt to be static in nature and do not tend to progress over time. A clinician must distinguish

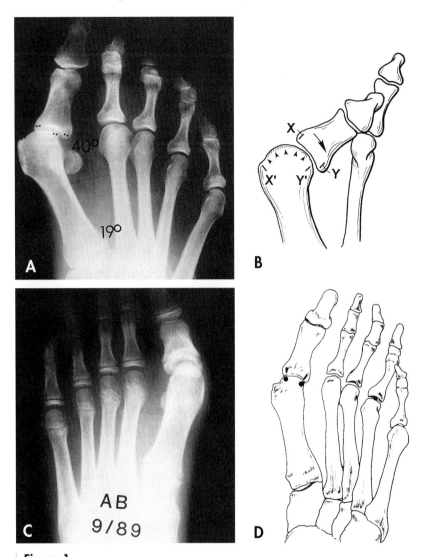

Figure 1

A and **B,** Radiograph and drawing of a subluxated metatarsophalangeal joint. Hallux valgus angle 40°, 1-2 inter-metatarsal angle 19°. **C** and **D,** Radiograph and drawing demonstrating hallux valgus with congruent MTP joint. (A and C, Reproduced with permission from Coughlin MJ: Juvenile bunions, in Mann RA, Coughlin MJ (eds): *Surgery of the Foot and Ankle*, ed 6. St. Louis, MO, Mosby Year Book, 1993, pp 297–337. Figures B and D, Copyright © Michael J. Coughlin, MD)

the base of the proximal phalanx in relationship with the first metatarsal articular surface. Mild subluxation may progress to a more severe deformity with time. This type of deformity may increase in severity either slowly or rapidly in contradistinction to a congruous joint, which does not tend to progress with time.

The hallux valgus angle (Fig. 3) is the angle formed by the intersection of the long axis of the proximal phalanx and the long axis of the first metatarsal. Normal is less than 15°, a mild deformity is less than 20°, a moderate deformity is 20° to 40°, and a severe deformity is greater than 40°. A juvenile hallux valgus deformity is characterized more frequently by mild and moderate hallux valgus deformities and it is uncommon for a severe hallux valgus angle to develop.

In the presence of a hallux valgus deformity, sesamoid subluxation may occur. Actually, it is the first metatarsal that migrates medially off of the sesamoid articulation, but by definition this is called sesamoid subluxation. Sesamoid subluxation is much less common in the juvenile with hallux valgus, just as pronation is much less common. With increasing magnitude of a hallux valgus deformity, the hallux may pronate or rotate because of the insertion of the conjoined adductor tendon on the plantar lateral base of the proximal phalanx. In a mild hallux valgus deformity, the lateral sesamoid is only uncovered approximately 25%. In a moderate deformity it may be uncovered 25% to 75%, and in a severe deformity it may be uncovered more than 75%. With any hallux valgus correction, the sesamoids must be relocated beneath the first metatarsal head.

whether the first MTP joint is congruous, as this will determine the appropriate surgical repair. An intra-articular repair, such as a distal soft-tissue reconstruction (modified McBride), in the presence of a congruent MTP joint is at high risk to develop postoperative stiffness or recurrence. An extra-articular repair is indicated in the presence of a congruent MTP joint.

A hallux valgus deformity with an incongruous first MTP joint is characterized by subluxation or lateral deviation of

Metatarsocuneiform Joint

Hallux valgus in the juvenile is often associated with an increased 1-2 intermetatarsal (IM) angle. The metatarso-cuneiform (MC) joint has a key role in the alignment of the first ray. An IM angle of greater than 9° is considered abnormal. It is difficult to determine the true orientation of the MC joint on routine radiographs. In one plane (anteroposterior) a radiograph may show an oblique orientation, and in another plane (posteroanterior) it may show a curved articulation.

Instability or hypermobility may allow increased medial angulation of the first metatarsal. A rigid MC joint may be characterized by an intermetatarsal facet between the proximal medial base of the second metatarsal and the proximal lateral base of the first metatarsal. This facet resists diminution of the IM angle with a distal soft-tissue repair. Regardless of the apparent angulation or radiographic appearance of the MC joint, an increased magnitude of the 1-2 intermetatarsal angle is associated with a hallux valgus deformity. Often, in the adult, as the hallux valgus angle increases, the intermetatarsal angle increases as well. It is felt that in the juvenile the intermetatarsal angle or metatarsus primus varus is often a primary deformity. The importance of this distinction is that flexibility of the MC joint can influence both the development of hallux valgus and the appropriate type of surgical repair used to correct the deformity. A fixed 1-2 IM angle is at risk for a recurrent

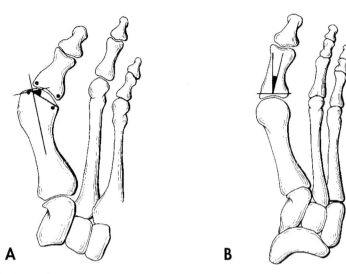

Figure 2

A, Distal metatarsal articular angle (DMAA) describes the angular relationship of the distal metatarsal articular surface to the longitudinal axis of the first metatarsal. (Copyright © Michael J. Coughlin, MD) **B,** The proximal phalangeal articular angle (PPAA) describes the relationship of the proximal articular surface of the proximal phalanx to the longitudinal axis of the proximal phalanx. (Reproduced with permission from Coughlin MJ: Hallux valgus, in Springfield DS (ed): *Instructional Course Lectures 46.* Rosemont, IL, American Academy of Orthopaedic Surgeons, 1997, pp 357-391.)

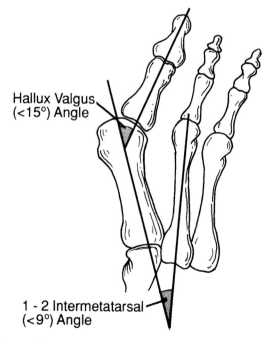

Figure 3

A hallux valgus angle of less than 15° and a 1-2 intermetatarsal angle less than 9° is normal. (Reproduced with permission from Coughlin MJ: Hallux valgus, in Springfield DS (ed): *Instructional Course Lectures 46.* Rosemont, IL, American Academy of Orthopaedic Surgeons, 1997, pp 357-391.)

hallux valgus deformity when only a distal soft-tissue repair is performed. A hallux valgus deformity that has occurred with progressive subluxation of the MTP joint and an increasing IM angle may be adequately corrected with a distal soft-tissue repair without a first metatarsal osteotomy. This inherent flexibility at the MC joint plays an important role in the success of a hallux valgus correction. Most MTP soft-tissue realignments, as well as distal metatarsal osteotomies, achieve some diminution of the 1-2 intermetatarsal angle because of flexibility at the MC joint.

The magnitude of the 1-2 IM angle depends on the orientation or angulation of the second metatarsal. When hallux valgus is associated with metatarsus adductus, the IM angle may be abnormally low. It is not unusual for a juvenile hallux valgus deformity to be associated with metatarsus adductus. This combination is difficult to treat, because there is a minimal amount of available space in which to realign the first metatarsal with an osteotomy.

Open Epiphyses

A juvenile hallux valgus deformity may be further characterized by the presence of open epiphyses at the base of the first metatarsal and at the base of the proximal phalanx. It has been speculated that a recurrent hallux valgus deformity may develop due to epiphyseal overgrowth, but this has not been substantiated. Epiphyseal injury with either a proximal phalangeal osteotomy or first metatarsal osteotomy is a distinct possibility. Consideration thus should be given either to postponing surgery or to the careful performance of an osteotomy. An open epiphysis is not a contraindication to surgical correction, but intraoperative identification of the epiphysis can help to avoid an epiphyseal injury. A hallux valgus deformity in a juvenile often requires an osteotomy in order to achieve correction. With the performance of an osteotomy, it is important to estimate the amount of growth expected in the first metatarsal postoperatively. An iatrogenic injury to the epiphysis can significantly reduce the overall length of the metatarsal. At age 12, in females, less than 1 cm in longitudinal growth remains in the foot. Less than half of this is present at the proximal metatarsal epiphysis. In adolescent males, at age 12, 3 cm of longitudinal foot growth remains, and at the proximal first metatarsal epiphysis approximately 1.5 cm of growth potential is present. In males growth is usually concluded in the foot by age 16.

Treatment

Conservative Care
Initially, nonsurgical care is often quite adequate to relieve most symptoms. While progression of deformity is an indication for surgery, a symptomatic bunion may be examined every 6 to 12 months by the treating physician. In the presence of a flexible flat foot deformity, an orthosis or arch support may be used. This also may be of advantage in the treatment of patients with a low collagen syndrome with an associated flat foot deformity. Roomy footwear may relieve symptoms, although typically a juvenile with a bunion deformity does not have an overly wide foot. Shoes that are characterized by a roomy toe box, low heel, and soft upper are helpful in diminishing symptoms. Footwear modifications may include stretching shoes in the area over the symptomatic bunion. While footwear modification may achieve significant relief for a symptomatic bunion, the use of sneakers or tennis shoes in this age group may be of great help in relieving symptoms. The use of high fashion footwear is uncommon in this age group and may be associated with increased symptomatology. When the use of roomy shoewear does not diminish symptoms, surgery may be considered. Surgery is infrequently needed on an emergent basis. It is important for the treating physician to distinguish between the cosmetic appearance of the foot and actual discomfort, such as pain over the bunion deformity. The juvenile and adolescent years can be a particularly difficult time for a patient, especially in compliance following surgical correction, and this further emphasizes the rationale for nonsurgi-

cal treatment. In preparing for the surgery, a careful decision-making process should be implemented in order to determine the most appropriate surgical procedure.

Decision Making
A physical examination is probably the most important step in preparing for correction of a juvenile hallux valgus deformity. The presence of an Achilles' tendon contracture, hyperelasticity, neurologic or neuromuscular abnormalities, or spasticity should be documented. Hindfoot valgus, pes planus, or even a cavus deformity may influence the success of a surgical correction.

Evaluation of radiographs helps to quantitate the magnitude of the deformity. The hallux valgus angle, the 1-2 IM angle, sesamoid subluxation, lesser metatarsal orientation (metatarsus adductus), the appearance of the MC joint, and MTP joint congruity are the major areas to be assessed on the radiograph.

After determining the magnitude of the deformity, the MTP joint shape (congruent versus subluxation) must be determined. In adults, congruity is present in approximately 9% of patients: in juveniles it is much more common, having been reported in one study to be present in 47% of patients. With a congruent (nonsubluxated) MTP joint articulation, a hallux valgus deformity is less likely to progress as compared to an MTP joint with subluxation. Nonetheless, a hallux valgus deformity with a congruent joint may require surgical correction. A soft-tissue realignment of the first MTP joint in the presence of a congruent joint (Fig. 4A) is contraindicated as it will create a noncongruous articulation. This situation may be at high risk either for postoperative recurrence of the deformity or for restricted range of motion and later degenerative arthritis. In the presence of a congruent joint, an extra-articular repair (phalangeal, metatarsal, or cuneiform osteotomy) is indicated (Fig. 4B). The magnitude of the hallux valgus angle or 1-2 intermetatarsal angle helps to determine the appropriate procedure. A combination of osteotomies (double or triple first ray osteotomies) may be considered. The major principle in treating a hallux valgus deformity with a congruent joint is the necessity for an extra-articular realignment. Osteotomies either in the proximal first metatarsal or proximal phalanx must be performed with care in order to prevent an epiphyseal injury. Intraoperative localization of the epiphysis is important.

In the presence of subluxation of the MTP joint with a mild deformity, a distal soft-tissue procedure or McBride repair may be indicated. With moderate and severe deformities, an MTP joint soft-tissue realignment with a proximal first metatarsal osteotomy may help to achieve complete correction.

Evaluation of the MC joint mobility is helpful in determining the presence of either rigidity or hypermobility of the metatarsal cuneiform articulation. Fixed obliquity of the MC joint is often associated with rigidity. A proximal first metatarsal osteotomy may be necessary in this case. Postoperative recurrence is greatly increased when an osteotomy is not performed in this situation. In the presence of hypermobility, an MC arthrodesis may help achieve reduction of the 1-2 IM angle as well as stabilization of the MC joint.

At the time of surgery, all elements must be corrected, including (1) increased hallux valgus angle; (2) increased 1-2 IM angle; (3) sesamoid subluxation; (4) pronation of the great toe; (5) enlarged medial eminence; and (6) MTP joint congruity.

Numerous surgical procedures have been reported for the correction of a juvenile hallux valgus deformity. The use of osteotomies to correct axial alignment is

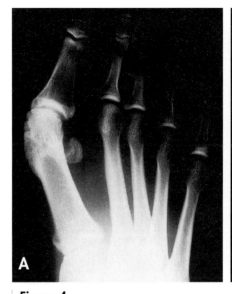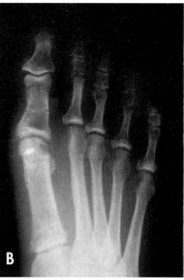

Figure 4

A, Radiograph demonstrating failed hallux valgus deformity with congruous joint. A simple bunionectomy was performed during adolescent years. **B,** Postoperative correction with triple osteotomy (phalangeal osteotomy, distal metatarsal closing wedge osteotomy, and proximal metatarsal crescentic osteotomy). (Copyright © Michael J. Coughlin, MD))

more frequent in the juvenile patient because of the higher incidence of a congruent MTP joint. The location of an osteotomy is often determined not only by the presence of an open epiphysis but also by the magnitude of the deformity. While a first metatarsal osteotomy is frequently performed, a distal or proximal location may depend upon the magnitude of the 1-2 IM angle. Use of algorithms is often helpful in the decision making process (Fig. 5). For a mild deformity, with a congruent MTP joint, a distal metatarsal osteotomy (chevron, Mitchell) may achieve an extra-articular correction. With an incongruent or subluxated MTP joint, a distal metatarsal osteotomy (chevron, Mitchell) or a distal soft-tissue realignment (modified McBride) may achieve correction. With a moderate hallux valgus deformity (Fig. 6) in the pres-

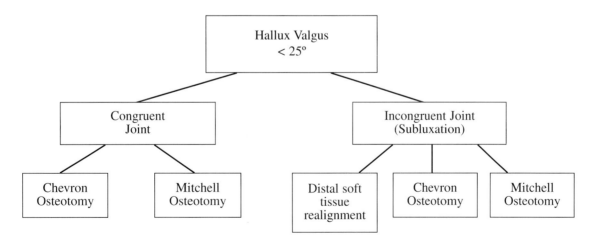

Figure 5

Algorithm for mild hallux valgus deformity with hallux valgus angle of 25° or less. (Reproduced with permission from Coughlin MJ: Juvenile bunion, in Mann RA, Coughlin MJ (eds): *Surgery of the Foot and Ankle*, ed 6. St. Louis, MO, Mosby- Year Book, 1993, pp 297–337.)

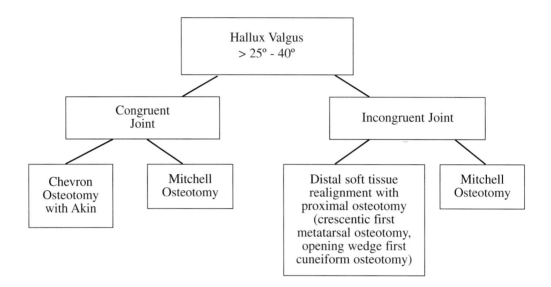

Figure 6

Algorithm for mild hallux valgus deformity with hallux valgus angle greater than 25°. (Reproduced with permission from Coughlin MJ: Juvenile bunion, in Mann RA, Coughlin MJ (eds): *Surgery of the Foot and Ankle*, ed 6. St. Louis, MO, Mosby-Year Book, 1993, pp 297–337.)

ence of a congruent MTP joint, a Mitchell osteotomy may achieve correction but a chevron osteotomy in and of itself often provides inadequate correction. A combined chevron and phalangeal osteotomy (Akin) may achieve complete correction. In the presence of an incongruent or subluxated MTP joint, again a Mitchell osteotomy may be used, or a distal soft-tissue realignment (McBride) in association with a proximal first metatarsal osteotomy may be performed. For severe deformities, decisions are made based on several factors (Fig. 7). In the presence of a hypermobile first MC joint, an arthrodesis of the MC joint is combined with a distal soft-tissue reconstruction. In the presence of a subluxated MTP joint, a distal soft-tissue realignment (modified McBride) may be combined with either a proximal first metatarsal osteotomy or a cuneiform osteotomy. A cuneiform osteotomy may be performed in the presence of an open first metatarsal epiphysis. With a congruent MTP joint, a double or triple osteotomy may be performed (Akin plus chevron, Akin plus proximal first metatarsal osteotomy, Akin plus first metatarsal plus cuneiform osteotomy, proximal plus distal first metatarsal osteotomy) may be performed (Fig. 8).

Akin Procedure A phalangeal osteotomy (Akin procedure) (Fig. 9) is mainly indicated in the presence of a hallux valgus interphalangeus deformity. Often there is an element of hallux valgus interphalangeus in the juvenile patient even if

there is more significant deformity proximally. Thus a phalangeal osteotomy may be combined with osteotomies in the first metatarsal or first cuneiform, achieving an extra-articular repair of a congruent MTP joint. The presence of an increased PPAA (proximal phalangeal articular angle) or hallux valgus interphalangeus deformity remain the major indications for a phalangeal osteotomy in association with a juvenile hallux valgus deformity. Care must be taken at the time of this procedure to avoid iatrogenic injury to the proximal phalangeal epiphysis.

Postoperative complications are unusual following this procedure. The use of internal fixations such as Kirschner wires are helpful in maintaining the surgical correction and in avoiding injury to the proximal phalangeal epiphyses.

Distal Metatarsal Osteotomy

Chevron Procedure Correction with a chevron osteotomy (Fig. 10) is based upon a medial eminence resection and distal metatarsal osteotomy. A chevron osteotomy achieves correction by lateral translation of the capital fragment of the distal metatarsal. A closing wedge medial osteotomy may be combined with the chevron osteotomy in order to achieve both lateral translation and realignment or correction of the increased distal metatarsal articular angle. Thus the chevron can be used for both a noncongruous (subluxated) MTP

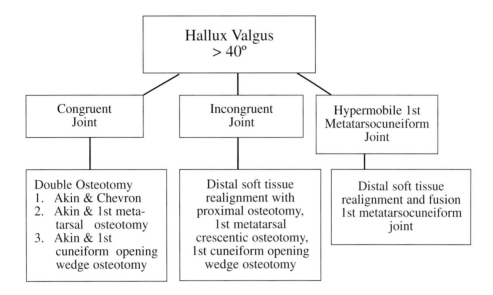

Figure 7

Algorithm for severe hallux valgus with hallux valgus angle greater than 40°. (Reproduced with permission from Coughlin MJ: Juvenile bunion, in Mann RA, Coughlin MJ (eds): *Surgery of the Foot and Ankle*, ed 6. St. Louis, MO, Mosby-Year Book, 1993, pp 297–337.)

joint with hallux valgus as well as in the presence of a congruous (nonsubluxated) articulation. The presence of an osteotomy in the distal metatarsal limits the correction that can be achieved and is indicated in the presence of a hallux valgus deformity less than 30°. Likewise, a biplanar osteotomy may achieve some correction of an increased distal metatarsal articular angle but, because of the location in the distal metatarsal, only approximately 10° of congruency can be corrected.

Internal fixation with a Kirschner wire is used to stabilize the osteotomy site and prevent recurrence. Internal fixation can be removed as early as 3 weeks following surgery. Excessive soft-tissue dissection should be avoided in order to minimize the risk of osteonecrosis. While a lateral release, including tenotomy of the adductor tendon, can be performed, significant soft-tissue stripping may increase the risk of osteonecrosis. A medial capsulorrhaphy and distal first metatarsal osteotomy disrupts both intraosseous circulation and the medial capsular circulation to the cap-

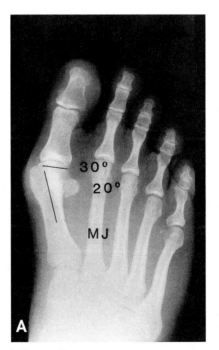
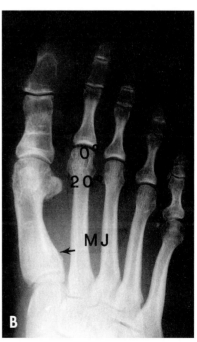

Figure 8

A, Hallux valgus deformity with preoperative hallux valgus angle of 30° and distal metatarsal articular angle of 20°. **B,** Postoperative radiograph following closing wedge phalangeal osteotomy and crescentic osteotomy. Note the correction of the deformity, which corrected 10° of hallux valgus at the MTP joint and included partial extra-articular correction. (Copyright © Michael J. Coughlin, MD)

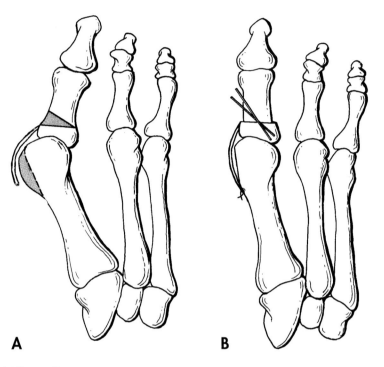

Figure 9

A, Proposed phalangeal osteotomy with medial eminence resection. **B,** Osteotomy is approximated with Kirschner wire fixation. The capsule is secured through drill holes in the metaphysis. With an open phalangeal epiphysis, care must be taken to avoid an intra-articular injury. (Reproduced with permission from Coughlin MJ: Hallux valgus, in Springfield DS (ed): *Instructional Course Lectures 46.* Rosemont, IL, American Academy of Orthopaedic Surgeons, 1997, pp 357-391.)

ital fragment. Thus, the last remaining circulation to the metatarsal head is delivered by lateral and dorsilateral capsular vessels. If a lateral capsular release and tenotomy is performed, it should be done with extreme care.

Mitchell Osteotomy A Mitchell osteotomy (Fig. 11), which achieves correction by lateral displacement and angulation of a distal metaphyseal osteotomy, is located slightly more proximal than a chevron osteotomy, thus allowing increased correction in comparison to the chevron procedure. A Mitchell osteotomy achieves an extra-articular correction of a hallux valgus deformity and can be used for hallux valgus deformities that are noncongruent or congruent.

The most common complication following a Mitchell osteotomy is postoperative metatarsalgia, which may occur in 25% to 40% of cases. The relative instability of this transverse osteotomy has made displacement or dorsal angulation possible, which can lead to the development of postoperative metatarsalgia. Osteonecrosis may occur following a Mitchell osteotomy as well. Plantar angulation at the osteotomy site

helps to reduce the incidence of postoperative metatarsalgia. Shortening at the osteotomy site is used to achieve correction. Rigid internal fixation of an osteotomy in this region helps to diminish recurrence as well as metatarsalgia.

Distal Soft-Tissue Realignment A distal soft-tissue realignment (Fig. 12) (modified McBride procedure) achieves correction as an intra-articular procedure. This correction relies on a lateral capsular and adductor tendon release, with freeing up (but not removal) of the lateral sesamoid medial eminence resection, and medial capsulorrhaphy. Although McBride initially described a lateral sesamoidectomy, this step has been eliminated in recent years due to the frequency of a postoperative hallux varus deformity. The eponym McBride has been eliminated because of the significant evolution of this procedure over the years. The indication for a distal soft-tissue realignment is a mild hallux valgus deformity with a subluxated (noncongruent) articulation. A proximal first metatarsal osteotomy, cuneiform osteotomy, or metatarsocuneiform arthrodesis also may be combined with a distal soft-tissue realignment.

While a distal soft-tissue realignment (DSTR) may be used in the presence of a mild deformity, its use in more severe deformities is accompanied by a high recurrence rate. In the presence of a flexible MC articulation, the 1-2 IM angle may be diminished with the use of a DSTR. However, the high failure rate with this procedure in the juvenile population has lead to its use in combination with a proximal osteotomy. The other significant complication associated with this technique is a hallux varus deformity, with a frequency varying from 4% to 11% of patients. Retaining the lateral sesamoid has diminished this complication.

Proximal First Metatarsal Osteotomy An opening or closing wedge osteotomy of the first metatarsal may be used depending upon the first metatarsal length. With a juvenile hallux valgus deformity, occasionally there is a long first metatarsal or a short first metatarsal, which may necessitate altering the length of the first metatarsal. When the first and second metatarsals are of similar length, neither lengthening or shortening is necessary. In this case, a curved or crescentic

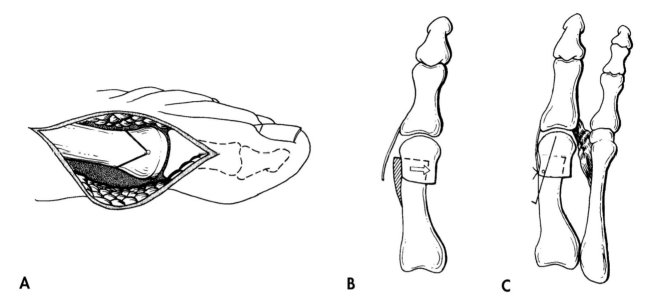

A   **B**   **C**

Figure 10

A, Chevron osteotomy demonstrated through medial approach. **B,** The capital fragment is translated laterally. **C,** The osteotomy is stapled with a Kirschner wire. The capsule is anchored with a suture through the metaphysis. (Reproduced with permission from Coughlin MJ: Hallux valgus, in Springfield DS (ed): *Instructional Course Lectures 46.* Rosemont, IL, American Academy of Orthopaedic Surgeons, 1997, pp 357-391.)

osteotomy will enable correction of the 1-2 IM angle without significant alteration of metatarsal length (Fig. 13). Localization of the osteotomy in the proximal metaphysis finds a broad contact area that allows rapid healing of the osteotomy. Care must be taken in the presence of an open epiphysis to avoid an iatrogenic epiphyseal arrest. Internal fixation may vary, depending on the presence of an open epiphysis. Screw fixation is used following epiphyseal closure, but stabilization of the osteotomy site with K-wires may be necessary in the presence of an open epiphysis. The use of a proximal first metatarsal osteotomy in combination with a distal soft-tissue realignment is indicated in the presence of a moderate or severe hallux valgus deformity with subluxation of the MTP joint. This procedure is versatile and can be used for moderate or severe deformities. Complications include hallux varus deformity or overcorrection. Care must be taken at the time of surgery to avoid overcorrection

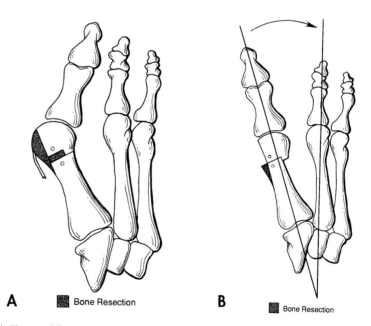

A   ■ Bone Resection   **B**   ■ Bone Resection

Figure 11

A, Proposed bone resection with a Mitchell osteotomy achieving shortening and angular correction. **B,** Following correction the osteotomy site is stabilized with a suture. The medial metaphyseal shelf is resected as well. (Reproduced with permission from Coughlin MJ: Hallux valgus, in Springfield DS (ed): *Instructional Course Lectures 46.* Rosemont, IL, American Academy of Orthopaedic Surgeons, 1997, pp 357-391.)

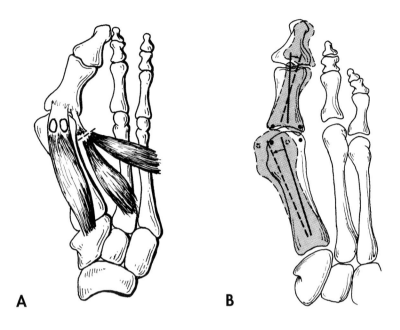

Figure 12

A, Illustration of a distal soft-tissue reconstruction. The conjoined tendon is released and secured to the lateral aspect of the metatarsal capsule at the conclusion of the procedure. (Reproduced with permission from Coughlin MJ: Hallux valgus, in Springfield DS (ed): *Instructional Course Lectures 46.* Rosemont, IL, American Academy of Orthopaedic Surgeons, 1997, pp 357-391.) **B,** With the release of contractures at the MTP joint, the intermetatarsal angle is reduced if there is flexibility at the metatarsocuneiform joint. (Copyright © Michael J. Coughlin, MD)

at the osteotomy site as well as an excessive medial eminence resection. An intraoperative radiograph or fluoroscopy helps to minimize the chance of overcorrection. Malunion at the osteotomy site may occur, as well as delayed union or nonunion, although these complications are uncommon. Epiphyseal injury may occur if the osteotomy injures the growth plate. This may lead to a short first metatarsal.

Metatarsocuneiform Arthrodesis An MC arthrodesis is indicated with an increased 1-2 intermetatarsal angle in order to stabilize this articulation in the presence of hypermobility. An MC arthrodesis may be used in the presence of severe MC obliquity greater than 30° as well. In the presence of generalized ligamentous laxity, an MC arthrodesis may achieve a more reliable repair than a metatarsal osteotomy. Typically, a distal soft-tissue realignment is combined with an MC arthrodesis. Rigid internal fixation and bone grafting may aid in achieving successful arthrodesis. Complications include delayed union and

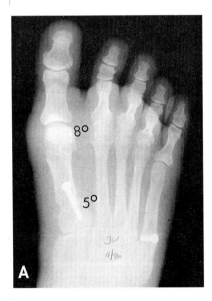
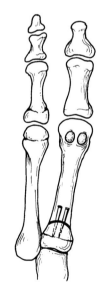
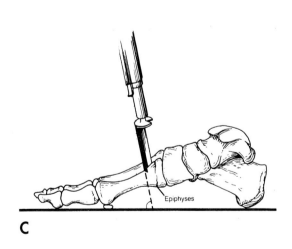

Figure 13

A, Postoperative radiograph demonstrating distal soft-tissue reconstruction with proximal first metatarsal crescentic osteotomy. The hallux valgus angle has been reduced to 8° and the intermetatarsal angle to 5°.(Copyright © Michael J. Coughlin, MD) **B,** Illustration of foot after distal soft-tissue reconstruction with a proximal osteotomy, and distal soft-tissue reconstruction. **C,** The proximal metaphyseal osteotomy should avoid an open epiphysis. (Figures B and C, Reproduced with permission from Coughlin MJ: Juvenile bunion, in Mann RA, Coughlin MJ (eds): *Surgery of the Foot and Ankle,* ed 6. St. Louis, MO, Mosby Year Book, 1993, pp 297–337.)

nonunion, which have been reported to vary from 9% to 75%. The difficulty of this procedure may lead to malunion or metatarsalgia due to dorsiflexion at the fusion site. Prolonged stiffness and pain at the arthrodesis site has been reported as well. The difficulty in fusing the MC joint is due to the resection necessary as well as the fact that excessive resection may lead to destabilization of this joint. Rigid internal fixation helps to diminish complications (Fig. 14).

First Cuneiform Osteotomy Although no series have been reported on the use of first cuneiform osteotomy in association with a hallux valgus deformity, the major indications for an opening wedge first cuneiform osteotomy are a juvenile hallux valgus deformity with a markedly increased 1-2 IM angle in the presence of an open first metatarsal epiphysis. Marked MC obliquity in association with an abnormally high 1-2 IM angle are further indications.

This procedure may be combined with other first ray osteotomies as well (Fig. 15). The first cuneiform osteotomy helps to achieve increased length in the first ray, and it may be combined with shortening or resection osteotomies in the first metatarsal or proximal phalanx. In performing this osteotomy, it is important to angulate the osteotomy in order to decrease the IM angle rather than to just lengthen the first ray at the osteotomy site. Therefore a triangular shaped graft is inserted at the time of the opening wedge

osteotomy. Frequently the graft is obtained from the iliac crest as the bone removed with a first metatarsal osteotomy often is not of sufficient width to achieve adequate distraction with this opening wedge osteotomy. The distraction at the osteotomy site along the medial border of the first cuneiform helps to diminish the 1-2 IM angle. Internal fixation often is performed with K-wires in order to prevent displacement of the osteotomy site or bone graft.

Double and Triple Osteotomies More recently, because of observed high rates of congruent MTP joints associated with juvenile hallux valgus deformities, multiple first ray osteotomies have been advocated (Fig. 16). In the presence of hallux valgus interphalangeus, a medial closing wedge phalangeal osteotomy may be performed. With an increased distal metatarsal articular angle (congruent MTP joint), a closing wedge distal metatarsal osteotomy may be performed. (A closing wedge distal metatarsal osteotomy is a modification of the Mitchell osteotomy.) It is performed in the distal first metatarsal metaphysis. The magnitude of the closing wedge depends upon the magnitude of the distal metatarsal articular angle. The goal is to orient the articular surface of the distal metatarsal as perpendicular as possible to the long axis of the first ray. By doing this, the articular surface of the first metatarsal can be rotated medially, thus correcting the DMAA.

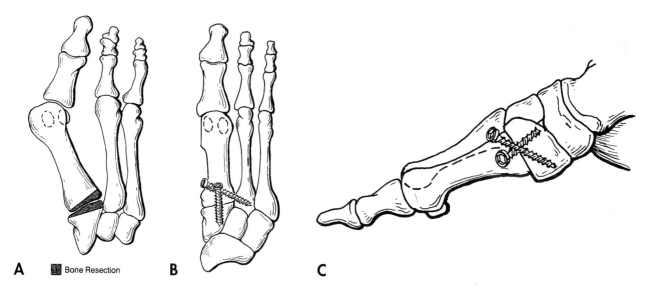

A   ▧ Bone Resection   B   C

Figure 14

A, Illustration demonstrating proposed bony resection for metatarsocuneiform fusion to diminish intermetatarsal angle. (Reproduced with permission from Coughlin MJ: Hallux valgus, in Springfield DS (ed): *Instructional Course Lectures 46.* Rosemont, IL, American Academy of Orthopaedic Surgeons, 1997, pp 357-391.) **B** and **C,** Illustration of screw fixation for metatarsocuneiform fusion. (Copyright © Michael J. Coughlin, MD)

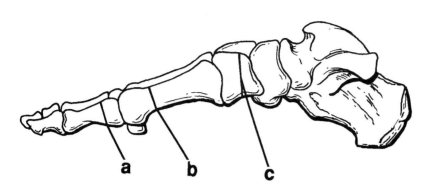

Figure 15

Multiple osteotomies. Lateral view, showing the locations of the osteotomies: **a,** phalangeal osteotomy; **b,** distal metatarsal osteotomy; and **c,** first cuneiform osteotomy. (Reproduced with permission from Coughlin MJ: Hallux valgus, in Springfield DS (ed): *Instructional Course Lectures 46*. Rosemont, IL, American Academy of Orthopaedic Surgeons, 1997, pp 357-391.)

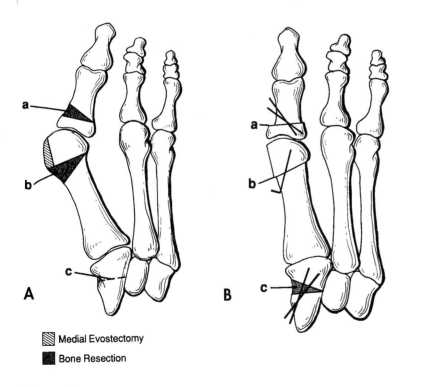

▧ Medial Evostectomy

▨ Bone Resection

Figure 16

Multiple osteotomies. **A, a,** A closing-wedge phalangeal osteotomy; **b,** a closing-wedge osteotomy of the distal end of the metatarsal with exostectomy of the medial eminence; and **c,** an opening wedge osteotomy of the first cuneiform. **B,** Appearance of the foot after a triple osteotomy. There is overall improved alignment of the first ray and the first metatarsophalangeal joint. (Reproduced with permission from Coughlin MJ: Hallux valgus, in Springfield DS (ed): *Instructional Course Lectures 46*. Rosemont, IL, American Academy of Orthopaedic Surgeons, 1997, pp 357-391.)

A medial closing wedge distal first metatarsal osteotomy may be performed to realign the articular surface of the distal first metatarsal. While this osteotomy will realign the articular surface at a more perpendicular orientation to the first metatarsal, it necessitates a proximal osteotomy to decrease the IM angle to make the entire first ray parallel with the second ray (Fig. 17).

In association with a phalangeal or distal metatarsal osteotomy, a proximal first metatarsal osteotomy may be performed. Most commonly, if length is to be maintained, a crescentic osteotomy may be performed. Another alternative may be an opening or closing wedge osteotomy depending on what osteotomy has been performed distally. When more than one osteotomy is performed in the first metatarsal, extreme caution must be maintained in any soft-tissue dissection. Devascularization of any portion of the first metatarsal may occur with extensive soft-tissue stripping. Likewise, multiple osteotomies of the first metatarsal may lead to an unstable situation with displacement and eventual malalignment or malunion of the first ray. An opening wedge first cuneiform osteotomy may be performed in combination with other distal osteotomies as well.

Multiple osteotomies are performed in order to diminish an increased proximal phalangeal articular angle (PPAA), distal metatarsal articular angle (DMAA), and increased 1-2 IM angle. Both Peterson and Coughlin, reporting on small series, have reported reliable correction of the juvenile hallux valgus deformity in the presence of a congruent MTP articulation.

Discussion

With a juvenile hallux valgus deformity, no single operation is sufficient to correct every deformity. Surgical versatility is most important in order that the various pathologic components present with dif-

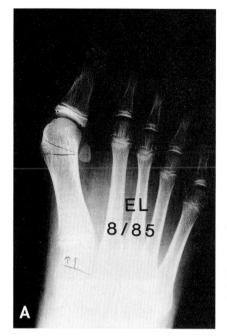 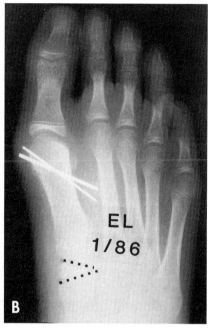 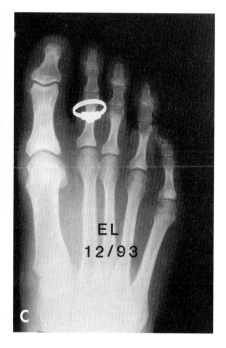

Figure 17

A, Preoperative radiograph demonstrates moderate/severe hallux valgus deformity with significant DMAA. **B,** Postoperative radiograph was taken after closing wedge distal metatarsal and opening wedge cuneiform osteotomy. **C,** Long-term follow-up demonstrating adequate alignment with congruent MTP joint. (Reproduced with permission from Coughlin MJ: Juvenile hallux valgus. *Foot Ankle Int* 1995;16:682–697.)

ferent deformities be completely corrected. With the initial patient physical examination, the presence of a pes planus deformity, contracted Achilles tendon, pes cavus, or hypermobility must not only be identified but may need to be corrected prior to the repair of any hallux valgus deformity. Radiographs must be assessed in order to quantitate the magnitude of the hallux valgus angle, 1-2 IM angle, and sesamoid subluxation. The presence of metatarsus adductus may affect the decision-making process as well. Significant metatarsus adductus may be difficult to correct, because an increased 1-2 IM angle may necessitate a proximal first metatarsal osteotomy. In the case of metatarsus adductus, a negative 1-2 IM angle may be created with a first metatarsal osteotomy. An alternative may be multiple lesser metatarsal osteotomies, although a surgeon must evaluate the magnitude of this surgery in comparison with the correction to be obtained at surgery. The presence of an increased 1-2 IM angle necessitates correction with an osteotomy. As the IM angle increases, a more proximal first ray osteotomy will achieve more correction than a distal metatarsal osteotomy. Likewise, the presence of an open phalangeal or metatarsal epiphysis may necessitate careful localization of a metatarsal osteotomy or a first cuneiform osteotomy.

Radiographic assessment of the MTP joint for congruency or subluxation (noncongruent joint) is equally important in determining whether an extra-articular or intra-articular correction is warranted. In the presence of hallux valgus interphalangeus, a phalangeal osteotomy may be performed. With a noncongruous (subluxated) MTP joint, a distal soft-tissue realignment may be performed with or without a proximal osteotomy. An MC arthrodesis may be combined with a distal soft-tissue realignment in the presence of severe MC obliquity or hypermobility.

More recently, in the presence of moderate or severe hallux valgus deformity with a congruous MTP joint, double and triple osteotomies have been advocated. Variations include a closing wedge phalangeal osteotomy (Akin procedure), a closing wedge distal metatarsal osteotomy (Mitchell procedure), Chevron osteotomy, an opening, closing, or crescentic metatarsal osteotomy, and/or an opening wedge medial cuneiform osteotomy. Multiple osteotomies have an increased risk for complications, due to increased dissection and increased instability. A surgeon must use care to avoid injury to an open phalangeal or metatarsal epiphysis with multiple osteotomies. When a double metatarsal osteotomy is performed, excessive soft-tissue stripping must be avoided.

Postoperative complications have been frequently reported following juvenile hallux valgus corrections. Recurrence following surgery is probably the most frequently reported complication and is likely due to the high rate of congruency associated with a juvenile hallux valgus deformity. The use of periarticular osteotomies appears to diminish recurrence rate. Likewise, the use of a single procedure to correct all juvenile hallux valgus deformities may lead to recurrence. Some juvenile hallux valgus deformities require only a simple soft-tissue realignment; others may require complex multiple first ray osteotomies to achieve acceptable realignment. As with an adult, any surgical procedure to correct a juvenile hallux valgus deformity must correct all components of the deformity, including an increased hallux valgus angle, increased 1-2 IM angle, enlarged medial eminence, sesamoid subluxation, pronation of the hallux, hypermobility or obliquity of the MC joint, and, at the same time, correct a subluxated or incongruous MTP joint. Different juvenile bunions present with different pathologic components and require considerably different surgical approaches to achieve successful correction. A surgeon must not stretch the indications for a particular hallux valgus surgical procedure. In the presence of a more severe deformity, a more aggressive surgical procedure should be used that can correct a more severe deformity. The variable success rate for hallux valgus procedures in the juvenile makes the case that no single surgery is suited as a standard correction for a juvenile bunion. The treating physician must vary the surgical technique depending upon the anatomic and pathologic factors present to achieve a consistently good success rate in treating the juvenile bunion.

Hallux Rigidus

Hallux rigidus presents with diminished motion of the MTP joint of the great toe. It occurs occasionally in juveniles and is primarily felt to be secondary to an osteochondritis dessicans lesion of the distal metatarsal articular surface. In adults, it is primarily degenerative arthritis although trauma may lead to the development of chondrolysis of the joint space and the formation of dorsal metatarsal-head exostosis.

On clinical examination, diminished range of motion (especially dorsiflexion) is noted, as well as a prominence over the dorsal aspect of the MTP joint. Patients tend to walk on the outer aspect of the foot to eliminate MTP joint dorsiflexion.

Radiographic examination may show a diminished joint space or a normal joint space. On the lateral radiograph, an exostosis is noted dorsally. Rarely are the sesamoids involved. In adolescent patients, an intra-articular loose body may be demonstrated.

Conservative treatment involves diminishing range of motion of the great toe. Shoe modifications such as a stiff sole (extended shank), or an enlarged toe box may accommodate the exostosis and joint swelling (synovitis). Non-steroidal anti-inflammatory medications (NSAIDs) and the occasional judicious use of an intra-articular steroid injection may diminish symptoms.

Where conservative care has failed, an arthrotomy of the MTP joint and chielectomy of the exostosis may lead to increased motion. On occasion, a dorsal closing wedge phalangeal osteotomy may increase dorsiflexion range of motion. Depending on the patient's age, a chielectomy (joint debridement) may give significant relief in the early stages of this disease process. At least 25% of the joint space should be present on the AP radiograph. The chielectomy is performed through a dorsal incision along the medial aspect of the extensor hallucis longus tendon. Thirty percent to 40% of the dorsal aspect of the metatarsal head is resected obliquely to permit dorsiflexion of 70° to 80°. Postoperatively, aggressive range of motion exercises are initiated. Often there is still diminished range of motion of the great toe following completion of the healing process.

With progressive degenerative arthritis, other options include an arthrodesis or a resection arthroplasty (Keller procedure). An arthrodesis in the younger patient gives good postoperative stability and durability. Women often desire motion at the MTP joint in order to accommodate various heel heights. In an older female, a Keller resection arthroplasty at the base of the proximal phalanx may give pain relief and allow continued motion. In some situations, a cock-up, shortened, or deformed toe may occur. In the younger patient, an excision arthroplasty is contraindicated. An interposition Silastic implant at the MTP joint, at this time, is felt to be controversial. Complications such as "silicone synovitis," loosening, and fracture of the prosthesis have been reported. The long term efficacy in the use of these implants has been questioned and they are contraindicated in younger, active patients.

Sesamoids

The MTP joint of the great toe is characterized by the medial and lateral sesamoids, which are contained in the dual head of the flexor hallucis brevis tendon. The medial sesamoid receives an attachment of the abductor hallucis and the lateral sesamoid receives an insertion of the adductor hallucis. The sesamoids tend to increase the strength of the plantar intrinsic muscles and protect the tendon of the flexor hallucis longus which courses between the two sesamoids.

Sesamoids can be injured by trauma, such as forced dorsiflexion, by repeated trauma, or by a fall from a height. On clinical examination, localized pain with palpation, diminished range of motion, and pain on range of motion are frequent complaints. Radiographs are important to evaluate sesamoid pathology. Sequential radiographs may show a change in the alignment or bony appearance of one of the sesamoids. Many patients have a bipartite medial sesamoid. It is uncommon to have a bipartite lateral sesamoid. Bilaterality is not consistent and is not helpful in making a diagnosis of a pathologic condition. A bone scan may be helpful in demonstrating an abnormal sesamoid with an otherwise normal radiograph.

Either acute or chronic inflammation of the sesamoids is termed sesamoiditis. Radiographs are typically negative. Treatment involves diminishing pressure beneath the sesamoids, nonsteroidal anti-inflammatory medications, and an occasional intra-articular steroid injection. Over a 3- to 6-month period, the discomfort may improve. When symptoms do not improve, a bone scan is indicated.

A fractured sesamoid may be difficult to differentiate from a bipartite sesamoid. Sequential radiographs and/or a bone scan may be helpful in making the diagnosis. Other diagnoses include chondromalacia of the sesamoid or osteochondritis. An acute fracture of a sesamoid is usually associated with a traumatic episode. Often patients will isolate their pain to the area of the medial or lateral sesamoid and radiographic examination may demonstrate a defect in the sesamoid. Casting is rarely helpful. Diminished range of motion of the MTP joint with taping, the use of a metatarsal pad, and a stiff-soled shoe is frequently sufficient. It may take several months for discomfort to subside, and often a fractured sesamoid may be associated with diminished range of motion. Again, where radiographs are negative and in the presence of chronic pain, a bone scan is indicated.

With the failure of conservative methods such as padding, orthotic devices, taping to restrict dorsiflexion excursion, and NSAID medication, excision of a sesamoid may be indicated. The medial sesamoid is excised through an inferiomedial incision, with care taken to protect the sensory branch of the medial plantar nerve. The lateral sesamoid is typically excised through a plantar incision just lateral to the lateral sesamoid. (Another alternative is to approach the lateral sesamoid from a dorsal/lateral first interspace incision, although this is often difficult.)

In either case, the sesamoid is excised subperiosteally and, when possible, the defect in the tendon of the flexor hallucis brevis is closed with interrupted 0 absorbable sutures. Both sesamoids should not be excised, because this can lead to a claw toe deformity. Postoperative diminished range of motion, continued pain, and progressive valgus or varus deformity may occur following sesamoid excision.

On occasion, an intractable plantar keratotic lesion (IPK) may develop beneath the medial sesamoid. Often the skin can be trimmed and symptoms will subside. When pain continues in the presence of an IPK, 50% of the sesamoid may be shaved surgically in order to reduce the bony prominence beneath the IPK. The medial sesamoid is approached through an inferior medial incision. Care is taken to protect the medial sensory nerve at the time of the surgical exposure. Postoperative care involves gauze and tape compression dressings changed weekly until adequate healing has occurred (usually after 6 weeks).

Annotated Bibliography

Coughlin MJ: Juvenile hallux valgus: Etiology and treatment. *Foot Ankle Int* 1995;16:682–697.

This long-term report assesses the results of the chevron distal soft-tissue procedure with proximal first metatarsal osteotomy and multiple first ray osteotomies in the treatment of juvenile hallux valgus. Probably the most comprehensive long-term study available, it describes the frequency of occurrence of congruent joints in the juvenile patient with hallux valgus.

Coughlin MJ: Hallux valgus, in Springfield DS (ed): *Instructional Course Lectures 46.* Rosemont, IL, American Academy of Orthopaedic Surgeons, 1997, pp 357-391.

This report analyzes the pathophysiology and surgical techniques, results, and complications of various procedures.

Coughlin MJ: Juvenile bunions, in Mann RA, Coughlin MJ (eds): *Surgery of the Foot and Ankle,* ed 6. St. Louis, MO, Mosby-Year Book, 1993, pp 297–339.

This chapter gives an in-depth review of surgical techniques to correct a hallux valgus deformity.

Coughlin MJ, Bordelon RL, Johnson K, Mann RA: Symposium: Presidents' Forum. Evaluation and treatment of juvenile hallux valgus. *Contemp Orthop* 1990;21:169-203.

This discussion by past-presidents of the American Orthopaedic Foot and Ankle Society regards their different methods of treatment and evaluation of juvenile hallux valgus.

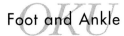

150   Juvenile Hallux Valgus and Other First Ray Problems

Coughlin MJ, Mann RA: The pathophysiology of the juvenile bunion, in Griffin PP (ed): *Instructional Course Lectures XXXVI.* Park Ridge, IL, American Academy of Orthopaedic Surgeons, 1987, pp 123–136.

This Instructional Course Lecture reviews the pathophysiology and treatment of juvenile bunions.

Hardy RH, Clapham JCR: Observations on hallux valgus: Based on a controlled series. *J Bone Joint Surg* 1951;33B:376–391.

This is a classic study on hallux valgus in associated deformities.

Mann RA, Coughlin MJ: Hallux valgus: Etiology, anatomy, treatment, and surgical considerations. *Clin Orthop* 1981;157:31–41.

This paper reports long-term results of the distal soft-tissue procedure as a treatment for hallux valgus.

Peterson HA, Newman SR: Adolescent bunion deformity treated with double osteotomy and longitudinal pin fixation of the first ray. *J Pediatr Orthop* 1993;13:80–84.

This paper gives an evaluation of multiple first ray osteotomies in the juvenile patient.

Piggott H: The natural history of hallux valgus in adolescence and early adult life. *J Bone Joint Surg* 1960;42B:749–760.

This classic study describes congruent versus subluxated metatarsophalangeal joints.

Simmonds FA, Menelaus MB: Hallux valgus in adolescents. *J Bone Joint Surg* 1960;42B:761–768.

This is a long-term study of the surgical treatment of hallux valgus deformity.

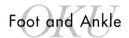

Chapter 12
Pathology of the First Ray

Hallux Rigidus

Hallux rigidus is the second most common pathologic condition of the hallux and many orthopaedists consider it to be the most disabling. It is primarily arthrosis of the first metatarsophalangeal (MTP) joint and is characterized by a painful loss of motion with the formation of prominent osteophytes. It is estimated to occur in up to 2.5% of the adult population and generally is seen in a younger population of patients than are other arthritides. First described by Davies-Colley in 1887 as what he termed hallux flexus, the term hallux rigidus was coined soon after by Cotterill and is the most common term used today. Other terminology includes hallux limitus, metatarsus primus elevatus, dorsal bunion, hallux equinus, hallux dolorosus, and metatarsus non-extensus.

Two age group subsets of patients have been described: adolescent (juvenile) and adult. The adolescent group is the least common and is characterized by localized chondral/osteochondral lesions in the articular cartilage of the metatarsal head. The adult type is more common and is characterized by a diffuse, more generalized degenerative arthrosis that increases in degree of involvement with increasing age. Chondral and osteochondral lesions can also be seen in adults after acute injuries.

The primary etiology of hallux rigidus is debatable. Many authors have noted predisposing conditions, such as a flat metatarsal head, a long first metatarsal, a dorsiflexed first metatarsal, improper shoe wear, a long slender foot, congenital deformities, pes planus, or a pronated foot. There is, however, no common predisposing factor. In general, hallux rigidus is a result of a degenerative process caused by a number of conditions, such as trauma, accumulated microtrauma secondary to eccentric loading, systemic diseases, osteochondritis dissecans, and infection. As the joint degeneration progresses, changes occur in the periosteum, synovium, and joint capsule. Impingement of the base of the proximal phalanx on the dorsal aspect of the metatarsal head with forced dorsiflexion leads to chondral and osteochondral injuries of the articular cartilage and metatarsal head with erosion and osteophyte formation. As osteophytes proliferate, the joint becomes more prominent and range of motion is limited mechanically by further impingement dorsally (Figs. 1, A and B and 2, A). Pain is secondary to movement of the degenerated joint surfaces, the synovitis from the joint degeneration, impingement of the osteophytes with dorsiflexion, and stretching of the inflamed synovium, digital nerves, and capsule over the dorsal osteophytes.

Findings

Most patients complain of the gradual development of a painfully swollen and stiff first MTP joint. Initially, their pain is activity related and progresses over time to a point where comfortable shoe wear is difficult, especially with elevated heels. Patients with osteochondral lesions after acute injuries may complain of a persistent clicking or catching sensation with range of motion. Their symptoms generally worsen over time.

On physical examination, the findings vary with the severity of the disease. Varying degrees of swelling and thickening of the first MTP joint can be seen and palpated. The key clinical finding is limited dorsiflexion with a sharp increase in pain at the end point. A hallux valgus or varus deformity is seen occasionally. Neuritic findings with paresthesias and pain with percussion along the dorsal lateral and, less commonly, the dorsal medial digital nerves, may be present. Because normal walking requires 15° of dorsiflexion, gait abnormalities are usually a late finding and include supination of the forefoot with lateral weightbearing and external rotation. In patients with early osteochondral lesions, the bony proliferative changes are not seen. Passive range of motion with compression across the joint can produce pain and clicking, which may be relieved with joint distraction during range of motion.

Radiographs range from totally normal to severe joint destruction as the disease progresses. The level of radiographic changes does not necessarily correlate to the degree of symptoms. Consequently, while some authors have presented radiographic staging criteria to develop treatment algorithms, others have not found these to be helpful. The anteroposterior (AP) view will show the amount of joint space narrowing and the medial and lateral osteophytes. Osteochondritic lesions are also best seen on the AP view. The lateral view profiles the dorsal osteophytes and any loose bodies that may be present. Also, with close inspection, the degree of joint space narrowing, which is usually worse dorsally, can be seen. Oblique views can be used to detect flat-

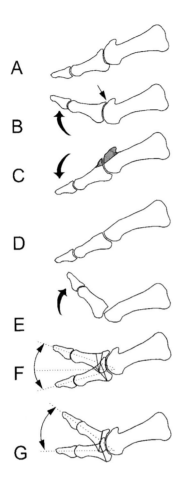

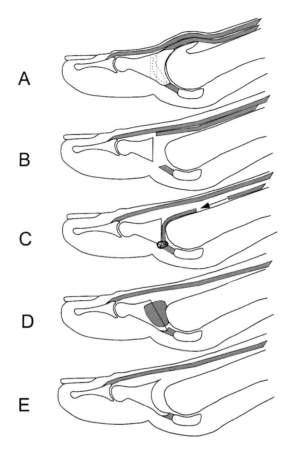

Figure 1

A, A hallux with joint space narrowing and dorsal osteophytes. B, Dorsiflexion of proximal phalanx and impingement of dorsal osteophytes (small arrow). C, Outline of bone to be removed with a cheilectomy. D, Hallux status post cheilectomy. E, Dorsiflexion without bony impingement following a cheilectomy. F, A hallux with limited dorsiflexion and preserved plantarflexion with arc of motion identified by arrows. Segment of bone to be removed from proximal phalanx is outlined. G, Hallux after Moberg dorsiflexion osteotomy of proximal phalanx. Note increased dorsiflexion without increase in arc of motion.

Figure 2

A, First toe with hallux rigidus with joint space narrowing and osteophyte formation. Dotted lines on proximal phalanx correspond with lines of bone resection for B, C, D, and E. B, Standard Keller resection arthroplasty with resection of 33% to 50% of proximal phalanx. C, Modified Keller resection arthroplasty with resection of less than 25% of the proximal phalanx with advancement and interposition of the dorsal capsule and extensor hallucis brevis. D, Modified resection arthroplasty with resection of dorsal base of proximal phalanx with preservation of plantar attachments and interposition of rolled plantaris tendon packet. E, Modified resection arthroplasty with resection of dorsal base of proximal phalanx with crescentic cut to preserve plantar attachments.

tening of the metatarsal head and determine the amount of joint space that is still remaining. Sesamoid involvement, which is rare, is best seen on the lateral and axial sesamoid views. Although it is seldom needed, a bone scan will detect an osteochondritic lesion or early degenerative changes before they are visible on plain radiographs. In rare instances, ultrasonography can be used to detect some chondral lesions and intra-articular loose bodies not visualized on routine radiographs.

Treatment

Conservative treatment is directed at preventing and relieving symptoms. Initially, shoe modifications with a wide/deep toe box and stiff sole along with nonsteroidal anti-inflammatory drugs (NSAIDs) are used. Although orthotics can be used to stiffen the sole and decrease motion, they can take up valuable room in the toe box and can cause increased symptoms from pressure over the dorsal osteophytes. A rocker bottom sole, metatarsal bar, or steel shanked shoe can also be used to decrease symptoms, but these are somewhat cumbersome and have a low degree of patient acceptance. Intra-articular steroid injections may provide temporary relief but should be used judiciously because their repeated use may accelerate the degenerative process.

If significant symptoms persist, surgical intervention should be considered. The ideal goal of surgical intervention is to alleviate pain, correct deformity, maintain or improve motion and stability, and preserve length. Multiple less than totally ideal surgical options exist, each with its own set of advantages and disadvantages. These options include open or arthroscopic synovectomy with debridement of chondral and osteochondral lesions, cheilectomy, dorsiflexion osteotomy of the proximal phalanx or metatarsal head, resection arthroplasty, prosthetic replacement, and arthrodesis. All of these procedures have been shown to have greater than 80% satisfactory results. The best procedure depends on the pathology present, the demands and expectations of the patient, and the experience of the surgeon.

For patients with few or no radiologic findings, but with symptoms of a loose body or a chondral or an osteochondral lesion, an open or arthroscopic synovectomy with debridement may be indicated. Studies have shown that arthroscopy can minimize the immediate postsurgical soft-tissue injury, but long-term results are not yet available.

In most patients with dorsal osteophytes and mechanical impingement, a procedure that simply removes these impinging osteophytes, a cheilectomy, is the primary procedure of choice. There is some controversy in the literature as to whether or not patients with significant joint space narrowing are candidates for a cheilectomy. The proper technique involves a dorsal or medial incision to expose the dorsal osteophytes so they can be removed (Fig. 1, C through E). It is important to explore the lateral joint and remove any bony osteophytes present. The amount of bone removed depends on the degree of pathology present. However, most authors suggest that 25% to 35% of the dorsal aspect of the metatarsal head be removed to allow 70° to 90° of dorsiflexion without bony impingement. Most poor results are related to insufficient bone removal. Postoperative range of motion will usually be less than that achieved at the time of surgery and depends greatly on the patient's compliance with early postoperative range-of-motion exercises. The procedure does not "burn any bridges" and will not preclude any further salvage procedure should it be necessary. If the patients are prepared for some postoperative arthritic pain symptoms, there is a high rate of satisfactory results.

For the rare patients with loss of dorsiflexion and preserved plantarflexion, a dorsiflexion osteotomy of the proximal phalanx (Moberg procedure) may be the procedure of choice

(Fig. 1, F and G). It can be combined with a cheilectomy if large dorsal osteophytes are present. A recent review, with an average follow-up of 12 years, of 10 patients following a dorsiflexion osteotomy and 20 patients following an arthrodesis for hallux rigidus, found that the patients with the dorsiflexion osteotomy had fewer complications and callosities. The authors concluded that the dorsiflexion osteotomy is an acceptable alternative to arthrodesis to preserve motion in patients with some remaining plantarflexion.

Resection arthroplasty, first popularized by Keller in 1904, works by decompression of the MTP joint by the removal of about one third to one half of the proximal phalanx (Fig. 2, B). A recent review, with a mean 9-year follow-up, showed the best results in patients who had 33% to 50% of the proximal phalanx resected. In the past, the Keller procedure was very popular for the treatment of severe hallux valgus and hallux rigidus but now is usually recommended only for elderly and inactive patients. Long-term follow-up evaluation has revealed a number of potential problems after resection of the base of the proximal phalanx and detachment of the plantar plate and insertion of the flexor hallucis brevis. The problems seen include a cock-up deformity of the first toe, weakness in push off, instability of the first ray, excessive shortening, valgus drift, and transverse metatarsalgia. In an effort to overcome these problems, there have been a number of recent modifications to the basic Keller procedure.

One recent modification removes less than 25% of the proximal phalanx, reattaches the short flexors to the base of the proximal phalanx, and interposes the capsule and extensor hallucis brevis between the metatarsal head and base of the proximal phalanx with reported good early results (Fig. 2, C). Another recent modification only removes bone from the dorsal portion of the proximal phalanx and interposes a rolled up section of plantaris tendon into a pocket made into the base of the proximal phalanx (Fig. 2, D). The authors state that this method gives good results because it relieves pain, corrects the deformity, provides good range of motion, avoids first ray shortening, and maintains joint stability. Still another recent modification describes using the crescentic saw blade to make a curved cut to remove bone from the base of the proximal phalanx and preserve the plantar attachments (Fig. 2, E). The author states that sufficient bone can be removed from the proximal phalanx to decompress the joint and still preserve the plantar attachments to maintain stability with this technique.

Prosthetic replacement gained popularity when Swanson presented his results with silicone implants in the toes in 1972. Several different types of implant designs have been developed over the years. Advantages include preservation of functional joint motion and length. Although short-term results are generally good, long-term results have been less than satisfactory. Problems include implant failure (excessive wear), soft-tissue foreign body reaction, joint stiffness, joint instability, transfer lesions, implant loosening, silicone synovitis, osteolysis, and progressive shortening of the hallux.

A recent survivorship analysis of first MTP joint implant arthroplasty identified young age as a significant risk factor for poor survival. Another recent review of single-stem silastic implants with an average follow-up of 9 years, showed that 36% of the patients were unhappy with the results. All the unsatisfied cases showed fragmentation of the implant with bone reaction around the implant. In a recent study of double-stem silastic implants with protective titanium grommets, after a 4-year follow-up it was concluded that the titanium grommets may protect the silicone implant and increase the durability. The authors did not recommend implant arthroplasty for young or active patients. Longer follow-up with the titanium grommets is pending. Recently, a 40-year review of a metallic resurfacing hemiarthroplasty with 95% good and excellent results in 279 patients was presented. In this study, a press-fit device was used to resurface the base of the proximal phalanx. The authors did not see the reactive synovitis or bone changes that have been observed with silastic implants. Additional studies with this design have not been presented.

Currently, the most widely used surgical solution for end stage hallux rigidus is arthrodesis of the first MTP joint. The main disadvantages are loss of motion, limitation of shoe wear, and time to recovery. The advantages include predictable pain relief, stability, and durability. Although there may not be much agreement on the best method for internal fixation, there is general agreement as to the alignment position for first MTP joint fusion. Most authors agree that the toe should be fixed in approximately 15° to 20° of valgus and 25° to 30° of dorsiflexion with respect to the first metatarsal and 10° to 15° of dorsiflexion with respect to the plantar aspect of the foot (Fig. 3).

Many different methods of internal fixation have been described. Methods include longitudinal Steinmann pins, compression screws, and dorsal plates. Recently, techniques using Herbert screws and tension band wiring have also been recommended. Steinmann pins and compression screws produce a stress riser at the insertion/exit site with the potential for stress fractures. The dorsal plates are bulky and have the potential to become irritating and require an additional procedure for removal.

One recent cadaveric biomechanical study compared the fixation strength of Steinmann pins, oblique compression screws, cannulated 4.5-mm Herbert screws, and dorsal quarter tubular minifragment plates. The minifragment plate was found to be significantly stronger than the compression screw

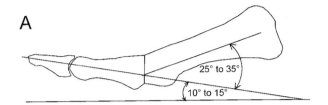

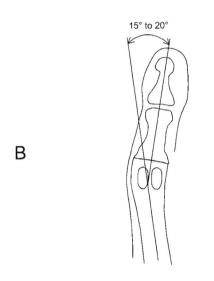

Figure 3

A, Lateral view of first metatarsophalangeal joint (MTP) arthrodesis with 25° to 35° of dorsiflexion with respect to the first metatarsal and 10° to 15° of dorsiflexion with respect to the plane of the sole of the foot. **B,** Anteroposterior view of a first MTP arthrodesis with 15° to 20° of valgus with respect to the first metatarsal.

in force to failure and initial stiffness. The authors concluded that a dorsal minifragment plate would provide sufficient fixation to allow early weightbearing. Another cadaveric biomechanical study compared the strength of fixation with crossed Kirschner wires (K-wires), a dorsal minifragment plate, and an interfragmentary compression screw with joint surfaces prepared with flat cuts to fixation with an interfragmentary compression screw with joint surfaces prepared by conical reaming. Although the conical reaming produced more shortening than the flat cuts, it was found to greatly increase the strength of the fixation. The lack of stiffness and the potential for hardware failure with the stainless steel minifragment plate has led to the development of a low profile Vitallium (Vitallium miniplate, Howmedica, East Rutherford, NJ) plate for use in first MTP fusions. The Vitallium plate is stiffer and stronger than the stainless steel minifragment plates and has no holes in the center of the plate over the fusion site, further adding to its strength. A recent article reported a 98% fusion rate with this plate and joint surfaces prepared with either cup shaped or conical reamers.

Hallux Varus

By definition, medial deviation of the first toe at the MTP joint is hallux varus. While not always painful, it is not well appreciated cosmetically and causes problems with shoe wear. Like hallux valgus, because the metatarsal head has no muscle insertions or origins, hallux varus is a result of an imbalance of the dynamic and static forces about the first MTP joint through the muscles, capsule, and ligaments that insert onto the base of the proximal phalanx.

Hallux varus is most commonly seen as a complication of bunion surgery but can be congenital, inflammatory, neurogenic, idiopathic, or posttraumatic in origin. It can be seen following all types of bunion procedures but is most commonly seen after a distal soft-tissue procedure or McBride type of bunionectomy. Factors that have been shown to increase the incidence of hallux varus include excision of the fibular sesamoid, excessive resection of the median eminence, over plication of the medial structures, excessive lateral capsular release, excessive varus postoperative dressing, and overcorrection of the intermetatarsal angle. When there is disruption of the lateral capsule and short flexor, the proximal phalanx migrates medially and dorsally. This produces a cock-up deformity as the extensor hallucis longus (EHL) migrates medially and becomes a deforming force for the varus deformity (Fig. 4, A). At the same time, the EHL loses its mechanical advantage to effectively dorsiflex the interphalangeal (IP) joint while the flexor hallucis longus (FHL) is stretched around the metatarsal head, increasing its flexion force on the IP joint. Over time, the toe stiffens with the MTP joint in extension and medial deviation and the IP joint in flexion. The deformity can occur early or may take months to years to develop.

Findings

Clinically, the deformities range from mild to severe and from flexible to fixed. Mild flexible deformities are rarely symptomatic and are more of a cosmetic problem. With time, more severe deformities range from an early flexible deformity to a later fixed deformity. Patients may complain of the obvious cosmetic deformities, painful motion, decreased motion, instability, weakness with push off, pain over the medial IP joint, and difficulty with shoe wear. Commonly, in cases of postsurgical deformities, the cosmetic complaints and difficulty with shoe wear are worse than with the original problem.

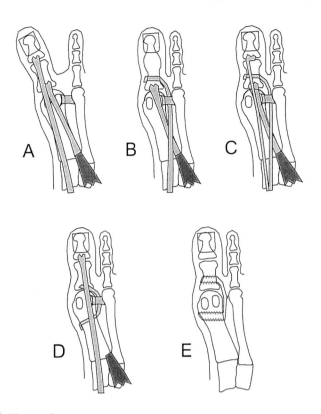

Figure 4

A, Hallux varus with medial subluxation of the extensor hallucis longus (EHL). **B,** Hallux varus reconstruction with transfer of EHL and arthrodesis of the interphalangeal (IP) joint. The EHL is detached distally and passed plantar to the transverse metatarsal ligament and secured to the proximal phalanx with enough tension to place toe into slight valgus. **C,** Modified hallux varus reconstruction using lateral two thirds of EHL to preserve the IP joint. **D,** Hallux varus reconstruction with extensor hallucis brevis (EHB) tenodesis. The EHB is detached proximally and is passed plantar to the transverse metatarsal ligament and secured to the first metatarsal with enough tension to place the toe into sight valgus. **E,** Hallux varus reconstruction with reconstruction of the lateral capsular ligament with a 1.5-mm elastic Ligapro suture passed through 2-mm drill holes in the first metatarsal and proximal phalanx. The suture is tied laterally in enough tension to place the toe into slight valgus.

Radiographically, the deformity is best seen and analyzed on the AP view. Cases with excessive resection of the median eminence, excessive lateral translation of the metatarsal head, or with resection or congenital absence of the fibular sesamoid are readily apparent. Joint space narrowing is often difficult to interpret because of the cock-up deformity and may be best appreciated on the lateral and oblique views.

Treatment

Very mild flexible deformities rarely require treatment other than a well-fitted shoe. In a recently published review of 13 patients (16 feet) with acquired hallux varus after bunion surgery with an average follow-up of 18.3 years and an average hallux varus angle of 10.1°, 9 patients (12 feet) were completely satisfied. All 4 of the unsatisfied patients had deformities greater than 15°. In this series, severe deformities greater than 15° were only noted after excessive resection of the median eminence.

In most cases, if the problem is recognized in the early postoperative period (within 4 to 6 weeks), taping the toe out of varus for 6 to 8 weeks to up to 3 months has been recommended as a possible early nonsurgical solution. Other than shoe modifications and taping or bracing, all other solutions are surgical. For the correction of flexible deformities, multiple surgical procedures have been described.

If the problem is detected early and is determined to be strictly one of soft-tissue imbalance without fixed deformities of the MTP or IP joints, a medial capsular lengthening with taping the toe out of varus for 6 to 8 weeks has been recommended. To be successful, the tibial (medial) sesamoid should be reduced and the deforming soft-tissue released to bring the toe into 15° of valgus. Overcorrection into increased valgus has not been a problem. Historically, for a well-established hallux varus deformity, surgical attempts at a static correction with medial capsular lengthening and lateral capsular repair have not met with long-term success. For most cases, the deforming forces are too great and a durable correction requires some type of reconstruction. Soft-tissue reconstructions are not indicated in cases with significant arthrosis, fixed deformities of the MTP joint, or after a very excessive median eminence resection. In these cases and in cases of hallux varus after failed implant or resection arthroplasty, first MTP arthrodesis has been shown to be the procedure of choice. In cases with a fixed deformity of the IP joint, an IP joint arthrodesis can be added to a soft-tissue reconstruction procedure.

Currently, the most frequently mentioned method of soft-tissue reconstruction involves the EHL tendon. The original description included a medial soft-tissue release with a transfer of the entire EHL tendon and arthrodesis of the IP joint. The EHL is detached distally, rerouted deep to the transverse metatarsal ligament from proximal to distal, and transferred to the base of proximal phalanx in proper tension to hold the toe in slight valgus (Fig. 4, B). A later modification included transferring only the lateral two thirds of the EHL to avoid fusion of the IP joint to preserve its motion in the event an arthrodesis would be required at a later date (Fig. 4, C). This procedure has produced about 80% satisfactory clinical results and has been shown to maintain 50% to 60% of first MTP joint motion.

Recently, an alternative reconstruction procedure which uses an extensor hallucis brevis (EHB) tendon tenodesis was presented with both a cadaveric biomechanical analysis and early postoperative clinical results. After the standard medial capsular release, this technique involves a proximal release of the EHB near its musculotendinous junction. The EHB is rerouted deep to the transverse metatarsal ligament from distal to proximal and is secured to the metatarsal shaft in proper tension to hold the toe in slight valgus (Fig. 4, D). The biomechanical analysis concluded that the EHB tenodesis restored the load displacement curves to that of the normal joint with a loss of 10° of passive dorsiflexion. Analysis of the clinical results in 6 patients with an average 28-month follow-up showed that an excellent correction was maintained in all patients, also with an average 10° loss of dorsiflexion.

Another technique recently presented uses a 1.5-mm diameter elastic polyethylene terephtalate suture to reconstruct the lateral ligament and capsule after a medial release. The elastic suture was specially produced for reconstruction and augmentation of ligamentocapsular structures. This technique weaves the suture through parallel 2-mm tunnels in both the metatarsal head and base of the proximal phalanx. The suture is tied in the first webspace under sufficient tension to correct the varus alignment (Fig. 4, E). In 5 cases with an average follow-up of 4 years, all patients had excellent results with an average hallux valgus angle of 10° with relief of pain and normal mobility. There was no evidence of intolerance of the elastic suture.

Claw Hallux

A claw hallux deformity is defined as hyperextension of the MTP joint with flexion of the IP joint. It results from a muscle imbalance between the long and short flexors and extensors (intrinsic minus deformity). It is seen in conjunction with a variety of disorders and infrequently occurs on its own as an idiopathic finding. Although it can occur after trauma or as an unintended iatrogenic result of surgery, it is most often associated with neurologic conditions or disorders that produce a neuromuscular imbalance. Neurologic conditions that can produce a claw hallux include Charcot-Marie-Tooth disease, cerebral palsy, multiple sclerosis, polio, spina bifida, spinal cord tethering, spinal cord and closed head injuries, brain abscesses, stroke, compartment syndromes, and lumbar radiculopathies. Other disorders that can produce a neuromuscular imbalance include diabetes, Hansen's disease, and tertiary syphilis. Acquired mechanical imbalances can occur with rheumatoid arthritis, hallux varus deformities, after resection or interposition arthroplasty, after sesamoid excision, and with flexor hallucis brevis (FHB) or tibialis anterior tendon lacerations or ruptures. With weakness of the tibialis anterior and/or contracture of the gastrocnemius-soleus complex, the long extensors will overpull and hypertrophy, producing claw toes.

Findings

Patients with a claw hallux often complain of the cosmetic deformity and difficulty with shoe wear. The key physical findings include either flexible or rigid contractures of the MTP and IP joints. Depending on the etiology, a number of other associated findings may include a cavus foot with a plantar flexed first metatarsal, a tight heel cord, and weakness of the tibialis anterior. Radiographs, for the most part, usually only confirm the physical findings except after trauma, when displaced sesamoid fractures or sesamoid migration after disruption of the plantar plate may be seen.

Treatment

Treatment for a symptomatic claw hallux depends upon the severity of symptoms, the etiology, and the associated findings. Nonsurgical treatment is limited to shoe wear modifications and therapy to stretch the gastrocnemius-soleus complex and strengthen the tibialis anterior. Surgical treatment includes possible tendon lengthening (EHL) and releases (EHB) for mild deformities, metatarsal or midfoot osteotomies for supple deformities, and tendon transfers and arthrodeses for more severe or fixed deformities. Rigid deformities in the presence of arthrosis are best treated with an arthrodesis.

The Robert Jones transfer of the EHL to the neck of the first metatarsal, modified to include an arthrodesis of the IP joint, has been used to treat patients with a claw hallux deformity with a flexible MTP joint. A recent review of 28 Jones transfers with a 5.5-year follow-up found that the procedure was 90% effective in relieving symptoms of the claw hallux but not for relieving pain under the metatarsal head. The authors recommended adding a basal dorsal wedge osteotomy to the Jones transfer to correct a plantarflexed first metatarsal with pain under the metatarsal head.

Turf Toe

In 1976, after correlating an increased incidence of soft-tissue injuries of the first toe to athletic competition on artificial turf, Bowers and Martin coined the term "turf toe." Since that time, sprains of the first MTP joint have been referred to as turf toe injuries whether or not they occur on artificial turf. Turf toe injuries have been found to have significant short-term and potential long-term morbidity and disability. In some studies, turf toe injuries have accounted for as much or more missed practice and playing time than ankle sprains

even though they occur less frequently. Because of the perceived trivial nature of the injury by players and coaches, prolonged disability often occurs after the return to athletic competition with insufficient recovery.

A number of different factors have been implicated in the increased incidence of turf toe injuries. Most often mentioned are the increasing hardness of artificial turf over time and the increased flexibility of turf shoe wear, which have been evaluated by numerous authors with mixed conclusions. Most agree that the more flexible soles of athletic shoes used on artificial surfaces place increased stresses on the MTP joints. Other factors implicated include increased shoe-turf traction, the sport, player position, weight, age, years of participation, increased range of ankle dorsiflexion, pes planus, restricted MTP motion, flat metatarsal head, and prior injury. First MTP joint sprains can occur in any sport or dance. Football has been noted to have the highest incidence of turf toe injuries, whereas an increased incidence of first MTP injuries has not been noted in soccer and lacrosse players competing with the same shoes and on the same playing surfaces. Offensive football players have been noted by some authors to have a higher incidence of turf toe injuries because they are more likely to have another player fall on the back of their foot and force their first MTP joint into hyperplantarflexion or dorsiflexion.

Most authors agree that the mechanism of injury is forced range of motion of the first MTP joint beyond normal for the individual. The normal range of motion of the first MTP joint varies significantly among individuals, with normal plantarflexion ranging from 3° to 43° and dorsiflexion ranging from 40° to 100°. For athletes with decreased motion to begin with, less motion is tolerated before soft-tissue/bony restraints are injured. The shape of the metatarsal head with its changing radius of curvature (cam effect) produces tension in various portions of the collateral ligaments during different stages of range of motion. Because of the cam effect, the normal sliding action of the proximal phalanx over the metatarsal head gives way to compression in full extension.

The most common turf toe injuries occur with hyperextension. Typically, a dorsiflexed foot with the forefoot fixed firmly to the ground is pushed further forward by an external force, driving the first MTP joint into further dorsiflexion. The plantar soft-tissue restraints are stretched and torn with the dorsal edge of the proximal phalanx compressed into the dorsal articular surface of the metatarsal head. The next most common mechanism is a hyperflexion injury, which can occur when a plantarflexed foot is struck from behind and the great toe is driven further into plantarflexion. With forced plantarflexion, the dorsal capsule is stretched and possibly torn while the plantar edge of the proximal phalanx is compressed into the plantar aspect of the metatarsal head. Valgus and varus stress injuries are less common and usually occur when the player decelerates and, with the foot firmly planted, rotates and pushes off to change direction acutely. With these injuries, the collateral capsular ligaments are stressed, with possible rupture or with avulsion fractures from the base of the proximal phalanx.

Findings

The spectrum of clinical findings for turf toe injuries varies widely. Injuries range from mild sprains to complete tears of the capsuloligamentous structures, subluxation to complete dislocation of the MTP joint, bruising to tearing of the articular cartilage, avulsion fractures, osteochondral fractures, sesamoid fractures, separation of bipartite sesamoids, and fracture dislocations of the MTP joint. A careful history and physical examination is essential to make an accurate assessment of the extent of the injury and the treatment required. A grading system based on the clinical complaints and physical findings has been devised for treatment and short-term disability prognostication.

Grade 1 sprains are a stretch injury with minor tearing of the soft-tissue restraints. Tenderness is localized to the specific area that was injured. There is minimal swelling and little to no ecchymosis. Range of motion is only mildly limited with mild pain with weightbearing. The athlete is usually able to participate with mild symptoms.

Grade 2 sprains represent a partial tear of the capsuloligamentous complex. Tenderness is more intense and diffuse. There is moderate swelling with ecchymosis and mild to moderate decreased range of motion. There is a moderate amount of pain with weightbearing, with a mild limp. The athlete is unable to perform normally.

Grade 3 sprains are more of a complete tear of the capsuloligamentous complex with avulsion of the bony attachments. Associated bony injuries can be seen. Pain and tenderness are more intense and diffuse. There is a significant amount of swelling and ecchymosis with a marked limitation of motion. The athlete is unable to bear weight normally and is unable to compete athletically.

In addition to a careful history and physical examination, radiographic evaluation can be used to further evaluate the extent of the injury. Some authors recommend radiographs only for grade 3 and some grade 2 sprains while others recommend them for all turf toe injuries. Radiographs can be used to determine joint congruity, detect fractures, and evaluate for preexisting intra-articular conditions. Serial radiographs can be used to evaluate for sesamoid migration, progressive widening of bipartite sesamoid, fracture healing, or subchondral bone resorption sometimes seen with chon-

dral injuries. Additional studies such as stress radiographs to check ligamentous stability; forced dorsiflexion views to check for joint subluxation, sesamoid migration, or separation; bone scans to check for sesamoid stress fractures; arthrography or magnetic resonance imaging (MRI) to evaluate the extent of the capsuloligamentous injury are occasionally indicated. A recent case report of the MRI findings of an acute turf toe injury showed that the MRI accurately confirmed the presence of a tear of the plantar metatarsophalangeal joint capsule. The authors felt that the MRI provided anatomic detail of the nature and extent of the soft-tissue injuries and substantiated the concept that the primary pathology of turf toe injuries is a plantar capsular sprain.

Treatment

The primary treatment of most turf toe injuries is nonsurgical and varies with the severity or grade of the injury. After an initial assessment is made to rule out fractures or dislocations, the treatment is then directed at protecting the soft-tissue injuries and to allow for functional rehabilitation. Initially the standard R.I.C.E. formula of rest, ice, compression, and elevation is indicated to be soon followed by early active range-of-motion exercises to limit loss of motion.

Rest is the key, is difficult to control, and is relative to the grade of the injury. As noted, returning too early can lead to prolonged disability. For grade 1 sprains, the athlete can return to participation as symptoms allow. Athletes with grade 2 sprains usually miss 3 to 14 days of playing time, while those with grade 3 sprains will require crutches for the first few days and are out from 2 to 6 weeks. Rest also includes taping or toe spacers to splint the first MTP joint in a fashion to protect the injured tissues. Equipment modifications, to reduce stresses across the forefoot by reducing the flexibility of the shoe wear and to limit first MTP joint movement, can be accomplished through inserts or structural shoe modifications.

Ice or cryotherapy is best instituted during the first 48 hours followed by contrast baths. Taping or wrapping with a compressive dressing prevents and reduces swelling. NSAIDs can be used to reduce pain and swelling also. Passive range-of-motion and progressive-resistance exercises are instituted as symptoms allow.

Surgical treatment of turf toe injuries is rarely necessary. Displaced intra-articular fractures and irreducible dislocations require acute surgical intervention. Ligamentously unstable avulsion injuries with displacement may require acute open reduction and internal fixation or excision of the avulsed fragment with repair of the ligament involved. Symptomatic loose bodies, osteochondritic lesions, or sesamoid nonunions may require surgical treatment after conservative

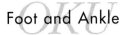
measures have failed. Acquired hallux valgus, varus, or rigidus may also require late surgical intervention.

Sesamoid Disorders

Disorders of the sesamoids of the first MTP joint are uncommon but can be a source of considerable pain and disability. The functions of the sesamoids are not well agreed upon or understood. Some of the presumed functions include protection of the FHL tendon, to serve as a fulcrum to increase the mechanical advantage of the FHB and FHL, to facilitate load transmission to the medial forefoot, to stabilize the first toe during stance to allow controlled and levered propulsion, and to disperse impact on the metatarsal head. The sesamoids are protected only by skin, a layer of adipose tissue, and, occasionally, a bursa. Because over 50% of the total body weight is transmitted through the first MTP complex, the sesamoids are vulnerable to athletic, traumatic, and repetitive stresses. Sesamoid injuries have been found to account for 12% of all first MTP joint injuries and 1.2% of all running injuries.

Over 30 separate etiologies have been attributed to cause pain over the sesamoids. Some of the most common conditions include sesamoiditis, chondromalacia, osteonecrosis, osteochondritis, acute fractures, stress fractures, diastasis of partite sesamoids, arthrosis, arthritis, infection, subluxation or dislocation, congenital absence, intractable plantar keratosis (IPK), FHL or FHB tendinitis, bursitis, and digital nerve compression. Because of its size and location, the tibial (medial) sesamoid is most frequently involved.

Findings
In general, the routine history and physical examination help localize the problem but are not usually sufficient to make a specific diagnosis. Although many patients may complain of pain after an acute injury or activity, most patients complain of a slow insidious onset of symptoms about the first MTP joint. Other complaints include swelling, tenderness, and decreased motion and strength. Symptoms are usually worse with weightbearing activities; especially with dorsiflexion of the first MTP joint at toe-off, with stairs, or high-heeled shoes.

On physical examination, there is invariably tenderness about the plantar aspect of the first MTP joint. Other nonspecific findings include swelling, erythema, decreased motion, decreased plantarflexion strength, and increased pain with forced dorsiflexion. Because of their close proximity, it is often difficult to localize the symptoms to a single sesamoid, the FHL, or digital nerves. More specific clinical findings include: marked erythema and warmth (infection,

arthritis, gout, and so forth), an IPK (exostosis), a painful digital nerve (nerve compression), and a painful bursa (bursitis, rheumatoid arthritis).

Radiographic evaluation includes routine standing AP and lateral views with a nonweightbearing oblique and an axial sesamoid view to outline the sesamoid articulations. Metallic markers can be taped over points of maximal tenderness to help localize the source of the symptoms. Like the history and physical examination, radiographs alone are often not sufficient to make a diagnosis. They will show the presence of an acute fracture (rough interdigitating edges) or a partite sesamoid (smooth noninterdigitating edges); however, the differentiation can often be difficult. Previous radiographs with intact sesamoids, when available, are very helpful in diagnosing acute fractures. Studies have shown that partite sesamoids occur in 25% of the general population, with 80% involvement of the tibial sesamoid. While the incidence of bilaterality is 90%, only 25% have identical findings in each foot, negating the value of comparison views. Other findings include joint space narrowing, bone fragmentation and collapse, and sesamoid migration. Serial radiographs can be used to follow fracture healing, partite sesamoid separation, and changes in bone composition (stress fracture, osteonecrosis, osteochondritis).

In cases in which physical findings and radiographs are equivocal, many authors advocate the use of radionuclide bone scans to corroborate or localize pathology about the sesamoids. Whereas bone scans are known to be highly sensitive for detecting bone pathology, they are not very specific, have a high rate of false positives, and often will not add more than location to the diagnosis. A recent study compared bone scans of the feet of asymptomatic active infantry recruits and asymptomatic sedentary adults. Mild to moderate increased uptake was found in the sesamoids of 29% (25 of 86) of the active infantry recruits and 26% (7 of 27) of the sedentary adults. The authors felt that their findings invalidated their hypothesis that increased uptake in the sesamoids in an active population is a physiologic response to demanding activity. They recommended the use of caution when determining the meaning of a positive bone scan based on mild to moderate increased uptake in the sesamoids.

Tomograms or computed tomography (CT) scans and MRI are also often recommended to further evaluate the sesamometatarsal joint. CT scans can be used to evaluate sesamoid fractures or the extent of arthrosis. MRI scans may be helpful in diagnosing sesamoid stress fractures, osteonecrosis, or osteomyelitis.

Treatment
Except for extreme circumstances, such as an open fracture

or a serious infection, the initial treatment for disorders of the sesamoid is nonsurgical. There is some controversy in treating patients with acute fractures in that some authors recommend cast immobilization for 3 to 6 weeks with a toe plate while others recommend stiff soled shoes with padding about the involved sesamoid until symptoms resolve. In general, while the treatment can be tailored to the specific diagnosis, an initial goal is to reduce weightbearing stress. Most patients can be treated initially with restricted weightbearing, shoe modifications (stiff sole, padding or custom molded arch support, and decreased heel heights), and NSAIDs. Athletes can also be taped rigidly to reduce symptoms during training and competition. If symptoms persist, an occasional local steroid injection or casting in a short leg walking cast for 3 to 6 weeks may be indicated. For patients with sesamoid enlargement and IPKs, periodic shaving and debridement of the keratotic lesion is helpful.

Surgical intervention is reserved for cases in which conservative measures have failed. Some authors advocate waiting up to a year before considering surgery, while others advocate waiting only 3 months for high performance athletes. The ultimate surgical option for all pathologic conditions of the sesamoid is excision. The medial approach is advocated for the tibial sesamoid; however, special care must be taken to avoid injury to the digital nerve. The dorsal or plantar approaches are used for the fibular sesamoid. It is important to maintain capsular and ligamentous integrity to avoid producing a valgus or varus deformity and to protect the digital nerves. The potential complications of sesamoid excision include decreased motion (plantarflexion), plantarflexion weakness, varus or valgus deformity, claw hallux, IPK over remaining sesamoid, neuroma formation, FHL or FHB injury, and inconsistent pain relief. A recent cadaveric biomechanical study determined that hemiresection or excision of a single sesamoid is unlikely to compromise the mechanical advantage of the FHB. Most authors recommend avoiding dual sesamoid excision.

Many authors advocate sesamoid sparing operations in selected cases as an attempt to avoid the problems associated with sesamoid excision. Some authors advocate partial sesamoid excision whereever possible. Because the extraosseus blood supply has been shown to enter the proximal pole, some authors advocate preserving the proximal pole whenever possible. A recent study showed good results with a technique for autogenous bone grafting of painful sesamoid nonunions using bone from the median eminence of the metatarsal head. In cases with persistent IPKs or nerve compression, many authors advocate sesamoid shaving or debridement to relieve pressure around the sesamoid.

Annotated Bibliography

Hallux Rigidus

Barca F: Tendon arthroplasty of the first metatarsophalangeal joint in hallux rigidus: Preliminary communication. *Foot Ankle Int* 1997;18:222–228.

The author presented a new method of resection arthroplasty, which preserves the plantar attachments of the proximal phalanx and uses the plantaris tendon as an interposition graft. The procedure was used in 12 feet with good results with an average 21-month follow up.

Easley ME, Anderson RB: Hallux rigidus in the adult and adolescent, in Adelaar RS (ed): *Disorders of the Great Toe*. Rosemont, IL, American Academy of Orthopaedic Surgeons, 1997, pp 23–32.

The authors review the symptoms, findings, and treatment options for adult and adolescent hallux rigidus.

Hamilton WG, O'Malley MJ, Thompson FM, Kovatis PE: Capsular interposition arthroplasty for severe hallux rigidus. *Foot Ankle Int* 1997;18:68–70.

This study presented the results of a modified resection arthroplasty, which uses the dorsal capsule and EHB as an interposition graft. The authors concluded that the procedure was a reliable method to reduce symptoms and improve motion in patients with severe hallux rigidus.

Harper MC: A modified Keller resection arthroplasty. *Foot Ankle Int* 1995;16:236–237.

The author presented a new technique for resecting the base of the proximal phalanx with a crescentic saw blade to preserve the insertion of the plantar plate. He felt that this technique allowed for sufficient bone resection to decompress and realign the joint.

Mann RA, Clanton TO: Hallux rigidus: Treatment by cheilectomy. *J Bone Joint Surg* 1988;70A:400–406.

This study evaluated the results of a cheilectomy on 25 patients with an average follow-up of 56 months. The authors concluded that the cheilectomy was a better treatment option for hallux rigidus than arthrodesis, resection arthroplasty, or implant arthroplasty.

Rongstad KM, Miller GJ, Vander Griend RA, Cowin D: A biomechanical comparison of four fixation methods of first metatarsophalangeal joint arthrodesis. *Foot Ankle Int* 1994;15:415–419.

The authors tested 4 methods of internal fixation for first MTP arthrodesis on 18 pairs of cadaveric great toes. They found that the dorsal miniplate was significantly stronger than the AO screw or Steinmann pin methods.

Sebold EJ, Cracchiolo A III: Use of titanium grommets in silicone implant arthroplasty of the hallux metatarsophalangeal joint. *Foot Ankle Int* 1996;17:145–151.

The authors evaluated the results of 47 double-stem silicone implants protected with titanium grommets in the first MTP joint for severe arthrosis in 32 patients with an average follow-up of 51 months. They concluded that the titanium grommets may protect the implant.

Shankar NS: Silastic single-stem implants in the treatment of hallux rigidus. *Foot Ankle Int* 1995;16:487–491.

This study followed 40 cases of hallux rigidus treated with a single-stem silastic implant for an average of 110 months. The author found that 36% of the patients were dissatisfied with their results. The author concluded that silastic hemiarthroplasty does not give an acceptable level of good results.

Hallux Varus

Donley BG: Acquired hallux varus. *Foot Ankle Int* 1997; 18:586–592.

This article reviewed acquired hallux varus. The author presented a review of the literature and discussed the anatomy, incidence, pathogenesis, evaluation, classification, and treatment options, both surgical and nonsurgical.

Juliano PJ, Myerson MS, Cunningham BW: Biomechanical assessment of a new tenodesis for correction of hallux varus. *Foot Ankle Int* 1996;17:17–20.

The authors presented a cadaveric biomechanical analysis of a new method to reconstruct the lateral capsule for the correction of hallux varus deformities using an EHB tenodesis. They found that the tenodesis restored the load displacement curve to that of the normal joint.

Myerson MS, Komenda GA: Results of hallux varus correction using an extensor hallucis brevis tenodesis. *Foot Ankle Int* 1996;17:21–27.

This study presented the early results of a new procedure to correct a hallux varus deformity with an EHB tenodesis. Six patients were followed up for an average of 28 months, with maintenance of an excellent correction with only a slight loss of dorsiflexion.

Tourné Y, Saragaglia D, Picard F, De Sousa B, Montbarbon E, Charbel A: Iatrogenic hallux varus surgical procedure: A study of 14 cases. *Foot Ankle Int* 1995;16:457–463.

The authors presented a new technique for the correction of iatrogenic hallux varus using an elastic suture to reconstruct the lateral capsular ligaments. In the 5 cases in which this technique was used, the results were excellent at an average 4-year follow-up.

Trnka HJ, Zettl R, Hungerford M, Muhlbauer, Ritschl P: Acquired hallux varus and clinical tolerability. *Foot Ankle Int* 1997; 18:593–597.

This retrospective study evaluated 19 feet in 16 patients with iatrogenic hallux varus with an average 18.3-year follow-up. The authors noted that only the patients with a greater than 15° hallux varus angle were dissatisfied with their results.

Claw Hallux

Tynan MC, Klenerman L: The modified Robert Jones tendon transfer in cases of pes cavus and clawed hallux. *Foot Ankle Int* 1994;15:68–71.

The authors presented a retrospective review of the modified Robert Jones tendon transfer in 24 patients and 28 feet. They concluded that the

transfer should be supplemented with a basal dorsal wedge osteotomy to treat first metatarsal head pressure pain.

Turf Toe

Bowman MW: Athletic injuries of the great toe metatarsophalangeal joint, in Adelaar RS (ed): *Disorders of the Great Toe.* Rosemont, IL, American Academy of Orthopaedic Surgeons, 1997, pp 1–22.

The author presented an extensive review of athletic injuries of the great toe, including a discussion of anatomy and biomechanics. He presented a classification system with treatment protocols.

Clanton TO, Ford JJ: Turf toe injury. *Clin Sports Med* 1994; 13:731–741.

This article reviewed turf toe injuries in athletes, using the authors' classification system. They emphasized that this was a significant athletic injury and that appropriate treatment should be tailored to the severity of the injury.

Tewes DP, Fischer DA, Fritts HM, Guanche CA: MRI findings of acute turf toe: A case report and review of anatomy. *Clin Orthop* 1994;304:200–203.

This case report reviews the MRI findings after an acute turf toe injury in a professional football player. The authors use these findings to validate previous descriptions of the soft-tissue anatomy of the injury.

Sesamoid Disorders

Anderson RB, McBryde AM Jr: Autogenous bone grafting of hallux sesamoid nonunions. *Foot Ankle Int* 1997;18:293–296.

The authors present a series of 21 patients who underwent autogenous bone grafting of symptomatic nonunions of the medial sesamoid with an average follow-up of 56 months. There were only 2 persistent nonunions both of which responded well to sesamoid excision. The authors concluded that this procedure was warranted to attempt to preserve the sesamoid.

Beaman DN, Saltzman CL: Disorders of the hallucal sesamoids, in Adelaar RS (ed): *Disorders of the Great Toe.* Rosemont, IL, American Academy of Orthopaedic Surgeons, 1997, pp 33–42.

The authors review the anatomy, biomechanics, evaluation, and treatment options for various disorders of the sesamoids of the great toe.

Chisin R, Peyser A, Milgrom C: Bone scintigraphy in the assessment of the hallucal sesamoids. *Foot Ankle Int* 1995; 16:291–294.

This study compared bone scans of the feet of asymptomatic active and sedentary individuals. The authors found increased uptake in the sesamoids of 29% of the active and 26% of the sedentary individuals and recommended using caution when determining the meaning of a positive bone scan.

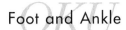

Chapter 13
Deformities of the Lesser Toes and Metatarsophalangeal Joint Disorders

Anatomy

Toes two through five are considered the lesser toes and serve as important adjuvants to balance and to pressure distribution on the sole of the foot. Normal position and function of these toes depends on passive and active stabilizers.

Active stabilization is a balance between the extrinsic muscles—extensor digitorum longus (EDL) and flexor digitorum longus (FDL)—and the intrinsic muscles—flexor digitorum brevis (FDB), extensor digitorum brevis (EDB), interosseii, and lumbricals. Passive stabilization occurs through the plantar fascia (aponeurosis), collateral ligaments, plantar plate, and joint capsule.

There are no significant direct tendon insertions on the proximal phalanx. The EDL and EDB combine to extend the metatarsophalangeal (MTP) joint through their pull on the extensor hood, and then continue distally to extend the proximal interphalangeal (PIP) and distal interphalangeal (DIP) joints. The FDL inserts on the plantar base of the distal phalanx and exerts a strong flexion force at the DIP joint, a moderate flexion force at the PIP joint, and a weak flexion force at the MTP joint. The lumbricals and interossei, which attach to the extensor hood, help to extend the PIP and DIP joints, but flex the MTP joint because of their position plantar to the center of rotation of the MTP joint. The interossei also have a small insertion on the bases of the proximal phalanges and the plantar plates. The FDB attaches to the middle phalanx and strongly flexes the PIP joint with weak flexion of the MTP joint (Fig. 1).

Passive stabilization at the MTP joint on the plantar side occurs through a very large, thick plantar plate, formed by the plantar capsule and plantar aponeurosis. Medial-lateral as well as some sagittal plane stability occurs through the collateral ligaments.

Extension forces at the MTP joint by upward ground pressure and the extensor tendons (EDB, EDL) are balanced by

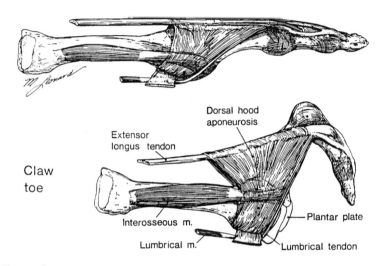

Figure 1

The anatomy of extrinsic and intrinsic musculature of the metatarsophalangeal joint. (Reproduced with permission from Myerson M: Claw toes, crossover toe deformity, and instability of the second metatarsophalangeal joint, in Myerson M (ed): *Current Therapy in Foot and Ankle Surgery.* St. Louis, MO, Mosby-Year Book, 1993, pp 19–26.)

weak flexion from the interosseii, lumbricals, FDB, and FDL, combined with strong resistance to extension by the plantar plate. Loss of balance because of dysfunction of any of these structures leads to deformity.

The plantar fat pad, another important forefoot structure, lies beneath the metatarsal head and is attached to the bases of the proximal phalanges. With extension deformities of the toes, it can become displaced distally, losing its protective cushioning effect on the sole of the foot (Fig. 2).

General Principles of Lesser Toe Deformities

Deformities of lesser toes are generally categorized into 3 types: mallet toe, hammer toe, and claw toe. All of these deformities are caused by intrinsic and extrinsic muscle imbalance, either alone or in combination with attenuation or contracture of passive restraints, which include the plantar aponeurosis, plantar plate, joint capsule, and collateral

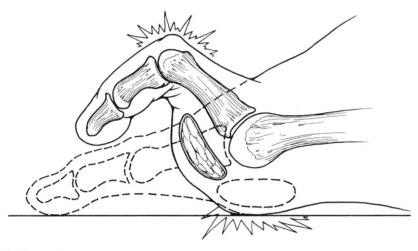

Figure 2

The fatty cushion is displaced dorsally with subluxation of the metatarsophalangeal joint. (Reproduced with permission from Mizel MS, Yodlowski ML: Disorders of the lesser metatarsophalangeal joints. *J Am Acad Orthop Surg* 1995;3:166–173.)

ligaments. These deformities may be caused by trauma, inflammatory processes, neurologic disorders, and such external deforming forces as poorly fitting shoes, or by some combination of the above. Temporary correction of flexible deformities is easy with manual manipulation; complete correction of fixed deformities cannot be achieved with manual manipulation.

The standard approach to treatment begins with accommodative shoewear (wide, deep toebox, or sandals), manual stretching exercises, padding painful areas (lamb's wool, foam, or silicone pads), and deformity-correcting devices (hammer toe restrictors, metatarsal pads, taping, or strapping).

Surgical treatment is indicated when conservative treatments fail to alleviate symptoms or are not tolerated by the patient. The actual surgical procedure will vary with the type and extent of deformity and includes soft-tissue release, tendon lengthening or transfer, resection arthroplasty, and arthrodesis. Skin contractures should not be overlooked when deformities are severe and inflexible. Bone resection to shorten the toe combined with Z-plasty incisions are often required. If neurologic conditions or inflammatory diseases are the source of the deformity, the rate of recurrence is likely to be higher. Joint resections or arthrodesis procedures should be used to lessen the chances of recurrent deformity.

Mallet toe is an isolated flexion deformity of the DIP joint (Fig. 3, *A*). Corns on the tip of the toe (end corn) or over the dorsum of the DIP joint can occur. If attempts at padding, tip elevation, or accommodative shoewear fail, surgical correction is indicated. Tenotomy of the FDL tendon works well for a flexible deformity, but sometimes leads to a hyperextension deformity or instability of the DIP joint. For fixed, flexible, or hyperextension deformities of the DIP joint, resection arthroplasty or DIP joint arthrodesis with or without FDL tenotomy are good surgical options.

Hammer toe is a flexion deformity of the PIP joint and is usually accompanied by a neutral or extended DIP joint (Fig. 3, *B*). Varying degrees of extension may occur at the MTP joint as well. It is not clear when hammer toe deformi-

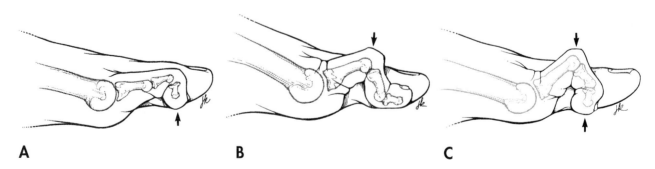

Figure 3

A, Mallet toe. **B,** Hammer toe. **C,** Claw toe. (Reproduced with permission from Alexander IJ: *The Foot: Examination and Diagnosis.* New York, NY, Churchill Livingstone, 1990, pp 68–71.)

ty is severe enough to be called a claw toe. Claw toe, classically considered to be caused by neurologic disorders, presents with extension at the MTP joint, flexion at the PIP joint, and flexion, extension, or neutral position at the DIP joint (Fig. 3, C). A severe nonneurologic hammer toe deformity thus may be called a claw toe. Eponyms aside, the treatment for nonneurologic and some neurologic deformities of this type are the same. Surgical correction requires a stepwise approach at each level of deformity. Correction of any MTP deformity should precede correction of PIP deformity in most cases. MTP joint correction begins with EDL tenotomy or Z-lengthening, EDB tenotomy, and progresses as necessary to dorsal capsulotomy, collateral ligament release, plantar plate and capsule elevation off of the metatarsal head, and metatarsal head arthroplasty (DuVries procedure) as the deformity becomes more severe. If partial resection is required, the surgeon should try to leave as much of the metatarsal head as possible so as to prevent a transfer metatarsalgia. Also, with severe deformities, skin Z-plasty should be performed.

PIP joint correction proceeds in a similar fashion with soft-tissue releases progressing to bony procedures as the deformity requires. An FDL transfer to the extensor hood through or around the base of the proximal phalanx may be chosen when the PIP joint is not contracted and can be easily passively corrected. This flexor-to-extensor transfer (Girdlestone-Taylor procedure) can also be done in combination with a resection arthroplasty or fusion of a contracted PIP joint. A PIP arthroplasty or fusion without the flexor-to-extensor transfer are also acceptable options in certain cases. Tenotomy of the FDL may also be necessary to relieve flexion forces at the PIP joint after a resection arthroplasty if the tendon has not been transferred.

If pin fixation is used to help stabilize the correction, a size 0.62 pin is generally believed to work best. Placement across the MTP joint is necessary for more severe deformities, especially MTP extension contractures and for flexor-to-extensor transfers. Pin removal is usually performed at 3 to 4 weeks. If pin fixation is not used, meticulous attention should be directed toward postoperative strapping.

Dissatisfaction with lesser toe procedures most commonly occurs when patients are not adequately educated and have inappropriate expectations. The patient should be made to understand the limitations of surgery, both functionally and cosmetically. With any toe surgery, patients should be warned of potential problems, especially prolonged swelling or a sausage toe, vascular embarrassment, recurrent deformities, stiffness, dysesthesias, and the appearance of a longer or shorter toe. To prevent soft-tissue complications, postoperative care, with appropriate passive stretching, massage, active exercises, and heat or ice treatments, is advisable. Early postoperative foot elevation should be stressed to all patients.

Second Toe Abnormalities

The second toe, because of its position adjacent to the great toe and its generally greater length, is usually subjected to higher stresses. This sets the stage for problems unique to the second toe.

Nonarthritic monoarticular synovitis of the second MTP joint is a common disorder that may have either a traumatic or nontraumatic source. Hallux valgus deformity is often present and allows stress shift to the second ray.

Nontraumatic monoarticular synovitis presents with painful swelling of the MTP joint. This chronic inflammation may lead to ligament attenuation, instability of the MTP joint, and progressive deformity. The MTP joint goes into extension, with dorsal subluxation and, sometimes, medial deviation with concomitant PIP flexion, creating what is often called a crossover hammer or claw deformity, in which the second toe overlaps the great toe.

Traumatic monoarticular synovitis caused by repetitive stress or acute injury affecting the plantar plate leads to pain, joint instability, and, often, but not always, joint swelling. Traumatic synovitis can progress to the same deformities noted with nontraumatic synovitis.

Physical findings besides joint swelling and tenderness include painful instability, as demonstrated by the dorsal drawer or MTP Lachman's test (Fig. 4), and painful passive flexion of the MTP joint, with reduced flexion excursion. Symptoms and signs of interdigital neuritis are common and can cause misdiagnosis. Inflammation or swelling from the involved joint may affect an adjacent interdigital nerve, or stretching of the nerve across the intermetatarsal ligament can occur because of joint instability and deformity.

Initial treatment should attempt to reduce inflammation and stress by off-loading or load transfer. Options include metatarsal pads, accommodative cushion shoes, metatarsal bars, rigid rocker soles, postoperative shoes, casting, and crutches or a walker with nonweightbearing. Nonsteroidal anti-inflammatory drugs are often of benefit. Corticosteroid joint injections can also be considered, but these injections can lead to more rapid or sudden MTP instability by causing further ligament attenuation. To prevent this complication, strapping of the toe or more aggressive off-loading should be considered for several weeks after the injection. Passive flexion exercises can reduce pain, improve flexibility, and decrease extensor deforming forces. Toe strapping or hammer toe restrictors also may be helpful.

Patients who do not respond to conservative treatment may require synovectomy. If deformity has occurred, correction is

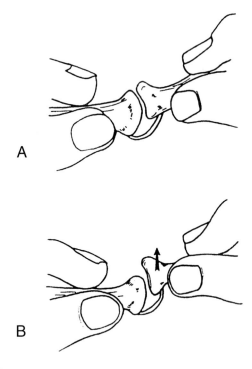

Figure 4

A, Instability of the metatarsophalangeal joint may be tested by grasping the base of the proximal phalanx. **B,** Manipulation in the dorsal-plantar plane may demonstrate increased laxity in an unstable joint. (Reproduced with permission from Coughlin MJ: Second metatarsophalangeal joint instability in the athlete. *Foot Ankle* 1993;14:309–319.)

performed as for hammer toes or claw toes. If interdigital neuritis is present, exploration of the interspace should be performed, with nerve resection or release of the intermetatarsal ligament as needed.

Direct ligament repair and collateral ligament reconstruction (Fig. 5), although technically demanding, can be used as alternatives to, or in combination with, traditional procedures such as the flexor-to-extensor transfer to correct MTP deformity. Basal proximal phalanx hemiphalangectomy has also been advocated and has been combined with a syndactyly to the adjacent toe. However, these procedures should be reserved for salvage situations, because good cosmetic and functional results are difficult to obtain.

Fifth Toe Deformities

The fifth toe, because of its border position, medially directed shoe pressure, and congenital anomalies, should be given special consideration. Cock-up, underlapping, and overlapping deformities occur commonly. The two-bone fifth toe has also been recognized as having a higher rate of deformity and callus formation. Soft-tissue contractures, especially of the skin, have been recognized as an integral part of the deformity, especially in the underlapping or overlapping fifth toe. Congenital variations of the tendinous anatomy have been demonstrated in some of these toes as well.

Symptoms usually involve painful callus formation caused by pressure from the adjacent toe or shoe. Conservative

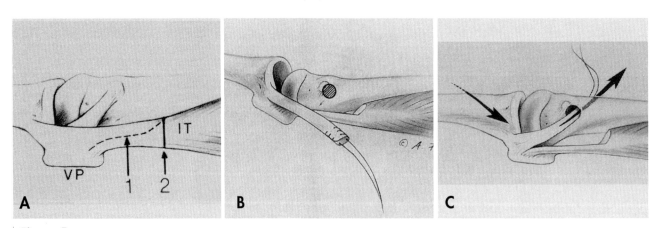

Figure 5

A, This anatomic drawing shows the relationship between the interosseous tendon (IT) and the volar plate (VP). The dotted line (1) indicates the outline of the dorsal portion of IT used when only part of the tendon is taken for graft, as has been done clinically. In this study, the entire thickness of the tendon was used at the level of the solid line proximally (2). Note the collateral ligament attaching to the dorsal tubercle of the metatarsal head. **B,** Hole for passage of graft. **C,** Passage of the graft with reduction of the proximal phalanx. More of the graft's volar plate attachment may be left intact or sutured to further strengthen the stability against dorsal subluxation. (Reproduced with permission from Deland JT, Sobel M, Arnoczky SP, Thompson FM: Collateral ligament reconstruction of the unstable metatarsophalangeal joint: An in vitro study. *Foot Ankle* 1992;13:391–395.)

treatment includes the same protective measures used for other lesser toe deformities to treat painful calluses.

The cock-up fifth toe, if the deformity is mild, can be treated surgically in the standard hammer toe fashion, addressing the contractures or deformities at both the MTP and PIP joints. If the deformity is more severe, that is, one with dorsal dislocation of the MTP joint, decompression by more extensive proximal phalanx removal will be required, as well as possible Z-plasty of the skin. The Ruiz-Mora procedure has been recommended to treat this deformity and combines proximal phalangectomy with plantar skin plasty. Problems with this procedure have mainly been cosmetic, as defined in a recent study of 12 patients interviewed more than 4 years after surgery. The author suggested that the patients be shown photos of the postoperative appearance prior to surgery. Toe floppiness has also been a common complaint with this procedure.

Underlapping and overlapping fifth toes may be congenital or acquired. Surgical treatment requires release of the medially contracted soft tissues and either dorsal (overlapping) or plantar (underlapping) structures as per the deformity. Skin rearrangement by VY-plasty (Wilson) or distal advancement of the lateral wound (DuVries) is recommended. The Lapidus procedure adds the transfer of the EDL, left attached to the distal phalanx, into the abductor digiti minimi to add a further restraint to medial deviation. The Thompson procedure is like a reversed Ruiz-Mora, with partial or total phalangectomy and Z-plasty of the dorsal skin. The Butler procedure, advocated as another acceptable treatment for these deformities, includes dorsal and plantar soft-tissue releases along with dorsal and plantar skin incisions.

Recurrent deformity, bunionette formation, floppy toe, and poor cosmesis are the main problems associated with these procedures. Salvage for recurrent deformity caused by instability or floppiness is syndactyly, which is considered by many patients to be cosmetically poor.

Bunionette

Bunionette, or tailor's bunion, is the abnormal lateral prominence of the fifth metatarsal head, usually accompanied by medial deviation of the fifth toe. Symptoms arise from shoe pressure on this prominence creating a painful lateral, or plantar lateral, callus.

Several anatomic variants of the fifth metatarsal have been identified as the underlying cause (Fig. 6). These are an enlarged or laterally prominent metatarsal head, a laterally curved or bowed fifth metatarsal, and a straight but laterally deviated fifth metatarsal creating a widened 4-5 inter-

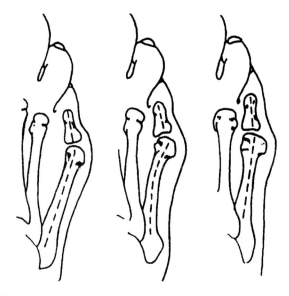

Figure 6

The variants of bunionette. (Reproduced with permission from Coughlin MJ: Etiology and treatment of the bunionette deformity, in Greene WB (ed): *Instructional Course Lectures XXXIX.* Park Ridge, IL, American Academy of Orthopaedic Surgeons, 1990, pp 37–48.)

metatarsal (IM) angle. The normal 4-5 IM angle has been reported to be from 6.2° up to 8°. A pronated foot and forefoot splaying, especially with hallux valgus, have been identified as associated factors.

Pressure relief by padding, shoe stretching, and wider soft leather shoes, along with paring of the callus, are appropriate initial forms of treatment. Correction of pronation by orthoses has also been described as a beneficial form of treatment.

Failure to control discomfort with conservative measures is an indication for surgery. The surgical procedure chosen should correct the underlying fifth ray deformity. Partial lateral condylectomy of the fifth metatarsal head and excision of the thickened deep soft tissues are appropriate treatment for a laterally prominent or enlarged metatarsal head (Fig. 7). Correction of any fifth MTP joint subluxation is necessary to prevent recurrence. This procedure may be combined with an osteotomy if more correction is necessary.

Osteotomies are appropriate for angular deformity of the fifth ray (widened 4-5 angle). Distal osteotomies are currently popular, especially the chevron type (Fig. 8). One study reported an average decrease of the 4-5 IM angle of 2.6°. Another reported an average forefoot width decrease of 0.6 cm. In both of these studies, all patients healed rapidly, and only one transfer lesion was noted. Other distal osteotomies have been advocated, such as the Hohmann-Thomasen, which is a peg-and-hole type procedure. Key factors for a successful distal osteotomy include

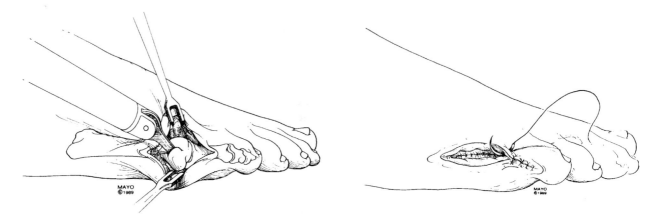

Figure 7
Condylectomy for the bunionette.

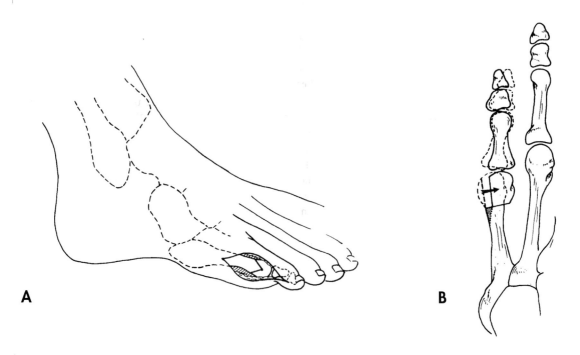

A   B

Figure 8
A, Lateral view of distal chevron osteotomy. **B,** Anteroposterior view of distal chevron osteotomy. (Reproduced with permission from Coughlin MJ: Etiology and treatment of the bunionette deformity, in Greene WB (ed): *Instructional Course Lectures XXXIX*. Park Ridge, IL, American Academy of Orthopaedic Surgeons, 1990, pp 37–48.)

stable fixation and minimal shortening of the osteotomy, along with stable repair of the lateral capsular structures to realign the fifth MTP joint. Midshaft or proximal osteotomies are recommended for a greater degree of divergence of the IM angle, but may be used for any increase of the 4-5 IM angle. As one would expect, a more proximal osteotomy will increase the ability to correct the IM angle to a greater degree. No delineation as to the appropriate osteotomy for differing IM angles has been clearly shown in the literature, unlike that for hallux valgus deformities. A midshaft oblique rotational osteotomy has been advocated and popularized by Coughlin. His results have shown excellent correction, with a low complication rate and a patient

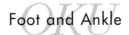
rating of excellent or good in 93% of the cases. More proximal fifth metatarsal osteotomies have been reported in the literature with varying success rates, but anatomic circulatory concerns have been raised as to the possible increased risks of delayed unions or nonunions. Lateral exostectomy, hypertrophic deep soft-tissue resection, and correction of the medially subluxated fifth metatarsal head should always be carried out along with a midshaft or proximal osteotomy.

Excision of the metatarsal head should be avoided because the complication rate is high, especially the formation of transfer lesions. Other complications of surgical correction by osteotomies include transfer lesions caused by shortening or elevation of the fifth metatarsal head and nonunion or delayed union, especially with more proximal osteotomies. Fixation is important to prevent loss of correction and to prevent healing problems, which have been noted to be very frequent with nonstabilized osteotomies.

Freiberg's Disease

Osteochondrosis of a lesser metatarsal head, usually the second or third, presents with activity-related pain and may appear normal on initial radiographs. Signs of inflammation are usually present, along with tenderness of the MTP joint and metatarsal head as the process progresses. When radiographs are normal, this condition can be confused with other entities, such as MTP joint synovitis syndrome. Follow-up radiographs, bone scan, and magnetic resonance imaging (MRI) will usually help with diagnosis. Much like other osteochondroses, repetitive trauma is believed to be the initiating cause for the problem, although this has not yet been proved. Disvascularity of the metatarsal head certainly seems to be an important part of the process.

Variable degrees of head involvement may lead to deformity, stiffness, and degenerative joint disease caused by loss of articular cartilage or metatarsal head articular cartilage deformity, as well as periarticular osteophytes. Early treatment is symptomatic to allow the process to resolve with as little deformity as possible. Nonsteroidal anti-inflammatory drugs, foot rest, and pressure relief for the involved metatarsal head are used to control symptoms and prevent deformity. Treatment may vary from metatarsal padding for pressure relief all the way to a walking cast or nonweight-bearing as maximum protection. Range of motion exercise to prevent stiffness may be of some benefit. A core decompression has been described for this condition in the case of one patient, with good long-term outcome. Dorsiflexion osteotomy has also been described as a treatment for early disease with persistent symptoms.

Symptomatic late disease usually manifests as pain and stiffness of the MTP joint. Treatment for these late problems includes the same pressure relief measures as for early symptomatic disease, as well as stiff-soled rocker bottom shoes and rigid forefoot orthotics similar to those used for hallux rigidus. Nonsteroidal anti-inflammatory medications and cortisone injections may occasionally be of benefit.

Surgical management for late disease depends on the severity of the condition and should strive to improve range of motion, especially extension, and relieve pain. A stepwise approach should be taken, starting with synovectomy and as much joint debridement as necessary for decompression. This may require as little as osteophyte removal, especially dorsally, to as much as a DuVries type arthroplasty. Interposition of capsular or other local tissues after joint debridement has been described as helpful when a great deal of the metatarsal head must be removed to help preserve toe length and MTP motion. A dorsal metatarsal head and neck closing wedge osteotomy has been used and reported in small series as a reasonable treatment for late problems, especially when the plantar aspect of the metatarsal head has been spared by the disease process. Resection of the base of the proximal phalanx, along with limited metatarsal head debridement and syndactyly of the involved toe to the adjacent toe, can be done, but this treatment leaves a more unstable situation, which can lead to further deformity or metatarsalgia. An attempt should always be made to preserve the normal weightbearing of the metatarsal head by resecting as little of a metatarsal head as possible in order to prevent transfer metatarsalgia, which may also occur with excessive dorsiflexion of neck osteotomies.

Intractable Plantar Keratosis

A persistent callus on the sole of the foot, usually beneath a metatarsal head or sesamoidal prominence, is termed intractable plantar keratosis (IPK). This epidermal proliferation in response to pressure may be diffuse or discrete, depending on the underlying cause. Pain with direct pressure helps to delineate discrete IPKs from plantar warts, which are generally tender to circumferential pressure. Paring of a plantar verruca will produce punctate bleeding; calluses have a dry base.

IPK may be primary caused by elongated central rays and cavus deformities or secondary as a result of previous surgery (especially on the first ray). Progressive toe deformities limiting flexion power, as seen with contracted or unstable metatarsophalangeal joints, or after deforming trauma of the forefoot, are also a common cause. Regarding appropriate treatment, these lesions are probably among the most problematic and controversial of all forefoot disorders.

Protection or off-loading of the callused areas along with reduction by sanding (pumice stone) or shaving (Credo device) should be tried first, especially for diffuse IPKs. Accommodative soft-soled shoes, pressure-relieving pads (metatarsal pads), and orthoses with appropriate posting and relief may also benefit the patient.

When conservative measures fail, surgery may be considered, but must be approached very carefully and with complete understanding of the cause. Very discrete lesions are usually easier to treat surgically than diffuse lesions. Radiographic evaluation with a metal marker on the discrete callus should include standard standing views, plus a metatarsal head axial view. If a prominent metatarsal head condyle is believed to be the source of the callus, a resection of this plantar condyle (modified DuVries procedure) should suffice (Fig. 9).

When there is a diffuse callus under one or more metatarsal heads, some form of osteotomy should be used after conservative treatment has failed. Various osteotomies have been described, including dorsal closing wedge, oblique shortening, and vertical chevron osteotomies. Any of these procedures can both shorten and elevate the ray to different degrees depending on the site of the osteotomy. More proximal osteotomies tend to displace the metatarsal head to a greater degree than a distal osteotomy performed in the same fashion. These procedures have been described with or without fixation, although fixation would seem advisable to help prevent nonunion or malunion. Proper position is critical and difficult to achieve. Excessive elevation of the metatarsal

can lead to transfer lesions. It is easier to overcorrect the deformity with more proximal osteotomies, because small changes proximally elevate the metatarsal head to a greater degree than distal osteotomies. Special care should be taken not to strip surrounding soft tissues or overheat the bone, which can lead to osteonecrosis of the metatarsal head for distal osteotomies and delayed union or nonunions at any site along the metatarsal. Diaphyseal osteotomies tend to take longer to heal and may carry a higher nonunion rate.

Multiple metatarsal osteotomies for diffuse calluses are even more difficult to perform properly. Obtaining and maintaining proper position of the metatarsal heads in relation to one another is challenging. Some surgeons advocate early weight-bearing without fixation to allow the metatarsal heads to seek their own level.

Postoperatively, regaining and maintaining full flexion of the MTP joint is important in order to maintain the normal toe lever push-off. If fixed MTP joint deformities exist, or if there is a significant limitation of flexion at the MTP joint, osteotomies should be avoided unless the toe deformity is also corrected. Simultaneous correction of a contracted MTP joint and deformed toe along with a distal osteotomy can lead to excessive soft-tissue stripping of the metatarsal head, leading to osteonecrosis and/or nonunion.

Because it is associated with a higher incidence of transfer lesions, removal of the metatarsal head should be avoided except in special cases. As a salvage procedure for failed previous surgery or severe diffuse calluses not amenable to standard procedures such as in rheumatoid deformities, removal of all the metatarsal heads along with first MTP joint fusion may provide pain relief, but function is sacrificed to variable degrees.

Success rates with different osteotomies have varied widely in the literature, with most studies being retrospective. With strict attention to detail and complete recognition of the pathology, it seems likely that good results can be achieved at least 80% of the time.

Corns

Pressure-induced hyperkeratotic lesions of the toes are termed corns (heloma, clavus). Corns are caused by poorly fitting shoes, toe deformities, or a combination of the two. Pressure on bony prominences causes the callus formation, which is not always painful.

The most common sites for a hard corn (heloma durum) are the dorsal lateral proximal interphalangeal (PIP) joint of the fifth toe, the tip of any lesser toe with mallet deformity, the dorsal aspect of PIP joints with hammer deformities, the nail folds of toes with thickened deformed or incurved toe-

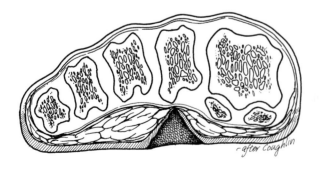

Figure 9

Cross section of the foot shows a discrete plantar keratosis beneath the prominent fibular condyle of a metatarsal head. (Reproduced with permission from Mizel MS, Yodlowski ML: Disorders of the lesser metatarsophalangeal joints. *J Am Acad Orthop Surg* 1995; 3:166–173.)

nails, and the area between adjacent toes distal to the bases. Soft corns (heloma molle) are found between adjacent toes deep in the webspace and are soft because of maceration from perspiration.

Treatment consists of pressure relief by accommodative shoes, stretching of shoes over the corn, padding (foam or silicone web spacers, donut pads, toe covers, lamb's wool) and callus reduction by sanding (with a pumice stone) or shaving. Special attention and care is extremely important for neuropathic conditions, which often require supervised or professional debridement.

Surgical treatment addresses removal of the offending bony prominence by partial condylectomy and occasionally total condylectomy (Fig. 10). Excessive bone removal may destabilize the toe. The adjacent toes should be strapped for approximately 6 weeks after the procedure to allow fibrous tissue stabilization. Often, bony resection of prominences on adjacent toes is required to prevent recurrence.

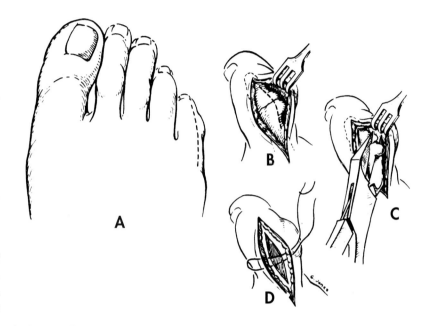

Figure 10

DuVries' technique for condylectomy of corn on fifth toe. **A,** Longitudinal incision over dorsolateral aspect of fifth toe. **B,** Skin and capsule retracted. **C,** Fibular condyles of phalanges amputated. **D,** Skin and capsule closed by mattress sutures. (Reproduced with permission from Mann RA (ed): *Surgery of the Foot,* ed 5. St. Louis, MO, CV Mosby, 1989, p 181.)

When the corn involves a nailfold with an abnormality such as incurved or thickened nail, a partial matrixectomy of the offending side of the nail, which acts like a bony prominence, usually cures the problem. Standard treatment for mallet and hammer toes usually resolves the corns dorsally at the PIP and DIP joints, as well as tip calluses.

Recurrent corns generally indicate inadequate bone removal or excessive bone removal with new deformity. Repeat surgery should address the cause and occasionally will require syndactyly as a salvage procedure.

Pedal Puncture Wounds

Puncture wounds of the foot are extremely common, and most of them are minor and are never reported. Because the literature to date has been anecdotal and retrospective, an accurate understanding of this condition is generally lacking, and undertreatment is very common. Children make up the largest group reporting puncture wounds, and most of these injuries occur during the warmer months. The most common source (98%) of puncture wound is a nail. Soft-tissue infection, the most common type of infection, ranges from 3% to 15% of all punctures. Pyarthrosis, osteomyelitis, and

osteochondritis occur in about 0.6% to 1.8% of puncture wounds. There are conflicting reports about the most common pathogens, but it appears that *Pseudomonas* is the predominant organism (up to 90%) causing pyarthrosis and osteomyelitis. There also appears to be a propensity for growth of *Pseudomonas* in cartilaginous tissue, thus increasing the risk of infection in children and around joints. Punctures involving shoes with synthetic or rubber-type soles seem to increase the risk of *Pseudomonas* infection. Most soft-tissue infections are polymicrobial, with *Staphylococcus* and *Streptococcus* the most common organisms, especially in adults. Other factors implicated in increasing the risk of infection include penetration beneath the plantar fascia, imbedded foreign bodies, lack of tetanus immunization, immunosuppression, and possibly even the use of prophylactic antibiotics that target specific pathogens such as *Pseudomonas*.

Treatment of established soft-tissue infections should be the same as for any soft-tissue infection of an extremity, and include exploration and debridement of the puncture tract, decompression of abscesses, removal of foreign bodies, and excision of granulomatous reactions. Pyarthrosis treatment requires arthrotomy, debridement, and drain placement. Osteomyelitis should be handled using well-recognized treatment protocols, which are beyond the scope of this review. Initial antibiotics should cover a broad spectrum and include *Pseudomonas* coverage, with adjustments made as cultures dictate.

Treatment of acute punctures has been less well defined, but guidelines have been recommended. Important factors guiding treatment include depth of penetration, type of shoewear, site of puncture, presence or absence of foreign body, type of object, condition of the object, and the health of the patient. Radiographs should be obtained if the presence of foreign bodies or deep penetration is suspected. If the puncture is not believed to have penetrated through the plantar fascia, simple superficial cleansing with an iodophor solution, followed by close observation, daily cleaning and off-loading of the injured foot for several days is recommended. Prophylactic antibiotics are not recommended if the fascia has not been penetrated.

Probing of a wound to determine depth is controversial because of the risk of pushing foreign material deeper into the foot. If the presence of a foreign object is suspected, or it is thought that the penetrating object has violated the plantar fascia, joint, or bone, formal wound exploration with debridement and irrigation is recommended. Most wound explorations can be carried out with an ankle block anesthetic in the outpatient setting. Antibiotic therapy after debridement has not been well delineated in the literature, but it would seem appropriate to treat these wounds after debridement as one would for any other extremity wound, based on the extent of contamination and structures involved. Tetanus immunization should also be included if appropriate.

Annotated Bibliography

Coughlin MJ: Operative repair of the mallet toe deformity. *Foot Ankle Int* 1995;16:109–116.

This is a long-term, retrospective study of resection arthroplasty for the treatment of symptomatic mallet toe deformity. There was an 86% subjective satisfaction rate, with 97% relief in pain in the 86 toes treated with this procedure.

Lehman DE, Smith RW: Treatment of symptomatic hammertoe with a proximal interphalangeal joint arthrodesis. *Foot Ankle Int* 1995;16:535–541.

This article addresses a specific technique for performing a peg-and-socket arthrodesis of the proximal interphalangeal (PIP) joint for symptomatic hammer toe deformities. There was a 95% radiographic fusion rate, 48% satisfaction without reservation rate, 37% satisfaction with reservation rate, and 15% dissatisfaction rate. This article helps to address the pros and cons of resection arthroplasty versus arthrodesis of the PIP joint for hammer toe deformities.

Mizel MS, Yodlowski ML: Disorders of the lesser metatarsophalangeal joints. *J Am Acad Orthop Surg* 1995;3:166–173.

This is an excellent general review covering the most common lesser metatarsophalangeal joint disorders. Explanations of disorders and treatments are complete and concise.

Myerson MS, Fortin P, Girard P: Use of skin Z-plasty for management of extension contracture in recurrent claw- and hammertoe deformity. *Foot Ankle Int* 1994;15:209–212.

The authors describe the use of a dorsal skin Z-plasty in the treatment of recurrent metatarsophalangeal joint extension contractures after a claw toe or hammer toe procedure.

Sarrafian SK: Correction of fixed hammertoe deformity with resection of the head of the proximal phalanx and extensor tendon tenodesis. *Foot Ankle Int* 1995;16:449–451.

The author describes a technique of hammer toe deformity correction by resection of the head of the proximal phalanx not requiring use of a Kirschner wire for fixation. This surgical technique is described in detail.

Second Toe Abnormalities

Bhatia D, Myerson MS, Curtis MJ, Cunningham BW, Jinnah RH: Anatomical restraints to dislocation of the second metatarsophalangeal joint and assessment of a repair technique. *J Bone Joint Surg* 1994;76A:1371–1375.

This cadaveric study demonstrates the level of instability occurring at the metatarsophalangeal joint by sequential transection of the volar plate and collateral ligaments simulating a hammer toe deformity. A flexor-to-extensor transfer was then performed to restore the low displacement curves to normal.

Fortin PT, Myerson MS: Second metatarsophalangeal joint instability. *Foot Ankle Int* 1995;16:306–313.

This is a complete review of the subject in a concise, complete form with extensive bibliography.

Mizel MS, Michelson JD: Nonsurgical treatment of monarticular nontraumatic synovitis of the second metatarsophalangeal joint. *Foot Ankle Int* 1997;18:424–426.

The authors describe a nonsurgical treatment regimen for treatment of monoarticular nontraumatic synovitis of the second metatarsophalangeal joint that was successful in 70% of the patients treated.

Fifth Toe Deformities

Dyal CM, Davis WH, Thompson FM, Bonar SK: Clinical evaluation of the Ruiz-Mora procedure: Long term follow-up. *Foot Ankle Int* 1997;18:94–97.

The authors did a retrospective review of 12 patients who underwent the Ruiz-Mora procedure for deformities of the fifth toe with an average 4-year follow-up. It was believed that this procedure was effective in dealing with cock-up fifth hammer toes, but did carry a high cosmetic dissatisfaction rate.

Thompson FM, Chang VK: The two-boned fifth toe: Clinical implications. *Foot Ankle Int* 1995;16:34–36.

The authors demonstrate the increased rate of pathology occurring in two-boned fifth toes. Sixty percent of fifth toes requiring surgery were of the two-bone type, but this anatomic variant was found in only 45% of a prospective controlled group.

Frieberg's Disease

Katcherian DA: Treatment of Freiberg's disease. *Orthop Clin North Am* 1994;25:69–81.

The author reviews the pathogenesis, diagnosis, and nonsurgical as well as surgical options for the treatment of this disorder, with emphasis on and description of a dorsiflexion osteotomy of the metatarsal head reported to give good results regardless of the stage of the disease.

Intractable Plantar Keratosis

Mann RA, Chou LB: Surgical management for intractable metatarsalgia. *Foot Ankle Int* 1995;16:322–327.

A review and demonstration of the metatarsal head resection and first ray stabilization as a salvage procedure for metatarsalgia.

Classic Bibliography

Coughlin MJ: Etiology and treatment of the bunionette deformity, in Greene WB (ed): *Instructional Course Lectures XXXIX*. Park Ridge, IL, American Academy of Orthopaedic Surgeons, 1990, pp 37–48.

Coughlin MJ: Second metatarsophalangeal joint instability in the athlete. *Foot Ankle* 1993;14:309–319.

Dreeben SM, Noble PC, Hammerman S, Bishop JO, Tullos HS: Metatarsal osteotomy for primary metatarsalgia: Radiographic and pedobarographic study. *Foot Ankle* 1989;9:214–218.

Harper MC: Dorsal closing wedge metatarsal osteotomy: A trigonometric analysis. *Foot Ankle* 1990;10:303–305.

Kinnard P, Lirette R: Dorsiflexion osteotomy in Freiberg's disease. *Foot Ankle* 1989;9:226–231.

Kitaoka HB, Holiday AD Jr: Metatarsal head resection for bunionette: Long-term follow-up. *Foot Ankle* 1991;11:345–349.

Kitaoka HB, Holiday AD Jr, Campbell DC II: Distal chevron metatarsal osteotomy for bunionette. *Foot Ankle* 1991:12:80–85.

Kitaoka HB, Leventen EO: Medial displacement metatarsal osteotomy for treatment of painful bunionette. *Clin Orthop* 1989; 243:172–179.

Leventen EO, Pearson SW: Distal metatarsal osteotomy for intractable plantar keratoses. *Foot Ankle* 1990;10:247–251.

Verdile VP, Freed HA, Gerard J: Puncture wounds to the foot. *J Emerg Med* 1989;7:193–199.

Chapter 14
Heel Pain

Introduction

Pain about the heel is a very common problem presenting to the orthopaedic surgeon. Multiple etiologies of heel pain have been described in the literature. Successful treatment requires proper identification of the cause of the pain and a treatment regimen tailored to that problem. A careful history and detailed physical examination are essential to the appropriate design of treatment protocols. Patients should be informed that their pain will not go away quickly and reminded that the goal is to treat the problem while allowing the patient to remain active. The length of time for the resolution of symptoms can be a great source of frustration to the patient and physician. Most authors recommend that conservative modalities should be employed for 9 to 12 months prior to consideration of surgical intervention. Heel pain can be divided into 2 main groups, subcalcaneal pain syndrome and posterior heel pain syndromes. Bordelon has suggested that although these heel pain syndromes are familiar to all orthopaedic surgeons they are probably fully understood by none.

Anatomy

The plantar aponeurosis arise off the medial tuberosity of the os calcis and extends distally in 3 parts. The central component of the plantar aponeurosis is the part most commonly involved in subcalcaneal pain syndromes. It extends from the medial tuberosity of the os calcis and inserts into the plantar plate of the proximal phalanges of the lesser toes and through the sesamoids into the great toe (Fig. 1). Verti-

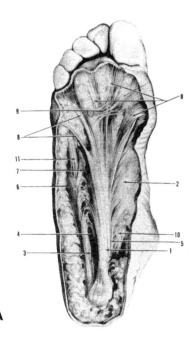

A

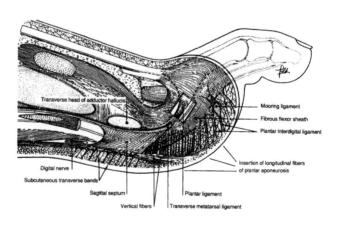

B

Figure 1

A, Plantar aponeurosis: (1) central component of plantar aponeurosis, (2) medial component of plantar aponeurosis, (3) lateral component of plantar aponeurosis, (4) lateral plantar sulcus, (5) medial plantar sulcus, (6) lateral crux of the lateral plantar component, (7) medial crux of the lateral plantar component, (8) superficial longitudinal tracts, (9) transverse superficial tract, (10) abductor hallicus muscle, (11) adductor hallicus muscle. **B,** Sagittal section through the second interspace showing the distal insertion of the plantar fascia. (Reproduced with permission from Sarrafian SK (ed): *Anatomy of the Foot and Ankle.* Philadelphia, PA, JB Lippincott, 1993.)

cal fibers from the plantar fascia extend into the skin of the forefoot. The windlass mechanism is produced by hyperextension of the toes and metatarsophalangeal joints, which tightens the plantar aponeurosis, raising the longitudinal arch of the foot, inverting the hindfoot, and leading to external rotation of the leg.

The plantar fat pad below the heel is a complex structure consisting of adipose tissues divided by multiple fibrous septae that extend from the calcaneus to the thickened keratinized skin. These U-shaped septae stabilize the adipose tissue and allow forces of direct compression and torsion to be absorbed, thereby protecting the underlying bone and soft-tissue structures.

The distal branches of the posterior tibial nerve have an intimate relationship with the subcalcaneal structures (Fig. 2). The medial calcaneal nerve separates from the posterior tibial nerve at the level of the medial malleolus and becomes superficial, providing innervation to the skin about the medial and inferior aspect of the heel. The posterior tibial nerve then splits into its medial and lateral branches. The first branch of the lateral plantar nerve passes deep to the abductor hallucis muscle and deep to the plantar aponeurosis, providing branches to the periosteum of the inferior portion of the calcaneus, to the flexor digitorum brevis muscle, and to the abductor digiti minimi muscle.

The medial and lateral plantar nerves then travel distally through foramen within the abductor muscle onto the plantar aspect of the foot. These distal branches can be considered as the distal extent of the tarsal tunnel.

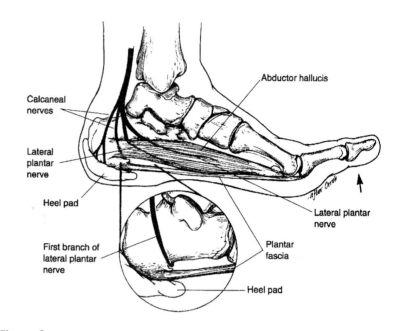

Figure 2

Location of nerves in proximity of the heel. Arrow indicates force of dorsiflexion. (Reproduced with permission from Gill LH: Plantar fasciitis: Diagnosis and conservative management. *J Am Acad Orthop Surg* 1997;5:109–117.)

History

Patients generally relate a history of a gradual insidious onset of pain without an acute episode of trauma. The pain is generally described as being along the plantar medial aspect of the heel without distal radiation or paresthesias. The pain is severe when arising out of bed in the morning, but as the patient begins to walk and stretch out the plantar structures, the pain often abates. It will be made worse with increasing activity through the course of the day. Patients also describe start-up pain after sitting for any extended period of time. In severe cases, patients can develop an antalgic gait and may describe pain with every step. A history of proximal or distal

radiation, numbness, or paresthesias is suggestive of nerve entrapment.

Subcalcaneal heel pain is more common in the middle-aged population and is not restricted to athletic individuals. It is generally unilateral but may be bilateral in up to 15% of patients. Subcalcaneal pain has been associated with obesity and prolonged standing in the nonathletic patient, suggesting that this is an overuse syndrome.

Many patients with heel pain are found to have some restricted dorsiflexion, with a contracture of both the plantar fascia and Achilles tendon. These contractures increase the load on the plantar fascia and may cause symptoms of overuse with normal activity levels. Once the plantar structures are inflamed, they will tighten at night while the patient sleeps, causing the foot and ankle to assume an equinus position. When the patient arises from bed and begins to walk with the foot and ankle in a neutral or dorsiflexed position, this contracted tissue is stretched, producing pain.

Physical Examination

The range of motion of the hindfoot should be assessed to determine the degree of dorsiflexion with the foot both adducted and abducted. Adduction of the forefoot while testing ankle dorsiflexion locks the transverse tarsal joint and eliminates the contribution of this part of the foot. Ankle dorsiflexion should be tested with the knee both extended and flexed so as to distinguish between tightness of the gastrocnemius and soleus muscles. Adduction of the forefoot reproduces the position of the foot in the gait cycle at the end of stance phase when the heel initially lifts off the ground. At this point in the gait cycle, pressure is transferred to the plantar fascia and its origin by the windlass mechanism.

The structures around the inferior and medial aspect of the heel should be carefully palpated. Atrophy of the plantar heel fat pad can cause tenderness directly over the inferior aspect of the calcaneus. Inflammation of the heel pad may also be present and evident with palpation and manipulation of the fat pad. The origin of the plantar fascia should be palpated to identify this as the source of pain. The compression over the first branch of the lateral plantar nerve just distal to the origin of the abductor muscle can reveal tenderness indicative of possible nerve entrapment (Fig. 3). In chronic cases, medial and lateral compression over the posterior inferior body of the calcaneus may produce significant pain suggestive of periostitis or stress fracture of the calcaneus. Percussion over the tarsal tunnel should be performed to rule out any component of tarsal tunnel syndrome. If the patient describes proximal or distal radiation of the pain, a straight leg raise test should be performed to rule out any component of sciatica.

The patient should be examined standing and while walking. Patients with a hypermobile supple flat foot may hyperpronate, which increases pressure on the windlass mechanism. Patients with a stiff cavus posture may be unable to dissipate the forces of impact because of the rigidity of their foot. Identification of these foot structures is an important step in devising an appropriate treatment plan. The plantar fascia should also be carefully palpated to identify any nodules suggestive of plantar fibromatosis. The fascia should be palpated with both the ankle and toes in extension to place the plantar fascia under stress. Dorsiflexion on the toes has been described as increasing the patient's symptoms in plantar fasciitis.

Radiographs

Standing, full weightbearing anteroposterior, lateral, and oblique radiographs should be obtained to demonstrate the bony architecture of the foot. The presence of a subcalcaneal heel spur is not indicative of this being the cause of pain. Heel spurs have been identified as being within the origin of the flexor hallicus brevis muscle. They have been identified in only 50% of patients with subcalcaneal heel pain syndrome, and are a normal finding in up to 15% of asymptomatic patients. Patients often have a larger spur on the asymptomatic opposite foot. The relationship between the heel spur and heel pain has not been clearly established. Radiographs may identify a fracture of this heel spur, which can be a cause of pain.

Technetium bone scans have been reported to show increased uptake at the insertion of the plantar fascia and the inferior portion of the calcaneus. The intensity of the uptake has been correlated with the severity of the patient's symptoms. Significant uptake, which may be indicative of severe periostitis or insufficiency fracture, often correlates with severe pain on medial and lateral compression of the calcaneus on physical examination. Other authors feel that this uptake is indicative of overuse syndrome and simply reflects the increased inflammation in this area.

The use of magnetic resonance imaging (MRI) in the investigation of heel pain remains controversial. MRI can demonstrate edema surrounding the plantar fascia as well as thickening of the fascia consistent with chronic inflammation. In addition, marrow edema has been identified at the insertion of the plantar fascia and in the inferior aspect of the calcaneus. In general, this correlates with the findings on physical examination, and the cost effectiveness of the use of MRI has yet to be determined. However, because of the confusing etiology of the subcalcaneal pain, MRI may prove useful in correlating distinct anatomic abnormalities with the findings on physical examination and patient history. Fur-

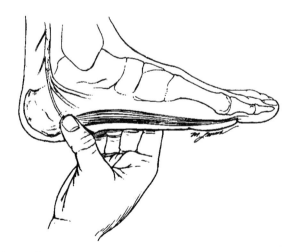

Figure 3

The point of maximum tenderness in a patient with entrapment of the first branch of the lateral plantar nerve. (Reproduced with permission from Schon L: Plantar fascia and Baxter's nerve release, in Myerson M (ed): *Current Therapy in Foot and Ankle Surgery.* Philadelphia, PA, CV Mosby, 1993.)

ther studies need to be performed to determine if this will become a useful modality.

Treatment

The majority of patients' symptoms with subcalcaneal heel pain will resolve with conservative management. The treatment protocol should be tailored to the precise diagnosis. In patients with severe fat pad atrophy or heel pad inflammation, the pain is caused by bruising of the underlying bone or inflamed soft tissue, and cushioning materials should be employed. These include visco heel cups, well-cushioned running shoes, and the avoidance of hard sole shoes. The patient's activities should be modified to avoid repetitive impact loading. These entities may be distinct or they may overlap and coexist with a diagnosis of plantar fasciitis.

In devising a treatment protocol for plantar fasciitis, the severity of the symptoms should be kept in mind. In general, an initial protocol includes stretching exercises to increase the flexibility of the heel cord and plantar fascia, activity modification to avoid impact loading activities, and the use of a well-padded running shoe and a visco heel cushion. Multiple modalities used at the same time appear to be more effective than the same modalities used individually. The patient should be instructed on the importance of compliance with home stretching and that the program should involve stretching with the forefoot in an adducted position to emphasize lengthening of the heel cord.

In patients who have severe pain with medial and lateral compression of the calcaneus or patients whose pain has not been relieved by the combined utilization of these other modalities, consideration of cast immobilization should be employed. In a review of 411 patients with chronic heel pain, Gill demonstrated that a period of cast immobilization proved to be the most effective modality when compared with 10 other conservative modalities (Outline 1). Once the symptoms have diminished, suggesting decreased inflammation, the other modalities of stretching and cushioning may prove more effective in completely resolving these symptoms and preventing recurrence.

It is important to inform the patient that it may take 6 months to 1 year for their symptoms to resolve completely. The importance of compliance with the multiple modalities suggested is critical for the ultimate resolution of symptoms.

The use of steroid injection can be considered if other conservative modalities are not successful. Care must be taken to not allow the steroid to infiltrate the plantar fat pad to avoid atrophy of these structures. Injections of the plantar fascia have been reported to cause an iatrogenic rupture and should

Outline 1

American Orthopaedic Foot and Ankle Society position statement on endoscopic and open heel surgery

1. Nonsurgical treatment is recommended for a minimum of 6 months and preferably 12 months

2. More than 90% of patients respond to nonsurgical treatment within 6 to 10 months

3. When surgery is considered for the remaining patients, then a medical evaluation should be considered prior to surgery

4. Patients should be advised of complications and risks if an endoscopic or open procedure is not indicated

5. If nerve compression is coexistent with fascial or bone pain, then an endoscopic or closed procedure should not be attempted

6. The AOFAS does not recommend surgical procedures before nonoperative methods have been utilized

7. The AOFAS supports responsible, carefully planned surgical intervention when nonsurgical treatment fails and workup is complete

8. The AOFAS supports cost constraints in the treatment of heel pain when the outcome is not altered

9. The AOFAS recommends heel padding, medications, and stretching prior to prescribing custom orthoses and extended physical therapy

10. This position statement is intended as a guide to the orthopaedist and is not intended to dictate a treatment plan

(Reproduced with permission from the American Orthopaedic Foot and Ankle Society.)

be given with significant caution. In general, steroid treatment should be limited to 2 injections given several weeks apart. If this is not successful, other modalities of treatment should be considered.

The patient should be reevaluated approximately 6 weeks after initial treatment has begun. If the symptoms are not responding, the addition of other modalities, such as casting, can be considered. If cast immobilization has been employed and the patient demonstrates decreased tenderness, then stretching, cushioning, and activity modification can be initiated. If these modalities have not proven successful, a dorsiflexion night splint can be used to prevent the foot from plantarflexing during sleep and to assist in maintaining increased flexibility of the plantar fascia and heel cord. These splints have been shown to relieve morning pain and to be an effective adjuvant in treatment. In recalcitrant cases, Mizel and associates have shown the use of a steel shank rocker bottom shoe to relieve the pressure on the plantar fascia by eliminating the windlass mechanism with walking to be effective.

It is generally recommended that these conservative modalities be continued for at least 1 year before considering surgical intervention (Fig. 4). The natural history of plantar fasciitis has been shown to be self-limiting. The patient needs to understand that prolonged use of conservative modalities will produce complete resolution of symptoms in close to 95% of cases. This includes the use of cast immobilization in recalcitrant cases. The use of cross-training to avoid impact loading of the heel is an important component of the treatment in an athletic individual. Having patients use a stationary bike rather than such activities as walking on a treadmill and jogging can increase the strength and flexibility of the lower extremity and assist in relieving their symptoms. If conservative modalities prove unsuccessful, surgical intervention can be considered.

The cause of failure of conservative modalities must be identified prior to consideration of surgery. In some instances recalcitrant plantar fasciitis is an expression of an underlying seronegative arthropathy, and a thorough rheumatologic evaluation should be undertaken. Seronegative spondyloarthropathies can produce chronic heel pain and can be bilateral. Medical management remains the treatment of choice in these instances.

In patients with severe fat pad atrophy, surgery should be avoided. The patient should be advised that this problem may be chronic but is best addressed by providing external cushioning under the heel. Visco heels, well-padded running shoes, and SACH modification to the heel should be used.

Acute rupture of the plantar fasciitis may be seen following trauma or multiple injections of steroid. Patients generally present with acute onset of pain, swelling, and tenderness following the sensation of a painful popping or snapping on the plantar aspect of the foot. Initial cast immobilization until the tenderness subsides, followed by modalities of stretching, will allow these symptoms to resolve.

Compression of the nerve to the abductor digiti quinti has been identified as a source of pain. Failure of conservative modalities to relieve the patient's symptoms may be an indication for surgical intervention. The patient generally identifies the pain as being on the medial aspect of the heel rather than on the plantar aspect of the heel.

On physical examination, the medial aspect of the plantar heel is tender just distal to the origin of the abductor muscle. The patient's pain generally can be reproduced by pressure exerted over the abductor hallucis origin where the nerve to the abductor digiti quinti passes deep to the muscle and the fascia. A positive percussion sign may be identified at the end of the abductor fascia in some patients. Surgical release of this nerve has been reported to give good results. Complete release of the nerve necessitates dividing the deep fascia of the abductor muscle as well as the medial edge of the plantar fascia. Excision of a heel spur, if present, has been advocated but has been shown to increase postoperative recovery time. Care must be taken to avoid direct injury to the nerve to prevent neuroma formation and numbness at the heel.

Multiple reports have outlined the results of surgical decompression for chronic plantar fasciitis. Careful review of the literature suggests that this decompression is indicated in

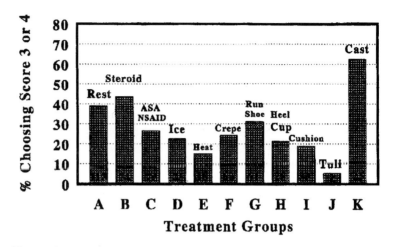

Figure 4

Response profile for patients with plantar fasciitis who had a favorable response to nonsurgical treatment. Bars represent the percentage of patients within each treatment group who chose mild moderate (score 3) or excellent improvement (score 4). The number of patients choosing score 3 or 4 is indicated in bars. (Reproduced with permission from Gill LH, Kiebzak GM: Outcome of nonsurgical treatment for plantar fasciitis. *Foot Ankle Int* 1996;17:527–532.)

only the 5% of patients who fail conservative modalities. Most authors agree that surgery should not be considered until after a minimum of 6 to 12 months of aggressive non-surgical treatment. Success in surgery has been reported in 50% to 100% of cases. Multiple techniques have been described and no control or comparative studies have been presented. Pitfalls of surgery include failure to relieve the patient's symptoms, postsurgical nerve entrapment and neuroma formation, persistent lateral foot pain with complete plantar fascia release, and long-term evidence of progressive collapse of the arch following complete release of the plantar fascia.

Both open and endoscopic release of the plantar fascia have been described. The risk of nerve injury has been suggested to be higher with endoscopic release. Complications seen with complete release of the plantar fascia with increasing lateral foot pain and collapse of the arch have led authors to recommend sparing the lateral band of the plantar fascia when surgical treatment is employed.

Posterior Heel Pain

Pain in the posterior portion of the calcaneus can have multiple causes. This pain should be distinguished from subcalcaneal heel pain by history and physical examination. Often there is a combination of entities causing this discomfort. These problems can stem from retrocalcaneal bursitis, Achilles insertional tendinitis, adventitial bursitis, or complications of Haglund's deformity.

Anatomy

The posterior aspect of the calcaneus has several landmarks as described by Pavlov and Heneghan. The bursal projection represents the superior tuberosity of the os calcis; the posterior tuberosity indicates the attachment of the Achilles tendon. A retrocalcaneal bursa lies between the Achilles tendon and the superior tuberosity of the calcaneus (Fig. 5). The retrocalcaneal bursa is a constant finding, but the size and shape of the superior tuberosity of the os calcis is variable. An adventitial bursa may be present between the Achilles tendon and the skin.

Diagnosis

Differential diagnosis of posterior heel pain is best determined by physical examination. The history of these symptoms is often quite similar, with patients complaining of pain with shoe wear infringing on the posterior portion of the heel. Morning pain as well as start-up pain after sitting is common and is experienced in the posterior aspect of the heel and distal portion of the Achilles tendon. These symptoms often lessen with light activity but worsen as the day

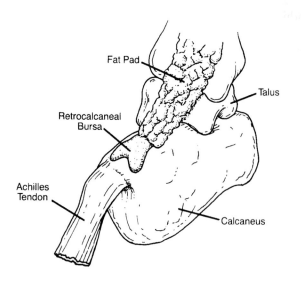
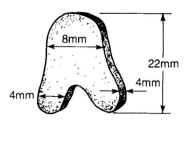

Figure 5

The retrocalcaneal bursa overlies the posterior superior tuberosity of the calcaneus. The average dimensions of the bursa are presented on the right. (Reproduced with permission from Frey C, Rosenberg Z, Shereff MJ, Kim H: The retrocalcaneal bursa: Anatomy and bursography. *Foot Ankle* 1992;13:203–207.)

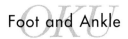

progresses. The onset may be insidious and can be caused by chronic irritation of shoewear or overuse. Acute symptoms may be caused by trauma.

Careful physical examination will assist in distinguishing between these various entities. Careful palpation of the Achilles tendon down to the area of insertion will allow identification of insertional tendinosis. The tendon insertion may be swollen and tender to palpation. In cases with significant inflammation, the area will be warm and boggy to palpation. If the tendon itself is neither swollen or tender, palpating the anterior border of the tendon both medially and laterally allows identification of retrocalcaneal bursitis. In some instances, ballottement of the bursa can be appreciated. This condition may coexist with insertional tendinosis, with thickening and swelling of the Achilles tendon. This must be differentiated from tendinosis within the body of the tendon itself proximal to the area of insertion. An adventitial bursa may be located between the skin and posterior portion of the Achilles tendon rather than deep to the tendon. Haglund's deformity can be palpated through the skin and may be associated with an overlying callus formation.

Range of motion of the ankle should be assessed to determine if an Achilles tendon contracture is increasing the tension at the insertion of the Achilles tendon on the os calcis. This testing is done with the knee in extension as well as flexion, and with the forefoot both in an abducted and an adducted position.

Standing radiographs should be obtained to identify the morphology of the posterior superior aspect of the calcaneus. In cases of insertional tendinosis, calcification may be identified within the distal aspect of the Achilles. Technetium bone scan will show an increased uptake in the posterior aspect of the calcaneus, and although sensitive, it is not specific. When concerns over degenerative changes of the insertion of the tendon exist, MRI examination can be helpful in delineating the extent of tendon that is damaged.

Treatment

Conservative management of these entities begins with modification of activity to decrease the load on the tendon. Modification of shoe wear to avoid direct pressure from the counter of the shoe onto the posterior aspect of the heel is helpful.

Padding of the area often assists in relieving the pressure. The use of nonsteroidal anti-inflammatory drugs and the initial use of a small heel lift have been described. Injection of steroid in this area can be used with great care. If degeneration of the Achilles tendon is present or if the steroid is injected into the tendon, the tendon may rupture. Careful injection into the retrocalcaneal bursa has been described. Night splints can be used to decrease morning pain and to improve the flexibility of the Achilles tendon. Stretching activities and the use of cross-training with a stationary bike may prove helpful.

In cases in which there is severe pain, significant tendinosis, or failure to respond to conservative modalities, cast immobilization can be employed. Patients can wear a short leg walking cast for a period of 4 to 8 weeks until the area is no longer tender to palpation. In treating existing tendinosis, prolonged immobilization with the use of a molded ankle-foot orthosis may allow healing over a 6- to 9-month period.

Surgical treatment may be employed after failure of conservative management. Surgery should address the specific etiologies producing symptoms in each patient. If the insertion of the Achilles tendon is within normal limits, excision of the retrocalcaneal bursa can be performed. At the time of surgery, the anterior aspect of the tendon should be carefully inspected for signs of degeneration. Debridement of the bursal protection of the calcaneus may be indicated if irritation of the anterior aspect of the Achilles tendon is observed. The anterior portion of the tendon should be repaired if degeneration of the tendon is observed. Similar principles should be employed when excision of an adventitial bursa is required.

If there is significant calcification of the distal portion of the Achilles tendon, this calcification should be debrided. The tendon should then be repaired. Depending on the degree of tendinosis and calcification present, reinforcement of the Achilles tendon with tendon transfer may be indicated. For patients with calcification that does not require tendon repair or transfer, Baxter has described a posterior splitting incision and has reported good results in patients below the age of 50. In patients above the age of 50, he recommends using a medial incision, and after thorough debridement of the calcification and the distal aspect of the Achilles tendon, employing a transfer of the flexor hallucis longus, as described by Wapner and associates, to augment the Achilles insertion. Following tendon repair or augmentation, postoperative immobilization should continue for 8 weeks, followed by gradual mobilization and progression to normal shoe wear.

Haglund's Syndrome

Enlargement of the posterior superior aspect of the calcaneus, first described in 1913, was later popularized by Haglund. An enlarged posterior superior bursal projection of the calcaneus impinges on the insertional fibers of the Achilles tendon and produces irritation over the bony prominence. In Haglund's

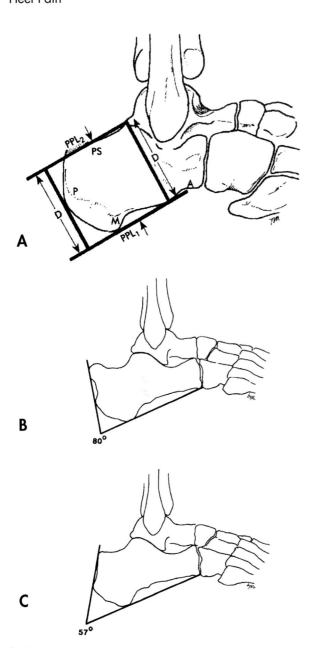

syndrome, the enlarged bursal prominence creates a combination of insertional tendinosis, retrocalcaneal bursitis, and adventitial bursitis. Pavlov reported on the use of the parallel pitch lines to identify patients at risk for Haglund's syndrome (Fig. 6). Radiographically, these reports described retrocalcaneal bursitis with loss of the lucent retrocalcaneal recess, Achilles tendinosis with an Achilles tendon measuring over 9 mm at a distance 2 cm above the bursal projection, and a prominent bursal projection with a positive pitch line. These findings were believed to be a more reliable indicator of Haglund's syndrome than the Fowler-Phillip angle.

Findings on physical examination include those listed previously for insertional tendinosis, adventitial bursitis, and retrocalcaneal bursitis. The posterior heel prominence is often warm, and the overlying skin may be thickened and inflamed. Radiographic findings are consistent with those described by Pavlov and associates. Initial conservative management uses the same modalities described for other types of posterior heel pain. If conservative modalities are unsuccessful, surgical intervention should be considered. Both a medial incision and combined medial and lateral incisions have been used. It is critical to remove enough bone so that there is no longer contact between the bursal projection of the os calcis and the Achilles tendon (Fig. 7). Once the bone and retrocalcaneal bursa are excised, the Achilles tendon must be carefully inspected. If significant tendinosis is present, debridement and either primary repair or augmentation should be employed. Following tendon repair or augmentation, postsurgical immobilization should continue for an 8-week period to allow adequate tendon healing.

Figure 6

A, The parallel pitch lines (PPLs) determine the prominence of the posterior superior tuberosity of the calcaneus (PS). The lower PPL (PPL1) is the baseline, constructed from the inferior line of the Fowler and Phillip angle. A perpendicular (D) is constructed between the posterior lip of the talar articular facet (T) and the baseline. The upper PPL (PPL2) is drawn parallel to the baseline at distance D. A posterior superior tuberosity touching or below the PPL2 is normal, whereas one extending above it is considered excessively prominent. (Reproduced with permission from Baxter DE (ed): *The Foot and Ankle in Sports.* St. Louis, MO, Mosby-Year Book, 1995, p 72.) **B** and **C,** Measurement of the Phillip and Fowler angle. Normal is considered to be less than 69°. **B,** an abnormal angle of 80°. **C,** normal angle of 57°. (Reproduced with permission from Drez D, DeLee J (eds): *Orthopaedic Sports Medicine: Principles and Practice.* Philadelphia, PA, WB Saunders, 1993.)

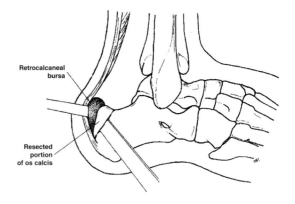

Figure 7

Resection of Haglunds deformity and retrocalcaneal bursa. (Reproduced with permission from Baxter DE (ed): *The Foot and Ankle in Sports.* St. Louis, MO, Mosby-Year Book, 1995, p 76.)

Annotated Bibliography

Geppert MJ, Mizel MS: Management of heel pain in the inflammatory arthritides. *Clin Orthop,* in press.

This review gives diagnostic modalities and presents the various inflammatory arthritides and treatment recommendations.

Gill LH, Kiebzak GM: Outcome of nonsurgical treatment for plantar fasciitis. *Foot Ankle Int* 1996;17:527–532.

Four hundred and eleven patients were followed over 10 years comparing 11 different treatment modalities, rating them for effectiveness in an outcomes review. Listed in descending order of effectiveness, the modalities tested were short-leg walking cast, steroid injection, rest, ice, runner's shoe, crepe soled shoe, aspirin or nonsteroidal anti-inflammatory, heel cushion, low profile plastic heel cup, heat, and Tuli heel cup.

Gill LH: Plantar fasciitis: Diagnosis and conservative management. *J Am Acad Orthop Surg* 1997;5:109–117.

This excellent review details the etiology and conservative modalities available for the management of plantar fasciitis.

Kitaoka HB, Luo ZP, An KN: Mechanical behavior of the foot and ankle after plantar fascia release in the unstable foot. *Foot Ankle Int* 1997;18:8–15.

This study suggests that plantar fascia release should be avoided in patients with pes planus to avoid further collapse of the arch after loss of the plantar fascia.

Mizel MS, Marymont JV, Trepman E: Treatment of plantar fasciitis with a night splint and shoe modification consisting of a steel shank and anterior rocker bottom. *Foot Ankle Int* 1996; 17:732–735.

Seventy-one feet in 57 patients with chronic plantar fasciitis were treated with a combination of a right splint and shoe with a steel shank and rocker bottom. Seventy-eight percent of patients had either resolution or significant improvement of their symptoms at average follow-up of 16 months.

Sammarco GJ, Helfrey RB: Surgical treatment of recalcitrant plantar fasciitis. *Foot Ankle Int* 1996;17:520–526.

Twenty-six patients underwent surgical release of the plantar fascia after an average of 21.5 months of failed conservative treatment. Satisfactory outcome was achieved in 92% of cases but the length of time to full recovery was varied from 3 to 30 weeks.

Classic Bibliography

Amis J, Jennings L, Graham D, Graham CE: Painful heel syndrome: Radiographic and treatment assessment. *Foot Ankle* 1988;9:91–95.

Anderson RB, Foster MD: Operative treatment of subcalcaneal pain. *Foot Ankle* 1989;9:317–323.

Baxter DE, Pfeffer GB: Treatment of chronic heel pain by surgical release of the first branch of the lateral plantar nerve. *Clin Orthop* 1992;279:229–236.

Baxter DE, Thigpen CM: Heel pain: Operative results. *Foot Ankle* 1984;5:16–25.

Bordelon RL: Heel pain, in Mann RA, Coughlin MJ (eds): *Surgery of the Foot and Ankle,* ed 6. St. Louis, MO, Mosby-Year Book, 1993, vol 2, pp 837–857.

Bordelon RL: Subcalcaneal pain: A method of evaluation and plan for treatment. *Clin Orthop* 1983;177:49–53.

Daly PJ, Kitaoka HB, Chao EY: Plantar fasciotomy for intractable plantar fasciitis: Clinical results and biomechanical evaluation. *Foot Ankle* 1992;13:188–195.

Fowler A, Philip JF: Abnormality of the calcaneus as a cause of painful heel: Its diagnosis and operative treatment. *Br J Surg* 1945;32:494–498.

Frey C, Rosenberg Z, Shereff MJ, Kim H: The retrocalcaneal bursa: Anatomy and bursography. *Foot Ankle* 1992; 13:203–207.

Jahss MH, Kummer F, Michelson JD: Investigations into the fat pads of the sole of the foot: Heel pressure studies. *Foot Ankle* 1992;13:227–232.

Jones DC, James SL: Partial calcaneal ostectomy for retrocalcaneal bursitis. *Am J Sports Med* 1984;12:72–73.

Leach RE, Seavey MS, Salter DK: Results of surgery in athletes with plantar fasciitis. *Foot Ankle* 1986;7:156–161.

Leach R, Jones R, Silva T: Rupture of the plantar fascia in athletes. *J Bone Joint Surg* 1978;60A:537–539.

Pavlov H, Heneghan MA, Hersh A, Goldman AB, Vigorita V: The Haglund syndrome: Initial and differential diagnosis. *Radiology* 1982;144:83–88.

Pfeffer GB, Baxter DE: Surgery of the adult heel, in Jahss MH (ed): *Disorders of the Foot and Ankle: Medical and Surgical Management,* ed 2. Philadelphia, PA, WB Saunders, 1991, vol 2, pp 1396–1416.

Rubin G, Witten M: Plantar calcaneal spurs. *Am J Orthop* 1963; 5:38–41,53–55.

Sarrafian SK: Functional characteristics of the foot and plantar aponeurosis under tibiotalar loading. *Foot Ankle* 1987;8:4–18.

Snider MP, Clancy WG, McBeath AA: Plantar fascia release for chronic plantar fasciitis in runners. *Am J Sports Med* 1983; 11:215–219.

Wapner KL, Sharkey PF: The use of night splints for treatment of recalcitrant plantar fasciitis. *Foot Ankle* 1991;12:135–137.

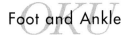
Chapter 15
Fractures of the Ankle

Introduction

The overall incidence of ankle fractures in the United States is estimated to be 250,000 per year, making this the most common injury treated by the orthopaedic surgeon. As longevity and participation in athletic endeavors increases, so does the incidence of ankle injuries. High speed vehicular accidents and the trend of larger, stronger athletes in contact sports has caused an increase in the severity of these injuries. As the results of long-term prospective studies become available, we have been better able to answer the important question of which injuries need surgical intervention and which will result in acceptable long-term function without surgery. This question can be answered only with a thorough understanding of normal ankle anatomy and biomechanics, and the correct interpretation of radiographic findings.

Anatomy and Biomechanics

The ankle joint is not a simple hinge joint. Although its motion is primarily in the sagittal plane, the complex interplay among the tibia, fibula and talus and their associated ligamentous connections allows rotation and even a small amount of translation. The tibia and fibula form the mortise in which the wedge-shaped talus resides. The distal articular surface of the tibia conforms to the talar dome with its surface being convex, the other concave, and both being wider anteriorly than posteriorly. The medial malleolus is an extension of the distal tibia. A longitudinal groove divides it into a large, anterior colliculus and a small, posterior colliculus. Its inner surface is covered with cartilage and articulates with the medial side of the talar body, thereby imparting medial bony stability. The fibula provides lateral bony stability. Its distal portion, the lateral malleolus, lies adjacent to the lateral border of the talar body and is covered with cartilage. Proximally, it sits in a groove at the lateral border of the tibia. There is no articular cartilage at this level although there is a small amount of motion between the two bones. The talus has multiple articulations with bones of the foot and ankle and is almost entirely covered by articular cartilage. Its neck has essentially no cartilage and serves as access for the blood supply. There are no muscular attach-ments to the talus, allowing it to serve as the intercalary bone connecting the ankle to the foot.

The ligaments of the ankle are divided into three distinct groups: medial collateral, lateral collateral, and syndesmotic. The medial ligamentous support is provided by the deep and superficial deltoid ligaments. The more important deep portion originates from both colliculi of the medial malleolus with its vertically oriented fibers inserting into the entire nonarticular surface of the medial talus. The superficial layer originates primarily from the anterior colliculus and inserts in three bands to the navicular bone and calcaneonavicular (spring) ligament, to the sustentaculum tali of the calcaneus, and to the medial tubercle of the talus.

The lateral ligamentous complex comprises the anterior talofibular ligament, calcaneofibular ligament, and posterior talofibular ligament. The anterior ligament is the weakest and is the structure injured in ankle sprains. This ligament prevents anterior subluxation of the talus by its attachments to the anterior fibula and neck of the talus. The midportion of this ligament is confluent with the joint capsule. The calcaneofibular ligament originates from the distal fibula and inserts on the posterolateral aspect of the calcaneus. Its function is to stabilize the subtalar joint and limit inversion. The posterior talofibular ligament is the strongest of the three and is the least commonly injured. It arises from the posteromedial fibula and inserts at the lateral tubercle of the talus.

The syndesmotic ligamentous complex maintains the anatomic relationship between the distal tibia and fibula. It comprises four ligaments, each of which contributes to the dynamic relationship between the bones. The anterior ligament originates from the anterior tibial tubercle and inserts at the anterior fibula. The posterior ligament originates from the posterolateral tibial tubercle and inserts on the posterior fibula. Disruption between the tibia and fibula at this level usually causes an avulsion fracture posteriorly due to the strength of the ligament. In contrast, the anterior ligament usually ruptures before the bone fails. The transverse tibiofibular ligament is located inferior to the posterior ligament and acts to deepen the posterior ankle joint. The remaining interosseus ligament is the primary restraint to transverse motion at the tibiofibular articulation. This ligament runs from the level of the plafond to the proximal tibiofibular joint where it meets the interosseus membrane. The complex arrangement and interaction of these ligaments allows for fibula rotation, translation, and proximal migration when the foot is dorsiflexed and the mortise "widens" to accommodate the anterior talar body. This dynamic relationship allows the fibula to carry approximately 16% of the axial load.

Multiple tendons and neural and vascular structures cross the ankle joint. The tendons are divided into four groups. The posterior tendons in the midline are the Achilles and plantaris with the tibialis posterior, flexor digitorum longus and flexor hallucis longus tendons passing medially and being innervated by the tibial nerve. The peroneus longus and brevis tendons pass posterior to the lateral malleolus and are innervated by the superficial peroneal nerve. The remaining tendons, the tibialis anterior, extensor hallucis longus, extensor digitorum longus and the peroneus tertius pass anterior to the ankle joint and are innervated by the deep peroneal nerve.

The anterior neurovascular bundle is composed of the anterior tibial artery and deep peroneal nerve. The posterior bundle is composed of the posterior tibial artery and tibial nerve. Three superficial sensory nerves cross the ankle joint. The saphenous nerve, along with the long saphenous vein, passes anteriorly to the medial malleolus and innervates the medial portion of the foot. The superficial peroneal nerve passes laterally to the midline and innervates the dorsum of the foot while the remaining sural nerve passes posteriorly to the fibula and supplies the lateral side of the foot.

Physical Examination

A thorough examination must begin with a good history. A patient's recounting of the injury may provide valuable information as to structures likely involved, the magnitude of the injury, and the possibility of associated injuries. Knowledge of any history of previous injury or systemic medical condition will also aid in diagnosis.

A systematic approach is needed to avoid overlooking important signs in the physical examination. Inspection begins with the skin and soft tissues. The presence of ecchymosis and swelling provides important information as to the location of an injury. Palpation includes examination of peripheral pulses and testing sensation, in addition to determining bone or joint line tenderness. When possible, ligaments should be tested. In the acute setting, sedation or a hematoma block is often needed. The anterior drawer maneuver is the equivalent of the Lachman maneuver in the knee. It evaluates the integrity of the anterior talofibular ligament and is performed with the patient in a seated or lying position. With the ankle in neutral or slight plantarflexion, the heel is cupped in one hand of the examiner with application of an

anteriorly directed force. The opposite hand of the examiner stabilizes the tibia with simultaneous application of a posteriorly directed force. Translation of greater than 8 mm between the opposite sides indicates injury to the anterolateral ligamentous complex.

If fracture or instability is suspected by history and physical examination, radiographs are obtained to identify the injury accurately and to guide the examiner in reducing the displaced fracture or dislocation. Immobilization in a well-padded splint prevents further soft-tissue injury, reduces swelling, and decreases pain. Elevation, gentle compression, and ice application all serve to further reduce swelling and discomfort.

Pathology of the Fractured Ankle

Basic orthopaedic tenets of joint stability, articular congruity, articular integrity, and near-anatomic alignment apply to the ankle joint as appropriately as to any other joint in the body. Accordingly, the goal in treatment of ankle fractures should be to achieve these tenets to better the chances of a good clinical result. Deficiency of any of these four principles can lead to a less favorable short-term result with early instability due to ligamentous injury or long-term failure due to arthrosis as a consequence of malalignment, malreduction, or cartilage damage. It is important to diagnose accurately those injuries that are likely to result in late clinical sequelae and to restore the anatomy as accurately as possible.

The need for anatomic reduction of the medial malleolus is well established, and resulting instability due to chronic deltoid ligament disruption has been shown to result in significant arthrosis. However, isolated lateral malleolus fractures have consistently been associated with good-to-excellent long-term results whether treated surgically or nonsurgically. This injury, once healed, does not significantly alter the relationship between the talus and distal tibia, thereby avoiding the complication of malalignment or joint incongruity. This differs from chronic lateral or syndesmotic ligamentous instability, in which the normal gliding motion between the talar dome and the distal tibia is altered. With anterolateral instability, shear forces may compromise articular integrity, causing premature arthrosis.

Malunion or shortening of the fibula results in malalignment of the ankle joint. The resulting decreased contact area of the articular surfaces causes an increase in surface pressure. Premature arthrosis may result due to cartilage degeneration.

There is a 49% incidence of injury to the articular cartilage of the talar dome in association with malleolar fractures. This damage, which usually cannot be detected on plain films, may be seen at the time of surgical fixation. Because of its high incidence, many authors advocate a complete joint inspection and debridement at the time of operation. The damage ranges from simple contusions to full-thickness injuries with exposure of subchondral bone. Even with immediate intervention, many of these injuries will progress to late arthrosis.

While poor reduction of ankle fractures with resulting malunion remains the most common factor in poor outcome after ankle fractures, instability and cartilaginous injury also contribute to the overall pathology.

Radiographic Evaluation

Ankle trauma is one of the most common presenting problems in North American emergency rooms. Of the five million radiographic series done per year to assess the ankle injury, only 20% of these examinations demonstrate a fracture. More exact and efficient criteria to determine the need for radiographic evaluation could reduce health care cost, radiation exposure, and waiting time in the radiology department. Using clinical findings as a guide rather than patient history alone would substantially decrease the number of negative films obtained for simple ankle trauma. Indications for radiographic evaluation include gross deformity, swelling and ecchymosis, localized bone tenderness, crepitus with motion, instability, and the inability to bear weight. Minor swelling without bone tenderness may occur with simple ankle sprains and does not often indicate significant pathology. The exception is a patient who immediately ices and elevates the injured extremity prior to evaluation. In this situation, the lack of swelling, pain, and ecchymosis may mask the extent of the injury.

Although the standard ankle trauma series in many offices and emergency rooms consists of an anteroposterior, a 15° internal oblique, and a lateral view, studies suggest that 95% of all ankle fractures may be detected with two views. The lateral combined with the anteroposterior or oblique view will detect most fractures. The oblique view is favored because it better demonstrates the ankle mortise.

There are two widely used ankle fracture classification systems. The Danis-Weber and the Lauge-Hansen systems vary

significantly in complexity, but both attempt to assist in selection of appropriate management although this ultimately depends on fracture and ankle stability. The Danis-Weber classification, now commonly referred to as the AO classification, is based on the level of the fracture of the fibula, with more proximal injuries indicating a greater risk of syndesmosis disruption and resulting ankle instability. There are three types, A through C, of fractures in the Danis-Weber system (Fig. 1). The AO modification further divides these types into three subtypes, 1 through 3 (Outline 1).

In a type A injury, the fibula fracture occurs due to supination of the foot. More extensive injury involves an oblique or vertical fracture of the medial malleolus and fracture of the posterior malleolus. The type B injury is characterized by an

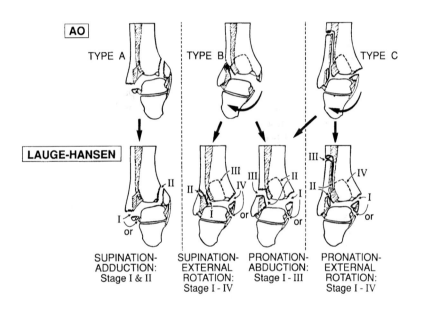

Figure 1

The Danis-Weber/AO and corresponding Lauge-Hansen classifications of fractures. (Reproduced with permission from Poss R (ed): *Orthopaedic Knowledge Update 3*. Park Ridge, IL, American Academy of Orthopaedic Surgeons, 1990, pp 613–624.)

oblique or spiral fracture of the fibula at or near the level of the syndesmosis. Again, the medial side of the ankle and posterior malleolus may be injured in more severe cases. In the type C injury, the fibula fracture occurs above the syndesmosis. The syndesmosis disruption is almost invariably associated with injury on the medial side of the ankle.

The Lauge-Hansen system (Fig. 1), introduced in 1950, classifies ankle fractures based on the position of the foot at the time of injury and the direction of the deforming force. It is

Outline 1
AO Classification of Malleolar Fractures

Type A: Fibula fracture below syndesmosis (infrasyndesmotic)

A1–Isolated

A2–With fracture of medial malleolus

A3–With posteromedial fracture

Type B: Fibula fracture at the level of the syndesmosis (transyndesmotic)

B1–Isolated

B2–With medial lesion (malleolus or ligament)

B3–With medial lesion and fracture of posterolateral tibia

Type C: Fibula fracture above syndesmosis (suprasyndesmotic)

C1–Diaphyseal fracture of the fibula, simple

C2–Diaphyseal fracture of the fibula, complex

C3–Proximal fracture of the fibula

estimated that more than 95% of ankle fractures can be placed into one of the four categories of injury. The most common ankle fracture patterns are those in the supination-external rotation (SE) group. The position of the foot is the same as that associated with lateral ankle sprains. Supination of the foot puts strain on the lateral ligamentous complex and bony structures of the ankle while the external rotation force at the tibia increases stress in this area. The result is a circular injury progression starting at the lateral ligaments and ending at the medial side of the ankle. The stage I injury is an anterior capsular and anterior tibiofibular ligament tear. Stage II includes a short-oblique or spiral fibular fracture. Stage III progresses to a posterior capsule tear or posterior malleolus fracture. Stage IV includes deltoid ligament disruption or a transverse medial malleolus fracture. In the pronation-external rotation (PE) group, the initial injury begins medially at the deltoid ligament or medial malleolus and progresses to finally include a posterior injury similar to that seen in supination-external rotation injuries. The major difference is the location of the fibular fracture. In PE injuries, the fibula fracture occurs above the syndesmosis and signifies syndesmosis disruption with ankle instability. The remaining fracture patterns in this system are supination-adduction (SA) stages I-II and pronation-abduction (PA) stages I-III.

Both Danis-Weber and Lauge-Hansen classifications are widely used and an understanding of both systems is important. The systems overlap somewhat in that the Weber "A" fracture corresponds to the Lauge-Hansen SA injury, the Weber "B" fracture corresponds to the SE injury of Lauge-Hansen, and the Weber "C" fracture corresponds to the PE or PA stage 3 injuries of Lauge-Hansen.

No one classification system can encompass all injury patterns, and both systems have their own merits and shortcomings. The Danis-Weber/AO system is simpler, emphasizes the importance of the fibula fracture, and describes the medial injury in type A and type B fractures. The original Danis-Weber system was too inclusive, was neither prognostic nor predictive of surgical treatment, and ignored the medial side of the ankle. The Lauge-Hansen system, although bulky and comprehensive, still misses 5% of fracture patterns. Its efficacy in SE patterns has been established with many studies supporting its prognostic and predictive value in planning surgical treatment. The system is a useful adjunct to the AO system because it characterizes both mechanism and sequelae of injury and emphasizes the ligamentous disruptions.

Although readers may prefer one system to the other or even exclusively use only one, the importance of both classifications is evident. Each features a different aspect of ankle injury and this information, along with a thorough examination of the patient, will lead to better care plans and outcomes.

In addition to radiographic classifications, other radiographic criteria have been established to aid in identifying potentially unstable ankle fracture patterns. These are useful in choosing the appropriate treatment and assessing the accuracy of reduction and final results. One of the most commonly used measurements is medial clear space. On the mortise view, this measurement is defined as the distance between the lateral border of the medial malleolus and the medial border of the talar dome as is shown in Figure 2, top. This space should be equal to the superior clear space between the talar dome and distal tibia. A space of greater than 4 mm is abnormal and indicates lateral talar shift.

Syndesmotic integrity may be assessed on an anteroposterior or mortise view. The syndesmotic space between the tibia and fibula is measured 1 cm proximal to the plafond. A normal space is defined by greater than 1 mm of overlap between the tibia and fibula on the mortise view. The tibiofibular clear space is defined as the distance between the medial border of the fibula and the medial border of the incisura fibularis, and should be, less than 6 mm.

Talar shift less than or equal to 2 mm is acceptable on plain radiographs (Fig. 2, bottom). In the absence of medial injury, acceptable lateral malleolar displacement ranges from 0 to 5 mm in any direction. The measurement is taken at the point of maximal fragment displacement. As is discussed in the section on isolated lateral malleolus fractures, the amount of displacement is often overestimated. The important factor in this injury is not fragment separation, but, rather, distal talofibular and tibiofibular integrity. With a fibula fracture at the joint line and an uninjured medial side, some of the distal ligamentous relationships remain intact, thereby preserving the normal anatomic relationship among the three bones of the ankle joint. In these injuries, fibular shortening does not usually occur. This problem may be detected by measuring the talocrural angle, which normally measures between 8° and 15°. A difference of 3° compared to the opposite side indicates fibular shortening (Fig. 2, top).

Occasionally, specialized studies are used to better evaluate ankle injuries. Stress films are used primarily to confirm suspected ligamentous instability. These films are rarely obtained in acute ankle fractures but may be important assessing resid-

ual instability after internal fixation or after a fracture has healed. Concomitant ligamentous injury may be missed at the initial presentation. Stress radiographs must always be compared to the unaffected side to accurately judge the importance of any seemingly abnormal findings.

Computed tomography (CT) is useful in evaluating the extent of comminuted or complex bony injuries and planning surgical intervention. It is most useful in pilon fractures and correction of malunions.

Magnetic resonance imaging (MRI) is most useful in evaluation of tendon or other soft-tissue injury. It is the best imaging modality for subtle fractures not discernable on plain films, for noting osteochondral lesions, and for documenting the changes of osteonecrosis.

Management of Specific Fractures

Nonsurgical Versus Surgical Management
The literature is replete with reports supporting both nonsurgical and surgical management of ankle fractures, regardless of type. Early reports advocate closed reduction with cast immobilization, often in long leg casts for lengthy periods of time. More recent literature strongly recommends surgical intervention for certain fracture patterns.

Early range of motion and weightbearing when symptoms and radiographs dictate are now standards of surgical management. The difficulty in interpreting early studies is the comparison of dissimilar fracture patterns and criterion of an acceptable closed reduction. It cannot be argued that an anatomic reduction of a displaced fracture treated successfully in plaster will do better in long-term follow-up than would a fracture treated by inadequate or improper open reduction and internal fixation.

Extraneous factors, such as the general health of the patient, obesity, skin condition and concomitant injuries, are also major factors in the decision to operate. Randomized prospective studies comparing closed to open management bring us closer to resolving the most difficult decision in treating ankle fractures: deciding which injuries require surgical intervention.

Isolated Lateral Malleolus Fractures
With rare exception, an isolated fracture of the lateral malleolus, not associated with concomitant medial injury or talar shift, is best managed by closed means. Clinical results of long-term studies on the stage II supination external rotation fracture have been uniformly excellent, and surgical treatment does not improve patient function or satisfaction in most cases.

Syndesmosis Radiographic Criterion
Mortise View

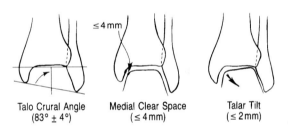

Talo Crural Angle
(83° ± 4°)

Medial Clear Space
(≤ 4 mm)

Talar Tilt
(≤ 2 mm)

Anterior Posterior View

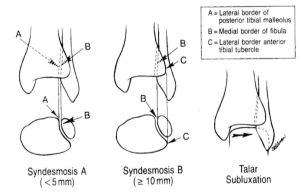

A = Lateral border of posterior tibial malleolus
B = Medial border of fibula
C = Lateral border anterior tibial tubercle

Syndesmosis A
(< 5 mm)

Syndesmosis B
(≥ 10 mm)

Talar Subluxation

Figure 2
Schematic diagram of radiologic criteria used in the evaluation of injuries to the syndesmosis. (Reproduced with permission from Stiehl JB: Ankle fractures with diastasis, in Greene WB (ed): *Instructional Course Lectures XXXIX*. Park Ridge, IL, American Academy of Orthopaedic Surgeons, 1990, pp 95–103.)

The tenet that mortise congruity is dependent on distal fibular position still remains. Recent studies using CT demonstrate that the relationships between the lateral malleolus, the medial malleolus, and the talus are usually preserved in these injuries, thereby maintaining essentially normal joint integrity. When evaluating radiographs, the abnormal relationship between the distal and proximal ends of the fibula fracture is often interpreted as distal fragment displacement. This radiographic abnormality is, in part, caused by internal rotation and medial displacement of the proximal fibula relation to the tibia. Healing of the fibula in this orientation does not lead to complications as evidenced by late clinical and radiographic results.

Shortening and/or displacement of fracture fragments are acceptable indications for surgical fixation of fractures. Various radiographic parameters have been proposed to assess these important findings in fractures of the distal fibula. Displacement of up to 5 mm and shortening, defined as less than 2° to 5° side-to-side difference of the talocrural angle, are published standards commonly referred to today. One CT study demonstrates slight widening of the lateral joint space, indicative of lateral translation of the distal fragment in 33% of the patients studied. In none of these patients was the medial joint space affected.

Based on current information, these fractures represent a stable injury pattern and can be managed by casting and early weightbearing. Open reduction and internal fixation is reserved for significant displacement, which may represent a more severe injury pattern than an SEII.

Isolated Medial Malleolus Fractures

Definitive management of the isolated medial malleolus fracture continues to be controversial. Although a common topic in the literature, most reports do not distinguish between displaced and nondisplaced fractures. The nonunion rate varies from 5% to 15% in fractures treated by closed methods, and several reasons have been cited for this unacceptably high percentage. Inadequate reduction, periosteal interposition, and even impaired blood flow have all been proposed, with most authors agreeing on the first two factors.

Displaced isolated medial malleolus fractures should be managed by anatomic open reduction and internal fixation, usually with parallel 4.0-mm lag screws. There are significant soft-tissue attachments to the medical malleolus, including the deltoid ligament, periosteum, and fascia. Any of these may be torn and become interposed in the fracture site, thereby inhibiting bony union. Although difficult to discern from the literature, the nonunion rate for these fractures treated with internal rigid fixation appears to be less than 1%. This is an acceptable rate and probably reflects other physiologic factors

in the development of nonunions. Inadequacy of blood flow to the medial malleolus has not been proven.

Nondisplaced, isolated medial malleolus fractures are managed differently. Initial displacement with possible soft-tissue interposition or nonanatomic reduction are not issues, and these fractures are expected to heal by closed methods. Adequacy of reduction and proper immobilization must be maintained. Variable periods of cast immobilization have been reported, but average 4 to 6 weeks. Time to weightbearing also varies but is usually started as the patient's clinical symptoms dictate and there is demonstrable healing by radiographs.

Symptomatic nonunions may occur at any level of the medial malleolus, but they usually occur at joint level. Management consists of open reduction with freshening of the fracture ends and compression via rigid internal fixation. Bone graft is usually not needed except in atrophic nonunions. Asymptomatic nonunions at any level are observed.

Bimalleolar Fractures and Deltoid Ligament Disruption

Unlike fractures that involve only one side of the joint, bimalleolar fractures and lateral malleolus fractures with disruption of the deltoid ligament often represent unstable injuries that require surgical fixation. These fracture patterns are likely to be displaced at the time of injury, thereby making anatomic reduction by closed means difficult. Even if the reduction is successful, maintaining it in a cast or splint is improbable due to variable swelling. As the swelling subsides, the fit of any external form of immobilization is compromised, and drift of the fragments with malalignment of the mortise is likely. Incomplete reduction of the lateral malleolus and residual talar tilt is commonly reported in symptomatic patients in the literature. This finding supports the view that the key to treatment of the displaced ankle fracture lies in anatomic reduction of the lateral malleolus. Three years after surgery, good results have been reported (85% to 90% of patients) following anatomic reduction of both the lateral and medial malleoli.

In a bimalleolar equivalent injury, disruption of the deltoid ligament is of secondary importance to the bony injury of the lateral malleolus. Anatomic reduction and fixation of the distal fibula obviates the need for repair of the deltoid ligament. At an average follow-up of 36 months, good results are seen in over 90% of these injuries treated by anatomic open reduction and internal fixation of the fibula. No residual instability was reported in these patients. The deltoid ligament heals adequately when the ends are apposed and the only indication for medial exploration is in the event of widening of the medial clear space after adequate reduction of the fibular fracture. In these cases, there may be soft-tissue entrapment of either ligament or tendon or osteochondral fragments interposed between the medial malleolus and the talar dome. All tissue must be removed to obtain normal alignment of the joint but the deltoid ligament need not be repaired. No reports have demonstrated clear clinical advantages to deltoid repair, and some have noted the disadvantage of decreased motion and discomfort after repair.

Trimalleolar Fractures

Fractures of the posterior malleolus are seen with severe external rotation or abduction forces. It is generally advocated that the posterior lip of the distal tibia fractures as a result of either avulsion of the posterior inferior tibiofibular ligament or direct pressure from the rotating talus. The vertical fracture pattern supports a ligamentous cause; the chondral lesions sometimes seen on the talus or tibia support the direct pressure theory.

It is generally accepted that fractures that comprise 25% or more of the articular surface as seen on a lateral plain film or those with greater than 2 mm of displacement require open reduction and internal fixation. These criteria are based on studies that demonstrate an increase in posterior subluxation of the talus when the fragment exceeded 25% of the articular surface. Other mechanical studies indicate that anatomic reduction of associated medial and lateral malleolus fractures provides enough stability to resist posterior subluxation. With anatomic stabilization of the fibula, involvement of 25% to 45% of the articular surface made no difference between the results obtained with or without internal fixation of the posterior fragment. The limitation of these studies is the accuracy of fragment measurement. A plain lateral radiograph usually overestimates the size of the fragment, and CT scan may be more beneficial.

Trimalleolar fractures should be approached in the same way as displaced bimalleolar fractures. Ligamentotaxis via the posterior tibiofibular ligament often reduces the posterior fragment when the lateral malleolus is reduced. Dorsiflexion of the foot may aid in reduction due to the posterior capsule attachment. The decision to internally fix the posterior fragment is based on size of the fragment, residual displacement, and overall stability of the ankle mortise once the medial and lateral malleoli are stabilized. Residual displacement of 2 mm or more should be addressed, and posterior subluxation must be corrected with rigid fixation of the posterior lip.

The posterior fragment may be secured directly through a posterolateral approach or by indirectly reducing the fracture and securing it with lag screws placed from anterior to posterior. The latter approach may be complicated by inadvertent displacement of the fracture by a drill bit or guide wire, or by

nonoptimal effect of the lag screws. Initial displacement and position of the fragment after closed reduction may offer some insight into whether the posterior malleolus will need to be addressed. In cases of severe displacement or substantial residual displacement after splinting, anatomic reduction and fixation may be difficult from a lateral approach and the surgeon may elect to make a posterolateral incision to better visualize the fracture.

Maisonneuve Fractures and Syndesmosis Injuries

Of all ankle injuries, the syndesmosis injury continues to cause the most controversy. Both the Maisonneuve fracture and pronation-external rotation patterns disrupt the syndesmosis and interosseus ligament, a primary component of instability and potential for long-term complications. Recent studies have addressed the main question—which injuries require fixation, and the best type, level, and duration of fixation.

While older studies propose the lateral malleolus to be the key to ankle alignment and stability, more recent biomechanical studies focus on the medial malleolus as the key to maintenance of mortise alignment. Significant diastasis of the ankle mortise as shown in Figure 3 has been commonly defined by the medial clear space, which should be less than 4 mm on good AP and mortise films. The joint space of the ankle should also be symmetrical medially, laterally, and superiorly. If these criteria are not met when analyzing a high fibular fracture, then syndesmotic injury must be suspected. The key to appropriate treatment is the medial injury. In cases of bony injury, anatomic fixation of the medial malleolus obviates the need for syndesmosis fixation, provided that there is no residual displacement of the fibula laterally. In the case of deltoid disruption, unless the deltoid is repaired, syndesmosis fixation is generally required for fractures that extend 3 to 4.5 cm above the joint line. Other studies have disputed the need for syndesmosis fixation in fractures up to 7 cm above the joint line. It must be stressed that these are general guidelines based on cadaver models, and each repair should be tested at the time of surgery. Stability may be tested by applying anterolateral traction to the internally fixed fibula. If it moves significantly or if an intraoperative radiograph demonstrates widening of the mortise, then a syndesmosis screw is needed.

If amenable, the syndesmosis screw should be placed after anatomic fixation of the fibula fracture. Maisonneuve fractures are often too high to safely be reconstructed with a plate. In these cases, the syndesmosis screw alone provides stability. The syndesmosis screw should be fully threaded (3.5 to 4.5 mm) and placed approximately 2 cm above the plafond to ensure that the screw is not placed into the ligamentous complex. The foot should be held in mild dorsiflexion to

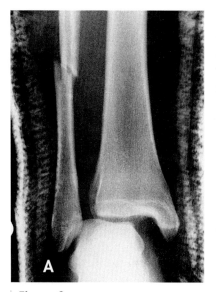 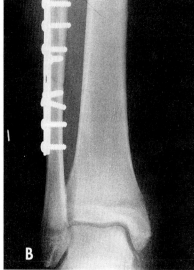

Figure 3

A, Stage 4 pronation-external rotation injury with deltoid ligament disruption and significant widening. **B,** The injury was treated with anatomic plating of the fibula only. This radiograph was taken 3 months after internal fixation. The mortise is preserved.

injuries are the result of motor vehicle accidents, and 10% result from gunshot wounds. These high-energy wounds require rapid surgical management with aggressive debridement of nonviable tissue along with anatomic rigid internal fixation of the injury. Second-look operations at 24 to 48 hours are advocated to address any nonviable tissue that declares itself later. Using these principles, along with appropriate and immediate antibiotic therapy, good-to-excellent results can be expected in 87% of grade I and II fractures. The increase in poor results in grade III fractures is attributed to the extent of the bony and soft-tissue injury, resulting in a high rate of nonanatomic reductions, articular damage, and deep infection.

Early skeletal fixation is the treatment of choice in grade I and clean grade II ankle fractures. Metal does not cause infection and, in fact, aids the body in prevention by providing an internal scaffolding for the soft tissues to heal. Grade III fractures represent a different type of injury. The use of minimal internal fixation along with meticulous soft-tissue handling is essential in caring for

bring the widest portion of the talus into the mortise. The screw is angled anteriorly 30° and placed through the fibula across the near cortex of the tibia only. The screw is not lagged. Compression across the syndesmosis will lead to pain and restriction of motion. If fibula fixation is not possible, two parallel screws will increase the strength and stability of the repair (Fig. 4).

Ligament healing does not occur before 6 to 8 weeks and syndesmosis fixation should not be removed prior to this time. Although syndesmosis fixation theoretically prevents normal motion of the fibula, crossing only one cortex of the tibia does allow some independent motion. Proximal and distal migration, in addition to external rotation, may still occur. Early weightbearing does not seem to adversely affect postoperative results and screw removal prior to ambulation is no longer thought to be necessary. Screw breakage is not often seen and is rarely a problem unless the head of the screw becomes prominent. Use of bioabsorbable screws may play a future role in these injuries in that they obviate the need for removal even in the case of breakage.

Open Fractures

As in other open fractures, the most important prognostic factor in open ankle injuries is the amount of energy absorbed and the damage to the soft-tissue envelope. Over 60% of these

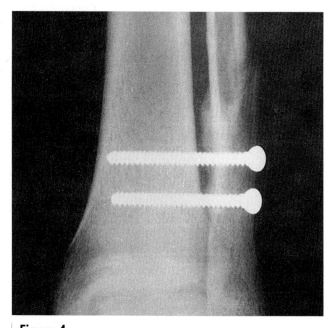

Figure 4

Fixation of a high, comminuted pronation-external rotation fracture with parallel, fully threaded screws.

these injuries. External fixation with traditional methods or small pin fiaxators is advocated. Surgical incisions may be closed but traumatic wounds should be closed after 5 days (usually enough time to declare themselves) or left to heal by secondary intention. The duration of antibiotic use is more controversial but should probably be continued at least 48 hours and preferably until the final culture result is obtained. Principles of postoperative weightbearing are unchanged and are determined by stability of fixation and clinical symptoms.

Principles of Fixation

Standard techniques and principles advocated by the AO group are used in the fixation of ankle fractures. A stepwise approach, usually starting with reduction and fixation of the fibula, ensures that all components of the injury are addressed and that each previous step facilitates the next.

The lateral malleolus is reduced first because it promotes easier reduction of any remaining fragments and provides instant stability to the joint as a whole. It may be approached from a direct lateral incision with full-thickness flaps or from a posterolateral incision. The latter may be more advantageous in the case of direct trauma with resulting soft-tissue injury, which may compromise wound healing. In the case of a large posterior malleolus fragment, the posterolateral incision provides direct visualization of the tibial fracture while still allowing easy fixation of the fibula. The fracture is fixed with a 3.5-mm cortical lag screw placed at a right angle to the oblique fracture line. The construct may then be neutralized by adding a laterally placed one-third semitubular plate secured with 3.5-mm cortical screws and 4.0-mm cancellous screws in the metaphyseal region of the bone. Care is taken not to drill or place screw threads into the ankle mortise. Alternatively, posterior plating of the fibula using the so-called "anti-glide" plate has also given excellent results. An unbent one-third semitubular plate is secured with one lag screw across the fracture site and other bicortical screws are placed above and below the fracture. This method has the advantage of less soft-tissue stripping, avoidance of intra-articular screws, and less palpable hardware. The disadvange is the development of per-

oneal tendinitis or a symptomatic lag screw necessitating the need for hardware removal. In the case of an isolated fibula fracture, the reduction of the bone and mortise is evaluated with an intraoperative radiograph. Any malalignment is addressed, and any residual talar tilt is corrected by removing the entrapped deltoid ligament from the ankle mortise. It is not necessary to repair the ligament. Fibular stability should be checked in high fractures to determine the need for a syndesmosis screw.

The medial malleolus is approached from a direct medial or anteromedial incision. The anteromedial incision allows inspection of the ankle joint with removal of intra-articular fragments, but this increases the risk of saphenous nerve and vein damage. Fixation is best accomplished with two parallel 4.0-mm lag screws or, in the case of a small or comminuted medial malleolus fragment, Kirschner wires and a figure-of-eight wire anchored by a superiorly placed 4.0-mm cancellous screw (Fig. 5). This wire construct is not a true tension band technique in that it does not rely on joint motion for compression.

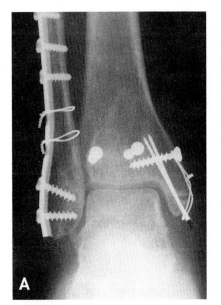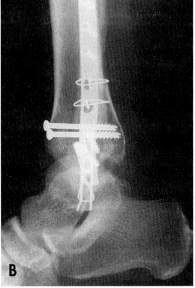

Figure 5

A, Severe supination-external rotation injury treated with several accepted fixation techniques. The fibula has been bridge-plated with cerclage wire around the comminuted diaphysis. The medial malleolus fragment was too small to fix with screws and required a Kirschner wire and figure-of-eight construct. **B,** The posterior malleolus was secured with anteroposterior lag screws.

Comminution, osteoporosis, and open injuries of the lateral malleolus may all present their own special challenges. When bone loss complicates an injury, anatomic length is restored by bridgeplating the fibula and filling the defect with bone graft obtained from Gerdy's tubercle or the iliac crest (Fig. 5). Use of the small AO distractor or tension device makes obtaining and holding the fracture out to length less difficult. Osteoporotic bone may be best fixed by use of the antiglide technique of posterior fibula plating with lag screws or by lateral plating with supplementary intramedullary Kirshner wires. While the antiglide plate often works well, intramedullary fixation alone has severe limitations. It does not allow for rigid fixation and cannot correct rotation or prevent shortening. It should be reserved for only the most extreme cases, in which open reduction and internal fixation is absolutely contraindicated.

Studies on absorbable implants show promise in treatment of ankle fractures. The previous problem of sterile abcesses secondary to polyglycolide polymer production has been reduced with the use of polylactic polymers. Their strength is equivalent to stainless steel screws in the treatment of the displaced medial malleolus.

Complications

Complications in the treatment of ankle fractures can begin at the time of initial presentation. Trauma management principles must be followed and a thorough history and physical examination done to determine the presence of injury at a remote site. It is easy to diagnose an injury when the patient has an acutely swollen, painful, ecchymotic lower extremity and radiographs demonstrate a displaced ankle fracture. Unfortunately, if a fall is the mechanism of injury, the obvious pathology may distract both physician and patient, leading to a failure to diagnose possible associated injuries of the knee, wrist, or spine.

More commonly, associated injuries occur near the ankle itself. Osteochondral fractures of the talar dome may occur after any type of trauma to the ankle, even the "simple ankle sprain." Concurrent osteochondral fractures have been reported to occur in 2% to 6% of acute ankle sprains and account for 1% of all talus fractures. They can be medial or lateral, with the latter more often associated with a history of trauma. This lesion is due to forceful inversion of the foot, which causes a shearing force as the lateral edge of the dome impacts the adjacent fibula. The medial lesion is believed to be a result of dome impaction against the tibial plafond or medial malleolus. Oftentimes, plain radiographs do not reveal these injuries. An anteroposterior radiograph in plantarflexion may increase visualization of medial injuries; lateral lesions are best seen on a mortise view in dorsiflexion.

These lesions must be suspected in the "ankle sprains" that are refractory to routine treatment. Small, nondisplaced lesions may heal spontaneously or displace and become loose bodies. Larger lesions or those that cause mechanical symptoms may require surgical intervention by open or arthroscopic methods.

Plafond fractures may also include osteochondral lesions with findings similar to those described above. They are a result of external rotation of a pronated foot. They are sometimes associated with an oblique fracture of the medial malleous. Their classification and treatment are described in a section to follow.

Deltoid ligament disruption is a recognized soft-tissue injury associated with lateral malleolus fractures. Lateral ankle ligaments may also be disrupted in high-energy injuries and must be evaluated during the treatment process. If the lateral malleolus is to be treated surgically, disruption of the ligamentous complex should be addressed simultaneously. If closed treatment is done, a thorough examination at the time of union is needed to determine symptomatic instability.

Seemingly simple avulsion fractures of the medial or lateral malleolus may signify important soft-tissue disruption of structures near the ankle. The retinacula surrounding tendons take a portion of their origin from bone. A small fragment near the tip of the medial malleolus may be more than a simple deltoid injury and may represent a disruption of the posterior tibial tendon and/or its sheath. This injury must be recognized and repaired primarily, if possible. If the tendon cannot be repaired, reconstruction, using a flexor tendon, is required to possibly prevent adult acquired flatfoot. A fragment posterior to the lateral malleolus suggests a disruption of the superior peroneal retinaculum, which can lead to peroneal tendon instability or dislocation. This condition may be treated nonsurgically if stable reduction in a cast can be maintained for 6 weeks. Open repair is required in unstable cases. Retinaculum repair with augmentation is usually successful. Fibular groove deepening is rarely required.

Prevention of wound complications begins at the time of presentation. Severely damaged soft tissues preclude immediate surgical intervention and preventive measures should be instituted immediately. Any dislocation should be expediently reduced and the extremity splinted, iced, and elevated to reduce swelling. Abrasions and blisters should be treated by gentle cleansing, sterile unroofing, and dressing to promote healing and epithelization of the skin. Once the soft tissues are deemed fit for incision, surgery should proceed without delay. Meticulous handling of the soft tissues, especially the skin edges, is essential. Minimizing tourniquet time, appropriately

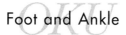
sized implants, gentle retraction, and wound closure without tension are fundamental tenents of wound healing and must be followed. Postoperative dressings should be supportive and provide gentle compression without being constrictive. Deferring surgery until the soft tissues are stable greatly reduces the risk of major complications. Marginal necrosis of skin edges occurs in approximately 3% of patients.

The infection rate in surgical treatment of closed ankle fractures with current techniques of internal fixation is less than 2%. This risk is decreased by attention to surgical principles outlined above. The use of perioperative antibiotics, usually a first-generation cephalosporin, such as cefazolin, can also aid in prevention of postperative infections. If, after internal fixation, an infection of the ankle is present, general orthopaedic principles of management apply. Cellulitis is treated with antibiotics and immobilization; deep infection is treated by surgical debridement as needed. If the fixation is stable, it should be left in place until the fracture heals. It is more difficult to treat an infected nonunion than an infected union. Deep cultures should be taken and the antibiotic coverage tailored to the bacteria identified.

Reflex sympathetic dystrophy may occur with minimal trauma to the ankle. Its incidence is difficult to discern as there is often a delay in diagnosis. It is charecterized by pain disproportionate to the injury, swelling, discoloration, and atrophy of the soft tissues and bone. Treatment begins with restoration of function and intervention designed to break the pain cycle. Physical threrapy and pharmacologic agents are used to restore appropriate responses to normal stimuli.

Malunion of an ankle fracture is usually a consequence of nonanatomic reduction of the fibula. The resulting rotatory deformity and/or shortening decreases the tibiotalar contact area, causing pain. The deformity may be difficult to diagnose if the talus remains in an anatomic position. A lateral radiograph may demonstrate incomplete reduction of the original fracture. Overt malunions are easily seen on mortise radiographs showing a widened medial clear space. The diagnosis is often delayed because the patient may be symptom-free for up to 5 years following the original injury. Once symptoms begin, fibular osteotomy is recommended. The bone is lengthened and derotated with the use of a distractor. The gap in the bone is filled with corticocancellous graft and the fibula plated. Its approximate length may be determined by radiographic evaluation of the noninvolved side. Good results are expected in 75% of patients. Neither preexisting arthritis nor duration from time of injury affect outcome.

Malunions of the medial and posterior malleoli also occur and may be amenable to osteotomy through a medial incision or posterolateral incision, respectively. If a medial malleolus fragment is too small, excision with advancement of the deltoid ligament is recommended. Posterior malleolus malunion often leads to arthritis and requires arthrodesis.

Ankle Fractures in Diabetic Patients

The incidence of diabetes mellitus in the adult population is 1%. Ankle fractures in these patients represent a complicated management issue in both diagnosis and treatment. The median time period between the initial symptoms attributable to fracture and diagnosis of the fracture is 5 weeks. Symptoms of deformity, swelling, and erythema are usually present. Unfortunately, absence or reduction of pain and unfamiliarity of the patients or their physicians with this problem may lead to delayed treatment.

The pathophysiology of fractures in diabetic patients has not been completely elucidated, but it is known that metabolism of bone and mineral is affected adversely by both the lack of insulin and accompanying renal disease that may be present. Insulin therapy corrects many of the cellular abnormalities that affect osteoblastic and osteoclastic activity, which explain why well-controlled insulin-dependent patients heal faster than patients on oral therapy. Sulfonylureas increase bone resorption and accelerate underlying bone demineralization.

In a study of 31 closed lower extremity fractures in diabetic patients, overall union time was 163% of expected (insulin-controlled patients, at 157% and oral hypoglycemic-controlled diabetics, 176%). Fractures treated by open methods are slower to union than those treated closed but this may be explained by the amount of initial displacement and resulting soft-tissue injury.

It may be difficult to rule out infection in diabetic patients presenting with swelling and erythema of the foot and ankle. Pain is variable and is not a reliable indicator in any process. A detailed history with particular attention to traumatic events, no matter how trivial, along with a thorough physical examination and proper radiographs will usually suffice to rule out infection. It is highly unlikely that a diabetic patient with a closed traumatic or atraumatic fracture has an infection. Additionally, changes of Charcot arthropathy are usually evident on radiographs. If there is still a question of infection, laboratory studies should be done. These include a comlete blood count (CBC) with differential, erythrocyte sedimentation rate, and C-reactive protein.

Recommendations in treatment of ankle fractures in diabetic patients vary widely. Some authors advocate closed treatment of nondisplaced fractures and displaced fractures amenable to closed reduction. Casting is done and nonweightbearing is maintained until there are radiographic and clinical signs of union. Other authors advocate open reduction and internal fixation of any displaced ankle fracture because of the delayed healing time and potential for late displacement in these patients. After union is achieved, long-standing protection of the involved extremity is recommended, with the use of a removable load-sharing orthosis.

Patients who undergo open reduction and internal fixation are at an increased risk of infection compared to the normal population. Proper surgical technique with careful handling of tissue and prophylactic antibiotic therapy are essential. Fixation may be difficult in diabetic patients. Reduction clamps should be avoided when possible. If fibular purchase is inadequate, the screws may be anchored into the tibia for better purchase, or supplementary intramedullary Kirshner wires may aid in fracture stability. Medial malleolus fixation may be supplemented in a similar fashion or with the use of small plates. Bone grafting is recommended for any loss of bone or comminution. Sutures or surgical staples are often left in place for up to 3 weeks to protect against wound dehiscence.

Diabetes is a systemic disease and the uninvolved ankle must also be protected. The increased strain of weightbearing on the unaffected limb may predispose it to injury, and prophylactic bracing, at least until weightbearing on the involved extremity is begun, is advised.

Charcot Arthropathy

Fractures of the foot or ankle in diabetic patients do not invariably lead to the development of a neuropathic joint. The overall incidence is 0.1% of 0.5% overall, with 11% of these changes located in the ankle joint. Delay in diagnosis and treatment appears to be the most important factor in the development of Charcot arthropathy. Immediate medical attention with immobilization in a nonweightbearing cast until evidence of clinical and radiographic loading is recommended.

In the case of established Charcot arthropathy, signs and symptoms often mimic infection. A detailed history, thorough examination and proper radiographs are all that is needed to make an accurate diagnosis. Swelling, warmth, and erythema in a diabetic patient without a clear history of trauma or open wound is invariably Charcot arthropathy, not osteomyelitis. Exceptions include lacerations or ulcerations of the skin of the foot or ankle or a history of sepsis. When the diagnosis is in doubt, 24 hours of rest and immobilization will relieve the symptoms of Charcot arthropathy while an extremity with

osteomyelitis will not improve. If there is still a question, laboratory studies including a CBC with differential, erythrocyte sedimentation rate and a C-reactive protein are indicated. A bone scan will invariably be positive and does not offer useful information. MRI may differentiate between inflammation and infection but is usually not needed.

Pilon Fractures

Tibial pilon or plafond fractures are relatively uncommon fractures of the distal tibia with extension into the ankle joint. They represent 7% to 10% of all tibial fractures and less than 1% of fractures of the lower extremity. These challenging fractures are a result of two separate mechanisms of injury. Lower energy fractures are primarily rotational, resulting from falls or sporting injuries. These fractures are less comminuted and significant soft-tissue damage is less common. Higher energy fractures are a result of a vertical compressive force with the talus being driven into the articular surface of the distal tibia. Comminution is often extensive, and soft-tissue injury common. These fractures are usually a result of a fall from a height or motor vehicle accidents. Fracture pattern is determined by the position of the foot at the time of impact.

The most frequently used classification scheme groups these fractures into three types based on the degree of articular and metaphyseal comminution and displacement (Fig. 6). A Type I fracture is an articular fracture without significant displacement. A Type II fracture has significant articular displacement with little comminution. Type III fractures have considerable comminution with gross incongruity of the articular surface. Several other classification schemes have been proposed. Some modifications of the one presented here and others that are much more extensive offer prognostic information. Although more specific, they are also more cumbersome to use. Generally, the prognosis for a poor result increases with the complexity of the fracture.

Because these fractures are often a result of high-energy trauma, there is a significant incidence of associated injuries. Any portion of the skeleton that is subject to axial load may be involved. It is essential to look for calcaneal, tibial plateau, pelvis, acetabular, and spinal fractures. The affected extremity must be carefully evaluated to assess the neurovascular status, swelling, and skin and soft tissue condition. Often, the soft-tissue involvement dictates the timing of any proposed treatment, especially surgical fixation. Preoperative calcaneal pin traction allows soft-tissue healing, restores some articular congruity through ligamentotaxis and prevents shortening. Radiographic studies should adequately identify

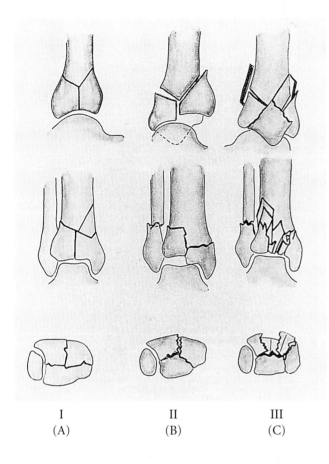

I
(A)

II
(B)

III
(C)

Figure 6

The Ruedi and Allgöwer classification of fractures of the tibial plafond. Type I fractures are minimally displaced; Types II and III show increasing articular displacement and metaphyseal comminution, respectively. (Reproduced with permission from Ruedi TP, Allgöwer M: The operative treatment of intra-articular fractures of the lower end of the tibia. *Clin Orthop* 1979;138:105–110.)

fracture patterns so that treatment may be based on a combination of clinical and radiological information. Often, plain radiographs do not adequately represent the true extent of injury, and CT must be used to delineate the extent of involvement. If surgery is contemplated, a detailed preoperative plan, including a representative drawing, should be made in order to better understand the fracture pattern and provide a template for planning of fixation.

Minimally displaced or nondisplaced pilon fractures may be amenable to closed treatment in plaster. The cast must be a well-molded, long-leg cast to control rotation and prevent displacement of the fracture. Any gap in the articular surface of more than 2 mm should be addressed, because patients with articular incongruity are more likely to develop post-traumatic arthritis. Type II and III fractures are not amenable

to simple plaster immobilization. Their displaced articular surfaces require open reduction and internal fixation, if possible. The use of large plates and screws has essentially been abandoned due to the high wound-complication rate. Combinations of limited internal and external fixation are popular, especially with the advent of the small pin fixator. Limited fixation of the tibia with bone grafting and fibular plating combined with external fixation is the preferred method of many experienced surgeons. It is imperative that the surgeon completely recognize the injury and the limitations of any technique proposed to address complex fractures. Treatment of the soft tissue begins in the emergency room and should be paramount at the time of surgery. Full-thickness incisions, atraumatic tissue handling and minimal dissection are essential to decrease wound complications. Indirect reduction methods preserve bone and limit soft-tissue stripping.

In fractures suited to open reduction and internal fixation, the initial step should be anatomic plating of the fibula through a posterolateral incision. This restores both fibular and tibial length. The posterolateral approach is used to maintain a wide skin bridge, at least 7 cm, between this and the anteromedial incision used to address the tibia. The articular surface should be reduced and preliminarily held with Kirschner wires or guide wires from an appropriately sized cannulated screw system. The bony defect is grafted as needed, and lag screws placed appropriately. Use of large buttress plates with extensive periosteal stripping is not advocated. Limited internal fixation is best neutralized by an external fixator. Closure must be tension free and may be delayed, as long as all bone is covered.

As in most musculoskeletal injuries, outcome and patient satisfaction rely primarily on the severity of the initial injury and the quality of the reduction. The orthopaedist must honestly and accurately assess his/her own expertise in these challenging fractures. Not all of these injuries can be made better with surgery. Major complications such as wound problems, infection, and loss of fixation are best avoided by limiting open treatment to properly selected plafond fractures.

Annotated Bibliography

Alioto RJ, Furia JP, Marquardt JD: Hematoma block for ankle fractures: A safe and efficacious technique for manipulations. *J Orthop Trauma* 1995;9:113–116.

Twenty-three patients undergoing closed reduction of displaced ankle fractures received a hematoma block with or without parenteral analgesics and/or sedation alone. Patients receiving the hematoma blocks related less pain at time of reduction. There were no complications.

Alpert SW, Koval KJ, Zuckerman JD: Neuropathic arthropathy: Review of current knowledge. *J Am Acad Orthop Surg* 1996;4:100–108.

The history, pathogenesis, diagnosis and treatment of neuroarthropathy is presented. The article summarizes these parameters for specific parts of the body commonly affected. Patterns of destruction in the foot and ankle are presented in addition to imaging modalities and treatment.

Baird RA, Jackson ST: Fractures of the distal part of the fibula with associated disruption of the deltoid ligament: Treatment without repair of the deltoid ligament. *J Bone Joint Surg* 1987;69A:1346–1352.

Twenty-one of 24 patients with lateral malleolus fractures and deltoid ligament tears were treated with fixation of the lateral malleolus only. At two year follow-up, 90% of these 21 patients had a good or excellent result. Patients with residual talar shift after fixation required medial arthrotomy to remove the deltoid ligament that had flipped into the joint. Those patients without deltoid repair did better than those with repair.

Belcher GL, Randomisli TE, Abate JA, Stabile LA, Trafton PG: Functional outcome analysis of operatively treated malleolar fractures. *J Orthop Trauma* 1997;11:106–109.

This retrospective review age-matched 40 patients, who 8 to 24 months previously had undergone open reduction internal fixation of closed, uncomplicated malleolar fractures, with normal patients with no history of ankle problems. The UCLA activity score and ankle score of the patients were significantly lower than that of the participants in the control group.

Boden SD, Labropoulos PA, McCowin P, Lestini WF, Hurwitz SR: Mechanical considerations for the syndesmosis screw: A cadaver study. *J Bone Joint Surg* 1989;71A:1548–1555.

This cadaver study established criteria for the use of syndesmosis fixation in simulated pronation-external rotation injuries. Based on mean widening of the syndesmosis after serially sectioning medial structures, a syndesmosis screw is not required if medial structures are intact and the fibula is anatomically reduced, or if medial disruption extends less than 3 cm above the plafond and the fibula is rigidly fixed. A syndesmosis screw is required if the syndesmosis disruption extends 4.5 cm above the plafond.

Brown TD, Hurlbut PT, Hale JE, et al: Effects of imposed hindfoot constraint on ankle contact mechanics for displaced lateral malleolar fractures. *J Orthop Trauma* 1994;8:511–519.

This cadaver study evaluated contact stress distributions on the tibial plafond with the use of pressure-sensitive film in Weber (AO) C fractures. The fibula offset progressed from 0 to 5 mm, but the increase in pressure was very modest. This work contrasts strikingly with the results presented by Ramsey and Hamilton with the authors concluding that Weber C fractures are forgiving in terms of accommodating articular incongruity.

Brumback RJ, McGarvey WC: Fractures of the tibial plafond: Evolving treatment concepts for the pilon fracture. *Orthop Clin North Am* 1995;26:273–285.

This comprehensive review summarizes the history and development of treatment strategies of pilon fractures. Operative goals and recent results support limited internal fixation with external fixation versus open plating. Complications and salvage procedures are presented.

Clohisy DR, Thompson RC Jr: Fractures associated with neuropathic arthropathy in adults who have juvenile-onset diabetes. *J Bone Joint Surg* 1988;70A:1192–1200.

This study of 18 patients, age 25 to 52 years, demonstrated a 5 week average delay in fracture diagnosis. Bilateral neuropathic arthropathy is common and prophylactic bracing of the contralateral, uninvolved extremity is recommended.

Franklin JL, Johnson KD, Hansen ST Jr: Immediate internal fixation of open ankle fractures: Report of thirty-eight cases treated with a standard protocol. *J Bone Joint Surg* 1984,66A:1349–1356.

This retrospective review of 38 cases of open ankle fractures treated with a standard protocol of emergent irrigation and debridement, rigid fixation, 48 hour antibiotic coverage and delayed primary closure at five days gave an overall excellent result in 26 cases. There were no deep infections, even in grade III injuries. Poor results were attributed to chondral damage sustained at the time of injury.

Harper MC: The short oblique fracture of the distal fibula without medial injury: An assessment of displacement. *Foot Ankle Int* 1995;16:181–186.

Eighteen patients with supination-external rotation stage II injuries were evaluated by plain films and computed tomography scan. Axial tomography confirmed the work of Michelson in which the relationship between the distal fibula and talus was undisturbed while the proximal fibula exhibited internal rotation. Occult avulsion fractures of the distal tibia were noted in 39% of cases.

Harper MC, Hardin G: Posterior malleolar fractures of the ankle associated with external rotation-abduction injuries: Results with and without internal fixation. *J Bone Joint Surg* 1988;70A:1348–1356.

Thirty-eight patients with posterior malleolus fractures comprising 25 percent or more of the articular surface underwent open reduction internal fixation of the medial and lateral malleoli. Fifteen patients had concomitant fixation of the posterior fragment while 23 did not. No posterior subluxation of the talus occurred in either group and there was no statistical difference in clinical result between these groups at 44 months follow-up.

Helfet DL, Koval K, Pappas J, Sanders RW, DiPasquale T: Intraarticular "pilon" fracture of the tibia. *Clin Orthop* 1994;298:221–228.

Thirty-four severe pilon fractures, including 18 open fractures, in 32 patients were retrospectively reviewed. Average follow-up was 16 months. Eighty-eight percent of fractures had united by 16 weeks. Poor results occurred in patients with malunion, articular incongruity and hardware failure.

Johnson EE, Davlin LB: Open ankle fractures: The indications for immediate open reduction and internal fixation. *Clin Orthop* 1993;292:118–127.

Twenty-two patients with primarily Gustillo grade II open fractures of the ankle were treated with irrigation-debridement, reduction and immediate stable internal fixation at an average of six hours from presentation. Excellent-to-good results were achieved in 87% of patients with no deep infections or nonunions.

Lantz BA, McAndrew M, Scioli M, Fitzrandolph RL: The effect of concomitant chondral injuries accompanying operatively reduced malleolar fractures. *J Orthop Trauma* 1991;5:125–128.

Sixty-three closed malleolar fractures were inspected for chondral injuries at the time of open reduction internal fixation. Forty-nine percent of patients had injuries to the talar dome. In a follow-up study of 26 patients at an average of 25 months after surgery, overall results were significantly poorer in patients with talar dome chondral injuries.

Loder RT: The influence of diabetes mellitus on the healing of closed fractures. *Clin Orthop* 1988;232:210–216.

In a review of 31 closed fractures of the lower extremity in diabetic patients, union time overall was prolonged to 163% of expected with insulin dependent patients at 157% and oral hypoglycemic-controlled patients at 176%. Non-displaced fractures healed in the normal time period while displaced fractures showed a prolonged union time.

Marsh JL, Bonar S, Nepola JV, Decoster TA, Hurwitz SR: Use of an articulated external fixator for fractures of the tibial plafond. *J Bone Joint Surg* 1995;77A:1498–1509.

This prospective study of 49 displaced fractures of the tibial plafond evaluated the results of an articulated external fixator placed medially across the joint. Forty ankles had limited internal fixation and 15 were bonegrafted. At 30-month follow-up, the ankle score averaged 67 points (range, 13 to 100 points). The theoretical advantage of early motion was not tested.

Michelson JD, Magid D, Ney DR, Fishman EK: Examination of the pathologic anatomy of ankle fractures. *J Trauma* 1992;32:65–70.

This prospective study of 26 patients with lateral malleolus fractures compared the amount of displacement seen on plain film with that demonstrated by computed tomography scan. While plain films demonstrated apparant malleolar displacement, CT images showed that the lateral fragment relationship to the talus was unchanged while the proximal fibula demonstrated internal rotation.

Miller SD: Late reconstruction after failed treatment for ankle fractures. *Orthop Clin North Am* 1995;26:363–373.

The author reviews radiographic criteria used in the evaluation of ankle fractures and the attempt to correlate them with clinical results. The article describes treatment options in malleolar malunion, syndesmosis widening, and degenerative changes.

Ovadia DN, Beals RK: Fractures of the tibial plafond. *J Bone Joint Surg* 1986;68A:543–551.

Fracture type, severity and quality of reduction were used as prognostic indicators in this retrospective study of 148 pilon fractures. Less severe fractures and those that were near anatomically reduced and rigidly stabilized did better. Complications were numerous and occurred in both patients treated both with and without internal fixation.

Phillips WA, Schwartz HS, Keller CS, et al: A prospective, randomized study of the management of severe ankle fractures. *J Bone Joint Surg* 1985;67A:67–78.

This randomized, prospective study of 138 patients with either a closed grade-4 supination external rotation or pronation external rotation ankle fracture proved anatomic open reduction with internal fixation to give

better long-term results than continued closed treatment of satisfactorily reduced fractures. Patients with a medial malleolus fracture and patients greater than 50 years old did significantly better with open reduction.

Schon LC, Marks RM: The management of neuroarthropathic fracture-dislocations in the diabetic patient. *Orthop Clin North Am* 1995;26:375–392.

The authors present an excellent, comprehensive review of the diagnosis and management of fracture-dislocations of the foot and ankle seen in diabetic patients with Charcot arthopathy. In select cases, initial aggressive management is needed to prevent or minimize the sequelae of neuroarthropathy.

Vangsness CT Jr, Carter V, Hunt T, Kerr R, Hewton E: Radiographic diagnosis of ankle fractures: Are three views necessary? *Foot Ankle Int* 1994,15:172–174.

Four attending physicians examined 123 sets of ankle radiographs. The first examination consisted of routine anterior posterior, lateral and mortise views while the second evaluation consisted of lateral and mortise views only. The overall accuracy of two views was within the 95% expected threshold of accuracy using three views.

Whitelaw GP, Sawka MW, Wetzler M, Segal D, Miller J: Unrecognized injuries of the lateral ligaments associated with lateral malleolar fractures of the ankle. *J Bone Joint Surg* 1989;71A:1396–1399.

The authors discuss the possibility of and necessity to test for anterolateral ligament injuries concomitant with lateral malleolus fractures. If ligament disruption is detected at operation, repair is indicated.

Wuest TK: Injuries to the distal lower extremity syndesmosis. *J Am Acad Orthop Surg* 1997;5:172–181.

Injuries to the tibiofibular syndesmosis are reviewed in this comprehensive article covering mechanism of injury, diagnosis, radiographic evaluation and treatment. The author's own approach to this problem is presented. Emphasis is on early recognition and obtaining and maintaining reduction.

Xenos JS, Hopkinson WJ, Mulligan ME, Olson EJ, Popovic NA: The tibiofibular syndesmosis: Evaluation of the ligamentous structures, methods of fixation, and radiographic assessment. *J Bone Joint Surg* 1995;77A:847–856.

External rotation torque was applied to 25 fresh-frozen cadaver ankles as the syndesmotic ligaments were incrementally sectioned. As expected, more extensive disruption of the syndesmosis resulted in greater instability. The stress lateral radiograph was more reliable than the stress mortise radiograph in the assessment of anatomic diastasis.

Yablon IG, Leach RE: Reconstruction of malunited fractures of the lateral malleolus. *J Bone Joint Surg* 1989;71A:521–527.

Twenty-six patients with malunion of the fibula and ankle pain at an average of six years after injury were treated with corrective osteotomy of the lateral malleolus. At an average of 7 years follow-up, 20 of 26 patients had no pain and had resumed normal activities. Two-thirds of the malunions were occult, exhibiting no talar shift but having residual shortening and external rotation deformity of the lateral malleolus.

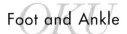

Chapter 16
Fractures of the Talus

Introduction

Treatment of fractures of the talus presents a challenge to orthopaedists because of the complex anatomy of the talus. A wide variety of injuries are encountered, most of which occur rarely. Outcomes related to these injuries are often poor because of the bone's unique function in the ankle mortise and the forces that must be transmitted across it.

General treatment principles apply to nearly all fractures of the talus. Immediate reduction of displaced fractures should be performed. Anatomic alignment of cartilaginous surfaces is paramount. Rigid internal fixation, when possible, seems to decrease postinjury complications.

Anatomy

The talus is key in the transition of forces between the foot and the leg and body. Its anatomy reflects its unique function as an intermediary, lacking either the origin or the insertion of any musculotendinous units. Seventy percent of the entire surface of the talus is covered with articular cartilage. The remaining 30% provides surface for important ligamentous attachments and the passage of blood vessels.

The talus is traditionally divided into 3 anatomic parts: head, body, and neck. The head articulates with the navicular through the talonavicular joint, and with the calcaneus through the anterior and middle facets of the subtalar joint. The body comprises the large talar surface that articulates with the tibia and fibula via the ankle joint and with the calcaneus via the posterior facet of the subtalar joint. The neck is the only part of the talus that is primarily extra-articular. It connects the head to the body in some degree of medial and plantar deviation. This inclination is variable from person to person, yet critical in maintaining normal function in all of the talar articulations.

The topographic anatomy of the body of the talus reveals several tubercles, which are often injured in talar trauma. The posterolateral and posteromedial tubercles form the sulcus for the flexor hallucis longus tendon. The posterolateral tubercle is the larger of the two, and may be associated with the os trigonum, a small accessory bone attached to it by ligaments. The lateral process of the talus and the deltoid tubercle medially are two other talar prominences that often lend themselves to injury.

Blood Supply

The blood supply to the talus enters from 6 major areas: the superior and inferior neck, the anterolateral and medial talar body, the posterior tubercle of the talus, and the deltoid ligament attachment. Many variations exist, but most would agree that the blood supply comes from 5 major vessel sources: the artery of the tarsal canal, the artery of the tarsal sinus, the superior neck vessels, the posterior tubercle vessels, and the deltoid branches of the posterior tibial artery. The volume of talus supplied by each of these arteries is variable, but is fixed in each individual such that loss of one branch cannot often be compensated for by the others, thus leading to focal areas of osteonecrosis. Figure 1 shows the intraosseous and extraosseous blood supply of the talus.

Understanding of the blood supply to the body of the talus is most critical because of the high incidence of osteonecrosis associated with talar neck injuries. The key principle is that blood flow to the body begins anteriorly at the neck and progresses posteriorly. The majority of this blood supply comes from an important anastomosis at the inferior talar neck between the artery of the tarsal canal (branch of the posterior tibial artery) and the artery of the tarsal sinus (variable contributions from the dorsalis pedis and peroneal arteries). This anastomosis functions much like the transverse arterial arches of the foot and hand, although if flow from one side is disrupted, the other side is often unable to completely fill the distribution of the injured side.

Osteonecrosis of the talar body is most dramatic, with injury to the artery of the tarsal canal. This artery is considered to be the primary arterial blood supply to the talus, providing blood flow to one half to two thirds of the talar body. Although the artery is well protected in an osseous tunnel, unfortunately, fractures of the talar neck with displacement easily lend themselves to injury of this artery.

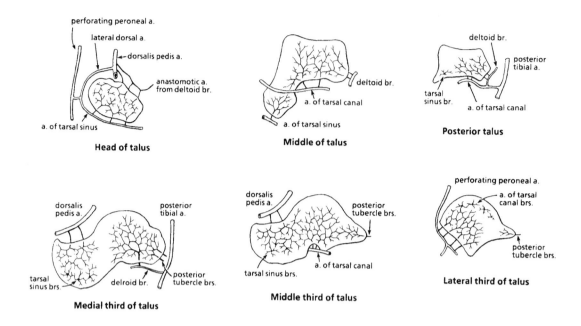

Figure 1

Extraosseous and intraosseous circulation of the talus. (Reproduced with permission from Adelaar RS: Fractures of the talus, in Greene WB (ed): *Instructional Course Lectures XXXIX*. Park Ridge, IL, American Academy of Orthopaedic Surgeons, 1990, pp 147–156.)

Fractures of the Talar Head

Fractures of the talar head comprise 5% to 10% of all talar fractures, and are believed to occur as the result of axial loading in plantarflexion or as a compression injury of the talar head against the anterior tibia in forced dorsiflexion. These

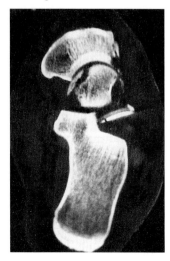

Figure 2

An osteochondral fracture of the talar head. Initial radiographs demonstrated a talar body fracture. CT scan was done to further define the fracture anatomy, when incidental note of the talar head fracture was made.

injuries are often associated with injuries to the transverse tarsal and midtarsal joints and can be associated with midfoot instability. Failure to recognize the full extent of these injuries can lead to secondary posttraumatic arthritis secondary to malalignment or chronic instability. The incidence of osteonecrosis of the talar head following these injuries is 10%. Osteochondral fractures of the talar head can also occur in subtalar dislocation, either as a direct result of the injury or iatrogenically as a result of reduction, as shown in Figure 2.

Physical examination leads to suspicion of the diagnosis. Radiographs can be helpful, but use of tomograms or computed tomography (CT) is sometimes necessary to further define fracture anatomy. Most talar head fractures are nondisplaced because of strong ligamentous attachments. Stress radiographs should be performed if clinically indicated by physical examination.

Nondisplaced fractures can be treated in a short leg nonweightbearing cast for 8 to 12 weeks. Healing should be confirmed radiographically before weightbearing is begun. Displaced fractures involving 50% of the talar head require internal fixation. Displaced fractures involving less than 50% of the talar head can be excised if no instability of the talonavicular joint can be demonstrated. Many of these fractures, despite their treatment, result in talonavicular arthritis, which may require arthrodesis.

Fractures of the Talar Neck

Mechanism of Injury
Three mechanisms reportedly lead to talar neck fractures. The most common is a dorsiflexion force to the foot that pushes the talus against the anterior lip of the tibia. The degree of injury correlates with the degree of force applied in the injury, resulting in a spectrum of injury from a nondisplaced fracture to extrusion of the body posteromedially. When the body is extruded, in many instances it remains attached only by residual fibers of the deltoid. This deltoid attachment is then its only source of remaining blood supply, and should be protected if open procedures are performed. Supination of the ankle causing impingement of the talus against the medial malleolus is a second mechanism of talar neck fractures. A direct blow to the talus is the third and most unusual mechanism of talar neck fractures.

Most talar fractures occur as a result of impact of the floorboard against the feet on the gas or brake pedal during motor vehicle accidents. Falls from a height are another common cause. Historically, these fractures were noted to occur during airplane accidents, giving rise to ther term "aviator's astragalus."

Associated Injuries
More than half of talar neck fractures are associated with other injuries; 25% are associated with malleolar fractures, with the medial malleolus most commonly involved. Fifteen percent to 20% of talar neck fractures are open injuries. Compartment syndrome of the foot must be considered because of the high-energy trauma that typically causes these injuries. Neurovascular injury is rare but careful evaluation is necessary, especially when posteromedial dislocation of the talar body is present.

Radiographic Evaluation
Because of the large number of associated injuries found with talar neck fractures, multiple radiographic views are often required to provide a thorough examination. A lateral view of the foot and ankle is perhaps most helpful in visualizing the fracture line along the talar neck. Anteroposterior (AP) and mortise views of the ankle are essential to confirm a diagnosis of associated medial malleolar fractures and to assess the position of the talus in the mortise. An AP radiograph of the foot is helpful to view the alignment of the talonavicular joint and to assess for associated talar head fractures. This view should be combined with an oblique view of the foot to exclude associated midfoot and forefoot trauma.

It is of primary importance to determine whether or not the neck fracture is displaced. Confirmation of subluxation of the subtalar joint can be difficult. Further information can be gained either by CT scan or conventional tomogram, or by a special radiographic view described by Canale (Fig. 3). The foot is placed in maximum equinus and 15° of pronation. The roentgen tube is directed cephalad at a 75° angle from the table top. This view is also helpful during surgery to determine adequacy of reduction.

CT scanning should be strongly considered in talar neck fractures, not only to assess displacement, but also to identify intra-articular loose bodies.

Classification
Talar neck fractures have been traditionally grouped into 3 types according to the Hawkins classification, which has been shown to correlate with overall prognosis of the fracture. Type I is a nondisplaced fracture of the talar neck. Type II is a neck fracture with displacement of the subtalar joint; the ankle joint is located. Type III is a fracture of the talar neck with displacement of both the subtalar and ankle joint. Canale describes a type IV talar neck fracture that has displacement at the talonavicular joint in addition to displacement of the subtalar and ankle joints. Few data exist on the overall prognosis of these fractures; however, it is most likely

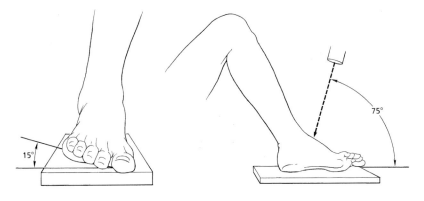

Figure 3

Talar neck view, as described by Canale. This intraoperative view helps assess the adequacy of reduction. (Reproduced with permission from Adelaar RS: Fractures of the talus, in Greene WB (ed): *Instructional Course Lectures XXXIX.* Park Ridge, IL, American Academy of Orthopaedic Surgeons, 1990, p 147–156.

poor. A recent article by Inokuchi and associates suggests that a type V category should be added for those fractures that can't be categorized into types I through IV. This category might include talar neck fractures in which the talar head was dislocated, but the subtalar and ankle joints were left intact.

Treatment

The goal of all treatment, regardless of type, should be anatomic reduction. All displaced fractures should be reduced as early as possible to minimize risk of postinjury complications.

Type I Fractures It is important to reemphasize that a type I fracture must be nondisplaced, by definition. A fracture that appears nondisplaced on radiograph should be judiciously scrutinized by CT scan or conventional tomography when possible, because small degrees of displacement will often be found with more specific testing methods. Most nondisplaced fractures are barely visible on radiographs and often are missed, particularly in the presence of a medial malleolar fracture. "Minimally" displaced talar neck fractures should be treated as type II fractures because even small degrees of displacement significantly increase the risk of malunion and posttraumatic arthritis. It is important that the patient be counseled appropriately.

Closed nondisplaced fractures without loose fragments in the subtalar joint can be treated with 8 to 12 weeks of casting. During the first 4 to 6 weeks, there should be no weightbearing, with the foot in slight plantarflexion. The cast is removed when the fracture is healed, and range of motion and strengthening exercises are begun. If radiographic evidence of osteonecrosisis is found, the period of no weightbearing would be extended past 6 weeks. This situation is found in approximately 13% of type I fractures.

Open fractures, fractures with loose fragments in the subtalar joint, and some closed fractures may require rigid internal fixation. This procedure prevents late displacement and allows for earlier range of motion, but subjects the patient to the risk of iatrogenic complications. Good clinical judgment is necessary in each case. Posterior-to-anterior screw fixation is the preferred form of internal fixation for this type of fracture.

Type II Fractures Displaced fractures of the talar neck are an orthopaedic emergency and require immediate reduction. Many surgeons advocate an attempt at closed reduction to determine if anatomic reduction can be achieved; others favor open reduction and internal fixation for all type II fractures.

If closed reduction is attempted, adequate anesthesia is given first. The foot is then pulled into plantarflexion, thus aligning the head with the body. Varus or valgus malalign-

ment is then corrected. Sometimes, pushing backward on a markedly plantarflexed foot while pulling forward on the tibia is helpful in difficult reductions. Repeated attempts at closed reduction are not advised. If the reduction if believed to be anatomic, the foot can be splinted in plantarflexion. Sometimes a pronounced degree of plantarflexion is required to maintain reduction, making internal fixation a better option because it allows the foot to be splinted in a neutral position.

Traditionally, an acceptable closed reduction was believed to be less than 5° of varus malalignment and 5 mm of displacement. Current views on this matter suggest that only anatomic alignment is an acceptable endpoint with closed reduction. It has also been suggested that 2 mm of displacement might be an intermediate position to these two viewpoints.

Open reduction, whether done initially or following closed reduction, should be performed in such a way that adequate visualization of the fracture is achieved without compromising the remaining blood supply to the talus. Exposure of the talar neck can be approached from either the medial or lateral side, or both, if necessary, to achieve anatomic reduction. The medial approach is generally preferred because it allows for fixation of the medial malleolus, if necessary, or osteotomy of the medial malleolus for better fracture exposure if required. Great care must be taken not to disrupt the deltoid ligament if the medial approach is selected, so as to preserve its blood supply to the talus. Screw fixation can be done either from anterior to posterior, or posterior to anterior, although it has been established that posterior-to-anterior fixation can achieve significantly better biomechanical fixation. Two 4.0-mm cancellous screws or one 6.5-mm cancellous screw are usually used for internal fixation.

Direct reduction of displaced talar neck fractures has also been described using an arthroscopically assisted method. The arthroscope allows for direct visualization of the fracture for reduction and for removal of loose fragments from the ankle and subtalar joint, while minimizing disruption of blood supply. Definitive fixation of the fracture can then be done from an anterior or posterior approach.

Postoperative treatment involves casting with the ankle at neutral. Early range of motion of the ankle and subtalar joint can be begun once the wound is stable, contingent on the patient's ability to manage such a routine. The patient remains nonweightbearing for at least 6 weeks. The decision to begin weightbearing is dependent on evidence of healing and the absence of evidence of osteonecrosis. Tomograms are often required to determine the progress of fracture healing.

Type III Fractures Type III talar neck fractures are rarely reducible by closed reduction techniques. Nonetheless, closed reduction may be indicated in some circumstances, particularly when there is neurovascular compromise or when the skin is severely tented, thus placing it at risk for delayed breakdown. The majority of these fractures require surgical treatment. The goals are the same as in type II fractures: anatomic reduction and rigid internal fixation, while preserving maximal blood flow. Over 50% of these fractures will be open, and strict adherence to the general principles of open fracture management should be followed. An example of a type III talar neck fracture and its subsequent reduction is shown in Figure 4.

If the body fragment is contaminated and stripped of its blood supply, treatment options can be a source of controversy. One option is that the body can be cleaned and replaced. If postoperative complications such as infection, nonunion, or osteonecrosis develop, the body can be removed later and tibiocalcaneal fusion or Blair fusion can be performed. Another option is to remove the fragment and allow wounds to heal; then perform early arthrodesis.

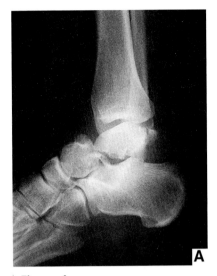
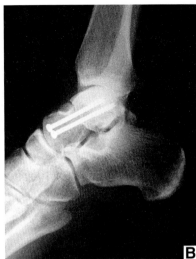

Figure 4

A, A Hawkins type III talar neck fracture, with dislocation of both the subtalar and ankle joints. **B,** The type III fracture after open reduction and internal fixation.

Prognosis and Complications

The prognosis for any talar fracture is guarded because of the potential for a variety of complex postinjury complications. Even type I fractures reportedly have an unsatisfactory outcome in 40% to 50% of cases.

Osteonecrosis Osteonecrosis is perhaps the best known postinjury complication in talar neck fractures. The incidence is correlated with the degree of displacement created by the injury. The Hawkins classification has some predictive value in assessing the risk of osteonecrosis. Type I fractures have been reported to have an incidence of up to 13%, type II fractures of 20% to 50%, and type III fractures of 50% to 100%. Type IV fractures occur so rarely that precise data are difficult to obtain; however, Canale has reported that fracture incidence is as high as 50%. With type IV fractures, it is important to recognize that osteonecrosis can occur in both the talar body and head. Recent studies report less incidence of osteonecrosis with immediate reduction and placement of rigid internal fixation.

Osteonecrosis can often be excluded at 6 to 8 weeks postin-

jury if the Hawkins sign is seen on routine radiographs. This sign is characterized by a thin rim of decreased radiodensity in the bone just under the cartilage of the talar dome, and is best seen on routine AP or mortise views of the ankle. The lack of a Hawkins sign does not confirm the presence of osteonecrosis, which otherwise may not be confirmed on plain radiographs until up to 3 months after the injury, when a clear increase in radiodensity in the body of the talus relative to the head of the talus can be seen, as shown in Figure 5. Technetium bone scanning has not been found to be a useful test in earlier diagnosis of osteonecrosis; magnetic resonance imaging (MRI) can be useful if titanium rather than stainless steel alloy screws are used.

The presence of osteonecrosis does not necessarily dictate a poor result. Osteonecrosis may increase the risk of delayed union, but it does not increase the risk of nonunion. In addition, only a small group of patients who develop osteonecrosis develop late segmental collapse; even so, many of these patients are still found to have a good functional result. Thus, the decision about when to begin weightbearing in a fracture with documented osteonecrosis remains controversial. Because complete revascularization can require 3 to 5 years, it can be argued that restricting weightbearing throughout this length of time is unreasonable. It also can be said that any degree of collapse could potentially lead to posttraumatic arthritis, and that some degree of protection is required until revascularization is complete.

In a recent study by Thordarson and associates, MRI was used to establish criteria for allowing a patient to begin

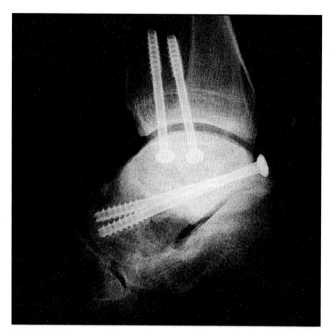

Figure 5

Radiograph of well-established osteonecrosis of the talar body. Note the sclerosis of the talar body relative to the talar head and neck.

Table 1

Classification of magnetic resonance signal changes in the body of the talus following fracture of the neck of the talus

Scan Type	Findings
Type A	Homogeneous bone throughout the body of the talus
Type B	Signal changes in up to 25% of the body of the talus
Type C	Signal changes in up to 25% to 50% of the body of the talus
Type D	Signal changes in more than 50% of the body of the talus

(Reproduced with permission from Thordarson DB, Triffon MJ, Terk MR: Magnetic resonance imaging to detect avascular necrosis after open reduction and internal fixation of talar neck fractures. *Foot Ankle Int* 1996;17:742–747.)

weightbearing. This study suggests that all type I and II fractures should be allowed protective weightbearing when radiographic evidence of healing at the fracture is present, because none of these patients in this study went on to develop late segmental collapse. It was recommended that in patients with type III fractures, MRI scans be done at 8 to 12 weeks postinjury to assess for osteonecrosis. The degree of osteonecrosis is then classified based on the percent of talar body affected by osteonecrosis, as shown in Table 1. In the protocol, all type A and B fractures are allowed to bear weight after fracture healing is complete because of a very low incidence of collapse. Type C fractures are kept nonweightbearing and the scan is repeated 6 to 12 months postinjury. If no progression of signal changes is noted, protected weightbearing is then allowed. Type D fractures are to remain nonweightbearing until radiographs are normal because of the higher risk of late collapse. Unfortunately, large outcome studies on this topic do not yet exist.

When osteonecrosis results in painful, late segmental collapse, surgical intervention often becomes necessary. Standard arthrodesis techniques of the hindfoot will rarely be successful because of the lack of blood supply to the body of the talus. Talectomy is a treatment option, but often results in residual pain, a short limb, and a deformed foot that is difficult to fit with a shoe. Standard tibiocalcaneal fusion can be accomplished, but this procedure also leads to a stiff ankle and foot with significant leg length discrepancy. Vascularized fibular strut grafts and Ilizarov techniques are two modified techniques of tibiocalcaneal fusion that minimize leg-length discrepancy. The Ilizarov technique is shown in Figure 6. Finally, a Blair fusion has become a popular method of salvage that maintains improved leg length, and maintains some degree of flexion and extension of the foot on the leg. This technique is shown and described in Figure 7. Modifications of the Blair fusion technique have also been described by Morris and associates, with the addition of a long pin from the plantar aspect of the foot up into the tibia to increase fixation, and by Lionberger and associates, with the use of a long lag screw from the posterior tibia into the talar neck and head and no anterior sliding graft.

Traumatic Arthritis

This is the most common postinjury complication of talar neck fractures, occurring in the subtalar joint in approximately one half of talar neck fractures, in the ankle joint in one third of talar neck fractures, and in both the subtalar and ankle joints in one fourth of talar neck fractures. It is important to remember that this complication can be generated not only by cartilage injury, fracture, and osteonecrosis, but by joint ankylosis following prolonged immobilization. It is believed that subtalar motion is the best indicator of clinical outcome, and efforts to begin early range of motion after rigid internal fixation may decrease the incidence of traumatic arthritis.

Initial treatment should be nonsurgical, with emphasis on activity modification, anti-inflammatory medication, and bracing where necessary. Subtalar arthritis can be braced with a molded hindfoot stabilizing brace, such as a UCBL type brace, whereas tibiotalar arthritis can be treated in a molded ankle foot orthosis (AFO) brace. Failed nonsurgical treatment may require tibiotalar, subtalar, or tibiocalcaneal (talo calcaneal) fusion. Selective anesthetic injection of either joint may be helpful preoperatively to ensure that the proper joint or joints are being fused.

Malunion

The surgeon has a direct role in minimizing malunion. As stated earlier, the goal of initial reduction and treatment must be nothing less than anatomic reduction. Failure to obtain this goal can increase significantly the risk of posttraumatic arthritis. In addition, dorsal displacement can limit ankle dorsiflexion.

Wound Complications and Infection

Skin overlying the talus can be compromised following dislocation, and immediate reduction is preferable in order to prevent a delayed slough. If sloughing occurs, timely debridement followed by local or flap coverage is necessary. Wounds from open fractures should be treated by standard open fracture algorithms with immediate debridement, prophylactic antibiotics, and delayed closure.

Infection in viable bone can be treated by standard methods with intravenous antibiotics, with or without debridement. Infection of osteonecrotic bone creates a difficult situation, and a sequestrum in the talar body can require excision. A tibiocalcaneal or Blair fusion may be necessary.

Delayed Union and Nonunion

Delayed union, defined as incomplete union 6 months after injury, occurs approximately 10% of the time. Nonunion is exceedingly rare and is defined by incomplete healing at 12 months postinjury. Nonunions will require a keyed corticocancellous bone graft with rigid internal fixation. Initial rigid internal fixation can lower the incidence of these postinjury complications.

Fractures of the Talar Body

Fractures of the body of the talus account for 13% to 23% of all talar fractures. Like talar neck fractures, these fractures are

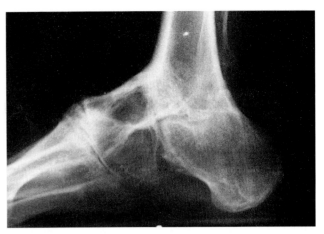

Figure 6
Radiographic example of tibiocalcaneal fusion accomplished by the Ilizarov technique.

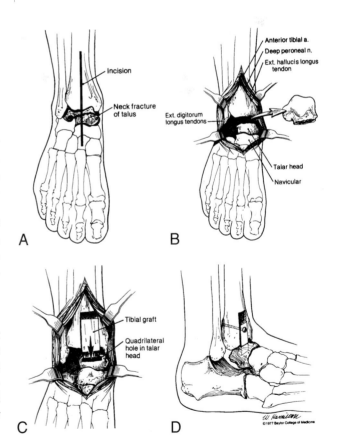

Figure 7
The Blair arthrodesis. **A,** The approach. **B,** Excision of the talar body. **C and D,** The sliding bone graft. (Reproduced with permission from Dennis MD, Tullos HS: The Blair tibiotalar arthrodesis for injuries to the talus. *J Bone Joint Surg* 1980;62A:104; Fig. D ©Baylor College of Medicine).)

associated with a high incidence of postinjury complications, and similar treatment principles apply.

In general, a talar body fracture has traditionally been distinguished from a talar neck fracture as being any fracture that involves the superior articular cartilage. Inokuchi and associates have suggested that the distinction between these fractures be made based on the exit site of the fracture on the inferior talar surface, as viewed on a lateral radiograph, rather than on the superior aspect of the fracture line, as previously believed. Neck fractures will exit through the tarsal sinus and body fractures will exit through the posterior facet of the subtalar joint, as shown in Figure 8. This distinction can be important in guiding the treatment and prognosis of these two independent fracture types.

There is no universally accepted classification system for talar body fractures that seems to correlate with outcome. Rather, body fractures seem to be grouped by recognizable fracture patterns. Fractures can be described as being vertical (sagittal or coronal) or horizontal (axial), as shown in Figure 9. There are also smaller body fractures that are described by their anatomic location, such as fractures of the lateral process of the talus, fractures of the posterior tubercle of the talus, and osteochondral fractures.

The mechanism of injury is the same in talar body fractures as in talar neck fractures, as is their clinical and radiographic evaluation. A complete set of ankle and foot radiographs is required for thorough evaluation of talar body fractures; CT scanning, shown in Figure 10, is a useful adjunct in talar body fractures to assist in selecting the proper treatment plan.

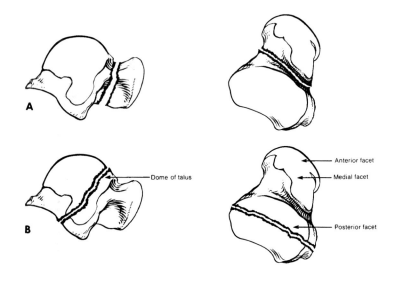

Figure 8

Distinction between talar body and talar neck fractures. **A,** This fracture exits inferiorly at the junction between the middle and posterior subtalar facets, making it a talar neck fracture. **B,** This fracture of the talar body exits inferiorly into the posterior subtalar joint. (Reproduced with permission from DeLee JC: Fractures and dislocations of the foot, in Mann RA, Coughlin MJ (eds): *Surgery of the Foot and Ankle,* ed 6. St. Louis, MO, CV Mosby, 1993, p 1551.)

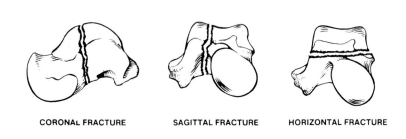

CORONAL FRACTURE   SAGITTAL FRACTURE   HORIZONTAL FRACTURE

Figure 9

Coronal, sagittal, and horizontal fracture planes in talar body fractures. (Reproduced with permission from DeLee JC: Fractures and dislocations of the foot, in Mann RA, Coughlin MJ (eds): *Surgery of the Foot and Ankle,* ed 6. St. Louis, MO, CV Mosby, 1993, p 1578.)

Subtalar dislocations, either recognized or occult, can cause talar body fractures that are often unrecognized if the subtalar dislocation is reduced. CT scanning is now recommended after subtalar dislocation to rule out associated intra-articular fractures.

Treatment principles of talar body fractures are also similar to those of talar neck fractures. Nondisplaced fractures can be treated with cast immobilization, and surgery is not general-

ly recommended. Internal fixation of nondisplaced fractures can allow early range of motion, but subjects the patient to iatrogenic risks. Displaced fractures can undergo a gentle attempt at closed reduction, but anatomic reduction is again the goal, and open reduction with rigid internal fixation is the norm. Lateral or medial malleolar osteotomy is sometimes required for exposure. Nonweightbearing is continued until union is documented.

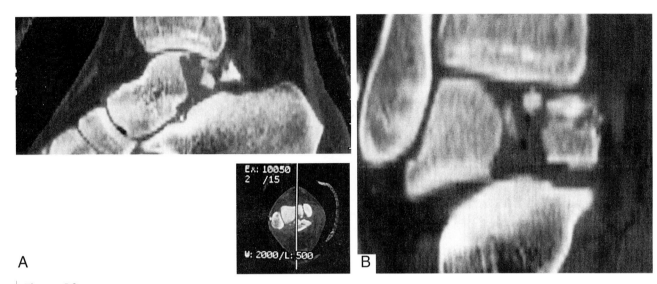

Figure 10

CT scanning with reconstruction. **A,** Coronal talar body fracture, **B,** Sagittal talar body fracture.

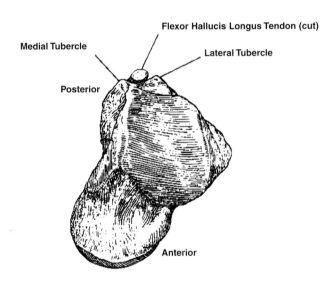

Figure 11

Anatomy of the posterior aspect of the talus. The flexor hallucis longus tendon rests in the groove between the medial and lateral tubercles of the posterior process of the talus. (Reproduced with permission from Ebraheim NA, Padanilam TG, Wong FY: Posteromedial process fractures of the talus. *Foot Ankle Int* 1995;16:734.)

Postinjury complications are similar, but generally worse for talar body fractures than for talar neck fractures. The risk of osteonecrosis is 25% to 50%, but tends to be higher in fractures associated with dislocation. Posttraumatic arthritis in either the ankle and/or subtalar joint is common, and arthrodesis treatment options are similar to those used for talar neck fractures.

Fractures of the Posterior Process of the Talus

The posterior process of the talus is comprised of 2 tubercles: posteromedial and posterolateral. Between them lies a groove in which the flexor hallucis longus resides, as shown in Figure 11. Both tubercles can be fractured, either simultaneously or individually; however, fractures of the posterolateral tubercle are the most common. These fractures can often be missed because they are difficult to image radiographically, and because of their similar radiographic appearance to the os trigonum. Technetium bone scanning is often useful in differentiating an acute fracture from an os trigonum if the distinction cannot be made by plain radiographs and physical examination.

Fractures of the posterolateral process of the talus have also been known as Shepherd's fractures. Two mechanisms are likely to create these fractures: avulsion of the lateral tubercle by the posterior talofibular ligament with excessive ankle dorsiflexion and/or inversion, and compression of the lateral tubercle between the posterior tibia and the talus. Physical examination reveals pain and swelling of the posterior ankle joint. Flexion and extension of the great toe will also create ankle pain in acute fractures of the posterolateral tubercle. Treatment of these fractures consists of a short leg nonweightbearing cast for 4 weeks, followed by a walking cast for 2 weeks. Continued tenderness can be treated by an additional 6 weeks of a weightbearing cast. It is recommended that patients with continued tenderness 6 months after injury undergo excision of the posterior fragment. Bone scanning should be considered prior to excision to verify the diagnosis. Injection of lidocaine into the area can also be useful in confirming the diagnosis.

Fractures of the posteromedial process of the talus have also been termed Cedell's fracture. This fracture is believed to be caused by an avulsion of the posterior talotibial ligament, which arises from the dorsal and distal parts of the medial malleolus. These fractures are also very difficult to image on plain radiographs and are often associated with talar dislocations, and a high index of suspicion is often necessary to identify this injury in a patient with medial talar tenderness after dislocation. CT scanning is recommended for better evaluation of the fracture fragments. Treatment of nondisplaced fractures or fractures without significant subtalar involvement can be 6 to 8 weeks in a short leg nonweightbearing cast. Excision is recommended for symptomatic nonunions of these fractures. Open reduction and internal fixation, although technically somewhat difficult, is recommended for fractures with significant subtalar joint involvement. Surgery can be performed through a posteromedial approach.

Fractures of the entire posterior process of the talus have only been reported in rare cases. They are believed to occur in plantarflexion with an inversion force applied to the subtalar joint. If the foot is not plantarflexed at the time an inversion force is applied, a simple medial subtalar dislocation would occur. Open reduction and internal fixation has generally been applied to the few fractures reported in case reports since articular surface is involved. Early range of motion is important to a good result.

Fractures of the Lateral Process of the Talus

Fractures of the lateral process of the talus are common and often missed on initial diagnosis. Physical examination often mimics that of lateral ankle sprains, with lateral tenderness and ecchymosis. Careful inspection of the talus on initial radiographs is necessary to increase the chance of making the diagnosis. Routine AP, mortise, and lateral views are often adequate, but extra detail can be obtained with a modified AP view, placing the foot in 30° of plantarflexion and 45° of internal rotation. A CT scan is often required to further define the fracture and the associated displacement. This fracture is currently known as "snowboarder's ankle," as a result of an increased incidence of this fracture since snowboarding has become a popular sport. This sport is per-

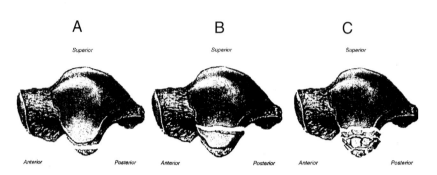

Figure 12

Hawkins classification of fractures of the lateral process of the talus: **A,** Type 1: avulsion. **B,** Type 2: large fragment fracture. **C,** Type 3: comminuted. (Reproduced with permission from McCrory P, Bladin C: Fractures of the lateral process of the talus: A clinical review. "Snowboarder's ankle". *Clin J Sport Med* 1996;6:126.)

formed in a soft-shell boot that is not rigid enough to prevent many ankle injuries.

Fractures of the lateral process of the talus are divided into 3 types, as described by Hawkins: a simple fracture line from the talofibular joint down to the subtalar joint; a comminuted fracture of the entire lateral process; and a "chip" fracture

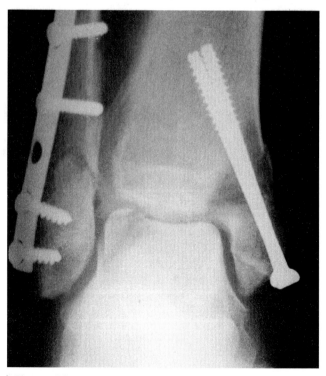

Figure 13

A missed osteochondral fracture of the lateral talar dome that was treated with open reduction and internal fixation. The talar dome lesion was not recognized until postoperative radiographs were renewed following completion of the case.

off the anterior portion of the lateral process, involving a tiny portion of the posterior facet of the subtalar joint. These 3 patterns are shown in Figure 12.

Successful treatment of this fracture is aided by early diagnosis and treatment. Nondisplaced fractures, as confirmed by plain radiographs or tomography, can be treated in a short leg nonweightbearing cast for 4 weeks, followed by 2 weeks in a walking cast. Displaced fractures require either open reduction and internal fixation or excision of the fragment. Open reduction is best performed with rigid fixation such as a 4.0-mm cancellous screw or a Herbert screw. The patient may be placed in a removable splint 2 weeks after surgery, allowing for early range of motion. The patient should not bear weight for 6 weeks, or until there is radiographic evidence of union. Missed fractures are generally not reducible after 12 weeks and immediate excision of the fragment with early range of

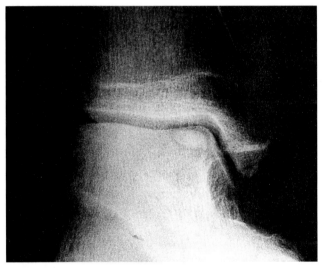

Figure 14
Radiographic appearance of a chronic osteochondral lesion of the medial talar dome.

motion is recommended. The patient may bear weight 3 weeks after excision.

Osteochondral Fractures of the Talar Dome

Osteochondral fractures are fairly common injuries because of their close association with ankle sprains. Osteochondral fractures can occur at any cartilaginous area of the talus, but are most commonly seen in the superior talar dome. Medial and lateral talar dome lesions occur with near-equal frequency. Many of these injuries are missed on initial exami-

nation because of the difficulty of identifying cartilaginous injuries on plain radiographs. Others are overlooked when they occur in conjunction with other major fractures because they are often small in size compared to the other fractures present (Fig. 13).

Many terms have been used to describe osteochondral lesions of bone. Most of the recent literature describes acute injuries as osteochondral fractures and chronic injuries as osteochondritis dissecans.

The etiology of these lesions has also been controversial. Some were believed to represent areas of spontaneous osteonecrosis whereas others were thought to be secondary to trauma. Current literature supports the theory that all of these lesions are traumatic, resulting from inversion sprains. Medial lesions, such as the one shown in Figure 14, result from inversion sprains in plantarflexion, whereas lateral lesions occur following inversion sprains in dorsiflexion. Because 6.5% of all ankle sprains result in osteochondral fractures, it is important to thoroughly evaluate the patient with a history of inversion sprain to the ankle with AP, mortise, and lateral radiographs.

Osteochondral fractures are traditionally described by the classification of Bernt and Hardy, which is based on the appearance of the lesion on plain radiograph. Stage 1 lesions involve a small area of compressed subchondral bone, without loosening of fragment. Stage 2 lesions demonstrate a partially detached fragment. Stage 3 lesions demonstrate a completely detached fragment that is nondisplaced. Stage 4 lesions are completely detached and displaced.

Radiographic evaluation of osteochondral injuries begins with plain radiographs. A CT scan would then be the next test of choice to more precisely define the nature of the lesion. MRI has also been helpful in identifying osteochondral injuries, particularly when they have not been identified by plain radiograph. Staging of lesions is more accurate with MRI than CT; more information is given about the interface between the fragment and the talus. Technetium bone scanning is a helpful test in identifying osteochondral injury in the patient who has continued ankle pain despite negative ankle radiographs.

Nonsurgical management is indicated in some types of acute osteochondral fractures. Stage 1 and 2 lateral lesions and stage 1, 2, and 3 medial lesions can be treated with a short leg nonweightbearing cast for 6 weeks. Casting may be continued up to 12 weeks if incomplete healing is seen on plain radiograph after 6 weeks of casting. If the patient remains symptomatic 4 to 6 months after the injury, surgical management may be necessary.

Surgical treatment is indicated in a variety of osteochondral injuries. In acute injuries, it is indicated for stage 3 lateral lesions and all stage 4 lesions, in addition to all acute lesions on which nonsurgical management has failed. Surgical treatment is also required in the majority of chronic lesions.

Surgical treatment can be performed either arthroscopically or by open ankle arthrotomy, with or without malleolar osteotomy. In either case, excision of the fragment and drilling of the base is required. Fixation of the osteochondral fragment can sometimes be performed with a countersunk AO cancellous screw, a Herbert screw, or absorbable pins. Osteochondral fractures involving greater than one third of the cartilaginous surface should be secured by internal fixation when at all possible. Bone grafting of some large lesions may also be necessary.

The prognosis of these fractures is fair to good. Post-traumatic arthritis is the most common complication. Decreased range of motion can also occur. Radiographic findings do not correlate with the degree of the patient's symptoms. Symptomatic improvement is often seen for up to 12 to 24 months after surgery.

Stress Fractures of the Talus

Recent literature has focused on the existence of stress fractures in the talus, which have been reported to occur in the talar neck, talar body, and even in the lateral process. Most have been described as the result of increased running, dancing, or military training. Stress fractures of the talar neck and body have been noted to occur in association with a planovalgus foot and calcaneonavicular coalition. Stress fractures of the lateral process of the talus have also been associated with a supinated foot in running injuries. Some fractures of the talus will occur simultaneously with stress fractures elsewhere.

Many of these injuries are associated with prolonged morbidity because of a delay in diagnosis. Stress fractures should be suspected in any athlete with chronic foot and ankle pain associated with decreased subtalar motion. Technetium 99 bone scanning is helpful in confirming the diagnosis. CT scan and MRI may also be of some benefit in early detection of stress fractures.

Decreased activity and time away from the sport will allow healing of some fractures, but other stress fractures, especially those of the talar neck, require a period of short leg casting to allow for healing. The prognosis for these fractures is generally poor, although early diagnosis may help to improve prognosis in future patients.

Annotated Bibliography

Talar Neck and Body Fractures

Baumhauer JF, Alvarez RG: Controversies in treating talus fractures. Orthop Clin North Am 1995;17:164–169.

This article is a concise review of the treatment of talar head, neck, and body fractures, and osteochondral fractures.

Bohay DR, Manoli A II: Occult fractures following subtalar joint injuries. Foot Ankle Int 1996;17:164–169.

This article suggests that CT scan should be done for all subtalar dislocations, whether known or suspected, because associated talar body fractures can be missed that will affect prognosis.

Ebraheim NA, Mekhail AO, Salpietro BJ, Mermer MJ, Jackson WT: Talar neck fractures: Anatomic considerations for posterior screw application. Foot Ankle Int 1996;17:541–547.

This article describes a cadaver and dry bone study examining the anatomic hazards of posterior screw placement in talar neck fractures. The study suggests that a single screw should be placed directly through the lateral tubercle of the posterior process of the calcaneus. A K-wire may be placed for rotational stabilization. The screw should be countersunk.

Frawley PA, Hart JA, Young DA: Treatment outcome of major fractures of the talus. Foot Ankle Int 1995;16:339–345.

The Szyszkowitz classification of talus fractures, combining talar body and neck fractures, is discussed and the principles of effective management of talus fractures emphasized. A wide variety of types of talus fractures and retrospective follow up are also discussed.

Inokuchi S, Ogawa K, Usami N: Classification of fractures of the talus: Clear differentiation between neck and body fractures. Foot Ankle Int 1996;17:748–750.

Redefinition of the distinction between talar neck and talar body fractures is presented. The distinction should be made by the fracture's location on the inferior rather than superior aspect of the talus.

Inokuchi S, Ogawa K, Usami N, Hashimoto T: Long-term follow up of talus fractures. Orthopedics 1996;19:477–481.

Retrospective analysis of 86 talar fractures is included. The paper describes a "type V" category for talar neck fractures to be used in conjunction with the old Hawkins-Canale classification system.

Khazim R, Salo PT: Talar neck fracture with talar head dislocation and intact ankle and subtalar joints: A case report. Foot Ankle Int 1995;16:44–48.

This article presents the second known description of a fracture not included in the standard Hawkins' classification system of talar neck fractures.

Marsh JL, Saltzman CL, Iverson M, Shapiro DS: Major open injuries of the talus. *J Orthop Trauma* 1995;9:371–376.

A retrospective analysis of 18 open talar fractures is presented, along with outcomes data. The study encourages early excision of extruded talar bodies to prevent subsequent infection.

Saltzman CL, Marsh JL, Tearse DS: Treatment of displaced talus fractures: An arthroscopically assisted approach. *Foot Ankle Int* 1994;15:630–633.

The surgical technique for a combined arthroscopic reduction of the talar neck fracture and limited open internal fixation is described.

Thordarson DB, Triffon MJ, Terk MR: Magnetic resonance imaging to detect avascular necrosis after open reduction and internal fixation of talar neck fractures. *Foot Ankle Int* 1996; 17:742–747.

Twenty-one patients with talar neck fractures are prospectively reviewed. An algorithm of treatment is suggested to manage the onset of weightbearing in these injuries based on magnetic resonance imaging findings.

Ankle and Tibiocalcaneal Arthrodesis

Mann RA, Chou LB: Tibiocalcaneal arthrodesis. *Foot Ankle Int* 1995;16:401–405.

The technique and outcome of direct tibiocalcaneal arthrodesis is reviewed.

Fractures of the Posterior Process of the Talus

Chen YJ, Hsu RW, Shih HN, Huang TJ: Fracture of the entire posterior process of talus associated with subtalar dislocation: A case report. *Foot Ankle Int* 1996;17:226–229.

A single case of a fracture of the entire posterior process of the talus treated with internal fixation using a miniscrew is presented.

Ebraheim NA, Padanilam TG, Wong FY: Posteromedial process fractures of the talus. *Foot Ankle Int* 1995;16:734–739.

General principles about the diagnosis and management of this rare injury are presented.

Kanbe K, Kubota H, Hasegawa A, Udagawa E: Fracture of the posterior medial tubercle of the talus treated by internal fixation: A report of two cases. *Foot Ankle Int* 1995;16:164–166.

This article discusses open reduction and internal fixation of isolated fractures of the medial tubercle of the posterior process of the talus. Good outcome is reported in two fractures.

Kim DH, Hrutkay JM, Samson MM: Fracture of the medial tubercle of the posterior process of the talus: A case report and literature review. *Foot Ankle Int* 1996;17:186–188.

Successful nonsurgical treatment of a single fracture of the medial tubercle of the posterior process of the talus is described.

Fractures of the Lateral Process of the Talus

McCrory P, Bladin C: Fractures of the lateral process of the talus: A clinical review. "Snowboarder's ankle". *Clin J Sport Med* 1996;6:124–128.

A thorough review of fractures of the lateral process is presented and its relationship to snowboarding injuries is reviewed. Recommendations for diagnosis and management are made.

Stress Fractures of the Talus

Bradshaw C, Khan K, Brukner P: Stress fracture of the body of the talus in athletes demonstrated with computer tomography. *Clin J Sport Med* 1996;6:48–51.

This article describes 4 case reports of stress fractures of the talar body. Empiric treatment of these patients is discussed.

Motto SG: Stress fracture of the lateral process of the talus: A case report. *Br J Sports Med* 1993;27:275–276.

A case report of stress fractures of the lateral process of the talus, resulting in prolonged disability is presented.

Umans H, Pavlov H: Insufficiency fracture of the talus: Diagnosis with MR imaging. *Radiology* 1995;197:439–442.

This article describes the appearance of several stress fractures of the talus or magnetic resonance imaging scans and provides a review of earlier reported cases.

Classic Bibliography

Berndt AL, Harty M: Transchondral fractures (osteochondritis dissecans) of the talus. *J Bone Joint Surg* 1959;41A:988–1020.

Canale ST, Kelly FB Jr: Fractures of the neck of the talus. *J Bone Joint Surg* 1978;60A:143–156.

Dennis MD, Tullos HS: Blair tibiotalar arthrodesis for injuries to the talus. *J Bone Joint Surg* 1980;62A:103–107.

Johnson EE, Weltmer J, Lian GJ, Cracchiolo A III: Ilizarov ankle arthrodesis. *Clin Orthop* 1992;280:160–169.

Lionberger DR, Bishop JO, Tullos HS: The modified Blair fusion. *Foot Ankle* 1982;3:60–62.

Morris HD, Hand WL, Dunn AW: The modified Blair fusion for fractures of the talus. *J Bone Joint Surg* 1971;53A:1289–1297.

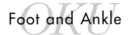
Chapter 17
Calcaneal Fractures

Introduction

The calcaneus is the most frequently fractured tarsal bone, accounting for 60% of all tarsal fractures. Approximately 75% are intra-articular, and occur because of an axial load. These fractures tend to be the result of high-energy injuries, frequently accompanied by associated pathology. Approximately 10% of patients have a fracture of the spine, 25% have extremity injuries, 10% are bilateral, and less than 5% are open. The majority of these fractures occur as a result of a fall from a height, usually in males 35 to 45 years of age, and are usually work-related. The intra-articular fractures frequently lead to long-term disability, with severe economic impact on the patient. Because of complex bony architecture and the frequently compromised soft-tissue envelope, open reduction and internal fixation remains a challenging and potentially complicated treatment option for displaced intra-articular fractures.

Although usually the result of an axial load from a fall, calcaneal fractures occasionally can occur secondary to an avulsion injury. A forceful contraction of the gastrocnemius-soleus complex is one type of avulsion injury involving the posterior calcaneal tuberosity. It can be either extra-articular or intra-articular with minimal joint surface damage and carries a better prognosis than fractures resulting from an axial load. Another avulsion injury can occur with an inversion injury of the ankle, which leads to an anterior process fracture.

Historically, the treatment of displaced intra-articular fractures has varied from nonsurgical treatment with or without reduction to open reduction and internal fixation via various means or primary arthrodesis. The impetus for nonsurgical treatment has been related to the onset of devastating wound complications and osteomyelitis in some patients. Recently, with improved exposure and surgical techniques, surgical treatment is now favored. A prospective randomized trial recently demonstrated superior results with surgical treatment of these fractures. This chapter will outline the mechanism of injury, radiographic evaluation and classification systems, and treatment for these fractures.

Mechanism of Injury

Two main mechanisms exist for the creation of calcaneus fractures: axial loading and avulsion injuries. Axial loading is the mechanism by which displaced intra-articular fractures occur and also carries the most serious prognosis. The majority of these fractures are caused by high-energy injuries that occur during a fall from a height. Axial loading can also occur occasionally when the foot makes contact with the floorboard of a motor vehicle during an accident. The posterior tuberosity of the calcaneus lies just lateral to the mechanical axis of the tibia and talus; thus, with an axial load, there tends to be an oblique shearing force that occurs through the calcaneus. This "primary" fracture line generally courses from the inferomedial wall of the calcaneus through a variable portion of the posterior facet in an anterolateral direction. The primary fracture line frequently enters the anterior process of the calcaneus. Recent reports have emphasized the importance of the anterior calcaneus fracture anatomy, with many of the fractures actually entering the calcaneocuboid joint.

A secondary fracture line also occurs in these fractures and can be classified as joint depression-type or tongue-type. In a joint depression-type fracture, the secondary fracture line extends from the primary fracture line and exits posteriorly along the dorsal aspect of the posterior tuberosity. The lateral joint fragment or fragments are impacted into the body of the calcaneus. In a tongue-type fracture, the lateral articular portion of the fracture has a secondary fracture that extends to the posterior aspect of the posterior tuberosity, and this entire fragment rotates into the body of the calcaneus. In both instances, there is generally a bulge of the lateral wall of the calcaneus as impacted bone displaces laterally as the heel shortens and widens. The lateral, displaced portion of the posterior facet frequently is found within the lateral wall. The widened calcaneus frequently leads to calcaneofibular abutment, peroneal tendon impingement, or, in extreme cases, sural nerve irritation.

Another mechanism of injury producing calcaneus fractures is avulsion injuries. An avulsion injury of the posterior tuberosity of the calcaneus, which can be an intra- or extra-articular fracture, can occur during a strong contraction of the gastrocnemius-soleus complex through the Achilles tendon, usually with a concurrent axial load, which causes an eccentric contraction of the muscle. The posterior tuberosity fracture is displaced proximally and, almost invariably, creates skin tension, necessitating immediate surgical fixation. Another avulsion injury of the calcaneus that can occur is of its anterior process. During an inversion/plantarflexion injury to the ankle, the bifurcate ligament, including the calcaneonavicular and calcaneocuboid portions, can avulse a fragment of the anterolateral aspect of the anterior process of the calcaneus. Both of these avulsion injuries carry a better prognosis than the axial loading injury because of the less severe involvement of the articular surface and less overall disruption of the calcaneal anatomy.

Regardless of the mechanism of the axial loading injury and subsequent fracture pattern, numerous problems result from the alteration of the calcaneal morphology in addition to the subtalar incongruity. Because of the decreased heel height, the talus sits relatively dorsiflexed within the mortise when the foot is in a plantigrade position, as opposed to its usual inclined orientation relative to the floor. This altered alignment decreases the range of dorsiflexion, which will lead to

anterior tibiotalar abutment during ambulation and subsequent degenerative changes in the ankle joint. In addition, the shortened hindfoot will bring the malleoli closer to the ground and thus lead to irritation with the heel counter of a shoe. The fracture also results in an elevation of the Achilles insertion, which results in a relative lengthening of the gastrocnemius-soleus complex. This lengthening decreases the available excursion and strength of the complex. The lateral bulging of the calcaneal wall will lead to peroneal impingement beneath the fibula and calcaneofibular abutment, and occasionally will result in sural neuritis. In addition, the widened heel will further compromise shoe wear. Finally, if there is any shortening of the calcaneus, this will decrease the lever arm of the gastrocnemius-soleus complex to the ankle, further weakening its function. These problems are summarized in Outline 1. Thus, any surgical fixation of the calcaneus will address all of these components of the fracture deformity instead of simply reconstituting the articular surface.

Radiographic Evaluation

Plain Radiography

The initial radiographic evaluation of all fractures is performed with plain radiographs. Anteroposterior (AP), lateral, and axial Harris views of the hindfoot should be obtained. Additional views include an oblique view of the hindfoot and a Broden view. The lateral projection is the most sensitive radiographic measurement of depression of the joint surface. A recent study has documented the underestimation of posterior facet displacement in fractures on CT evaluation in up to one third of all cases. The lateral plain radiograph allows one to classify the fracture as either a tongue-type or a joint depression-type of fracture. The lateral view also allows a numeric measure of the Böhler angle as a quantitative assessment of the shortening of the hindfoot. This angle is formed by a line drawn from the superior aspect of the posterior tuberosity of the calcaneus to the superior aspect of the posterior facet, and a second line drawn from the superior aspect of the posterior facet to the superior aspect of the anterior process of the calcaneus. This angle is typically between 30° and 35°. Frequently, extension of the anterior component of the fracture line into the calcaneocuboid joint will be visible on the lateral projection. The Harris axial view allows visualization of the amount of varus misalignment of the posterior tuberosity fragment, shortening of the medial wall of the calcaneus, and the amount of medial wall offset. Occasionally, the fracture line can be visualized through the posterior facet, but is better visualized with a computed tomography (CT) scan. An AP view of the hindfoot is useful for visualiz-

---

Outline 1

Problems associated with unreduced intra-articular calcaneus fracture

Arthritis/arthrosis of the subtalar +/- calcaneocuboid joint

Peroneal tendon impingement +/- calcaneofibular impingement

Widened heel with subsequent shoe-fitting problems

Malleoli closer to ground with heel counter irritation by shoe

Decreased ankle dorsiflexion caused by relative dorsiflexed position of talus, leading to anterior tibiotalar abutment and subsequent arthritic changes

Elevated Achilles tendon insertion, leading to weakened gastrocnemius-soleus complex

Limb-length discrepancy

Shortened calcaneus with decreased lever arm to gastrocnemius-soleus complex, thus weakening it

ing extension of the fracture into the calcaneocuboid joint. Occasionally, an oblique view of the hindfoot is useful to better visualize the calcaneocuboid joint.

Some authors recommend obtaining Broden views to visualize the posterior facet. This view is obtained by internally rotating the foot approximately 45° with the ankle in neutral position and angling the x-ray beam in 10° increments from 10°, 20°, 30°, and 40° from vertical. Each projection provides an evaluation of a different portion of the posterior facet from anterior to posterior. However, Broden views have essentially been replaced with CT scanning to define the articular surface anatomy; they can be useful intraoperatively to assess the reduction under fluoroscopic control.

Computed Tomography

CT scanning has vastly improved the ability to visualize the anatomy of the fracture. CT scans are typically obtained in both coronal and transverse planes through the calcaneus. The coronal cuts allow visualization of the posterior facet articular surface so that the number of articular fragments can be determined. In addition, the coronal cuts allow an overall evaluation of the fracture morphology. The transverse CT cuts allow assessment of the amount of shortening of the calcaneus and whether there is calcaneocuboid joint involvement. The CT scans allow for better preoperative decision-making as to whether a fracture will be amenable to surgical fixation and to determine the direction of the fracture lines and the best placement of hardware intraoperatively.

Spiral scanning CT machines, which can provide 3-dimensional reconstructions of the calcaneus fracture, are now available. These images are operator-dependent, as other bony structures such as the talus must be subtracted from each image in order to avoid obscuring the articular surface of the posterior facet. Although these scans make understanding of the fracture anatomy easier, the same information can be obtained from the 2-dimensional CT scan.

Classification Systems

Although the first system for classifying calcaneal fractures relied on the plain radiographic appearance (joint depression- versus tongue-type), the advent of CT scanning has led to further refinement of the calcaneal fracture anatomy and thus new, superior classification systems.

Sanders developed a CT classification of calcaneus fractures that has both treatment and prognostic significance (Fig. 1). On a coronal cut through the posterior facet of the subtalar joint, the articular surface is divided into 3 equal columns. These 3 columns are separated by a potential

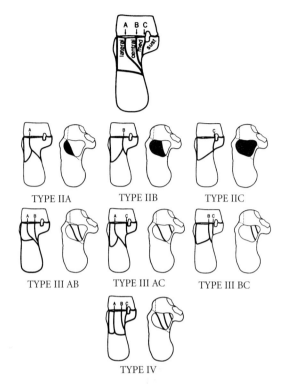

Figure 1

Computed tomographic scan classification of intra-articular calcaneal fractures. It is important that the coronal section analyzed includes the widest point of the articular surface (the sustentaculum tali). (Reproduced with permission from Sanders R: Intra-articular fractures of the calcaneus: Present state of the art. *J Orthop Trauma* 1992;6:252–265.)

fracture line, A (laterally) or B (medially). A third potential fracture line at the base of the sustentaculum tali also exists. The posterior facet can thus be characterized as having anywhere from 2 to 4 or more articular fragments. All nondisplaced articular fractures, regardless of their location, are classified as a type I. Type II fractures are 2-part fractures of the posterior facet. The fracture is further classified as A, B, or C, depending on the location of the fracture line. Type III fractures have 3 articular fragments, with the central fragment frequently being depressed. These fractures are similarly classified by the location of the fracture lines but have 2 fracture lines added (that is, III A-B or III A-C). Type IV fractures have 4 or more articular fragments with high comminution. This classification system allows determination of whether surgery is indicated and, if so, whether the patient would be a candidate for open reduction and internal fixation or possibly a primary fusion. In addition, the classification system has prognostic importance, as higher grades of fractures understandably have a poorer prognosis.

Treatment of Avulsion Fractures

Anterior Process Fractures

An anterior process fracture occurs with a plantarflexion/inversion injury of the ankle, causing an avulsion of a variable size piece of the anterior process of the calcaneus attached to the bifurcate ligament. These fractures can generally be visualized on a lateral radiograph. If the anterior process of the calcaneus is not visible on a lateral radiograph, an oblique radiograph of the hindfoot can be obtained to bring it into profile and demonstrate the fracture line. Although these patients will present complaining of an "ankle sprain," their tenderness will be located more distally over the anterior process of the calcaneus instead of over the lateral ankle ligament complex. Generally, these fractures involve a small piece of bone measuring less than 1 cm in diameter and are nondisplaced. These fractures can be treated the same as an ankle sprain, with rest, ice, compression, and elevation. Occasionally, a patient will develop a symptomatic nonunion of a small anterior process fracture, and if conservative treatment fails, excision can be done.

Less frequently, the fragment is large, measuring more than 1 cm in diameter, and involves a significant portion of the articular surface of the calcaneocuboid joint. In these instances, open reduction and internal fixation should be performed if the fragment is displaced. A longitudinal incision is made overlying the displaced fragment, and the fracture can be secured with a single cancellous screw.

Avulsion Fracture of Posterior Tuberosity

A posterior tuberosity fracture usually occurs during a strong contraction of the gastrocnemius-soleus complex with axial loading of the foot, creating failure of and tension on the calcaneus. The bony fragment displaces superiorly with the attached Achilles tendon. The fracture line can exit dorsally through the posterior tuberosity of the calcaneus and be extra-articular, or it can enter the posterior facet of the calcaneus. A nondisplaced fracture, although relatively rare, can be treated in plantarflexion in a cast for approximately 3 to 4 weeks until initial fracture tenderness subsides, and a walking cast can be used for an additional 2 to 4 weeks. The majority of these fractures have significant displacement, with the posterior aspect of the fragment tenting the posterior skin. In these cases, the fracture must be treated urgently as the skin will slough if there is no relief of underlying bony tension. The skin is frequently blanched upon initial presentation. In less serious cases, blistering will occur if the fracture is not reduced promptly. In more serious cases, full-thickness necrosis can occur, which can make free muscle transfer necessary to allow for bony coverage.

The usual surgical approach for an avulsion injury is a longitudinal incision along the medial aspect of the Achilles tendon. The fracture can be reduced with plantarflexion of the foot and pressure applied along the superior aspect of the fracture fragment and secured with 1 or 2 large cancellous screws. An intra-articular posterior tuberosity avulsion fracture is generally approached through the L-shaped extensile lateral approach. The longitudinal portion of this approach can be used to reduce the fracture without exposing the entire lateral aspect of the calcaneus first. If the reduction does not appear anatomic upon radiographic imaging, then the entire lateral approach is used and the lateral aspect of the joint surface exposed. A bony tenaculum can then be placed across the fracture to maintain the reduction while one or two large cancellous screws are placed in a lag fashion across the fracture.

Postoperatively, the foot should be immobilized in mild plantarflexion until the wound is healed. After wound healing, which usually occurs 1 to 2 weeks after surgery, the sutures are removed and range of motion exercises of the ankle and subtalar joints are commenced. Subtalar range of motion exercises are more important in the patients who have intra-articular fractures. These patients should not bear weight for approximately 4 to 6 weeks after surgery until initial fracture healing is evident radiographically; a short-leg walking cast can be employed for an additional 2 to 4 weeks.

Treatment of Intra-articular Calcaneus Fractures

Nonsurgical Treatment

Despite the plethora of problems following a displaced calcaneus fracture (Outline 1), many fractures are still treated nonsurgically. Nonsurgical treatment of calcaneus fractures should include initial elevation with placement of a bulky compressive Jones dressing. A splint is used to maintain the ankle in neutral position until swelling begins to resolve, which can take from less than a week in low-energy injuries to up to 3 weeks in severe, comminuted fractures, depending on severity of injury. Once edema is controlled, patients are switched to some type of removable splint, and active and passive range of motion of the ankle and hindfoot is begun. Nonweightbearing continues until healing has occurred, which generally requires approximately 6 to 8 weeks. Weightbearing is then advanced as tolerated at that time.

Different types of fractures are treated nonsurgically for various reasons. Nondisplaced (type I) fractures should be treated nonsurgically in every instance because surgery cannot correct nondisplacement. Markedly comminuted (type IV) fractures generally are not considered amenable to open reduction and internal fixation. Therefore, many surgeons now treat these fractures nonsurgically although primary fusion is now being advocated. Some surgeons still advocate nonsurgical treatment in type II and III fractures because of potential complications of surgical treatment and the contradictory data regarding the results of surgical versus nonsurgical treatment.

Surgical Treatment

The condition of the soft tissue frequently dictates the timing and necessity for surgical management. Clearly, open fractures of the calcaneus, which account for less than 5% of all calcaneus fractures, mandate urgent surgical treatment. Irrigation and debridement should be standard. The open wounds are generally along the medial aspect of the calcaneus where the sharp medial wall fragment lacerates the skin from within, and irrigation and debridement should be performed until the wounds are clean and free of devitalized tissue. In Gustilo type III B fractures, some type of free-tissue transfer will be necessary to cover the bone. Patients with significant soft-tissue wounds are probably best treated nonsurgically with regard to the management of their fracture. Some surgeons will treat type I and some type II open fractures with surgical reduction via a lateral approach after the medial wound has healed.

Another soft-tissue condition mandating urgent surgical treatment is a compartment syndrome. The foot has five main compartmental spaces that are susceptible to compartment syndrome in high-energy injuries. The calcaneal compartment is separate and frequently has increased compartmental pressures following a calcaneus fracture because of the soft-tissue trauma and bleeding associated with these fractures. These patients will complain of severe pain and require larger doses of narcotics despite immobilization and elevation of the foot. Compartment pressures should be measured in patients in whom compartment syndrome is suspected, or in those with severe swelling of the foot and altered mental status. If any doubt exists as to the presence of a compartment syndrome, the compartments should be released and the surgical wounds left open to prevent this potentially devastating complication. The wounds can subsequently be closed secondarily or skin grafting done if excessive edema remains.

Although open calcaneal fractures and compartment syndromes are relatively uncommon, all calcaneus fractures are complicated by varying degrees of soft-tissue edema. One of the most important decisions regarding treatment of these fractures is the appropriate timing of surgery. Patients with excessive edema must wait until edema has begun to resolve before risking surgical intervention and the possibility of wound dehiscence; the most serious complications occur

following wound dehiscence and include subsequent infection. Patients are usually placed in a bulky Jones compressive dressing and the foot elevated until the time of surgery to reduce edema. Recently, the use of intermittent pneumatic pedal compression (foot pumps) has been demonstrated to markedly reduce preoperative edema when used in patients with calcaneus fractures and is generally well tolerated. These devices can be used both in the hospital and in the outpatient setting.

As a rule, patients with fracture blisters should not undergo surgery until the blisters have healed. Most patients are considered to have adequate edema resolution to allow for surgery when they have a positive "wrinkle test." A wrinkle test is performed by dorsiflexing and everting the ankle. The skin over the lateral aspect of the ankle and hindfoot should wrinkle with this maneuver. If tense edema is present and the skin does not wrinkle, then surgery should be delayed until such time that the skin wrinkles.

Closed Reduction and Percutaneous Fixation

Essex-Lopresti described placing a large percutaneous pin through the posterior aspect of a tongue fracture fragment, performing a closed reduction maneuver, and subsequently placing the pin across the fracture site into the anterior aspect of the calcaneus. The advantage to this approach is that there is less morbidity because of the absence of a surgical incision. However, this maneuver is rarely indicated, as it can only be used in a tongue-type fracture or avulsion fracture of the posterior tuberosity and does not address the deformity of the calcaneal body. The maneuver cannot be used in joint depression fractures because no bone is attached to the posterior aspect of the articular surface that could be used to reduce the articular surface with this percutaneous pin. Because of the inaccuracy of this reduction technique, it has been abandoned by most surgeons.

Open Reduction and Internal Fixation

Although some authors continue to recommend nonsurgical treatment of intra-articular calcaneus fractures, surgical treatment of these fractures is again coming into favor. Most surgeons who advocate surgical treatment of displaced intra-articular calcaneus fractures recommend repairing those with adequate soft tissues and 2 or 3 major articular fragments (Sanders type II and III fractures) and reconstructing the remainder of the calcaneal morphology. The advocates of surgical treatment attempt to restore the normal anatomy of the calcaneus to prevent as many as possible of the problems presented in Outline 1.

Various surgical approaches to the calcaneus have been described. Some surgeons advocate a medial approach to the calcaneus because it provides excellent visualization of the medial wall. The disadvantages of this approach are the increased risk of damage to the neurovascular structures along the medial side of the hindfoot (especially the calcaneal branches to the heel pad) and the fact that it affords very poor visualization of the posterior facet. Other surgeons have advocated a lateral approach to the calcaneus to allow better visualization of the posterior facet and the lateral wall of the calcaneus. One approach is to make a gentle curved incision overlying the peroneal tendons, open the tendon sheath, and subsequently expose the underlying calcaneus to gain access to the posterior facet in this fashion. Although this approach does allow improved visualization of the posterior facet, there is a higher likelihood of postoperative peroneal tendon instability and risk of sural nerve injury, and some surgeons have noted an increased risk of delayed wound healing with this approach.

Other surgeons have advocated a limited approach to the lateral side via a sinus tarsi incision. This approach markedly limits the ability to visualize the posterior facet but involves less morbidity and swelling because of the smaller incision. In addition, the amount of hardware that can be placed in the wound is markedly limited.

The most popular approach to the calcaneus at this time is the extensile, L-shaped approach (Fig. 2). This surgery involves elevating the entire soft-tissue envelope off the lateral aspect of the calcaneus with the flap containing the per-

oneal tendons and sural nerve. It allows excellent visualization of the entire lateral wall of the calcaneus and of the posterior facet of the subtalar joint. Retraction pins can be placed in the fibula, talus, and cuboid to allow for a "no touch" technique of flap retraction. The disadvantage to this extensile approach is that it causes more swelling and pain than the less extensive incisions. In addition, the medial wall is not visualized directly, although it can be indirectly reduced.

Some surgeons advocate a combined medial and lateral approach to the calcaneus to allow direct visualization of both the medial wall fracture and the posterior facet. The disadvantage of this approach is the greater soft-tissue trauma to the foot and thus greater pain, swelling, and risk of wound-healing problems.

Various types of internal fixation devices have been described for securing surgical reduction of these fractures. Most surgeons now use low-profile plates over the lateral aspect of the calcaneus combined with small fragment or mini-fragment screws. The use of staples has been described in the past, especially to support the medial wall fragments, but these are unable to provide any type of lag fixation. A variety of plates have been developed by various manufacturers specifically for the treatment of calcaneus fractures. The results with various types of these plates have been reported and all appear to provide adequate fixation strength. The most important feature of these plates is that they are low-profile and thus minimize the chance of subsequent peroneal tendon and shoe wear irritation.

Another aspect of the surgical treatment of calcaneus fractures that is controversial among treating surgeons is the use of bone graft. The lateral, displaced portion of the posterior facet of the calcaneus is usually impacted into a relatively osteopenic area of the calcaneus known as the neutral triangle. After reduction of the articular surface and the overall calcaneal alignment, a bony defect is usually present beneath the anterior portion of the posterior facet. Some surgeons routinely bone graft this defect. Others, including Sanders, routinely leave this bony void because it is in an area that normally is osteopenic. In patients who are compliant with the postoperative nonweightbearing regimen, displacement of the fracture in patients who have not had bone graft has not been problematic.

Surgical Technique

The patient is placed in a lateral decubitus position with the affected side placed upright on a beanbag. In bilateral fractures, the patient is placed prone, and access to the lateral side of the calcaneus is achieved by externally rotating the hip. A pneumatic tourniquet is placed around the thigh to improve visualization intraoperatively. The lateral, L-shaped extensile

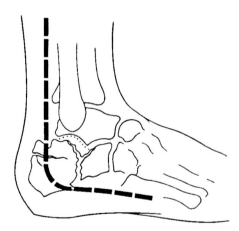

Figure 2

The extensile right angle lateral approach to the calcaneus. The longitudinal limb is made just anterior to the Achilles tendon to avoid damage to the sural nerve. The inferior limb of the incision is made at the junction of the plantar and dorsal skin and ends just proximal to the base of the fifth metatarsal. (Reproduced with permission from Sanders R, Hansen ST, McReynolds IC: Trauma to the calcaneus and its tendon, in Jahss M (ed): *Disorders of the Foot and Ankle: Medical and Surgical Management,* ed 2. Philadelphia, PA, WB Saunders, 1991, pp 2326–2360.)

approach allows maximum exposure of the lateral aspect of the calcaneus and the subtalar joint (Fig. 2). The superior aspect of the incision is made along the anterior aspect of the Achilles tendon to avoid injury to the sural nerve. The incision is angled relatively acutely at the junction of the plantar and dorsal skin in the hindfoot region and then is extended anteriorly to 1 cm proximal to the base of the fifth metatarsal. The incision is then carried down to bone at the angle of incision and the entire flap elevated off the lateral wall of the calcaneus with a scalpel. Blunt dissection should be performed in the proximal and distal aspects of the wound to avoid injury to the sural nerve if it crosses the wound in these locations. The peroneal tendons are generally visualized in the distal aspect of the wound after they exit the peroneal tendon sheath, which will have been sharply elevated from the lateral side of the calcaneus. Fibrous bands course obliquely through the superior aspect of this incision, and these must be divided to facilitate visualization of the posterior aspect of the subtalar joint. The entire posterior and lateral aspects of the posterior facet should be visualized. The bifurcate and intraosseous ligaments can be sharply divided while exposing the anterior aspect of the calcaneus. Dissection is carried distally until the calcaneocuboid joint is visualized.

Pins are placed to maintain the exposure with a "no touch" technique of retraction of the flap. A 0.062 Kirschner wire (K-wire) is placed across the tip of the fibula after subluxating the peroneal tendons superior to this level. A second K-wire is placed into the lateral neck of the talus and a third is placed into the cuboid. During the reduction of the calcaneus, a narrow Homan retractor can be placed over the anterior process of the calcaneus to improve visualization of the anterior calcaneus and calcaneocuboid joint. A deep retractor, such as an Army/Navy, can be placed along the posterior aspect of the subtalar joint to improve visualization in this area.

After exposure of the lateral wall of the calcaneus, the fracture anatomy can then be delineated. A small elevator, such as a Freer, can be inserted into the fracture lines in the lateral wall of the calcaneus. The lateral articular fragment will generally be found to be impacted into the body of the calcaneus up to 2 cm. The fracture planes should be mobilized with this small elevator via blunt dissection using the CT scan as a guide to the location of the fracture planes. Generally, the lateral articular fragment can be rotated on its posterior soft-tissue attachments and displaced laterally to allow better visualization of the medial fracture anatomy. During visualization across the subtalar joint, the articular surface of the sustentaculum tali fragment (constant fragment) will be seen to be anatomically aligned with the undersurface of the talus medially.

At this time, either the posterior aspect of the calcaneus or the anterior aspect of the calcaneus can be reduced. Surgeons have differing preferences as to which requires treatment first.

Prior to reducing the posterior facet articular fragment, the posterior tuberosity of the calcaneus must be reduced indirectly to reestablish the normal heel height and the normal varus-valgus alignment of the heel. Then the lateral articular fragment can be reduced to the medial "constant fragment." A preoperative CT scan will frequently demonstrate a wedge-shaped superior aspect of the tuberosity fragment between the 2 or 3 major articular fragments of the posterior facet. Once this wedge-shaped bone is reduced into its normal position, it no longer precludes the anatomic reduction of the lateral to the medial aspect of the posterior facet.

Various methods have been described for indirect reduction of the posterior tuberosity fragment. A large threaded pin can be placed into the posterior-inferior aspect of the posterior tuberosity fragment and used to indirectly pull the posterior tuberosity fragment out of varus to reestablish medial wall height and reduce the lateral displacement (Fig. 3). Another method is blunt dissection through the fracture plane extending into the medial wall and direct reduction of the medial wall fragment by levering the posterior tuberosity fragment with a large periosteal elevator through the body of the calcaneus. After reduction of the posterior tuberosity fragment with either method, the reduction can be temporarily maintained by placement of a percutaneous K-wire through the medial column of the tuberosity fragment into the "constant fragment" of the calcaneus.

After the posterior tuberosity fragment is reduced, anatomic reduction of the lateral articular fragment(s) of the posterior facet to the medial, nondisplaced articular fragment should then be possible. This component requires the most accuracy and is the most technically demanding. A biomechanical study has demonstrated that an articular step-off of as little as 2 mm causes significant changes in the joint contact stresses. The accuracy of the reduction can be facilitated by completely visualizing the lateral and posterior aspect of the posterior facet. The undersurface of the talus can be used as a reduction template for the lateral articular fragment. After reducing the fragment, it should be held provisionally with an anterior and posterior K-wire. Prior to insertion of the definitive screw fixation, the reduction can be checked by placing the flat end of the Freer elevator over the articular surface to palpate the fracture for any step-off or diastasis. In addition, intraoperative Broden's views can be obtained fluoroscopically to further assess the reduction. After the articular reduction is achieved, 2 subchondral cortical lag screws can be placed beneath the articular surface of the posterior facet. The amount of medial calcaneal cortex available for

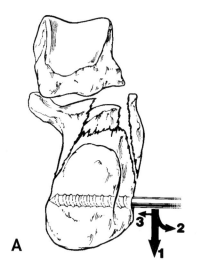

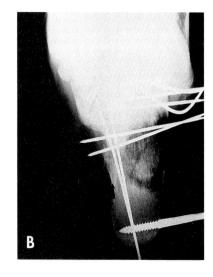

Figure 3

A, The reduction technique used to reduce the tuberosity of the calcaneus. A Schanz pin has been placed in the tuberosity fragment. Three arrows indicate the relative motion of the Schanz pin. The 3 components of the reduction are demonstrated, thus bringing the tuberosity fragment plantarly, medially, and in a slight valgus position to reestablish its normal alignment. **B,** An intraoperative axial radiograph demonstrating the maneuver in the schematic. The medial wall is reduced indirectly (arrow) and held provisionally with two Kirschner wires directed from the heel upward into the sustentaculum. (Reproduced with permission from Sangeorzan BJ, Benirschke SK, Carr JB: Surgical management of fractures of the os calcis, in Jackson DW (ed): *Instructional Course Lectures 44*. Rosemont, IL, American Academy of Orthopaedic Surgeons, 1995, pp 359–370.)

placing these screws can be seen on the coronal CT sections. Great care must be exercised in placing all of the screws because the neurovascular and tendinous structures are in close proximity to the medial cortex.

The anterior aspect of the calcaneus can then be reduced. The entire lateral and superior aspect of the calcaneocuboid joint should be visualized if there is any articular involvement. After reduction of the joint surface, provisional K-wire fixation can be placed. The lateral wall of the calcaneus can then be reconstructed. An appropriate low-profile plate should be contoured to fit the lateral aspect of the calcaneus and achieve secure screw fixation. The combination of the subchondral screws and the screws placed through the lateral plate should reestablish continuity between the posterior tuberosity, the anterior portion of the calcaneus, and the sustentacular fragment. After placement of the definitive fixation, the range of motion of the subtalar joint can be assessed and a smooth, gliding motion with uniform movement is noted between these 3 main portions of the calcaneus. Intraoperative lateral and axial Harris views should be obtained to assess the fracture reduction, placement of the hardware, and length of the screws. Preoperative and postoperative radiographs of a typical patient are presented in Figure 4.

As long as stable bone-to-bone contact is present between the main fragments of the calcaneus which are held with the plate and screws, the author does not believe that cancellous bone grafting is necessary. Some surgeons will routinely use bone graft in order to buttress the posterior facet, but the compressive strength of morsellized cancellous bone graft is marginal.

Occasionally, an interposed flexor hallucis longus tendon may be noted along the medial aspect of the subtalar joint. These tendons can be reduced by simply pushing them out of the subtalar joint. If reduction cannot be achieved or subluxation into the joint occurs after this reduction maneuver, a small medial incision can be made to isolate the flexor hallucis longus tendon to prevent its displacement back into the joint.

Meticulous wound closure is essential in these patients. A suction drain is placed beneath the flap to prevent accumulation of a hematoma, which could place added tension on the wound margins. Interrupted, buried absorbable subcutaneous sutures are placed along the length of the wound. A monofilament, nonabsorbable suture is used to close the skin. Although some surgeons advocate a running suture, which therefore is "self-tensioning," I prefer multiple interrupted vertical mattress sutures along the length of the wound. Modified horizontal mattress sutures (Allgower-Donati) can be placed at the apex of the wound such that no sutures cross the tip of the flap. Patients are placed in a compressive dressing and posterior splint postoperatively.

Once the wound has sealed postoperatively, which generally occurs by 5 to 7 days after surgery, the patient is placed in a removable splint to allow for ankle and subtalar range of motion exercises. Stiffness of the subtalar joint is an accepted occurrence following this fracture but must be minimized to improve the eventual functional result. These patients are kept strictly nonweightbearing for the first 10 weeks following surgery. Between weeks 10 and 12, the patients are allowed to begin weightbearing as tolerated in a walking boot. After 12 weeks, the patients are advanced from ambulating with a cane and a walking boot to unprotected walking. Most patients have progressive improvement in their symptomatology for 1 year after surgery. Up to 50% of laborers do not return to the same type of work following this severe

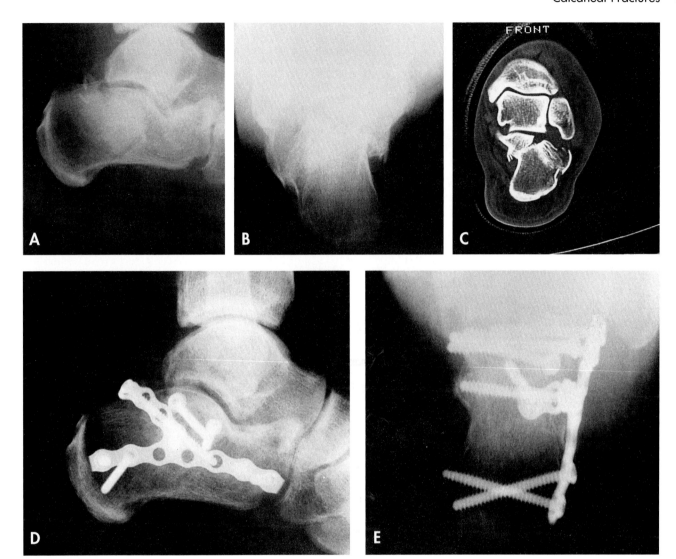

Figure 4

A, A preoperative lateral radiograph demonstrating a displaced intra-articular calcanceus fracture in a man who fell 8 feet from the top of a ladder. Note that the anterior aspect of the posterior facet is depressed approximately 1 cm into the neutral triangle of the calcaneus. Böhler's angle is approximately zero. **B,** Preoperative Harris axial radiograph demonstrating varus impaction of the tuberosity fragment with approximately a 1-cm medial wall offset and 1 cm of medial wall shortening. **C,** Preoperative CT scan demonstrating a Sanders type IIA fracture with depression and rotation of the lateral articular fragment. Note how the tuberosity fragment has been impacted between the 2 articular fragments, thus precluding their reduction to each other until it has been reduced. The peroneal tendons are being impinged between the lateral wall of the calcaneus and the inferior aspect of the fibula. **D,** Postoperative lateral radiograph demonstrating anatomic reduction of the posterior facet and reestablishment of Böhler's angle. A contoured Y-plate along with small fragment screws has been used to maintain the reduction. **E,** Postoperative Harris axial view demonstrating reestablishment of medial wall alignment and appropriate length of screws.

injury. All patients must be counseled about the devastating nature of this injury before surgery. The author emphasizes to all patients that their foot will never be the same again.

Primary Subtalar Fusion

Some patients have marked articular surface comminution (Sanders type IV fracture), which can make obtaining an anatomic reduction difficult or impossible. In addition, other patients will be noted at the time of surgery to have a marked degree of cartilaginous damage as a result of abrasion by the fractured bony surface. Some surgeons have begun to report relatively good initial results with primary subtalar fusion in these patients with marked joint surface disruption. One recent report evaluated the results of 14 patients treated with a primary subtalar arthrodesis for a comminuted calcaneus fracture. Eleven of 12 working patients did return to work. According to the Foot and Ankle Society hindfoot score, the average postoperative score was 72.4, which correlated to a good functional result. These results were believed to be superior to those of the nonsurgical treatment of these severe fractures.

The general treatment principles are the same as open reduction and internal fixation of these complex fractures. Adequate soft-tissue edema resolution must occur prior to surgery, because these patients have a worse soft-tissue injury and are therefore at higher risk of delayed postoperative wound healing and infection. The same lateral, extensile approach is made to the calcaneus. Although the body of the calcaneus is comminuted, there are enough large fragments that can be reduced together that the overall calcaneal morphology can be approximately reestablished. After the articular surface has been confirmed to be markedly disrupted, any remaining cartilage that is evident on the calcaneal side is removed. The cartilage is then removed from the posterior facet of the talus. These patients require autogenous iliac crest bone graft to fill the void at the arthrodesis site. In general, small fragment screws are used to maintain the reduction of the calcaneal morphology with or without a lateral plate. One or two large fragment cancellous screws are used to transfix the fusion site. Fully threaded cancellous screws can be used to try to prevent impaction of the body of the calcaneus and arthrodesis site.

Complications

Wound dehiscence with subsequent infection remains the most common and feared complication following the surgical treatment of calcaneus fractures. As mentioned previously, prevention, by postponing surgery until adequate edema resolution has begun, can be one of the most important aspects of treatment. The angle of the incision is the site of greatest risk for wound breakdown. It is for this reason that some authors advocate using modified horizontal mattress sutures such that none of the sutures cross the tip of the skin flap. Despite taking precautions, some patients will develop wound complications. The rate of wound complications generally ranges from 5% to 30% in most series. If a wound complication occurs, it must be treated aggressively to prevent the devastating complication of osteomyelitis. These patients must be immobilized until their wound heals despite the subsequent development of stiffness of the subtalar joint. With small wound-healing problems, local debridement, dressing changes, and antibiotics as needed can be employed. With large wound problems, aggressive debridement and free soft-

tissue transfer with the assistance of a microvascular surgeon are essential. In general, patients with significant wound complications will develop a stiff subtalar joint, but this is unavoidable because of the period of immobilization that is necessary to allow for the wound to heal.

Subtalar arthrosis or arthritis are also frequently present to a varying degree. Because of the intra-articular nature of these fractures, most patients develop some degree of postoperative stiffness. My personal experience is that the average patient loses approximately one third to one half of the normal subtalar motion despite aggressive postoperative rehabilitation. The stiffness can be caused by a nonanatomic reduction of the joint or, more commonly, intra-articular adhesions or chondral damage incurred at the time of the initial injury. Despite an anatomic reduction, some patients will continue to complain of pain that may need to be lessened with an arthrodesis.

The lateral approaches to the hindfoot place the sural nerve at risk for injury. Sural nerve injuries are common following the curved, peroneal tendon-mobilizing approach to the calcaneus. The sural nerve is injured much less frequently with the L-shaped extensile approach to the calcaneus. The author advocates blunt dissection through the subcutaneous tissues in the proximal and distal aspects of the wound to minimize the risk of damage to this nerve. If the nerve is damaged, then a proximal resection of the nerve in the distal leg is necessary to place the neuroma in a less irritable location.

Results of Surgical Treatment

A contradictory body of literature exists regarding the results of surgical versus nonsurgical treatment of calcaneus fractures. Some studies have reported superior results with nonsurgical treatment, others with equivalent results between surgical and nonsurgical treatment, and others have reported superior results with surgical treatment. Most authors are in agreement that nonsurgical treatment of calcaneus fractures leads to persistent functional deficits. One recent study evaluated 27 patients with a unilateral calcaneus fracture treated nonsurgically. Seventeen of the patients had a fair or poor result, and gait abnormalities were noted in the 16 patients analyzed. It was concluded that despite the lack of subsequent surgical treatment, these patients generally had persistent pain and a functional deficit.

Only two studies have compared the results of surgical versus nonsurgical treatment in a prospective randomized fashion. Other studies have retrospectively evaluated nonrandomized series of patients or used case control studies. In one of the prospective randomized trials, Parmar and associates reported on a series of 66 patients with displaced intra-articular calca-

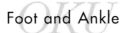
neus fractures who were randomized to conservative or surgical treatment. The nonsurgical group was treated with early mobilization. The surgical group underwent open reduction and internal fixation with subchondral K-wires as the sole method of fixation and were placed in a cast for 6 weeks. The authors noted no significant difference between their treatment groups with regard to pain or function, but clearly the surgical results would have been compromised by 6 weeks of immobilization. Thordarson and Krieger reported on a series of 30 patients with displaced intra-articular calcaneus fractures who were randomized to surgical versus nonsurgical treatment. The nonsurgical treatment included early mobilization, whereas the surgical treatment included current fixation methods via an L-shaped extensile approach and early mobilization. At early follow-up, they noted far superior results in the group treated with surgery. That study is the only prospective randomized trial evaluating the results of current surgical treatment methods and aggressive postoperative mobilization.

Initial results of patients treated with primary fusion for markedly comminuted fractures have been promising. Nonsurgical treatment of these massively comminuted fractures frequently leads to fair or poor results. Delayed surgical treatment of these patients requires a complex reconstruction, which can necessitate a distraction arthrodesis with its increased morbidity from tricortical iliac crest bone grafting and a high risk of varus malunion. Also, complex calcaneal osteotomies, which attempt to reestablish the original fracture planes, are another reconstructive method. A successful primary fusion can obviate the need for subsequent, complex reconstructive surgery of these fractures.

Conclusion

Although the generally poor results following nonsurgical treatment of calcaneus fractures have been well documented, it is hoped that longer term results of surgical treatment will soon be available. Most surgeons are currently reporting superior results with surgical treatment. It is hoped that results will continue to improve with increased expertise in treatment. The role of primary arthrodesis for severely comminuted fractures does appear to be promising in certain cases and will hopefully be delineated with further studies. The use of foot pumps will hopefully allow for more rapid preoperative reduction of edema and decrease the incidence of wound healing complications in upcoming years.

Because of the tenuous initial fracture stability, patients are kept nonweightbearing for an extended period of time, which contributes to the prolonged disability experienced with

these fractures. A new in situ setting cancellous bone cement is being investigated in Europe and has shown promising results in the treatment of a small series of calcaneus fractures with this substance, since rehabilitation was much faster. More study is needed to further define the possible role of this substance in the treatment of these fractures.

Annotated Bibliography

Albert MJ, Waggoner SM, Smith JW: Internal fixation of calcaneus fractures: An anatomical study of structures at risk. *J Orthop Trauma* 1995;9:107–112.

This article evaluates the structures at risk in 10 fresh cadaveric specimens. Wires placed in the subchondral bone of the posterior facet or anterior to the critical angle of Gissane were found to increase the risk of injury to the medial neurovascular structures and flexor hallucis longus tendon.

Buch BD, Myerson MS, Miller SD: Primary subtalar arthrodesis for the treatment of comminuted calcaneal fractures. *Foot Ankle Int* 1996;17:61–70.

The results of 14 patients who underwent primary fusion for a comminuted calcaneus fracture are reviewed. A 100% union rate was noted, with 11 of 12 employed patients returning to work at an average of 8.8 months after injury.

Crosby LA, Fitzgibbons TC: Open reduction and internal fixation of type II intra-articular calcaneus fractures. *Foot Ankle Int* 1996;17:253–258.

The authors reviewed the results of 23 calcaneus fractures and noted an average score of 91.4 versus an unmatched series of 10 fractures treated nonsurgically with an average score of 70.

Ebraheim NA, Biyani A, Padanilam T, Christiensen G: Calcaneocuboid joint involvement in calcaneal fractures. *Foot Ankle Int* 1996;17:563–565.

The radiographs of 48 surgically treated calcaneus fractures were reviewed and calcaneocuboid joint involvement was 38.7%. This involvement was evident in 18 of 19 patients with plain anteroposterior or oblique radiographs of the hindfoot. Involvement was noted more often in patients with joint depression-type fractures.

Ebraheim NA, Biyani A, Padanilam T, Paley K: A pitfall of coronal computed tomographic imaging in evaluation of calcaneal fractures. *Foot Ankle Int* 1996;17:503–505.

Thirty-six CT scans of patients with intra-articular fractures were evaluated, and in 9 patients the CT scan underestimated the displacement of the posterior facet program. The lateral plain radiograph was more accurate in determining the degree of displacement.

Kitaoka HB, Schaap EJ, Chao EY, An KN: Displaced intra-articular fractures of the calcaneus treated non-operatively: Clinical results and analysis of motion and ground-reaction and temporal forces. *J Bone Joint Surg* 1994;76A:1531–1540.

Twenty-seven patients with displaced intra-articular calcaneus fractures that had been treated nonsurgically were evaluated on average of 6 years following injury. There were 5 excellent, 5 good, 7 fair, and 10 poor results. Gait analysis revealed altered ground reaction force and decreased proportion of single limb support of the involved side.

Kundel K, Funk E, Brutscher M, Bickel R: Calcaneal fractures: Operative versus nonoperative treatment. *J Trauma* 1996; 41:839–845.

This article presents a retrospective analysis of 33 nonsurgically and 30 surgically treated cases that were selected from a much larger group of fractures treated during the period of the study. There was a minimal difference between the 2 treatment groups, but open reduction and internal fixation of these fractures can benefit patients if a near anatomic reconstruction is achieved.

Laughlin RT, Carson JG, Calhoun JH: Displaced intra-articular calcaneus fractures treated with the Galveston plate. *Foot Ankle Int* 1996;17:71–78.

Thirty-three calcaneus fractures were treated with surgery and evaluated an average of 21 months later. Seventy percent of patients had no pain or only occasional pain, with 78% having a good or excellent clinical result.

Lowery RB, Calhoun JH: Fractures of the calcaneus: Part I: Anatomy, injury mechanism, and classification. *Foot Ankle Int* 1996; 17:230–235.

Lowery RB, Calhoun JH: Fractures of the calcaneus: Part II: Treatment. *Foot Ankle Int* 1996;17:360–366.

A brief, concise review of the treatment of extra-articular and intra-articular fractures of the calcaneus is presented.

Melcher G, Degonda F, Leutenegger A, Ruedi T: Ten-year follow-up after operative treatment for intra-articular fractures of the calcaneus. *J Trauma* 1995;38:713–716.

Sixteen patients managed with open reduction and internal fixation were reviewed on average more than 10 years after surgery. Seventy-five percent of these patients had an excellent or good functional result with none requiring a secondary arthrodesis. Some patients had slowly progressing posttraumatic subtalar osteoarthritis. The subjective results were clearly better than 3 years after surgery.

Monsey RD, Levine BP, Trevino SG, Kristiansen TK: Operative treatment of acute displaced intra-articular calcaneus fractures. *Foot Ankle Int* 1995;16:57–63.

Eighteen fractures were treated surgically and the results compared to a different series of patients treated nonsurgically. A significant difference was noted between surgical and nonsurgical treatment in more comminuted fractures.

O'Farrell DA, O'Byrne JM, McCabe JP, Stephens MM: Fractures of the os calcis: Improved results with internal fixation. *Injury* 1993;24:263–265.

The authors reviewed a series of 12 fractures treated surgically and compared them to 12 fractures treated nonsurgically in a prospective study. The patients were treated by two different surgeons, one of whom preferred surgical treatment. Superior results were noted in the group that had surgery.

Parmar HV, Triffitt PD, Gregg PJ: Intra-articular fractures of the calcaneum treated operatively or conservatively: A prospective study. *J Bone Joint Surg* 1993;75B:932–937.

A prospective randomized series that evaluated 66 patients with displaced intra-articular calcaneus fractures who were randomized to conservative or surgical treatment is presented. The nonsurgical group was treated with early mobilization. The surgical group had open reduction and subchondral Kirschner wires as the sole method of fixation, and the foot was subsequently placed in a cast for 6 weeks. There was no significant difference in pain or function between the treatment groups.

Sanders R, Gregory P: Operative treatment of intra-articular fractures of the calcaneus. *Orthop Clin North Am* 1995; 26:203–214.

This article presents a review of the surgical treatment of calcaneus fractures and details some of the authors' own results. The authors advocate surgical treatment of type II and III fractures. Reduction or primary fusion (as indicated) are suggested for the type IV fractures. It is also noted that a learning curve exists and that a surgeon can expect significant improvement after approximately 35 cases.

Sangeorzan BJ, Ananthakrishnan D, Tencer AF: Contact characteristics of the subtalar joint after a simulated calcaneus fracture. *J Orthop Trauma* 1995;9:251–258.

A 2-part intra-articular calcaneus fracture was created in 9 cadaveric specimens. The contact area of the posterior facet was significantly decreased with 2, 5, and 10 mm of displacement. The authors recommended that a calcaneus fracture be reduced to within 2 mm to decrease the alteration of contact area and pressure.

Sangeorzan BJ, Benirschke SK, Carr JB: Surgical management of fractures of the os calcis, in Jackson DW (ed): *Instructional Course Lectures 44*. Rosemont, IL, American Academy of Orthopaedic Surgeons, 1995, pp 359–370.

A review of the surgical management of fractures of the os calcis emphasizing the surgical technique is presented.

Thordarson DB, Krieger LE: Operative vs. nonoperative treatment of intra-articular fractures of the calcaneus: A prospective randomized trial. *Foot Ankle Int* 1996;17:2–9.

A prospective randomized study of 30 patients with displaced intra-articular calcaneus fractures was evaluated. All patients had Sanders type II or III fractures. Nonsurgical treatment involved early mobilization, whereas surgical treatment involved an extensile L-shaped approach with rigid internal fixation and early mobilization with delayed weightbearing. In the surgical group, there were 7 excellent, 5 good, 2 fair, and 1 poor result. In the nonsurgical group, there was 1 excellent, 3 good, 1 fair, and 6 poor results. This study is the first prospective randomized trial to demonstrate the superior results of current surgical treatment with early mobilization compared with nonsurgical treatment.

Tornetta P III: Open reduction and internal fixation of the calcaneus using minifragment plates. *J Orthop Trauma* 1996; 10:63–67.

Thirty-five intra-articular fractures of the calcaneus were treated with mini fragment plates and small fragment screws. Anatomic reduction was achieved in 91% of patients. Seventy-seven percent good or excellent results were achieved.

Classic Bibliography

Bohler L: Diagnosis, pathology, and treatment of fractures of the os calcis. *J Bone Joint Surg* 1931;13:75–89.

Buckley RE, Meek RN: Comparison of open versus closed reduction of intraarticular calcaneal fractures: A matched cohort in workmen. *J Orthop Trauma* 1992;6:216–222.

Sanders R: Intra-articular fractures of the calcaneus: Present state of the art. *J Orthop Trauma* 1992;6:252–265.

Chapter 18
Soft-Tissue Injuries of the Ankle

Soft-tissue injury to the ankle predominantly involves sprains to the lateral ankle ligaments, the most common injury in sports. Approximately 27,000 ankle sprains occur daily in the United States but despite this incidence, there is significant variety in treatment protocols and recommendations. Though 80% to 90% of all ankle sprains will heal with satisfactory functional results following nonoperative treatment, about 20% to 40% of patients will have residual pain sufficient to limit their activities after a grade III ankle sprain. The persistently symptomatic "failed ankle sprain" is one of the more difficult challenges to the foot and ankle or sports medicine specialist. Ankle sprains dominate a discussion of trauma to this region but differential diagnosis of ankle injury must include injury to the tibiotalar and subtalar joints, the syndesmosis, the medial ankle, and to regional tendons. Accurate diagnosis of ankle soft-tissue injury is predicated on a detailed knowledge of anatomy.

Anatomy

The ankle joint is a uniaxial, composite joint consisting of the syndesmotic (distal tibia and fibula) and mortise (tibiotalar and talofibular) articulations. Inherent bony stability is due to the truncated body of the talus being wider anteriorly than posteriorly so that the talus is "locked" into the mortise in dorsiflexion, and more mobile and therefore susceptible to injury in plantarflexion. The malleolus of the tibia constitutes the medial buttress. Laterally, the fibula articulates with the lateral wall of the talus and extends distally to the calcaneus. The plafond is the distal end of the tibia that, irrespective of the position of the foot, articulates with only two thirds of the talus.

The ligaments of the lateral ankle are divided from superior to inferior into 3 anatomic groupings: the distal tibiofibular interosseous ligaments, the lateral ligament complex, and the lateral subtalar ligaments. The lateral ligamentous complex is the primary structure involved in soft-tissue injury of the ankle and comprises the anterior talofibular ligament (ATFL), the calcaneofibular ligament (CFL), and the posterior talofibular ligament (PTFL) (Fig. 1).

The ATFL is the most frequently injured ligament in the body and is the weakest of the three components of the lateral ligamentous complex. The ATFL is a flat, broad ligament that originates on the anterior border of the fibula between the inferior border of the anterior tibiofibular ligament and

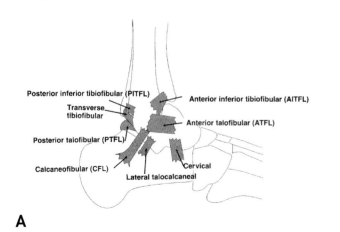

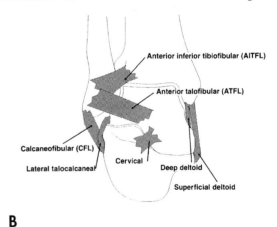

A   **B**

Figure 1

A, Lateral view of the ligaments of the ankle and subtalar joint. **B,** Anterior view of the ligaments of the ankle and subtalar joint. (Reproduced with permission from Lutter LD, Mizel MS, Pfeffer GB (eds): *Orthopaedic Knowledge Update: Foot and Ankle.* Rosemont, IL, American Academy of Orthopaedic Surgeons, 1994, pp 241–253.)

above the CFL. Intimately blending with the capsule of the talofibular joint, the ATFL inserts on the talar body anterior to the lateral articular surface. In the neutral position of the ankle, the ligament approximates a horizontal position.

The CFL is the second component of the lateral ligament complex. It originates just inferior to the ATFL on the anterior surface of the lateral malleolus and courses beneath the peroneal tendons inserting on a small tubercle on the lateral wall of the calcaneus, posterior and superior to the peroneal tubercle. Increasing importance is accorded the CFL as a subtalar joint stabilizer. Some anatomy texts draw the CFL as 90° perpendicular to the ATFL though its course is variable and usually directed posteriorly. Rarely injured, the PTFL is the strongest of the lateral ligaments and inserts lateral to the flexor hallucis longus groove on the lateral tubercle of the talus.

Much less attention has been directed to the 5 components of the lateral subtalar ligament complex, divided into a superficial, intermediate, and deep layer. In addition to the CFL, the superficial layer is composed of the inferior extensor retinaculum and the lateral talocalcaneal ligament, which connects the body of the talus to the lateral wall of the calcaneus. The intermediate layer comprises the intermediate portion of the inferior extensor retinaculum and the cervical ligament. The latter is the strongest connection between the talus and calcaneus, lying within the sinus tarsi connecting the 2 bones. Between the posterior and middle facets lies the interosseus talocalcaneal ligament, which coupled with the deep portion of the inferior extensor retinaculum, comprises the deep layer of the lateral subtalar ligament complex.

The distal tibiofibular syndesmosis consists of 3 ligaments: anterior inferior tibiofibular ligament (AITFL), the posterior inferior tibiofibular ligament (PITFL), and the interosseous ligament (IL). The IL is continuous with the interosseous membrane, is located between the AITFL and PITFL, and is considered the primary component of the syndesmotic complex.

The medial collateral or deltoid ligament is a fan-shaped ligament composed of a superficial and deep layer. The superficial portion connects anteriorly to the navicular (tibionavicular ligament) then to the sustentaculum and spring (plantar calcaneonavicular ligament) as the calcaneotibial ligament, and posteriorly to the talus as the posterior talotibial ligament. The deep portion originates on the intercolliculus and the posterior colliculus of the tibia and inserts on the nonarticular medial wall of the talus as the talotibial ligament.

Although ankle injury is most often sustained by ligaments, knowledge of the regional anatomy helps localize diagnosis to nonligamentous structures. Medially, the posterior tibial, flexor digitorum longus, and flexor hallucis tendons are restrained in separate sheaths by the laciniate ligament. Laterally, the inferior and superior peroneal retinaculum restrains the peroneal tendons in their groove in the retrofibular region.

Biomechanics

Ankle motion consists of a gliding motion of the tibia over the talar dome, with bony anatomy supplementing ligamentous structures as static restraints. Ligamentous injury occurs when physiologic loads are exceeded, or during movement when the contribution of osseous stability is minimized. Classic ligamentous sectioning studies have attempted to clarify the contribution of each individual ligament to stability. Unfortunately, the all-or-none nature of ligament sectioning studies cannot recreate the pathologic ankle with abnormal secondary or other primary ligamentous restraints. Additionally, most of the earlier ligamentous sectioning studies were done without an applied axial load. Subsequent studies found that axial rotation and/or talar tilting decreased with increasing axial load so that it was concluded that the articular surfaces provided the main constraint to talar tilting. These bench studies are limited because axial rotation or inversion was constrained during testing. In an elegant recent study using computed tomography, axial load, and neither inversion nor external rotation constraints, no talar tilting occurred with isolated sectioning of the ATFL or CFL alone. Talar tilt occurred in all specimens when both ligaments were sectioned. It appears likely that earlier ligamentous sectioning studies, by constraining motion and/or not using axial loading, overstated both the role of the articular surfaces and individual ligaments such as the CFL as a restraint to inversion.

Classic studies by Inman revealed the obliquity of both the ankle and subtalar axes with respect to their anatomic axes so that inversion consists of external rotation of the leg and adduction of the hindfoot. External rotation of the leg unlocks the subtalar joint allowing further inversion. Newer studies emphasize the coupling of the ATFL and CFL to limit external rotation of the leg and thereby secondarily keep the hindfoot "locked" to prevent further inversion. Ankle instability appears to be a combination of axial rotation and talar tilting in the mortise.

Biomechanical strain gauge studies have indicated that the ATFL is weakest, least stiff, and has the greatest strain to failure of all the ankle ligaments. It is the primary restraint to anterior displacement, internal rotation, and inversion of the talus at all flexion angles. Strain in the CFL has been shown to increase from plantarflexion to dorsiflexion.

Etiology, Pathology, and Mechanism of Injury

Attenuation or rupture of ankle ligamentous structures can lead to mechanical or ligamentous instability. The muscular or dynamic restraints to ankle instability may compensate in an ankle with ligamentous instability to provide a functionally stable ankle. In the injured ankle, proprioceptive deficits and prolonged reaction times of the peroneal muscles have been electromyographically demonstrated. Conservative, nonsurgical ankle rehabilitation protocols attempt to improve proprioceptive function and peroneal reaction time by taping, bracing, proprioceptive training, and strengthening. It has been postulated that repetitive minor sprains can lead to a mechanical or ligamentous instability.

Surgical exploration of acute lateral ligamentous injury indicates that the majority of ankle injuries are midsubstance tears to the ATFL, occurring with a 60% to 70% frequency, followed by a 20% incidence of combined ATFL/CFL injury. Syndesmotic, deltoid, isolated CFL or PTFL, and subtalar ligament injuries make up the remaining 10% of ankle injuries.

Despite the limitations of extrapolating bench studies mentioned previously, the ATFL is most probably injured with inversion, plantarflexion, and internal rotation forces, whereas the CFL is injured with inversion and dorsiflexion.

Diagnosis of Ankle Ligamentous Injury

A detailed history with particular attention to mechanism of injury, combined with a competent physical examination provides the basis for accurate diagnosis of ankle ligament injuries. Exactly where the ankle hurts, the position of the foot and direction of force, and the functional capability following injury are key elements in the history. The elicitation of point palpation tenderness warrants plain radiographs to rule out a fracture.

Early initial examination prior to diffuse swelling and ecchymosis is important to pinpoint which structures are injured. The determination between tenderness over the lateral collateral ligaments versus the inferior tibiofibular ligaments helps distinguish a lateral ankle ligament injury from a syndesmotic injury. The entire fibula should be palpated to clinically detect a deltoid injury with fracture or dislocation of the fibula. Retrofibular tenderness or subluxability of the peroneal tendons may indicate a superior peroneal retinaculum or peroneal tendon injury. Associated injuries should be clinically ruled out by the systematic detection of point pal-

pation tenderness at the sinus tarsi, base of fifth metatarsal, Chopart joint, anterior ankle, posterior talus, subtalar region, and Achilles tendon.

Ligamentous stress testing is controversial and probably unreliable without anesthesia in the acute or subacute setting as a result of protective spasticity. Mechanical instability should be documented through stress radiographs only if it will help clarify the specific structures affected and the extent of tissue injury and thereby affect treatment protocol. When the talus is neutrally positioned, excessive inversion motion or pain may indicate subtalar instability, although this is a difficult diagnosis to quantitate and detect. It is recommended that the anterior drawer be performed in slight plantarflexion with the fingers of one hand placed on the talus. If the test is positive and the talus does not move, then subtalar rather than tibiotalar instability theoretically exists though this is difficult to demonstrate clinically. It is estimated that approximately 10% of patients with lateral instability of the ankle will have coexistent subtalar instability. Comparison with the contralateral limb is important because ligamentous instability may not be pathologic if the ankle is functionally stable.

Provocative tests for syndesmotic injury include the squeeze test. Pain at the ankle region with the squeezing of tibia and fibula in the mid-calf is suggestive of a syndesmotic injury. Painful external rotation of the neutrally positioned ankle with the knee flexed to 90° also indicates a probable syndesmotic injury.

Diagnostic Imaging and Procedures

In today's climate of health-care cost containment, it is important to distinguish between what can and should be ordered. The initial evaluation of significant ankle ligamentous injuries should routinely consist of and probably be limited to radiographic images. Injury confined to the ankle region at a minimum should consist of a mortise view to demonstrate uniform joint spacing and a lateral view of the foot (weightbearing, if possible). An anteroposterior (AP) view completes the series and helps reveal fractures of the lateral process of the talus. If clinically indicated by point palpation tenderness, an AP of the foot will reveal avulsion fractures of Chopart joints, unsuspected midfoot injuries, and fifth metatarsal fractures. Oblique radiographs of the foot reveal an anterior process of the calcaneus fracture in addition to confirming alignment of the tarsometatarsal joints.

Stress radiographs help document clinical tests for mechanical instability, although anatomic studies report wide variability in measurement of talar tilt and anterior ankle translation in normal asymptomatic ankles. Utility of stress radiographs is diminishing, and they should be confined to specific instances in which the clinical treatment regimen may be affected. Relative indications for stress radiographs may be in the elite athlete where prognosis, duration, and intensity of rehabilitation and other factors are important although the diagnosis of mechanical instability is primarily a clinical one.

Definitions of abnormal talar tilt vary from 3° to 15° greater than the contralateral limb, or an absolute value greater than 9°, thereby limiting radiographic exposure to the abnormal ankle. Similarly, an absolute value of 5 to 10 mm forward translation on lateral view of the talus or 3 mm more than the contralateral limb indicates ligamentous (mechanical) instability. Because of the anatomic position of the ligaments, an abnormal anterior drawer and talar tilt in ankle plantarflexion correlates with an ATFL injury and a talar tilt in dorsiflexion with CFL injury although a combined continuum of injury to both ligaments probably exists. Attempts to standardize forces and positioning with special devices to apply a uniform stress have not proven clinically useful.

Because of its anatomic alignment, the CFL is felt to be a restraint to abnormal motion of both the tibiotalar and the subtalar joint. A 40° stress Broden's view recommended to detect subtalar instability is more difficult to document and more controversial than the talar tilt images for ankle instability. Loss of parallelism of the posterior facet or > 3 mm anterior translation on the lateral view indicate subtalar instability. A recent study challenged these claims, detecting significant variability in subtalar radiographs in an asymptomatic, uninjured population. In cadaveric studies, to detect significant changes on subtalar stress views, the tibiotalocalcaneal ligament must be sectioned correlating with a severe subtalar injury. Also, considerable anatomic variability in the orientation of ligaments, especially the CFL, may help explain the large ranges of different stress radiographic measurements.

Plain weightbearing radiographs help evaluate the syndesmotic region for injury. A reliable indicator is the measurement of the clear space between the medial border of the fibula and the lateral border of the posterior tibia at the incisura fibularis measured at 1 cm above the plafond. This measurement should be 6 mm or less on both the AP and mortise views. Equal distances between the tibiotalar and medial space should also exist. A common error is to have the foot plantarflexed during imaging, which artificially increases the medial clear space, again indicating the importance of standing radiographs.

Ankle arthrograms have been shown to have a near 100% reliability for the diagnosis of acute ATFL rupture if performed within the first week of injury. The usefulness of this test is diminishing as the indication for immediate surgical treatment of ankle ligament injury is similarly decreasing. Similarly, peroneal tenograms may document injury to the peroneal sheaths but are primarily of historical interest.

High resolution computed tomography (CT) or magnetic resonance imaging (MRI) can document osteochondral injury, ligamentous injury, and tendon injury, but the cost can be prohibitive in the acute setting. In the acute setting, a delayed physical examination 5 days after injury was found to be 84% specific and 90% sensitive for the detection of complete ankle ligament rupture. Physical examination was found to be superior to arthrography, stress radiographs, and ultrasonography in this study, although the MRI was not evaluated as a diagnostic modality. In another study, physical diagnosis detected 100% of grade III ankle injuries but only 25% of grade II injuries. MRI detected grade II ankle sprains that were not picked up on physical examination, but the authors recommended MRI as an imaging modality only for ankle injuries failing initial conservative measures. For suspected cases of osteochondral injury, the MRI has a major role. In the chronic setting, if surgical intervention is planned and the treatment, diagnosis, or surgical approach may be altered based on information provided by those imaging techniques, then these tests may be considered for greater definition of the pathologic process.

Classification of Soft-Tissue Injuries of the Ankle

The easily understood single ligament injury classification (grade I, stretch, intact ligaments; grade II, partial tear; grade III, complete rupture) does not correlate well with a description of injury to the 3 ligaments of the lateral ligament complex. Because of the prevalence of injuries to the lateral ligament complex, grade I ankle sprain is commonly described as a mild injury to the lateral ankle ligament complex with minor swelling and tenderness, with slight or no functional loss. The ankle is mechanically stable with negative stress test findings. Normal activity is possible but painful, and the pathology is believed to be limited to, at most, a partial tear of the ATFL and minor strain of the CFL.

A grade II injury is a moderate ankle injury with diffuse swelling, tenderness, and difficult weightbearing. Functional activity is significantly limited, and the ankle is partially unstable. A partial to complete injury of the ATFL provides a mildly positive anterior drawer in plantarflexion but the par-

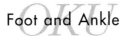

tial tear of the CFL provides a negative talar tilt stress examination. Grade III ankle sprains represent severe double ligament injury, usually with complete rupture of the ATFL and CFL. Weightbearing is not usually tolerated, and there is marked tenderness, swelling, and pain. Both anterior drawer and talar tilt tests in dorsiflexion and plantarflexion are clinically and radiographically positive. Injury to the PTFL is rarely present and is not a clinically significant injury pattern.

Complete syndesmotic rupture in the absence of fractures or plastic deformation of the fibula is rare. Although there is a continuum of injury from grades I to III, the most clinically useful classification scheme uses the terms latent and frank diastasis. A frank diastasis is a complete (grade III) rupture of the syndesmosis evident on plain radiographs. A latent diastasis requires stress radiographs to demonstrate the complete syndesmotic injury. Grade I and II injuries to the syndesmosis are clinically stable. The utility of stress radiographs for this injury to distinguish a grade II (stable) from a grade III (latent diastasis) is important, because the treatment recommendations are significantly different. Other classification schemes include a temporal element (acute, subacute, or chronic) and the presence or absence of tibiotalar arthritis and synostosis.

The acute isolated deltoid injuries are generally classified as grade I or II ligament sprains. Though complete rupture of both the superficial and deep deltoid is not uncommon, this grade III ligament sprain is virtually always associated with a fracture and is documented through ankle fracture classification schemes.

Injury to the superior peroneal retinaculum may accompany deltoid ligamentous injury due to the common mechanism of injury of dorsiflexion, eversion, and external rotation. Retrofibular tenderness, subluxability of the peroneal tendons, and a radiographic "fleck sign" of an osteochondral bone fragment that anchors the retinaculum indicates a superior peroneal retinacular injury. Classification systems for chronic injury exist but more important than a particular classification system is the early recognition of the injury, because treatment regimens vary depending upon whether the injury is acute or chronic.

Subtalar ligament injuries are of recent note, interest, and controversy. Through clinical experience and ligament sectioning studies of the interosseous, CFL, and cervical ligaments, subtalar instability has been demonstrated. Whether isolated subtalar instability exists or is seen as a continuum of ankle injury is uncertain. Subtalar instability is considered to exist when clinically present and radiographically confirmed with stress radiographs. At present, classification is limited to a temporal basis of acute or chronic subtalar instability.

Treatment of Acute Ankle Injuries

The most important step in determining an ankle injury treatment regimen is to define precisely the structures injured and the severity of injury. The majority of soft-tissue injuries to the ankle can be initially treated with the conservative PRICE regimen (Protection, Rest, Ice, Compression, and Elevation) to limit the extent of injury, to control edema, and to minimize pain. Anti-inflammatories have a definite role during the acute injury phase. Grade I and II lateral ankle injuries are mechanically stable but may benefit from short-term immobilization or protection in a stirrup-type brace or fracture boot until nonprotected weightbearing is relatively pain-free. During the protection period, nonweightbearing ankle range-of-motion exercises should be performed gradually, progressing to increasing weightbearing, strengthening, proprioception, and, ultimately, agility training. Crutch use should be continued until there is an adequate reciprocal gait with minimal limp. Formal physical therapy for early range of motion, edema control, proprioception, and peroneal strengthening is clearly helpful in shortening the period of disability, but a carefully supervised home program can be equally successful. Most ankle sprains should be reexamined in the office to ensure adequate progress, to confirm the diagnosis, to counsel for further strengthening and rehabilitation, and to rule out an untoward process such as reflex sympathetic dystrophy. Generally, a grade I ankle sprain should be nearing full return at 1 to 2 weeks and a grade II at 2 to 3 weeks, but the recovery in some instances may be significantly longer. Injuries to the syndesmosis (high ankle sprain) are often underrecognized, mislabeled as lateral ankle ligament injuries, and these may account for some prolonged recovery periods. Residual symptoms, subsequent instability, or prolonged recovery periods are related to the severity of injury and are more commonly seen with grade III ankle injuries.

Because of the mechanical instability (by definition) of grade III ligament injuries, varied treatment regimens have evolved. In the high level athletes, it was previously believed that a grade III injury mandated surgical repair. Prospective randomized studies comparing various treatment protocols are helping to clarify the controversy. A recent prospective study found nearly identical eventual results with surgical versus nonsurgical treatment of grade III ankle sprains in the acute setting, but the surgical group had a longer recovery time, more complications, and a slightly higher rate of residual symptoms. Most recent prospective studies indicate the success of a nonsurgical protocol, so that the indications for early surgical intervention are decreasing.

The nonsurgical treatment of grade III ankle sprains is slightly controversial because of the mechanical instability of the ankle ligaments. Options include functional bracing and mobilization versus resting and immobilization. Functional bracing implies a removable brace with progressive weight-bearing, range of motion, strengthening, and proprioception training. Proponents of cast treatment advocate 4 to 6 weeks of casting in slight dorsiflexion and eversion to anatomically reapproximate the ligaments; then begin the range of motion and functional rehabilitation described above. Recent MRI studies have indicated that grade III ligament ruptures will heal in continuity even if there is early mobilization. Presently, in the United States, short-term immobilization in a cast for grade III injuries is a widespread treatment protocol. A recent review of all prospective randomized treatment protocols for grade III ankle sprains involving cast immobilization, functional mobilization, and surgery indicated functional rehabilitation to be the preferred protocol in terms of cost, rapidity of recovery, stability, improved mobility, and fewer complications. Rapid mobilization with functional rehabilitation should replace the short-term cast immobilization protocols currently used.

Orthopaedists are often asked when, following an ankle injury, sport activity can be resumed. Successful performance of simple tests such as the ability to run, cut, jump 10 times onto the single injured foot, and to stand on one foot with the eyes closed for a minute without excessive pain provide general and adequate guidelines for safe return to sports activity. If Biodex testing is available, eversion strength should be at least 80% of the contralateral limb prior to allowing unrestricted activity. Protection in an ankle stirrup or taping primarily provides proprioceptive feedback and some physical support and should be continued until the ankle is asymptomatic and free of any swelling. Recent studies indicate that these supportive devices or taping have no measurable impact on athletic performance.

Syndesmotic Injuries

Syndesmotic or "high ankle sprains" are infrequent injuries but frequently misdiagnosed. Various reports indicate 1% to 15% of "ankle sprains" involve injury to the syndesmosis, with football and skiing being particularly high-risk sports. History and physical examination are keys to the diagnosis, because plain radiographs are often reported normal. In this suspected injury, use of stress examinations can be important to distinguish between a stable strain of the syndesmosis and deltoid versus an unstable or latent diastasis. A stable injury can be rapidly mobilized, whereas a latent diastasis should be protected and immobilized for 6 to 8 weeks.

Unstable frank diastasis injuries may be associated with plastic deformation of the fibula, posterior subluxation of the fibula, dislocation of the talus, or medial entrapment of the deltoid ligament. Treatment recommendations include open reduction and internal fixation with placement of a non-lagged syndesmotic screw engaging three cortices, which must be placed with the foot dorsiflexed. Fibular osteotomy may be indicated in instances of fibular plastic deformation. Weightbearing, removal of screws, and use of resorbable screws all are controversial, although redisplacement with screw removal prior to 8 weeks has been reported. Symptomatic calcification of the intraosseous membrane has been reported, but most studies indicate a good long-term prognosis with appropriate reduction and treatment of syndesmotic widening.

Deltoid Ligament Injuries

Significant injuries to the deltoid without lateral fractures or syndesmotic injury are extremely rare and should trigger proximal fibular radiographs and stress external rotation view to rule out occult syndesmotic injury or fibular fracture. Adequate maintenance of the medial clear space in a cast or fracture brace coupled with appropriate ankle rehabilitation should provide adequate results, although medial injuries tend to take longer to heal than lateral injuries.

Subtalar Injuries

Subtalar injuries can be reproduced in the laboratory setting with sectioning of the CFL and other ligaments of the subtalar ligament complex. Their incidence, prevalence, and concomitant existence with lateral ankle ligament injuries is controversial. One prospective arthrographic study revealed that 80% of acute lateral ankle sprains had significant subtalar injury indicated by leakage of the dye with subtalar injection. The recommendation to use stress Broden views to indicate subtalar instability has been challenged recently. A study comparing stress Broden views taken under fluoroscopic guidance failed to detect any radiographic difference between symptomatic and asymptomatic feet. Further studies regarding the diagnostic criteria for subtalar instability are needed to help clarify these issues.

Failed Ankle Sprain

The primary cause of a persistently painful sprained ankle is unrecognized peroneal weakness. Inadequate rehabilitation should be addressed while determining whether continued symptoms are due to pain or instability. A painful lateral ankle may "give way," mimicking instability; or a mechanically unstable ankle can invert and cause pain. Mechanical

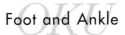

instability is simply defined by an excessive ankle mobility beyond physiologic norms determined by physical signs (drawer, talar tilt) or stress measurements. This ankle may or may not be symptomatic. Functional instability, on the other hand, is a subjective feeling of the ankle giving way during an activity. A mechanically stable ankle (normal static ligament restraints) can be functionally unstable. The exact pathophysiologic factors responsible for functional instability are not defined and may represent a combination of mechanical, functional, and neuromuscular defects. Etiologies may include injury to the lateral ligaments, proprioceptive defects, peroneal (dynamic stabilizer) weakness, and subtalar instability. Repetitive sprains from a functional instability may later result in mechanical instability. Extensive rehabilitation may compensate for a functional or mechanical instability but will probably not alleviate the "giving way" episodes resulting from a painful intra-articular stimulus.

Documented mechanical instability that does not respond to appropriate rehabilitation can be effectively treated with surgical techniques for the chronically unstable ankle. A mechanically stable ankle that is persistently painful is a more difficult entity to treat, and the surgeon must critically rule out potential missed diagnoses. A history of chronic ankle instability is characterized by asymptomatic periods between episodes of "sprain," whereas other causes of chronic ankle pain tend to fluctuate in severity but are constant in nature. In addition to inadequate peroneal rehabilitation and chronic ankle instability, the differential diagnoses of the persistently painful sprained ankle include intra-articular pathology, subtalar instability, syndesmosis injury, posterior impingement syndrome, sinus tarsi syndrome, tendon disorders, stress fracture, arthritis, reflex sympathetic dystrophy, nerve injury, tumors, and undetected epiphyseal injuries in the skeletally immature. A review of all prior studies, performance of stress radiographs, and consideration of selective injection, a bone scan, or more sophisticated imaging techniques such as the MRI should be considered if clinically indicated or to further clarify the specific anatomic injury.

In the painful ankle with no documentable instability, the anterior inferior aspect of the fibula will often be tender in the region of the anterior talofibular ligament (ATFL). Almost half a century ago, an internal derangement of fibrocartilaginous scar tissue was reported and later termed the "meniscoid lesion." This scar tissue is readily evident arthroscopically and can result from the inferior slip of the anterior tibiofibular ligament, synovial hypertrophy, or partial tear of the ATFL. Intra-articular steroid injections coupled with anesthetic at the site of maximal tenderness should provide a good diagnostic/therapeutic test. A recent prospective study of arthroscopically confirmed soft-tissue anterolateral impingement lesions revealed competent clinical examination to be superior to the MRI to detect these lesions. If no other causes of symptoms can be determined, arthroscopy via noninvasive distraction should be performed at 6 months for a persistently painful but mechanically stable ankle.

Treatment of Chronic Ankle Instability

The distinction between functional and mechanical instability tends to blur on a temporal basis and coexists in the chronically unstable ankle. Failing appropriate proprioceptive training and peroneal strengthening, the documentation of mechanical instability may be by clinical examination or stress radiographs described previously. Inversion instability may be of subtalar origin and needs to be considered.

The nonsurgical treatment of chronic ankle instability includes restriction of activities and various shoe or brace options. The pedorthic treatment of chronic ankle instability includes a lateral heel wedge, a flared sole, reinforced counter, avoidance of high heels, and use of high top sneakers or a chukka boot. Bracing measures include a University of California, Berkeley, orthosis, an ankle-foot orthosis (AFO), or a hinged AFO. All these measures can prove effective in the well-selected patient.

The multiple techniques for the surgical treatment of lateral ankle instability fall into one of two categories: anatomic repair or nonanatomic reconstruction. The former involves a recreation, imbrication, or repair of the anatomic ankle ligaments as a nonaugmented ankle reconstruction. The latter involves a substitution of an endogenous tendon or other material to replace mechanically insufficient ligaments as an augmented ankle reconstruction.

The anatomic, nonaugmented, direct repair of lateral ankle ligaments with recurrent instability was originally advocated by Broström some 30 years ago and has been modified by Peterson, Gould, and others (Fig. 2). A principal advantage is the maintenance of anatomic ligament attachment sites with the preservation of dynamic stabilizers (peroneal tendons). Range of ankle motion should theoretically be maintained if the ankle ligaments are anatomically reconstructed. This preservation of ankle motion coupled with stability is crucial for elite ballet dancers and other athletes and is a major factor in the selection of this surgical technique. Theoretically, return of a more normal tension to the anatomic ligaments may improve proprioceptive training, shorten rehabilitation time, and result in preservation of peroneal tendons. Variations in technique include surgical incision, augmentation with regional tissues (osteochondral flaps), extensor retinacular reinforcement, and suture anchoring techniques. Originally, a transverse oblique incision was advocated, whereas a

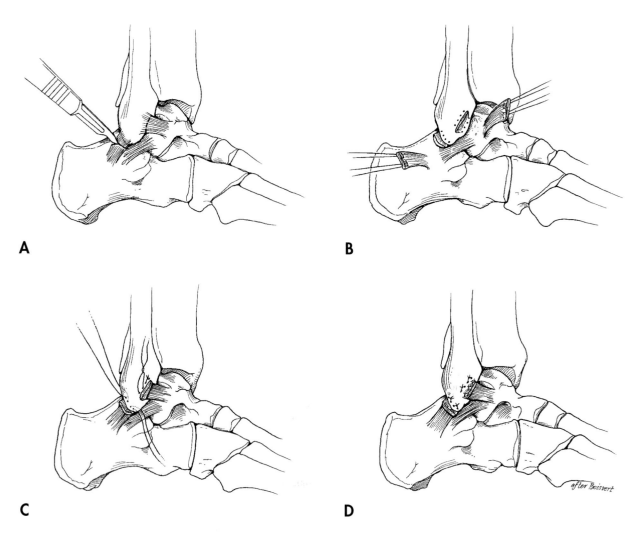

A

B

C

D

after Boissert

Figure 2

Anatomic reconstruction of chronic ankle ligament instability according to Peterson. **A,** Elongated ligaments are divided 3 to 5 mm from insertion on the fibula. **B,** Bone surface of the distal end of the fibula is roughened to form a trough to promote ligament healing. Holes are drilled through the distal fibula. **C,** Mattress sutures are used to fix the distal stump of the ligaments and the capsule to the fibula. The sutures are tightened while the foot is held in dorsiflexion and eversion. **D,** The proximal ends of the ligaments are imbricated over the distal portion. (Reproduced with permission from Renström PAFH: Persistently painful sprained ankle. *J Am Acad Orthop Surg* 1994;2:270–280.)

longitudinal incision allows inspection of the peroneal tendons, the subsequent use of the peroneal tendons for an augmentation technique if necessary, and a decreased incidence of iatrogenic injury to branches of the superficial peroneal nerve. Earlier reported failures of anatomic ligamentous reconstruction techniques were thought to be caused by failure to reconstruct the CFL. Relative contraindications to an anatomic reconstruction include failed prior surgery, longstanding (> 10 years) instability with severely attenuated tissues, connective tissue disorders with hyperlaxity, and fixed heel varus.

The modified Broström technique involves the addition of the extensor retinaculum as a reinforcement to the repair and has been gaining popularity with reports of excellent functional results (Fig. 3). A recent prospective comparison of the direct repair of ankle ligaments versus the modified Broström technique with augmentation of the inferior extensor retinaculum revealed no difference in functional outcome. One of the few prospective studies comparing anatomic reconstruction with various check-rein procedures revealed equivalent functional results with decreased complications from the anatomic reconstruction.

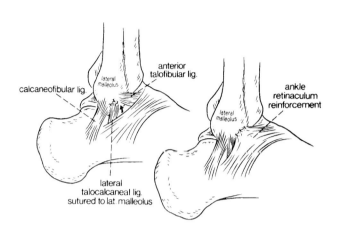

Figure 3

Modification of the Broström reconstruction includes an imbrication of the inferior extensor retinaculum to reinforce the repair. (Reproduced with permission from Gould N: Technique tips: Footings. Repair of lateral ligament of ankle. *Foot Ankle* 1987;8:55–58.)

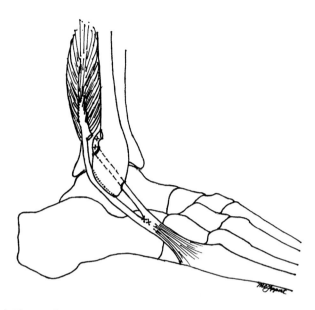

Figure 4

Modified Evans technique utilizing half the peroneus brevis tendon.

Numerous check-rein procedures exist that use local tendons for the replacement or the augmentation of incompetent ligaments. The majority of the most popular procedures report 80% to 90% good and excellent results, but critical evaluation of range of ankle motion and reporting of residual pain varies considerably in these reports. Residual stiffness following check-rein reconstructions may be due to the biomechanical differences between tendons and ligaments. Biomechanical studies of intact lateral ankle ligaments and tendons indicate that the split peroneus tendon graft has a greater load to failure than the ATFL and is approximately as strong as the CFL. Unfortunately, the tendon grafts were significantly stiffer (less strain) and had much less strain to failure (stretchability) than ligaments. Graft placement therefore is critical because inaccurate placement can result in significant loss of motion (ankle stiffness) or tendon graft failure.

Substitute materials for the peroneal tendon include allografts, synthetic materials, extensor digitorum longus or plantaris tendon, partial Achilles tendon, and a portion of the fascia lata. No distinct advantage to any of these materials has yet been evidenced in a long-term study. Until such documentation, the primary surgical option for ligamentous ankle reconstruction includes either an anatomic reconstruction (Broström) or one of several peroneus brevis check-rein techniques.

The simplest check-rein technique is the commonly used Evans technique, which involves placing a split peroneus brevis graft through the resultant vector of the ATFL and CFL (Fig. 4). Originally, the technique involved using the entire peroneus brevis graft, but biomechanical studies indicate that the split peroneus tendon graft is of adequate strength to serve as a ligament replacement. Subsequent revision surgery in cases using half of the peroneus brevis tendon indicated that the retained (split) peroneus brevis appears to hypertrophy and maintain its role as a dynamic ankle stabilizer so that augmentation techniques should not sacrifice the entire peroneus brevis tendon.

The Watson-Jones technique involves a tenodesis of the peroneus brevis tendon to the fibula with anterior routing through the fibula to reconstruct the ATFL (Fig. 5). This technique has been demonstrated to control internal rotation and anterior displacement but is less effective in controlling talar tilt as it reconstructs only the ATFL. The third major and most frequently used nonanatomic reconstruction is the Chrisman-Snook modification of the Elmslie reconstruction (Fig. 6). This technique uses one half of the peroneus brevis tendon to reconstruct the ATFL and CFL. All three of these techniques have been criticized for substituting for the function of, but not accurately recreating, the ATFL or CFL. Frequently, illustrations of these techniques vary in the orientation of drill holes, fixation of tendons, and the exact tendon weaving technique. All of these techniques have been shown in clinical studies to effectively stabilize the ankle, but they have been associated with restricted inversion. In addition to subtalar stiffness, a frequent complaint of residual pain is reported in most series of augmented

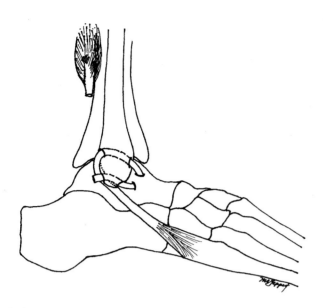

Figure 5

Watson-Jones technique utilizing the entire peroneus brevis tendon.

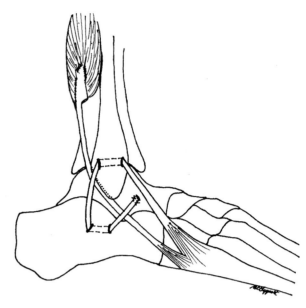

Figure 6

Chrisman-Snook technique with half the peroneus brevis tendon.

reconstructions. Subsequent modifications of these techniques involve an attempt to more anatomically recreate the location of the ATFL and CFL. A recent technique reported by Colvile most accurately recreates the anatomy of the injured ligaments and effectively provides functional stability but is accompanied in a limited series with residual complaints of ankle pain.

Comparison of augmented and nonaugmented techniques has some intrinsic limitations. Bench cadaveric studies compare the biomechanical strength of tissues but ignore the contribution of dynamic stabilizers, which are preserved in nonaugmented reconstructions. Despite this limitation, the modified Broström reconstruction was shown in a recent cadaveric study to provide a greater mechanical restraint to anterior drawer and talar tilt displacement than either the Watson-Jones or Chrisman-Snook technique. A biomechanical comparison between the Evans, Watson-Jones, and Chrisman-Snook techniques revealed the Evans procedure to provide the most consistent increase in stability with the least abnormal reduction in subtalar motion. The Chrisman-Snook provided good stability but restricted subtalar motion significantly more than an ankle with intact ligaments.

Multiple clinical studies of ankle reconstructions indicate satisfactory short-term results for all techniques. Anatomic reconstructions originated in Europe and have a longer clinical history there. The tradition of nonanatomic reconstructions originated in the United States and continues so that clinical prospective studies are needed to make more definite

recommendations between and within augmented and nonaugmented techniques. A recent prospective randomized comparison of Chrisman-Snook and modified Broström procedures revealed similar stability in greater than 80% of the patients but a significantly higher complication rate with the more extensive Chrisman-Snook procedure. A European study by Wallenboch found improved long-term results after anatomic reconstruction over both the Watson-Jones or Evans procedures and a long-term study of the Evans tenodesis indicated satisfactory results in less than 50% of cases.

Currently, indications and recommendations for surgical management of a clinically unstable ankle would include: (1) failed complete peroneal and proprioceptive training; (2) preferred anatomic reconstruction with some variations of a Broström technique if adequate tissue exists; (3) combined calcaneal osteotomy for excessive heel varus; (4) augmentation with the inferior extensor retinaculum or slip of peroneus brevis tendon if there is severe attenuation of tissue; and (5) primary augmentation techniques in ankles with severe ligamentous laxity.

Failure of Ankle Ligament Surgery

Every surgical approach to ankle ligament reconstruction must consider the potential need for surgical revision or change in technique if local tissues prove inadequate and augmentation techniques are subsequently required. For this

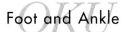

reason, longitudinal incisions are preferred for the anatomic reconstructions. Additionally, inspection of peroneal tendons for concomitant pathology is more easily performed through longitudinal incisions, and iatrogenic injury to the regional superficial peroneal branches is less likely to occur.

The primary complications to consider are an ankle that has become "too stiff" or "too loose" following reconstruction. Excessive stiffness may be due to inadequate rehabilitation, prolonged immobilization, or fixing the reconstructed, augmented tissues too tightly. The anatomic reconstructions appear to have a lesser incidence of subtalar rigidity (loss of inversion movement) than the augmented techniques. Arthroscopic lysis of adhesions and manipulation should be used following failed rehabilitation and prior to revising a ligament reconstruction.

Recurrent instability following reconstruction is most often caused by inadequate rehabilitation, but if an ankle is unstable or becomes unstable following reconstruction, a change in surgical technique should be considered. Successful repeat Broström revisions have been reported, but these most often occur if the index procedure was successful and the patient sustained a significant reinjury.

Unrecognized heel varus, connective tissue disorders with generalized laxity, or inadequate tissue or technique often results in recurrent instability. Corrective heel osteotomy may be indicated; the region explored and possibly an additional augmentation technique used if anatomic reconstruction has failed. The addition of a peroneus brevis slip to the resultant vector of the ATFL and CFL, as in an Evans procedure, is my personal choice when potential stiffness is traded for recurrent instability. Adequate attention to restoring the scarred CFL and ATFL is necessary for success. This approach is particularly expedient if faced with an oblique/transverse incision, which limits safe exposure for the additional dissection needed for a more complicated augmentation technique.

Prevention

Because of the prevalence of lateral ankle ligament injury, a great emphasis has been placed on prevention. A prospective twofold decrease in the incidence of ankle sprains among high-level volleyball players was attributed to an injury prevention program. Theoretically, correction of predisposing conditions such as weak extrinsics, weak peroneals, proprioceptive defects, midfoot varus, inadequate shoe wear, and other factors should decrease the incidence of ankle injury but critical controlled studies are lacking.

In addition to these, rule changes such as breakaway bases, a return to natural turf, and a change in cleat pattern should reduce the incidence of injury. The role of protective devices, such as taping or bracing, to prevent ankle injury remains controversial. Braces are reusable, adjustable, washable, more cost effective, and their use requires minimal time or expertise. Taping, on the other hand, although it is more time consuming and expensive, and rapidly loses its effectiveness, is the traditional athlete's preference. One study indicates that strong active evertor muscles are the most effective form of ankle protection. Braces, taping, or high-topped shoes, however, are the most effective forms of protection from inversion injury when the evertor muscles are inactive.

Athletic performance has been tested and found not to be affected by the wearing of ankle braces. In a clinical prospective study, ankle stabilizers were demonstrated to significantly reduce the frequency but not the severity of ankle injury. It is thought that both taping and bracing provides a shortened reaction time, thereby affecting the proprioceptive function of the ankle. The reaction time for reflex activation of the dynamic stabilizers has, however, been determined to be too slow in the case of unanticipated sudden inversion stresses. Protection from ankle injury may require anticipated preinversion muscle activity. Bracing or taping enhances exterior support to reinforce the static stabilizers and enhance proprioceptive awareness, in addition to preloading the ankle.

Bracing clearly has advantages over taping in terms of cost and ease of use. Braces have not impeded physiologic performance in several studies, although the psychological effects of bracing may interfere with patient compliance. Semirigid braces clearly have resulted in a decreased incidence of ankle injury in contact injuries. Athletes with prior ankle injury or ankle reconstructions, who have a higher incidence of reinjury than those with noninjured ankles, are the most appropriate candidates for prophylactic bracing.

Annotated Bibliography

Review Articles

Bennett WF: Lateral ankle sprains: Part I. Anatomy, biomechanics, diagnosis, and natural history. *Orthop Rev* 1994;23: 381–387.

This article is a review of the essential fundamentals of ankle sprains.

Renstrom PA, Konradsen L: Ankle ligament injuries. *Br J Sports Med* 1997;31:11–20.

This is the most current and comprehensive review of ankle ligament injuries, and includes an extensive bibliography.

Anatomy and Biomechanics

Burks RT, Morgan J: Anatomy of the lateral ankle ligaments. *Am J Sports Med* 1994;22:72–77.

A more precise description of the anatomic attachments of the ATFL and CF ligaments allows a more anatomic (isometric) ligament reconstruction.

Cass JR, Settles H: Ankle instability: In vitro kinematics in response to axial load. *Foot Ankle Int* 1994;15:134–140.

This important study used computed tomography and permitted free axial rotation in ligamentous sectioning studies to demonstrate that the ATFL and CFL work in tandem to prevent tilting of the talus. This study disputes prior reports that attribute primary stability in version stress to the articular surfaces.

Earll M, Wayne J, Brodrick C, Vokshoor A, Adelaar R: Contribution of the deltoid ligament to ankle joint contact characteristics: A cadaver study. *Foot Ankle Int* 1996;17:317–324.

Significant changes in peak pressures and joint contact characteristics result before significant radiographic changes in medial talar tilt are present, indicating that greater attention to the medial side of the ankle may be required to restore normal biomechanics to the ankle.

Ogilvie-Harris DJ, Reed SC, Hedman TP: Disruption of the ankle syndesmosis: Biomechanical study of the ligamentous restraints. *Arthroscopy* 1994;10:558–560.

The anterior inferior tibiofibular, deep posterior inferior tibiofibular, and interosseous ligaments are the primary restraints of the syndesmosis. The latter ligament can be visualized arthroscopically.

Mechanism of Injury

Miller CD, Shelton WR, Barrett GR, Savoie FH, Dukes AD: Deltoid and syndesmosis ligament injury of the ankle without fracture. *Am J Sports Med* 1995;23:746–750.

Diagnosis of tears of the deltoid and syndesmotic ligaments without fracture requires a high index of suspicion, including possible stress radiographic analysis.

Roberts CS, DeMaio M, Larkin JJ, Paine R: Eversion ankle sprains. *Orthopedics* 1995;18:299–304.

The diagnosis, treatment, and rehabilitation of stable eversion ankle sprains are reviewed.

Veltri DM, Pagnani MJ, O'Brien SJ, Warren RF, Ryan MD, Barnes RP: Symptomatic ossification of the tibiofibular syndesmosis in professional football players: A sequela of the syndesmotic ankle sprain. *Foot Ankle Int* 1995:16:285–290.

Symptomatic ossification of the syndesmosis was successfully treated by excision with a full painless return to sports by 2 professional athletes.

Xenos JS, Hopkinson WJ, Mulligan ME, Olson EJ, Popovic NA: The tibiofibular syndesmosis: Evaluation of the ligamentous structures, methods of fixation, and radiographic assessment. *J Bone Joint Surg* 1995;77A:847–856.

This article convincingly argues that the stress lateral radiograph appears to provide a more reliable assessment of the syndesmosis than the more familiar stress mortise view.

Physical Examination and Diagnostic Studies

Frey C, Bell J, Teresi L, Kerr R, Feder K: A comparison of MRI and clinical examination of acute lateral ankle sprains. *Foot Ankle Int* 1996;17:533–537.

Physical examination alone is sufficient to diagnose grade III ankle ligament injuries but is far less sensitive than the MRI for grade II injuries.

Liu SH, Nuccion SL, Finerman G: Diagnosis of anterolateral ankle impingement: Comparison between magnetic resonance imaging and clinical examination. *Am J Sports Med* 1997; 25:389–393.

Competent physical examination is superior to the MRI for the diagnosis of anterolateral impingement.

Marder RA: Current methods for the evaluation of ankle ligament injuries, in Jackson DW (ed): *Instructional Course Lectures 44.* Rosemont, IL, American Academy of Orthopaedic Surgeons, 1995, pp 349–357.

The author reviews the current physical examination and radiographic techniques for the evaluation of ankle injuries.

van Dijk CN, Lim LS, Bossuyt PM, Marti RK: Physical examination is sufficient for the diagnosis of sprained ankles. *J Bone Joint Surg* 1996;78B:958–962.

Accuracy in the detection of ankle ligament injury improved with a delayed (5 days postinjury) examination of the injured ankle.

van Dijk CN, Mol BW, Lim LS, Marti RK, Bossuyt PM: Diagnosis of ligament rupture of the ankle joint: Physical examination, arthrography, stress radiography and sonography compared in 160 patients after inversion trauma. *Acta Orthop Scand* 1996;67:566–570.

Delayed physical examination is superior to all modalities listed in terms of sensitivity, specificity, cost, and patient comfort. This study did not evaluate the MRI as a diagnostic modality.

Nonsurgical Treatment

Eiff MP, Smith AT, Smith GE: Early mobilization versus immobilization in the treatment of lateral ankle sprains. *Am J Sports Med* 1994;22:83–88.

Early mobilization allows earlier return to work and is more comfortable than an immobilization protocol.

Lofvenberg R, Karrholm J, Lund B: The outcome of nonoperated patients with chronic lateral instability of the ankle: A 20-year follow-up study. *Foot Ankle Int* 1994;15:165–169.

Nonoperative treatment of a chronically unstable ankle did not lead to significant arthrosis and was felt to be a major hindrance requiring further treatment in only 3 of 37 patients.

Surgical Treatment

Colville MR: Reconstruction of the lateral ankle ligaments, in Jackson DW (ed): *Instructional Course Lectures 44.* Rosemont, IL, American Academy of Orthopaedic Surgeons, 1995, pp 341–348.

This good review of ligamentous reconstruction favors anatomic over augmented reconstructions for the well-selected patient.

Hamilton WG, Thompson FM, Snow SW: The modified Broström procedure for lateral anklo instability. *Foot Ankle* 1993;14:1–7.

Excellent results are reported in the elite athlete—the professional ballet dancer—allowing a full range of motion and normal peroneal function with the Broström procedure.

Hennrikus WL, Mapes RC, Lyons PM, Lapoint JM: Outcomes of the Chrisman-Snook and modified-Broström procedures for chronic lateral ankle instability: A prospective, randomized comparison. *Am J Sports Med* 1996;24:400–404.

This prospective randomized study resulted in good to excellent results in 80% of patients with either procedure, but a statistically significant greater proportion of complications occurred in patients treated with the Chrisman-Snook procedure.

Hollis JM, Blasier RD, Flahiff CM, Hofmann OE: Biomechanical comparison of reconstruction techniques in simulated lateral ankle ligament injury. *Am J Sports Med* 1995;23:678–682.

This cadaveric study revealed superiority of both the Evans and Chrisman-Snook over the Watson-Jones procedure for increased ankle stability. The Chrisman-Snook procedure restricted subtalar motion to an excessive degree compared to the preferred Evans technique.

Kaikkonen A, Hyppanen E, Kannus P, Jarvinen M: Long-term functional outcome after primary repair of the lateral ligaments of the ankle. *Am J Sports Med* 1997;25:150–155.

Two thirds of patients had good or excellent results 6 to 8 years following primary repair of the lateral ligaments of the ankle. The overall long-term results were acceptable in the majority of patients.

Karlsson J, Eriksson BI, Bergsten T, Rudholm O, Sward L: Comparison of two anatomic reconstructions for chronic lateral instability of the ankle joint. *Am J Sports Med* 1997;25:48–53.

The Broström and modified Broström reconstruction technique produced equivalent functional results and mechanical stability in this prospective randomized study.

Liu SH, Baker CL: Comparison of lateral ankle ligamentous reconstruction procedures. *Am J Sports Med* 1994;22:313–317.

The modified Broström procedure produced greater mechanical restraints to anterior drawer and talar tilt than the Watson-Jones and Chrisman-Snook procedures performed in this cadaveric study.

Liu SH, Jacobson KE: A new operation for chronic lateral ankle instability. *J Bone Joint Surg* 1995;77B:55–59.

A new reconstructive technique involving a lateral shift of the lateral capsule-ligament complex and proximal advancement of the talocalcaneal ligament and inferior extensor retinaculum is described. Results were satisfactory in 92% of patients with 9 of 11 collegiate and 25 of 28 recreational athletes returning to their preinjury level of function.

Rosenbaum D, Becker HP, Sterk J, Gerngross H, Claes L: Long-term results of the modified Evans repair for chronic ankle instability. *Orthopedics* 1996;19:451–455.

Ten-year follow-up of Evans reconstruction resulted in a significant incidence of arthrosis, limited inversion, and residual pain despite a subjective 79% good or excellent result.

Sammarco GJ, Carrasquillo HA: Surgical revision after failed lateral ankle reconstruction. *Foot Ankle Int* 1995;16:748–753.

Results of revision ankle reconstruction compared favorably to primary ankle reconstruction in this first report of revision ankle reconstruction.

Failed Ankle Sprain

Montella BJ, O'Farrell DA, Furr WS, Harrelson JM: Fibular osteochondroma presenting as chronic ankle sprain. *Foot Ankle Int* 1995;16:207–209.

A rare osteochondroma of the proximal fibula resulted in a peroneal palsy and recurrent ankle sprains.

Renstrom PAFH: Persistently painful sprained ankle. *J Am Acad Orthop Surg* 1994;2:270–280.

This is an excellent review of the multiple potential causes of a persistently painful sprained ankle, the most common being incomplete rehabilitation. Evaluation, diagnosis, and management of the failed ankle sprain are outlined.

Subtalar Instability

Ishii T, Miyagawa S, Fukubayashi T, Hayashi K: Subtalar stress radiography using forced dorsiflexion and supination. *J Bone Joint Surg* 1996;78B:56–60.

A new lateral stress view measuring the anterior transposition of the lateral process of the talus at the posterior subtalar joint is described.

Louwerens JW, Ginai AZ, van Linge B, Snijders CJ: Stress radiography of the talocrural and subtalar joints. *Foot Ankle Int* 1995;16:148–155.

A wide range of subtalar motion was found in symptomatic and asymptomatic feet in this fluoroscopically controlled study of the stress Broden view.

Pisani G: Chronic laxity of the subtalar joint. *Orthopedics* 1996; 19:431–437.

MRI documentation of abnormalities of the interosseous talocalcaneal ligament is described in addition to the results of reconstruction of this ligament in 47 surgeries.

Prevention

Ashton-Miller JA, Ottaviani RA, Hutchinson C, Wojtys EM: What best protects the inverted weightbearing ankle against further inversion? Evertor muscle strength compares favorably with shoe height, athletic tape, and three orthoses. *Am J Sports Med* 1996; 24:800–809.

Fully activated and strong ankle evertor muscles are the most effective form of ankle protection and foot strike.

Bahr R, Lian O, Bahr IA: A twofold reduction in the incidence of acute ankle sprains in volleyball after the introduction of an injury prevention program: A prospective cohort study. *Scand J Med Sci Sports* 1997;7:172–177.

An injury prevention program including technique training, an injury awareness session, and a balance board training program effectively reduced the incidence of ankle sprains.

Callaghan MJ: Role of ankle taping and bracing in the athlete. *Br J Sports Med* 1997;31:102–108.

This current literature review of this controversial topic includes an extensive bibliography. Taping restricts ankle motion more than bracing but is rapidly stretched out, both serve a proprioceptive role.

Konradsen L, Voigt M, Hojsgaard C: Ankle inversion injuries: The role of the dynamic defense mechanism. *Am J Sports Med* 1997; 25:54–58.

The reflex reaction pattern to counteract a sudden ankle-foot inversion was too slow to prevent ankle ligament overloading in this experimental study.

Pienkowski D, McMorrow M, Shapiro R, Caborn DN, Stayton J: The effect of ankle stabilizers on athletic performance: A randomized prospective study. *Am J Sports Med* 1995; 23:757–762.

Braces had no effect on the athletic performance of male high school basketball players.

Sitler M, Ryan J, Wheeler B, et al: The efficacy of a semirigid ankle stabilizer to reduce acute ankle injuries in basketball: A randomized clinical study at West Point. *Am J Sports Med* 1994;22:454–461.

Ankle injuries were significantly decreased in frequency but not severity in this large prospective study.

Chapter 19
Injuries to the Midfoot and Forefoot

The increased recognition of the variable and sometimes subtle injury patterns of the midfoot have led to improved treatment outcomes for this patient population. Enhanced imaging techniques have greatly helped in the evaluation of patients. Accurate reduction of intra-articular injuries with stable fixation methods has been the hallmark of successful treatment.

Navicular Injuries

Fractures of the tarsal navicular represent relatively uncommon foot fractures. Of these, fractures of the dorsal lip and tuberosity make up the majority of injuries. Fractures of the body of the navicular are less frequent but are potentially debilitating injuries that warrant careful evaluation. Stress fractures of the navicular are an important consideration in the differential diagnosis of midfoot pain in athletes.

The navicular bone provides an important articulation between the talus and the cuneiforms, as well as the cuboid and calcaneus. Its large articular surface limits blood flow to the dorsal and plantar aspects. Vascular perfusion studies have shown that blood flow is diminished at the central third of the bone.

Initial radiographic evaluation of injuries involving the midfoot requires a minimum of anteroposterior, lateral, and oblique views of the foot. Weightbearing views should be obtained when possible. Potential instability patterns may require stress views to complete the examination. Bone scans also provide useful screening tools for occult bone injury. Recently, magnetic resonance imaging (MRI) has been helpful in the diagnosis of occult stress fractures and in evaluating the symptomatic accessory navicular.

Chip Fractures of the Dorsal Lip

Avulsion fractures of the dorsal lip of the navicular are the most common fracture pattern. These fractures are usually related to excessive plantarflexion forces with eversion or inversion components. Most are associated with adjacent capsular sprains and potential instability that needs to be sought out during the examination. Stable injuries respond well to conservative care with brief immobilization using a cast or boot brace followed by soft compressive support for swelling.

Significantly displaced fragments may need excision. Larger fragments (greater than 25% of the articular surface) may need reduction and internal fixation to prevent late arthrosis.

Tuberosity Fractures

The navicular tuberosity may be avulsed during eversion stress and contraction of the posterior tibial tendon. Most fractures are nondisplaced and respond to immobilization and conservative care. A nonunion does not always indicate residual symptomatology. When a symptomatic nonunion is present, removal and repair of the posterior tibial tendon is indicated. Displaced fractures should be repaired acutely to prevent posterior tibial tendon dysfunction.

This fracture is also occasionally associated with other midfoot injuries including subluxation or compression fractures (nutcracker fracture) of the cuboid. An accessory navicular, which is present in 12% of the population, should be distinguishable by its regular smooth borders on plain radiographs. Bone scan or MRI may be helpful in cases in which radiographs are not diagnostic.

Body Fractures

Although body fractures do not occur frequently, they have the highest morbidity, with potential for posttraumatic arthritis and foot deformity. Navicular body fractures are generally divided into 3 types, based on the direction of the fracture line and pattern of disruption of the adjacent joints.

Type I body fractures result in a fracture line in the coronal plane producing dorsal and plantar fracture fragments of the navicular. There is no associated deformity of the foot. When displaced, the fracture can be repaired through an anteromedial incision between the anterior tibial and posterior tibial tendons. A small external fixator or distractor may be useful for indirect reduction, followed by internal fixation with compression screws from the dorsal side.

The type II body fracture is the most common type. It occurs as a result of axial compression with a dorsomedial force, causing an oblique fracture that runs from dorsal-lateral to plantar-medial. There may be an associated adduction deformity of the forefoot. Reduction is more difficult and may require stabilizing the larger medial fragment to the cuneiforms. Emphasis is placed on alignment and protecting the talonavicular joint during fixation. Residual stiffness from screws or pins crossing the relatively immobile navicular-cuneiform joints is better tolerated than stiffness of the talonavicular joint.

Type III body fractures result from an axial load, with lateral compression forces causing central or lateral comminution and compression of the navicular. There may be an abduction deformity through the midfoot along with associated injuries of the cuboid or anterior calcaneus. Again, displaced fractures should be treated surgically with direct and indirect reduction techniques along with bone grafting when needed. It is often necessary to stabilize the larger medial fragment to the cuneiforms. In severely comminuted injuries, consideration should be given to primary arthrodesis with bone grafting to maintain length of the medial column of the foot. Postoperative care is based on the severity of injury. Most patients require no weightbearing in a short leg cast for at least 6 to 8 weeks followed by gradual resumption of weightbearing based on roentgenographic healing. Salvage of a malunion or posttraumatic arthritis requires single or multiple arthrodeses of the involved joints.

Stress Fractures
Stress fractures of the navicular have been increasingly recognized in the differential diagnosis of midfoot pain in athletes such as track and field participants. The diagnosis is based on a high index of suspicion and localized tenderness at the midnavicular, which has been referred to as the "N" spot (Fig. 1). This area corresponds to the usual location of the stress fracture, which is predictably in the sagittal plane, beginning at the dorsal border of the navicular near the talonavicular joint. These findings are occasionally confused with anterior tibial tendinitis. Stress fractures, however, are generally most painful during activity rather than afterward. Radiographs are usually not diagnostic. A bone scan is the most sensitive screening tool but MRI can be useful as well. Tomograms or computed tomography (CT) scans provide more information in terms of evaluating the extent of the fracture and potential displacement.

Treatment for early, incomplete, nondisplaced fractures requires 6 weeks of nonweightbearing cast immobilization followed by 6 weeks of gradual resumption of activity. Old fractures, evidenced by cystic changes on radiographs, or displaced fractures should be managed surgically with curettement and possibly bone grafting with internal fixation.

Cuboid and Cuneiform Injuries

Isolated injuries to the cuboid or cuneiform tarsal bones are unusual. The secure support of the adjacent tarsal bones and

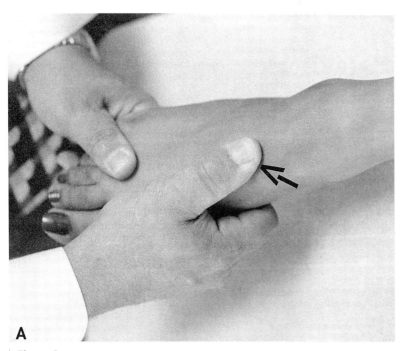
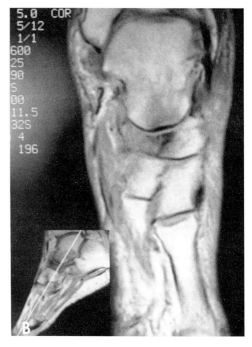

Figure 1
A, The usual location of tenderness with navicular stress fractures. **B,** Magnetic resonance image of a navicular stress fracture.

strong ligaments minimizes associated displacement. Most isolated fractures are from direct blows to the foot. The most common fractures are simple chip or avulsion injuries of the cuboid associated with ankle inversion sprains.

One exception is the compression injury of the cuboid, or nutcracker fracture, that occurs from wedging of the cuboid between the metatarsals and calcaneus with forced abduction of the forefoot. When this fracture is identified, other adjacent midfoot injuries should be sought out as well. Often these include injury to the cuneiforms, navicular tuberosity, and subtalar joint areas. A bone scan or CT scan can be helpful in fully identifying the extent of this injury.

Significantly displaced fractures or subluxations often require surgical intervention for optimal results. Direct and indirect reduction techniques are applicable. Often an external fixator or similar bone distractor is needed to restore lateral column length during surgery. The bone grafting of the cuboid can be performed and alignment maintained with internal or external fixation after surgery. Recently, circular external fixators have been used as an adjunct for complex midfoot trauma.

The goal of surgery should be to maintain lateral column length. In severely comminuted cases, primary or delayed calcaneocuboid arthrodesis may be necessary. Because of the importance of maintaining mobility at the fourth and fifth tarsometatarsal joints, arthrodesis of these 2 joints should be avoided if possible. Prolonged protection is needed postoperatively because of slow ligamentous healing in this area. Usually 6 to 8 weeks of immobilization with limited weightbearing followed by a period of gradual loading is recommended.

Subluxations and dislocations of the cuneiform and cuboid bones are unusual. Most cuneiform instabilities are associated with Lisfranc-type injuries and are treated as such. Isolated dislocation of the cuboid is quite rare but requires open reduction and internal fixation when discovered. Occult subluxation of the cuboid in either a plantar or dorsal direction has been reported. These injuries are most often associated with relatively minor inversion sprains and are also seen in ballet dancers. Patients complain of persistent pain at the cuboid articulations and exhibit antalgia. Occasionally, a depression on the dorsal aspect of the cuboid is visible or the height of the fourth metatarsal head appears decreased relative to the normal foot. This condition has been described as a "locked cuboid." Manual reduction techniques have been described.

Stress fractures of the cuboid have been reported in athletes. Treatment is straightforward and based on rest and protected ambulation for a period of 6 weeks. Predictable healing is expected.

Tarsometatarsal Injuries (Lisfranc Fracture Dislocation)

Injuries to the tarsometatarsal joints of the midfoot are not unusual and constitute approximately 0.2% of all skeletal fractures. In the past, as many as 20% of these injuries were either missed or misdiagnosed. Increasing recognition, particularly regarding more subtle instabilities, will raise the importance of this injury group. Understanding the special anatomy of the tarsometatarsal joints helps in treating these injuries. Stability is based on bony architecture as well as supporting ligaments. The cuneiform and tarsal bones, along with the medial 3 metatarsal bases, have a trapezoidal configuration that is wider on the dorsal aspect. This is similar to the effect of a "Roman arch," which aids in resisting collapse. Similarly, the recessed second metatarsal base between the medial and lateral cuneiforms results in a "keystone" mortise that greatly adds to stability in the transverse plane. Additional stability comes from the strong plantar intertarsal ligaments at the base of the second through fifth metatarsals. Although there is no direct connection between the first and second metatarsals, the important Lisfranc ligament traverses the base of the second metatarsal to the medial cuneiform. This results in a less rigid relationship between the first and second metatarsals, allowing the frequently observed divergent injury in this area. The insertions of the peroneus longus and posterior tibial tendons also add dynamic support to this region.

From a clinical perspective, the tarsometatarsal joints may be divided into 3 columns. The medial column involves the first ray, the middle column involves the second and third rays, and the lateral column involves the fourth and fifth rays. Because of the keystone positioning of the second metatarsal base, injuries that are forceful enough to create displacement usually result in fracture of the second metatarsal. Occasionally only a subtle "fleck sign" is seen on radiographs because of avulsion of the Lisfranc ligament from the second metatarsal base (Fig. 2A).

The mechanism of injury is either direct or indirect. Direct injuries include crushing or direct blows to the foot that can result in dorsal or plantar dislocations. The indirect mechanism is more common. Dorsiflexion or plantarflexion injuries as a result of mishaps on stairs or in motor vehicle accidents are usual causes. In athletes, "pile on" injuries or twisting during quick turns can result in an abduction force applied to the forefoot by the anchored cleated shoe.

Diagnosis and Classification

Diagnosis of tarsometatarsal injuries requires a high index of suspicion. In polytrauma patients, midfoot swelling and tenderness should alert the examiner to possible midfoot insta-

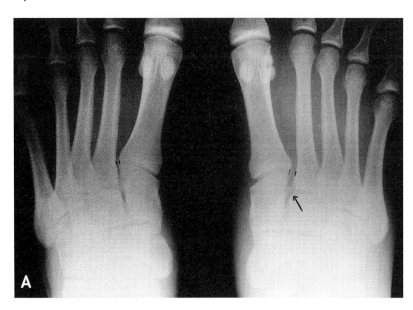
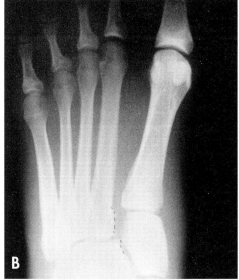

Figure 2

A, Occult instability evident on weightbearing radiographs. Note the widening of the first and second intermetatarsal space and the "fleck sign" representing Lisfranc ligament avulsion fracture (arrow). **B,** Lisfranc instability is evident when the medial border of the second metatarsal is not continuous with the medial border of the middle cuneiform on the anteroposterior view.

bility. Compartment syndromes are associated with Lisfranc injuries and need to be evaluated by pressure measurement when swelling is significant.

Radiographic evaluation requires a minimum of 3 views: anteroposterior (AP), 30° internal oblique, and lateral. When possible, weightbearing views may increase diagnostic yield. Subtle injuries of the first and second metatarsals are best seen on standing AP views of both feet together. When stability is in question, stress views are necessary. An ankle block anesthetic may be helpful in obtaining standing or stress view films. Useful, consistent radiographic parameters that help in the evaluation include continuity of the medial border of the second metatarsal and medial border of the middle cuneiform on the AP view (Fig. 2B). In addition, the intertarsal space between the metatarsals and cuneiforms should be aligned and similar between the right and left sides. On the oblique view, the medial border of the fourth metatarsal should be aligned with the medial border of the cuboid. Similarly, the lateral border of the third metatarsal is continuous with the lateral border of the lateral cuneiform. On the lateral view, there should be a continuous unbroken line of the dorsal tarsometatarsal relationships. CT scans are useful in evaluating comminution of the tarsometatarsal joints and identifying subtle malalignments. Bone scans may also be helpful in screening for injury when no displacement is evident radiographically. Although the ligaments are identifiable

on MRI, this method does not offer any significant advantages in determining treatment for these patients. The examiner should be alert to other concomitant injuries including the cuboid compression or "nutcracker" fractures as well as intercuneiform instabilities and posterior tibial tendon injuries that are frequently associated with Lisfranc injuries.

Classification is difficult because of the multiple variations of displacement. The systems available are not always useful for prognostication but do help in understanding of and preoperative planning for the injuries. The most accepted classification describes three basic types of injury with accompanying subtypes: total incongruity, partial incongruity, and divergent (Fig. 3).

Treatment

Treatment is based on establishing a stable anatomic reduction. In stable, nondisplaced injuries, nonsurgical treatment is possible. Cast immobilization and protected weightbearing for a minimum of 6 weeks is advised. Unstable injuries require internal fixation to achieve satisfactory healing. Surgery is most effective when done acutely but may be delayed to improve soft-tissue conditions. Surgery after 6 weeks is associated with a poor prognosis. Pin fixation is useful when closed reduction is stable and anatomic. Open reduction with

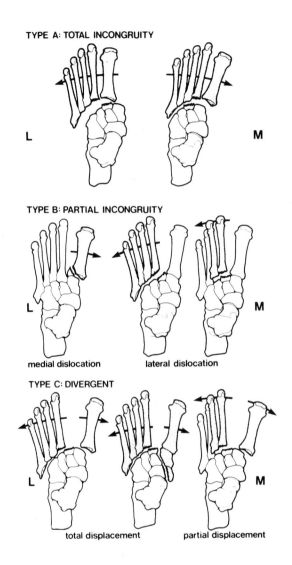

TYPE A: TOTAL INCONGRUITY

L   M

TYPE B: PARTIAL INCONGRUITY

L   M

medial dislocation   lateral dislocation

TYPE C: DIVERGENT

L   M

total displacement   partial displacement

Figure 3

Diagram illustrating the classification of tarsometatarsal dislocations. L=Lateral; M=Medial. (Reproduced with permission from DeLee JC: Fractures and dislocations of the foot, in Mann RA, Coughlin MJ: *Surgery of the Foot and Ankle*, ed 6. St. Louis, MO, Mosby 1993, pp 1465-1703; Adapted from Hardcastle PH, Reschauer R, Kutscha-Lissberg E, Schoffmann W: Injuries to the tarsometatarsal joint: Incidence, classification and treatment. *J Bone Joint Surg* 1982;64B:349-356.)

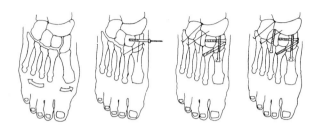

Figure 4

Diagram illustrating the sequence of repair for reduction and stabilization of tarsometatarsal fracture dislocations. The sequence of repair should follow 3 steps. Stabilization of the first ray by alignment of the metatarsal, medial cuneiform, and navicular; stabilization of the Lisfranc ligament by accurate alignment of the second metatarsal to the medial cuneiform as well as the medial and middle cuneiforms; and alignment and stabilization of the third through fifth metatarsal rays. Cannulated screws replace pins as needed for stability and compression. (Reproduced with permission from Trevino SG, Kodros S: Controversies in tarsometatarsal injuries. *Orthop Clin North Am* 1995;26:229–238.)

screw fixation is preferred for unstable injuries. Opening the joints allows debridement of the interposed tissue and debris as well as direct anatomic reduction.

The sequence of repair is outlined in Figure 4. Rigid fixation with screws across the medial 3 tarsometatarsal or intertarsal joints is not associated with any adverse clinical affects.

Because of the importance of maintaining mobility through the fourth and fifth tarsometatarsal joints, temporary pin fixation is preferred.

Postoperatively, weightbearing is limited for 6 to 8 weeks. Supplemental Kirschner wires (K-wires) are removed by 6 to 8 weeks and the patient is allowed to ambulate in a walking brace. After approximately 16 weeks, the intertarsal screws can be removed. Arch support and a rigid soled shoe are helpful until the patient is asymptomatic.

Subtle minor instabilities of the first or second tarsometatarsal joints are increasingly recognized in athletic injuries. Minimum malalignment can result in a good functional outcome with protected casting and limited weightbearing for 4 to 6 weeks. Displacements greater than 2 mm are more consistently treated with reduction and screw fixation to compress the diastasis and improve healing of Lisfranc's ligament in a more anatomic position.

Posttraumatic arthritis occurs in a significant percentage of injured patients. Orthoses as well as stiff-soled shoes with a rocker bottom offer adequate conservative care for many patients. Reconstruction of the painful degenerative arthritic joints is possible by arthrodesis. Generally, fusion is directed to the first, second, and third tarsometatarsal areas with an attempt to spare the important mobility of the fourth and fifth joints. In mildly displaced injuries, in situ fusion is best. With larger deformities, realignment and iliac grafting along with rigid internal fixation are desirable. Recovery is slow, with maximum improvement often occurring 9 to 12 months after surgery.

Forefoot: Metatarsal Fractures

Fractures of the metatarsals are among the most frequent of foot injuries. They usually result from injury forces such as direct blows from a falling object. Most are relatively stable injuries that heal with conservative treatment. In contrast to prolonged immobilization and nonweightbearing, progressive postoperative activity in a stiff-soled type of shoe or walking cast can result in improved outcome.

Evaluation requires careful assessment of radiographs. Although transverse fracture displacements are generally well tolerated, plantar or dorsal angulation may alter plantar weightbearing loads, which may result in metatarsalgia or hyperkeratosis at the injured or adjacent metatarsals. Closed or open reduction and stabilization should be considered for angulation in the sagittal plane of more than 10° or displacement more than 3 to 4 mm. Intramedullary or crossed K-wires as well as small fragment plates have been used successfully.

Metatarsal Stress Fracture

Stress fractures occur most often in the metatarsal bones. The bone fails when the fatigue process exceeds the reparative process. Bone failure is based on the amount of load and degree of repetitive stress, as well as the frequency of loading. Patients present with forefoot swelling and pain of insidious onset that increases with weightbearing activity. Examination will reveal point tenderness over the fracture site. Early radiographs are not always diagnostic but will usually indicate the healing fracture site with callus development by 3 to 4 weeks from the onset of symptoms. Bone scans are a more sensitive screening tool but are not necessary to initiate treatment and should be reserved for atypical cases.

All patients should be assessed for the possible etiology of the stress fracture. Incorrect training technique is a common cause in athletes. The alignment of the foot should be assessed as well. A short hypermobile first ray or bunion may predispose to stress fractures of the second or third metatarsals. There may have been a change in the footwear, such as an increased heel height or increased weightbearing demands in the work environment. Injury or residual deformities that alter gait may also predispose to metatarsal stress fractures. In patients with osteopenia, bone densiometry and metabolic evaluation may be appropriate.

Treatment for most patients is based on reduced activity and protective footwear. A stiff-soled postoperative shoe usually suffices. Most patients are well on their way to healing by 6 to 8 weeks. Gradual return to activity should be allowed after 8 to 12 weeks while avoiding the training errors that may have caused the problem to begin with. If significant angulation in the sagittal plane develops, indications for open reduction and internal fixation are the same as for acute fractures.

Fifth Metatarsal Fractures

The fifth metatarsal has several predictable injury patterns, each with unique healing properties. The most proximal fractures are at the tuberosity. These fractures are associated with inversion injuries resulting in direct as well as indirect forces applied to the bone by the peroneus brevis tendon and strong supporting ligaments in this area. Significant separation of the fracture fragment is unusual. Even displaced fractures have a favorable prognosis with nonsurgical care. When an intra-articular fracture is displaced more than 2 to 3 mm in an athletic individual, surgical repair is considered. However, good results are reported without surgery and the majority of patients are treated nonsurgically. Most patients do best with symptomatic care with clinical evidence of healing expected within 6 to 8 weeks. One recent study demonstrated earlier return to function using soft dressings instead of casts. Radiographic union may be delayed or absent but does not always correlate with outcome. The rare, painful nonunion should be excised. Familiarity with the appearance of the accessory bones in this area reduces the occasional confusion with the os peroneum and os vesalianum in adults and the tuberosity apophysis in children.

Fractures of the metaphyseal-diaphyseal junction (Jones fracture) are less predictable. Careful evaluation of this injury is needed to optimize treatment. Clinical history and radiographs are used to determine acute, chronic (stress), or combined fracture types. A history of prodromal symptoms combined with intramedullary sclerosis and a widened fracture line indicates a preexisting stress fracture of the metatarsal. This group is associated with delayed healing or nonunion. Nonweightbearing immobilization is recommended as the first treatment for 6 to 8 weeks in most patients. Early intervention with a 4.5-mm intramedullary screw correlates with an earlier, more predictable return to activity in athletes. This is also a preferred treatment for fractures that fail to heal with cast immobilization. Poor results have been associated with the use of screws other than 4.5-mm ASIF malleolar type (Fig. 5).

The acute, nondisplaced Jones fractures may be treated with limited weightbearing and immobilization for 4 to 6 weeks followed by protected weightbearing in a boot brace until complete healing occurs. Delayed unions or nonunions are treated by bone graft or screw fixation. Acute displaced fractures usually require early open reduction and internal fixation.

Fractures of the distal shaft and neck area of the fifth metatarsal rarely require surgical intervention. The so-called

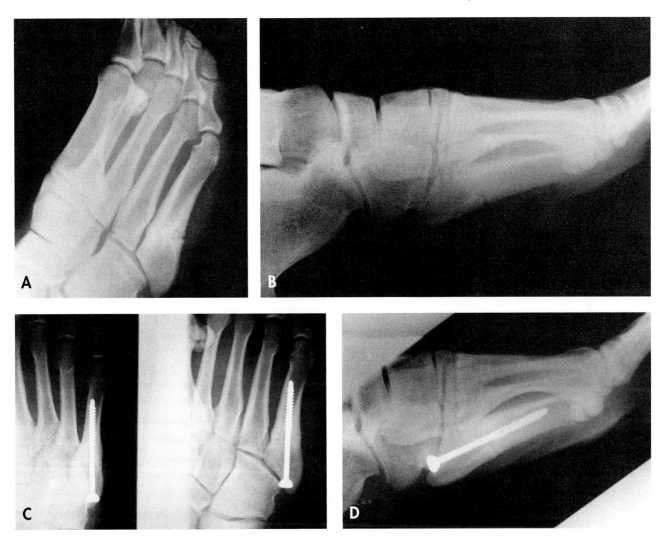

Figure 5

A, Preoperative and **B,** postoperative radiographs of a Jones stress fracture that failed to unite with conservative care. **C** and **D,** Postoperative films approximately 10 weeks after surgery.

"dancer's fracture" occurs with loading on the plantarflexed foot and may result in a long oblique fracture in this area. Although separation of the fracture fragments is frequently seen on the AP and oblique radiographs, sagittal alignment is usually satisfactory. Nonsurgical care is recommended with use of a stiff-soled postoperative shoe until the fracture heals, usually in 8 to 12 weeks. Open reduction and internal fixation is considered for severely displaced injuries (Fig. 6).

Injuries

Phalangeal fractures of the lesser toes are common. Most are related to direct trauma from falling objects or direct blows, such as the "night walker's fracture." Middle and distal phalanx fractures and most proximal phalanx fractures can be treated with supportive taping of the adjacent toes. When the proximal phalanx is significantly displaced, closed manipulation is indicated. A fracture treated with closed manipulation that is not improved to the degree that surgical repair is justified is extremely rare. Very few fractures that are treated conservatively will require late reconstruction (usually by exostectomy).

Fractures of the first toe warrant closer scrutiny. Significantly displaced intra-articular fractures of the interphalangeal or metatarsophalangeal joint should be reduced, and pinned with K-wires or small screws when unstable. Crush injuries to the distal phalanx may benefit from sterile decom-

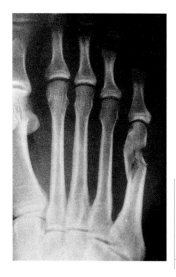

Figure 6

Illustration of a typical dancer's fracture of the fifth metatarsal. Prompt healing occurred after 6 weeks in a postoperative shoe.

pression of the subungual hematoma. Early weightbearing has been shown to improve outcome and healing time in patients with phalangeal fractures.

Fractures of the sesamoids occur from direct trauma as well as indirect injuries such as acute hyperdorsiflexion of the first toe. The medial sesamoid is involved most often. Patients exhibit tenderness over the sesamoid as well as accentuated pain with dorsiflexion. The fracture can be visualized on radiographs but must be differentiated from bipartite sesamoids. The latter are usually larger with smooth sclerotic borders, whereas the fractured sesamoid has an irregular appearance at the fracture line.

Sesamoid fracture treatment can be difficult. Protected weightbearing in a cast with a peg to prevent weightbearing on the toes, or using a toe plate that prevents dorsiflexion is advised for 3 to 4 weeks. Stiff-soled footwear with metatarsal pads are used afterward. If symptoms persist past 6 months, excision or repair is considered. Recently, bone grafting has been used successfully in these injuries.

Stress fractures of the sesamoids are treated similarly, although casting and protection from weightbearing is usually longer, 6 to 12 weeks. Surgical treatment options are similar for those used in symptomatic fracture nonunions.

Dislocations

Dislocations of the lesser toes are unusual. They occur primarily at the metatarsophalangeal joint from hyperextension injuries resulting in dorsal dislocations. Frequently, there are other associated foot injuries. In approximately one third of patients, the plantar plate is interposed in the joint space, preventing closed reduction. This condition may appear as a wide separation between the metatarsal head and phalanx on the AP radiographic view. When closed methods fail, an open dorsal approach to achieve reduction is recommended to prevent late pain sequelae.

Dislocation of the interphalangeal joint is even less common but deserves a similar approach, because the plantar plate can prevent closed reduction there also. Again, residual pain and deformity is more likely when the joint is left unreduced.

First metatarsophalangeal joint injuries are usually sprains associated with hyperdorsiflexion injuries of the toe, often called turf toe. This term arises from the relative frequency of this injury in football players, especially those playing on artificial turf. This injury may take weeks or months to resolve but usually responds to protected activity within 3 weeks, and an orthosis or stiff-soled shoe can reduce dorsiflexion during convalescence.

Frank dislocations are usually dorsal. These injuries result in disruption of the plantar plate sesamoid complex. In type I injuries, the sesamoid complex is interposed into the joint space dorsal to the metatarsal head. These injuries are often irreducible by closed means and require open reduction, preferably through a dorsal approach.

Type II injuries involve disruption of the sesamoid complex with separation of the sesamoids medially and laterally (type IIA) or fracture through the sesamoids and displacement distally (type IIB). The latter type II injury is usually amenable to closed reduction, although fracture fragments that will require removal may be left within the joint. Protection in a cast or stiff-soled shoe is advised for 4 weeks after the injury.

Open Wounds

Midfoot and forefoot trauma often result in open wounds to the foot. The principles of wound care, including debridement of the foreign material or necrotic tissue, copious irrigation, cleansing, and adequate skeletal stabilization, must be followed to obtain satisfactory results. Local as well as systemic antibiotics are indicated. The potential for compartment syndromes must be recognized and addressed promptly.

Gunshot Wounds

Gunshot wounds need to be assessed in terms of energy delivery to the tissues. Most handguns are of low velocity and energy (1,000 to 2,000 ft/sec). Rifles tend to develop higher velocities and energy (greater than 2,000 ft/sec). Close range shotgun injuries also deliver high energy injuries despite a relatively low velocity and should be treated accordingly.

Recent reports indicate that simple debridement and first-generation cephalosporin antibiotic therapy is all that is needed for low velocity gunshot wounds to the foot. Use of intravenous or oral antibiotics remains controversial but 3-day minimum coverage is advised.

Higher velocity (energy) wounds are best managed by inpatient care. Broad-spectrum intravenous antibiotic therapy with serial wound debridements to produce a healthy environment prior to internal fixation or soft-tissue free flaps is recommended.

Lawnmower Injuries

Lawnmower injuries occur when children play too close to or fall off of a lawnmower. Injuries in adults usually involve mowing over an inclined area on a wet, slick surface. The tremendous energy of these injuries requires extensive debridement of foreign material and devitalized tissue. Repeat procedures are usually necessary and major reconstructive procedures should be delayed until wounds are stable. Early split-thickness skin grafting is a useful adjunct in stabilizing open wound areas.

Intravenous antibiotics should include broad spectrum coverage for a minimum of 72 hours. Use of first-generation cephalosporins combined with an aminoglycoside has been recommended. With severe dirt contamination, penicillin should be added to protect against clostridium. Local antibiotic delivered by irrigant or polymethylmethacrylate beads may be useful as well.

Annotated Bibliography

Midfoot

Beaman DN, Roeser WM, Holmes JR, Saltzman CL: Cuboid stress fractures: A report of two cases. *Foot Ankle Int* 1993; 14:525–528.

Mooney M, Maffey-Ward L: Cuboid plantar and dorsal subluxations: Assessment and treatment. *J Orthop Sports Phys Ther* 1994;20:220–226.

The authors describe the diagnosis and treatment of the "locked cuboid" syndrome. Case studies and reduction techniques are highlighted.

Davis CA, Lubowitz J, Thordarson DB: Midtarsal fracture-subluxation: Case report and review of the literature. *Clin Orthop* 1993;292:264–268.

The authors emphasize the importance and potential sequelae of navicular tuberosity avulsions. They suggest that early intervention for displaced injuries may improve the prognosis.

Khan KM, Brukner PD, Kearney C, Fuller PJ, Bradshaw CJ, Kiss ZS: Tarsal navicular stress fractures in athletes. *Sports Med* 1994; 17:64–76.

This article reviews evaluation and treatment of navicular stress fractures.

Steinbronn DJ, Bennett GL, Kay DB: The use of magnetic resonance imaging in the diagnosis of stress fractures of the foot and ankle: Four case reports. *Foot Ankle Int* 1994;15:80–83.

This article highlights the use of magnetic resonance imaging (MRI) in evaluating stress fractures of the foot and ankle when other studies had been inconclusive.

Lisfranc

Curtis MJ, Myerson M, Szura B: Tarsometatarsal joint injuries in the athlete. *Am J Sports Med* 1993;21:497–502.

The authors review the treatment and outcome of 19 patients with tarsometatarsal joint injuries that occurred during athletic activity. They advocate early diagnosis and treatment by screw fixation for injuries with diastasis not believed to be stable under fluoroscopic examination.

Groshar D, Alperson M, Mendes DG, Barsky V, Liberson A: Bone scintigraphy findings in Lisfranc joint injury. *Foot Ankle Int* 1995;16:710–711.

Bone scan as a sensitive tool in identifying the degree of involvement in nondisplaced Lisfranc injuries is highlighted in this case report.

Lu J, Ebraheim NA, Skie M, Porshinsky B, Yeasting RA: Radiographic and computed tomographic evaluation of Lisfranc dislocation: A cadaver study. *Foot Ankle Int* 1997;18:351–355.

The authors correlate computed tomography (CT) scans with anatomic dissections. They recommend CT scanning as a more sensitive tool than plain radiography for detecting minor amounts of Lisfranc displacement.

Mantas JP, Burks RT: Lisfranc injuries in the athlete. *Clin Sports Med* 1994;13:719–730.

This review article describes Lisfranc instabilities that occur in athletes, as well as indications and techniques for surgical management.

Preidler KW, Wang YC, Brossmann J, Trudell D, Daenen B, Resnick D: Tarsometatarsal joint: Anatomic details on MR images. *Radiology* 1996;199:733–736.

This article highlights the capabilities of magnetic resonance imaging in assessing the tarsometatarsal joints and correlates findings with anatomic specimen.

Rosenberg GA, Patterson BM: Tarsometatarsal (Lisfranc's) fracture-dislocation. *Am J Orthop* 1995;(suppl):7–16.

This review article discusses classification, diagnosis, and treatment methods for tarsometatarsal injuries.

Shapiro MS, Wascher DC, Finerman GA: Rupture of Lisfranc's ligament in athletes. *Am J Sports Med* 1994;22:687–691.

The authors reviewed 9 first-second tarsometatarsal injuries in athletes that were treated conservatively. The diastasis ranged from 2 to 5 mm. They indicated good results with nonsurgical treatment using cast immobilization with partial-weightbearing for 4 to 6 weeks. In most patients, it took 4 months to return to athletic activities.

Trevino SG, Kodros S: Controversies in tarsometatarsal injuries. *Orthop Clin North Am* 1995;26:229–238.

The authors detail their approach to diagnostic and surgical management of tarsometatarsal injuries with emphasis on surgical technique and postoperative care.

Metatarsals

Eisele SA, Sammarco GJ: Fatigue fractures of the foot and ankle in the athlete. *J Bone Joint Surg* 1993;75A:290–298.

This review article discusses presentation, etiology, and treatment of stress fractures in the foot.

Glasgow MT, Naranja RJ Jr, Glasgow SG, Torg JS: Analysis of failed surgical management of fractures of the base of the fifth metatarsal distal to the tuberosity: The Jones fracture. *Foot Ankle Int* 1996;17:449–457.

According to this article, complications correlated with use of other than a 4.5-mm ASIF malleolar screw. Undersized corticocancellous grafts or incomplete medullary reaming correlated with failure in treating fifth metatarsal Jones fractures. Slow return to vigorous activity is recommended.

Wiener BD, Linder JF, Giattini JF: Treatment of fractures of the fifth metatarsal: A prospective study. *Foot Ankle Int* 1997;18:267–269.

The authors compared recovery time for fifth metatarsal tuberosity fractures using a soft dressing and stiff shoe versus a cast and found return to activity was significantly faster by an average of 13 days with soft dressing treatment methods. The prognosis for both treatment groups was good.

Toes

Anderson RB, McBryde AM Jr: Autogenous bone grafting of hallux sesamoid nonunions. *Foot Ankle Int* 1997;18:293–296.

The authors performed autogenous bone grafting for 21 patients with sesamoid nonunions. Nineteen of 21 lesions united, at an average time of 12 weeks postoperatively. Seventeen of 18 patients available for postoperative evaluation returned to their preinjury activity level, including participating in running sports. Repair of the nonunion in an otherwise healthy sesamoid is believed to be a good alternative to excision, which may result in deformity or weakness.

Brunet JA, Tubin S: Traumatic dislocations of the lesser toes. *Foot Ankle Int* 1997;18:406–411.

This article is a review of the author's experience with 31 dislocations of the metatarsophalangeal and proximal interphalangeal joints of the toes. Neglected dislocations correlated with residual symptoms whereas reduced injuries remained pain free.

Schenck RC Jr, Heckman JD: Fractures and dislocations of the forefoot: Operative and nonoperative treatment. *J Am Acad Orthop Surg* 1995;3:70–78.

This article is a review of evaluation and treatment of tarsometatarsal and toe fracture dislocations.

Open Wounds

Boucree JB Jr, Gabriel RA, Lezine-Hanna JT: Gunshot wounds to the foot. *Orthop Clin North Am* 1995;26:191–197.

The authors reviewed 101 patients with gunshot wounds to their feet. Wound infections were associated with higher velocity injuries. Complications were believed to be minimized by frequent debridement and delayed skeletal fixation as well as prolonged antibiotic coverage. The lower velocity injuries were adequately treated with simple debridement and 72 hours of antibiotic therapy.

DeCoster TA, Miller RA: Management of traumatic foot wounds. *J Am Acad Orthop Surg* 1994;2:226–230.

An overview of various foot wounds and their treatments is presented.

Vosburgh C, Gruel CR, Herndon WA, Sullivan JA: Lawn mower injuries of the pediatric foot and ankle: Observations on prevention and management. *J Pediatr Orthop* 1995;15:504–509.

The authors studied lawnmower injuries to 25 children ranging in age from 2 to 19 years to determine factors leading to increased morbidity. Ride-on mower injuries resulted in the most severe wounds. Injury to the posterior and plantar aspect of the foot and ankle resulted in higher morbidity. Thorough surgical debridement and staged treatments were emphasized.

Chapter 20
Tendon Problems
of the Foot and Ankle

Achilles Tendon

Achilles tendon ruptures are the third most frequent major tendon disruptions. A healthy tendon will rupture only under very severe conditions; the mechanism of injury is commonly acceleration-deceleration secondary to forceful dorsiflexion of a plantarflexed ankle. The expected extreme stresses in the lateral tendon fibers during such a movement are a possible starting point for a rupture.

Some patients have symptoms of preexistent tendinitis. Chronic steroid therapy, gout, and fluoroquinolone antibiotics are associated with Achilles tendon ruptures, and a case of bilateral partial Achilles tendon ruptures has been associated with ciprofloxacin therapy. Treatment with fluoroquinolones should be discontinued at the first sign of tendon inflammation in order to reduce the risk of subsequent rupture. In this situation, magnetic resonance imaging (MRI) is useful in distinguishing between Achilles tendinitis and partial tendon rupture. Tendinitis usually resolves within weeks of discontinuing fluoroquinolone therapy.

Diagnosis

Frequently, patients feel as if they have been hit with an object in the heel or calf area. Often, they described a pop or snap. Diagnosis is made by the Thompson test, which is performed by squeezing the calf with the patient prone and the ankle free. The foot will plantar flex if the Achilles tendon is intact. Tenderness is also often elicited at the site of rupture. Chronic pain in the region of the Achilles tendon is a common problem and often a sign of progressive degeneration, which may lead to its rupture.

Ultrasonography (US) and MRI can be of value if the diagnosis is in question. US can detect the disappearance of the tendon within its normal pathway with hematoma formation. MRI shows a heterogeneous signal instead of the normal black appearance of the tendon. US can determine the tendon's thickness and echotexture. A spontaneous rupture was noted in 28% of the patients who described chronic pain and demonstrated thickening and circumscribed lesions of the echotexture. Patients without sonographic changes had substantially better clinical outcomes from conservative treatment.

The surgical findings and histopathology have been correlated with preoperative US and MRI in patients with chronic Achilles tendinopathy. US was positive in 21 of 26 cases and MRI in 26 of 27 cases. Severe intratendinous abnormalities and a sagittal tendon diameter > 10 mm suggested a partial rupture. Assessment of the paratenon was unreliable with both US and MRI.

US is of limited value in evaluating functional results after surgical repair. Sonographic morphology was studied in 60 patients an average of 11 years after surgical repair of Achilles tendon rupture. Extensive functional subjective and objective parameters were evaluated using an Achilles tendon score. There was no statistical correlation between US morphology and clinical outcome.

Treatment

Surgical treatment of ruptured Achilles tendons is preferable for active patients, with the goal of returning them to their preinjury level of activity. Surgical treatment has a lower incidence of rerupture and results in increased strength of push off, less calf atrophy, and better motion through restoration of the normal tendon length. However, there are surgical risks, which include infection, skin slough, sural nerve injury, and complications of anesthesia. Nonsurgical management is indicated for patients with compromised skin or wound-healing ability (patients with peripheral vascular disease, diabetes mellitus, or corticosteroid or chemotherapy, such as methotrexate) or those who are less active.

The goal of primary surgical repair is restoration of normal resting tendon length. The noninjured leg also should be prepped and draped to facilitate comparison with the operated side. Meticulous soft-tissue handling is required. The plantaris tendon can be unwrapped and placed around the repair, as well. However, the plantaris tendon is missing in approximately 30% of the population and 5% of Achilles tendon ruptures also have simultaneous rupture of the plantaris.

A cadaver study tested the ultimate strength of repaired tendon "ruptures" in 18 fresh-frozen human Achilles tendons

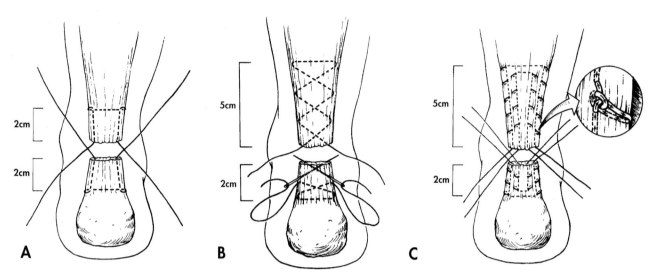

Figure 1

A, A standard Kessler repair configuration was performed on group 1 specimens. **B,** A standard Bunnel repair configuration was used to repair group 2 specimens. **C,** A locking loop repair method, used for group 3, has four suture strands: an outer and inner suture in both tendon stumps. Inset shows the course of the suture passing through the tendon substance creating the locked loop. (Reproduced with permission from Watson TW, Jurist KA, Yang KH, Shen KL: The strength of Achilles tendon repair: An in vitro study of the biomechanical behavior in human cadaver tendons. *Foot Ankle Int* 1995;16:191–195.)

using the Kessler, the Bunnell, and the locking loop methods (Figs. 1 and 2). Under uniform and standardized laboratory conditions, the specimens were loaded to failure. The locking loop suture method was substantially stronger than the other two. There was no significant difference between the strength of the Kessler and Bunnell repairs.

The optimal time from injury to repair has been evaluated. One study reported greater satisfaction among patients treated surgically within 72 hours of injury. Unfortunately, this injury is not always diagnosed and has been overlooked in as many as 25% of patients. Retraction of the proximal portion of the tendon can make surgical repair a formidable task. Often, a primary repair still can be performed several weeks after injury, provided intraoperative longitudinal traction can be maintained on the tendon end. A study comparing 11 patients who had late reconstruction for Achilles tendon rupture with 10 patients who had immediate repair (mean follow-up, 8 years for both groups) found that patients with late reconstruction had outcomes comparable to those patients undergoing immediate repair.

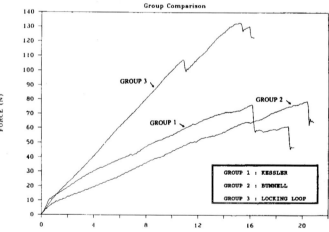

Figure 2

The graph represents an average of all trials of each method tested. The variations, as noted in the double peak in group 1, are the result of averaging the number of all trials when some trials were zero secondary to previous failure. This graph represents each test method for comparison. (Reproduced with permission from Watson TW, Jurist KA, Yang KH, Shen KL: The strength of Achilles tendon repair: An in vitro study of the biomechanical behavior in human cadaver tendons. *Foot Ankle Int* 1995;16:191–195.)

Different surgical techniques may be used in the late repair of Achilles tendon rupture (Figs. 3 and 4). One retrospective study identified 11 patients who were treated for late Achilles

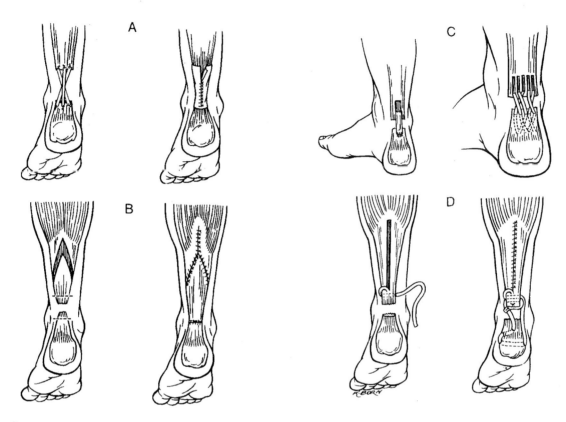

Figure 3

Fascial repairs of chronic ruptures of the Achilles tendon. **A,** Free fascia lata. The fascia lata is harvested through a separate incision. Three strips are sewn across the defect (**left**). The remaining piece of fascia lata is wrapped around the repair to create a tube and is secured with suture (**right**). B, V-Y advancement flap. The gastrocnemius-soleus fascia and muscle are incised in a V shape. The distal portion of the proximal half of the tear is advanced distally to allow for end-to-end repair (**left**). The incision is then closed with interrupted sutures to create a Y (**right**). **C,** Gastrocnemius-soleus turndown. One central slip of gastrocnemius-soleus fascia is turned down and sutured across the defect (**left**). Multiple strips of gastrocnemius-soleus fascia are turned down across the defect and sutured (**right**). Pullout wires may be used to strengthen the repair. **D,** Gastrocnemius-soleus weave. One long central slip gastrocnemius-soleus fascia is turned down and woven through the end of the tear (**left**). The harvested site is repaired side-to-side (**right**). (Reproduced with permission from Dalton GP: Chronic Achilles tendon rupture. *Foot Ankle Clin* 1996;16:225.)

tendon rupture (repair ≥ 4 weeks and ≤ 12 weeks from injury) by proximal release of the gastrocnemius-soleus complex, imbrication of the early fibrous scar without excision of any local tissue, and primary repair of the tendon ends. With follow-up periods ranging from 1.5 to 5.8 years, there were no reruptures and all patients returned to a preinjury level of activity at a mean of 5.8 months. There was no significant difference in subjective and objective outcome when compared with acute repairs by the same surgeon.

During the repair, the site and extent of pathology should be identified. If there is an old rupture with minimal retraction, the tendon is plicated with a long oblique incision. Another option includes mobilization of the central half of the Achilles tendon. If substantial tendon retraction prevents reapposition of the tendon ends, then reconstruction with a

flexor digitorum longus (FDL) or flexor hallucis longus (FHL) tendon is indicated.

Insertional tendinosis often presents with a boggy and grossly abnormal tendon. If the lesion is small and localized, the tendon resection can allow for primary repair. If the lesion is large, the central half of the Achilles tendon is mobilized and attached to either the distal remaining stump or the calcaneus with suture anchor technique. Another option includes transfer of the FDL and FHL tendons to add strength and promote revascularization to the resected area of Achilles tendon.

The FHL has been advocated as a tendon transfer of choice for Achilles reconstruction. It facilitates surgical repair due to its contiguous anatomic location and it has a similar axis of contraction dynamically in phase with the gastrocnemius-

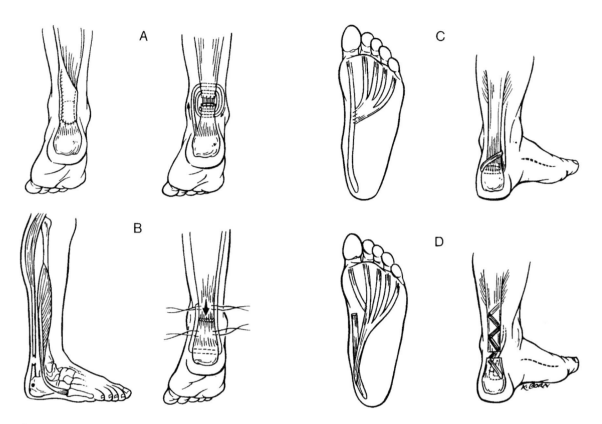

Figure 4

Tendon transfers for repair of chronic Achilles tendon ruptures. **A,** Plantaris tendon repairs Technique of Lynn (**left**). The Achilles tendon is repaired end-to-end. The plantaris tendon is "fanned out," wrapped around the tendon repair, and sutured. Technique of Quigley (**right**). The plantaris tendon is divided proximally, and the free end is woven clockwise (arrows) through the torn ends of the tendon. **B,** Peroneus brevis tendon repair. The tendon is harvested through a separate incision over the base of the fifth metatarsal and pulled through the lateral septum into the posterior incision (**left**). The tendon is passed through a drill hole in the calcaneus laterally to medially. The peroneus brevis tendon is secured to the Achilles tendon (arrow) by horizontal sutures (**right**). **C,** Flexor digitorum longus (FDL) tendon repair. The tendon is harvested through a separate incision in the midfoot. The distal stump is tenodesed to the flexor hallucis longus (FHL) tendon (**left**). The FDL tendon is brought lateral and posterior to the neurovascular bundle and then through the septum into the posterior incision. The tendon is brought through a drill hole in the calcaneus and secured into the proximal portion of the ruptured Achilles tendon. **D,** Flexor hallucis longus tendon repair. The tendon is harvested through a separate incision in the midfoot and the distal stump is tenodesed to the FDL tendon (**left**). The FHL is retracted through an incision in the septum into the posterior incision. The tendon is passed through a drill hole in the calcaneus and woven through the distal and proximal ends of the ruptured Achilles tendon (**right**). (Reproduced with permission from Dalton GP: Chronic Achilles tendon rupture. *Foot Ankle Clin* 1996;16:225.)

soleus complex. The FHL is the strongest plantarflexor next to the gastrocnemius-soleus. The low-lying, distal muscle belly of the FHL also brings in additional vascularity to the tendo-Achilles complex.

One author advocated surgical treatment of chronic ruptures of the Achilles tendon with FHL reconstruction after finding subjective satisfaction and no poor results (all patients returned to work with no reruptures) in 7 patients with a mean follow-up of 17 months. Most patients had excellent or good return of function. Conversely, another author reported good results as well with the FDL tendon.

A skin slough can result in the loss of the repaired tendon

complex. Skin slough is a reconstructive challenge to the orthopaedic surgeon because of the relative absence of viable tissues and the inherent avascularity of the Achilles tendon. The skin along the distal medial portion of the leg is very thin and is easily compromised. Meticulous soft-tissue handling is crucial, and tension on the wound edges must be avoided. One report described 4 patients treated by soft-tissue expansion prior to tendon repair to allow tension-free wound closure. The authors recommended using a soft-tissue expander to facilitate skin closure and provide increased local blood flow.

After a skin slough, treatment options include local and free-tissue transfers. The island adipofascial flap can provide a durable and thin coverage for the Achilles tendon as well as a good vascularized bed for skin grafting. Radial forearm and lateral arm flaps, composite flaps, (free tissue transfer with microvascular anastomoses), and the dorsalis pedis island flap can also be used. One study reported 2 patients in whom a radial forearm-palmaris longus composite free flap was used to reconstruct full-thickness defects of the heel and tendo-Achilles. Rapid healing and return of function were obtained without substantial donor site deficit. Another series described 10 patients with exposed Achilles tendons in whom the island adipofascial flap successfully preserved the exposed tendon and provided a gliding surface. Another study reported the long-term functional results following free-tissue coverage in 4 patients who developed wound complications after surgical treatment of Achilles tendon rupture. Three radial forearm flaps and 1 lateral arm flap were used. All patients were able to return to their preoperative level of activity within a year and the aesthetic outcome was good in all cases. Although these various methods can be successful, no specific technique for reconstruction can be advocated due to the limited numbers of patients reported in these published studies.

Postoperative Regimen

Traditionally, the postoperative regimen includes rigid immobilization for 6 to 8 weeks. Several studies have reported that early range of motion after Achilles repair is safe with no increased risk of rerupture in compliant patients. The patients achieved a good return of plantarflexion strength, power, and endurance.

Careful controlled passive motion stimulates intrinsic repair, improves early tendon material properties, and reduces adhesion formation. The duration, intensity, and frequency of passive or active motion necessary for optimal Achilles tendon healing has yet to be determined. Conversely, immobilization achieves tendon healing through hematoma to collagen proliferation and maturation and may be associated with atrophy, weakness, stiffness, and deep venous thrombosis.

Flexor Hallucis Longus

Introduction

The passage of the FHL through various tunnels and pulleys predisposes it to more pathology than any other flexor tendon. Pathology includes tendinitis, stenosing tenosynovitis, tendon degeneration, development of nodules, and partial and complete rupture. Pathology can occur proximal to flexor retinaculum, medial malleolus, distal border of the tarsal tunnel, sustentaculum tali, intersesamoid region, and distal phalangeal insertion of the great toe.

Anatomy

The FHL tendon originates from the muscular tendinous juncture and crosses lateral-to-medial through a fibro-osseous tunnel at the posterior aspect of the talus to the sole of the foot. It courses behind the medial malleolus with the FDL and peroneal tendon within a fibro-osseous sheath grooving the os calcis. Distally, it crosses the FDL. Both tendons are bound to the vault of the arch by a common tendon sheath, the master knot of Henry. Just distal to the knot, the FHL usually gives off an interconnecting tendon to the FDL after its separation into individual tendons. The FHL courses through another fibro-osseous tunnel formed by the two heads of the flexor hallucis brevis and sesamoids under the metatarsal head along its pathway to the distal phalanx.

En bloc dissection of the second muscle layer of the sole of the foot demonstrated the existence of intratendinous connections (78%) arising from the fibular side of the FHL to the FDL. Seldom were there no connections evident. In addition, the tendons of the FDL often are reinforced by tendinous connections from the flexor accessorius. While reciprocal interconnections do exist between the FDL and FHL tendons, they do so to a lesser extent (only 29 of 86 cases). The anatomic location of the FDL and the minimal donor deficit following its harvest supports its use as the tendon transfer of choice for posterior tibia reconstruction. The FHL is ideal for late Achilles tendon reconstruction because of its relative strength, anatomic location, and length.

Stenosing Tenosynovitis

Stenosing tenosynovitis occurs in any part of an extremity where a tendon muscle pulls through a pulley system. The first pulley system for the FHL is behind the medial malleolus and grooving the os calcis and the second is between the sesamoids. After trauma, the tendon sheath becomes inflamed and heals with constriction. Triggering of the great toe has been reported due to constriction in several locations: proximal to the hindfoot sheath, callus adhesion/incarceration after ankle/os calcis fracture, and distally between the sesamoids.

Previous surgery (ie, bunion), trauma (ie, sesamoid fracture), or local injury (ie, laceration) can influence the development of stenosing tenosynovitis, as well as an aberrant muscle belly in the region of the flexor retinaculum. Successful treatment includes surgical exploration versus tenolysis of the sheath (by tendon sheath insufflation with 1% lidocaine). In a series of 9 patients, 3 responded to sheath insufflation with 1% lidocaine; the remainder required tenolysis.

Partial Tears of the FHL

Partial tears of the FHL recently have been identified at the level of the knot of Henry (n = 3), involving the intertendinous connections between FHL and FDL. Often chronic pain was present for 1 to 3 years. Each patient had exquisite point tenderness at the knot of Henry and increased pain associated with passive extension of the FHL. A partial or longitudinal tear of the FHL remains a clinical diagnosis, because no imaging study (including MRI) easily identifies the exact nature of the pathology. Surgical treatment depends on the location; however, treatment requires adequate exposure, release of the knot of Henry, excision of tendinous interconnection, and repair of tendon split. Often, tenolysis, tenosynovectomy, and excision of distal muscle fibers may be necessary.

FHL Tendon Ruptures

Acute Open Lacerations Most disruptions of the FHL are caused by open lacerations. Although a previous study concluded that repair of an acute laceration is not necessary (even in athletes), this concept has been challenged recently. Possible loss of windlass mechanism and function have raised concerns about long-term outcome. Secondary complications include loss of great toe motion and the development of secondary hallux hyperextension. Severe deformity usually is associated with a combined FHL/flexor hallucis brevis (FHB)

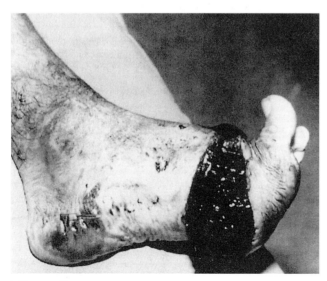

Figure 5

This patient sustained an industrial injury to the plantar aspect of the MTP joints. Notice the hyperextension of all the toes, indicative of laceration of the FHL, FDL, flexor hallucis brevis, and flexor digitorum brevis. (Reproduced with permission from Bell W, Schon L: Tendon laceration in the toes and foot. *Foot Ankle Clin* 1996;1:355.)

laceration (this may require tenodesis of FHL to FHB) (Fig. 5). Of the 5 nonrepaired cases in 2 series, only 3 did well. Another indication for surgical repair is the high incidence of documented nerve injuries; approximately 50% had an associated nerve injury and over 13% of the nerve injuries were not identified in the emergency room. None of the patients who underwent primary surgical repair developed secondary deformity, and most (60%) regained active interphalangeal (IP) flexion.

Atraumatic Rupture Spontaneous atraumatic rupture of the FHL is extremely rare and is most likely to occur in high-performance athletes (eg, marathon runners) who perform repetitive activities.

The mechanism for atraumatic FHL rupture is related to its function and tendon vascularity. The FHL is associated, specifically, with push off upon a dorsiflexed first MTP joint, to propel the limb forward. The tendon is completely ensheathed from its decussation to its insertion at the distal phalanx. Several studies reported the FHL blood supply consists of either a single or double mesomembrane. During dorsiflexion, the increased tension secondary to muscle contraction and compression about the first metatarsal head may result in vascular compromise. Inadequate healing or recovery time secondary to repetitive activities may result in FHL rupture. Additional mechanical factors (such as pseudarthrosis of the talus or os trigonum) also can lead to FHL rupture. A majority of atraumatic FHL ruptures occur proximal to its insertion to the distal phalanx (0.5 cm) or intersesamoid metatarsal head region. Other locations include under the sustentaculum tali, as well as the groove of the posterior process of the talus. The mechanism is a secondary failure with retraction and disruption of the supportive soft-tissue structure. Operative findings include a frayed and bulbous tendon end, which may be less amenable to repair.

Surgical options depend on the location of the rupture. For distal FHL rupture (distal phalanx insertion or metatarsal intersesamoid region), primary repair with early active motion should be attempted. If necessary, the distal FHL tendon remnant can be secured to the FHB muscle belly. For rupture about the hindfoot or under the sustentaculum, the tendon is often retracted proximally. Options include exploration with FHL tenodesis to the FDL proximally and distally.

Due to the small number of cases reported, only certain trends have been identified. After primary repair of a closed FHL rupture distal near its insertion, active motion at the IP joint did not return. Stiffness did develop but was not disabling. After an FHL rupture in the hindfoot (sustentaculum), active flexion was recovered with some disability.

Isolated Stenosing Tenosynovitis/Posterior Impingement Syndrome

Recent attention has been directed to dancers who sustain either stenosing tenosynovitis of FHL (dancer tendinitis) and/or posterior impingement syndrome of the hindfoot. These disorders primarily affect professional-level ballet dancers and are rarely seen in the general athlete population. Although distinct entities, they often coexist and must be considered in patients (especially dancers) who present with vague hindfoot discomfort. The nonanatomic, rigidly defined positions at the extreme joint range of motion place substantial functional demands on ballet dancers' tendons. One author describes the moving from flat foot to *demi pointe* or *en pointe* position as predisposing the dancer to "stenosing tendinitis of FHL."

Clinical hallmarks of these two disorders allow differentiation between dancer tendinitis and a posterior impingement syndrome. Dancer tendinitis is characterized by recurrent posteromedial pain and swelling over the tarsal tunnel, directly posterior to the medial malleolus. Often this entity is confused with posterior tibial tendinitis. The triggering and crepitus of the FHL commonly is reproducible, especially with great toe actions similar to its movement while dancing. A painful crepitus of the FHL with active motion can lead to "functional hallux rigidus."

Dancer tendinitis is thought to be an inflammatory process that occurs at the proximal margin of the fibro-osseous tunnel beneath the sustentaculum tali. Chronic inflammation and hypertrophy of the muscular tendinous junction occur, leading to a painful stenosing tenosynovitis (Fig. 6). Other

mechanisms include a secondary impingement of the aberrant muscle belly.

In one series, the symptoms of pain and tenderness were present for a mean of 6 months. Exacerbated by jumping, the symptoms caused all dancers to lose their ability to stand *en pointe*. Crepitus was noted in half the patients and triggering in one fourth of the patients. None had pain in the posterolateral aspect of the ankle with forced plantarflexion, which would suggest an os trigonum.

Pain in the posterior ankle when a dancer assumes *demi pointe* or *en pointe* position suggests the diagnosis of posterior impingement syndrome. Reproduction of the pain with passive plantarflexion of the relaxed foot (the plantarflexor test) is one objective test. The diagnosis can be confirmed by pain relief after injecting an anesthetic agent in the region of os trigonum. Other clinical findings consistent with posterior impingement syndrome are an enlarged talar process (Steida process), prominence of posterior process of calcaneus, loose bodies, and an os trigonum. Although the size of the anatomic findings has not been associated with symptom severity, the etiology of the symptoms is compression of the talofibular ligament and the posterior capsule with passive plantarflexion.

Other diagnoses should be considered in patients with posterior hindfoot pain. For patients with pain in the posteromedial aspect of the ankle, the differential diagnosis includes FHL tendinitis, posterior deltoid ligament strain, osteochondritis dissecans (OCD) of the talus dome, soleus syndrome, posterior tibial tendon (PTT) dysfunction, and tarsal tunnel syndrome. For patients with pain in the posterolateral aspect

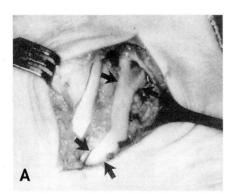 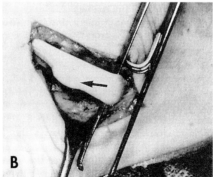 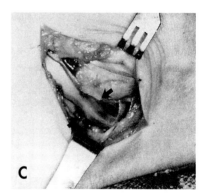

Figure 6

A, Operative photograph showing the flexor hallucis longus to be constricted at the entrance of the fibro-osseous tunnel (arrows). The tendon is completely free with the ankle and the great toe in the neutral position. The flexor digitorum longus is anterior to the flexor hallucis longus. **B,** Operative photograph showing a large nodule (arrow) within the fibro-osseous tunnel. Despite the size of the nodule, there was free excursion of the tendon after release of the tunnel. **C,** Operative photograph showing that the distal insertion of muscle fibers (arrows) into the tendon within the tunnel creates a mass effect contributing to the tendinitis of the flexor hallucis longus. (Reproduced with permission from Hamilton WG, Geppert MJ, Thompson FM: Pain in posterior aspect of the ankle in dancers: Differential diagnosis and operative treatment. *J Bone Joint Surg* 1996;78A:1491–1500.)

of the ankle, the differential diagnosis includes posterior impingement syndrome, fracture of the os trigonum, Achilles tendinitis, peroneal tendinitis, and retrocalcaneal bursitis.

MRI may be useful in diagnosing FHL tenosynovitis. One case report documented an increased signal on T2-weighted image representing fluid completely surrounding the tendon 5 months after injury. Surgery confirmed a partial FHL tear. However, specificity of the MRI, theoretically, is limited by the typical presence of fluid in the tendon sheath of asymptomatic individuals. Sensitivity is obscured by synovial proliferation, which can displace the fluid surrounding the tendon. Advanced radiographic study with bone scan or CT scan rarely is indicated. However, one series documented a previously missed osteoid osteoma in the posterior aspect of the talus using a CT scan.

Treatment

Initial nonsurgical treatment of dancer tendinitis and posterior impingement syndrome involves activity modifications, muscle strengthening, and correction of the patient's dance technique. Training can continue but without the *en pointe* exercise and turnout should be reduced so that the weight of the body is centered over the foot. Other conservative measures include a nonsteroidal inflammatory medication and physical therapy (stretching, massage, ice, ultrasound, contrast bath).

Steroids are not advocated. Risk of tendon rupture and difficulty of accurate steroid placement as well as the contiguous nature of the posterior tibial tendon preclude its routine use. In one series, 13 of 32 patients had injections of local anesthetics and steroids into the posterior lateral aspect of the ankle without relief. Failure to respond to nonsurgical therapy (range, 5 to 21 months) was an indication for surgery. One author believed that failure to respond after 3 months of nonsurgical therapy was an indication for operative treatment.

Several surgical approaches exist for FHL tendinitis and posterior impingement syndrome. For patients with both diagnoses, a medial approach is advocated. A lateral approach should be used to treat only the isolated posterior impingement syndrome.

One retrospective review assessed surgical outcomes of stenosing tenosynovitis of the FHL tendon and posterior impingement syndrome in 37 dancers (41 operations). Twenty-six operations were performed for tendinitis and posterior impingement syndrome, 9 for isolated tendinitis, and 6 for isolated posterior impingement syndrome. Thirty ankles had good or excellent results, 6 had fair results, and 4 had poor results after 7 years. One interesting finding was a good or excellent outcome in 28 of 34 professional dancers, as compared with only 2 of 6 amateur dancers.

Another series described 13 female ballet dancers who had surgical release of the FHL tendon because of isolated stenosing FHL tenosynovitis. After 6.5 years, all 13 had returned to dancing at a mean of 5 months, and 11 of 13 reached a level of full dancing participation without restrictions.

Results of these two clinical series indicated that surgical release of the FHL tendon is effective for the treatment of isolated stenosing tenosynovitis at the level of the ankle after failure of conservative treatment. This can be useful for ballet dancers who place a high demand on the ankle and foot. In contrast, it appears that surgical treatment in amateur dancers rarely meets their expectations.

Posterior Tibial Tendon

Anatomy

The posterior tibial tendon (PTT) courses behind the medial malleolus, posterior to the axis of the ankle and medial to the axis of the subtalar joint. It inserts into the plantar and medial aspect of the navicular, plantar aspects of three cuneiforms, and the base of second, third, and fourth metatarsals. By virtue of its anatomic location and strength, the PTT is considered a plantarflexor as well as an invertor of the foot. The PTT is critical in inverting the hindfoot and locking the transverse tarsal joint for normal gait and ambulation. When the hindfoot is everted, the transverse tarsal joints are unlocked and become parallel. This allows the hindfoot joint to remain supple. Conversely, when the hindfoot is inverted, the axes of the transverse tarsal joint become divergent and the subtalar complex becomes rigid. This biomechanical relationship is critical in allowing the gastrocnemius-soleus complex to flex the foot as a rigid lever arm during the push off phase of gait.

Posterior Tibial Tendon Dislocation

Although subluxation/dislocation of the peroneal tendons is a well-recognized phenomenon, a similar disorder of the PTT rarely is recognized. In a series of 7 patients with PTT dislocation diagnosed by symptoms, physical examination, and MRI (n = 2), surgical findings included tenosynovitis in 3 patients, a shallow or incompetent flexor groove in 5 patients, and a tear or absence of flexor retinaculum in all 7 patients. MRI was useful in documenting dislocation in the 2 patients. The surgical treatment consisted of flexor retinaculum reconstruction with an occasional groove-deepening procedure.

Posterior Tibial Tendon Dislocation and Incarceration

PTT dislocation with incarceration is an uncommon phenomenon after fracture-dislocation of the ankle. Although rare, PTT entrapment can occur in patients with a pronation eversion injury of the ankle. It is theorized that the site of entrapment is dependent upon the energy involved and the degree of lateral talar subluxation. With a low-energy injury and minimal subluxation, the PTT becomes entrapped in the medial malleolar fracture or medial joint space. Ten reported cases of PTT entrapment demonstrated a ruptured PTT with interposition into the gutter or into the medial malleolus fracture. With a high-energy injury, as seen with severe talar subluxation/dislocation, further displacement of the PTT results in entrapment within the syndesmosis. The inability to achieve an anatomic reduction of the joint, medially or at the syndesmosis, is an indication for exploration for soft-tissue interposition.

Posterior Tibial Tendon Dysfunction

PTT dysfunction refers to a spectrum of changes involving varying amounts of pathology. Often there is a flexible or fixed deformity of the subtalar and transverse tarsal joints. At surgery, the PTT changes can range from paratenonitis without intratendinous deterioration to a pure tendinosis and, finally, to a frank tendon rupture. In addition, the static constraints (ie, spring ligament) can be involved without substantial PTT pathology.

In patients with PTT dysfunction, the ability to invert the hindfoot is diminished by the gastrocnemius-soleus complex acting upon the talonavicular joint. In addition, loss of PTT function results in an unopposed peroneus brevis muscle, with a dynamic abduction eversion force. Through these dynamic forces, gradual attenuation of the medial static constraints of the longitudinal arch occurs. Loss of the secondary soft-tissue constraints (deltoid ligament, talonavicular capsule, spring ligament) allows a progressive deformity to develop, including flattening of the arch, medial subluxation/plantarflexion of the talus, valgus alignment of the calcaneus, and increased abduction of the forefoot. As the heel assumes an increased valgus alignment, the Achilles tendon aligns lateral to the axis of rotation of the subtalar joint. This shortened position results in a secondary Achilles tendon contracture. Secondary changes may develop over time, with chronic malalignment of the transverse tarsal (forefoot abduction and supination) as well as hindfoot articulations (valgus angulation of the heel with horizontal orientation of the subtalar joints). Although initially flexible and reducible, this chronic malalignment leads to a fixed deformity with development of secondary arthritis. Further progression with valgus angulation of the heel results in a lateral impingement of the calcaneus and fibula (creating pain and discomfort in the lateral aspect of sinus tarsi) as well as the development of arthritis in the tibiotalar articulation.

PTT dysfunction has been attributed to numerous factors. Although initially described in obese, middle-aged women, one study of 67 patients (average age, 57 years) with ruptured PTT found that 47 of the patients (60%) had additional medical problems including hypertension, obesity, diabetes, steroid exposure, and/or previous surgery or trauma about the medial aspect of the foot. The authors concluded the prevalence of PTT rupture parallels the degenerative changes associated with aging.

The origin of PTT pathology has been attributed to extrinsic and intrinsic factors. One extrinsic factor is local injection of steroids. In one series, 3 of 10 patients with a spontaneous rupture of PTT had received a local injection of corticosteroid in and about the area. Another series documented that corticosteroid injection about the PTT or oral intake was associated with increased risk of PTT rupture. Although rare, traumatic injuries such as an ankle fracture or fracture/dislocation have been associated with PTT rupture and incarceration.

However, it is likely that most PTT dysfunction is secondary to an intrinsic abnormality of the tendon. Two theories have been postulated: hypovascular theory and inflammatory process. Due to the lack of the mesotenon in that region, hypovascularity of the PTT can predispose the tendon to degeneration after injury. A cadaveric study found a relative zone of hypovascularity that begins approximately 1.0 to 1.5 cm distal to the medial malleolus and extends 14 mm distally around the PTT's excursion about the medial malleolus. PTT dysfunction also has been linked to several inflammatory processes. Of 76 patients with PTT dysfunction, 47 also had seronegative spondyloarthropathy (ie, Reiter syndrome, spondylosing arthropathy, and psoriasis). In these patients, multiple sites of enthesopathy as well as oral ulcers, conjunctivitis, colitis, and especially psoriasis, were common.

Clinical Presentation and Diagnosis

Patients usually deny any major, acute traumatic event and describe a gradual onset of flatfoot deformity. The classic description is an elderly woman with vague discomfort about the ankle. While obtaining a history, it is useful to elicit any information concerning a systemic inflammatory process (eg, seronegative inflammatory arthropathy).

Initially, it may be difficult for patients to localize the discomfort. Tenderness can occur along the medial aspect of the ankle, especially upon stress with activities. Discomfort along the PTT tendon sheath may also be elicited along its attachment on the undersurface of the navicular. When localized, the site of tenderness usually corresponds to the area of PTT involvement. Upon further progression, substantial discomfort can be elicited laterally in the sinus tarsi secondary to lateral impingement and the development of secondary subtalar arthritis.

In a weightbearing situation, the physical examination may reveal a classic triad of foot deformity associated with advanced PTT dysfunction. First, a "valgus alignment of the hindfoot and increased abduction of the forefoot" is commonly present. As a result of these deformities, a flatfoot appearance develops. Upon observing the patient from behind, there is the appearance of "too many toes" on the involved foot. This triad, in conjunction with the inability to perform a single heel rise, is consistent with the diagnosis of PTT dysfunction.

Although PTT dysfunction can be identified easily in its advanced stages, early diagnosis is often difficult. A recent study described a new, simple clinical test, the first metatarsal rise sign, to recognize early PTT dysfunction. The test is performed by externally rotating the shank of the affected foot with one hand or passively aligning the heel of the affected foot into varus position. The head of the first metatarsal will rise in presence of a PTT dysfunction and will remain on the floor if PTT function is normal. In a prospective series of 19 patients and 21 consecutive feet, the first metatarsal rise sign was positive in all cases of PTT dysfunction, while other clin-

ical signs (too many toes sign, single heel rise, and double heel rise) were negative in 20% to 35%. This simple clinical test may be the earliest finding of PTT dysfunction and can enable the clinician to recognize and treat the PTT dysfunction prior to its progression.

Care should be taken to exclude other causes of flatfoot deformity. The differential diagnosis includes a neuropathic arthropathy, or posttraumatic deformity (ie, status post-Lisfranc dislocation). Other considerations for acquired adult flatfoot include secondary arthritis of the ankle, talonavicular, or tarsal metatarsal articulation.

Classification of PTT Dysfunction

PTT pathology can occur at several anatomic sites: tendon insertion, a mid-substance rupture, incontinuity tears, as well as an isolated tenosynovitis. A wide range of PTT dysfunction exists; therefore, clinical staging of PTT dysfunction is critical to determining an optimal treatment protocol (Table 1). The original three stages are based on the presence or absence of the hindfoot or transverse tarsal deformity and the ability to achieve a flexible reduction of the involved articulation. Recent modification of the classification added a fourth stage: progression of the PTT dysfunction leading to an

Table 1

Treatment of dysfunction of the posterior tibial tendon

		Treatment	
Stage	**Characteristics**	**Nonoperative**	**Operative**
Tenosynovitis	Acute medial pain and swelling, can perform heel-rise, seronegative inflammation, extensive tearing	Anti-inflammatory medication, immobilization for 6 to 8 weeks; if symptoms improve, ankle stirrup-brace; if symptoms do not improve, operative treatment	Tenosynovectomy, tenosynevectomy + calcaneal osteotomy, or tenosynovectomy + tenodesis of flexor digitorum longus to posterior tibial tendon
Rupture			
Stage I	Medial pain and swelling, hindfoot flexible, can perform heel-rise	Medial heel-and-sole shoe wedge, hinged ankle-foot orthosis, orthotic arch-supports	Debridement of posterior tibial tendon, flexor digitorum longus transfer, or flexor digitorum longus transfer + calcaneal osteotomy
Stage II	Valgus angulation of heel, lateral pain, hindfoot flexible, cannot perform heel-rise	Medial heel-and-sole wedge, stiff orthotic support, hinged ankle-foot orthosis, injection of steroids into the sinus tarsi	Flexor digitorum longus transfer + calcaneal osteotomy or flexor digitorum longus transfer + bone-block arthrodesis at calcaneocuboid joint
Stage III	Valgus angulation of heel, lateral pain, hindfoot rigid, cannot perform heel-rise	Rigid ankle-foot orthosis	Triple arthrodesis
Stage IV	Hindfoot rigid, valgus angulation of talus	Rigid ankle-foot orthosis	Tibiotalocalcaneal arthrodesis

(Reproduced with permission from Myerson MS: Adult acquired flatfoot deformity: Treatment of dysfunction of posterior tibial tendon, in Springfield DS (ed): *Instructional Course Lectures 46.* Rosemont, IL, American Academy of Orthopaedic Surgeons, 1997, pp 393–405.)

increasingly progressive talar subluxation and valgus angulation, which leads to degenerative arthritis of the tibiotalar articulation.

Imaging

Classic radiographic findings suggesting PTT rupture include a collapse of the talocalcaneal angle seen on lateral radiographs or an increase in the talocalcaneal angle seen on the anteroposterior (AP) radiographs of the foot. The AP view can also show lateral subluxation of the talonavicular joint and on the lateral view, sagging of the talonavicular, navicular cuneiform, or medial metatarsal cuneiform joint with increased talocalcaneal overlap. While these findings may confirm a flatfoot deformity, these changes are seen late in the disease process. Often, the radiographic findings observed in conjunction with PTT dysfunction are not directly related to the extent of the PTT degeneration. One series reported that only 3 of 21 consecutive feet in patients with surgically proven PTT dysfunction had any significant increase in the talocalcaneal angle. Another study found similar results (3 of 19 feet had increased talocalcaneal angle).

Ultrasonography has demonstrated an increasing role in the diagnosis of tendon pathology. Advantages of real-time US include the ability to confirm PTT rupture in vague clinical scenerios, the ability to differentiate between intratendinous and peritendinous structural changes, noninvasive follow-up without risk of radiation, objective means to assess effect of conservative and surgical treatment, and the ability to provide US-guided aspiration. In addition, dynamic assessment of tendon function is possible under real-time conditions. Using a 10 MHz linear array transducer, normal PTTs appear hyperechoic and oval, with an average diameter of 7.8 mm ˇ 3.7 mm at the medial malleolar level. Degenerated PTTs appear hypoechoic and swollen (9.8 mm ˇ 5.0 mm). Peritendinitis presents as a hypoechoic rim on a longitudinal sonogram and a "target" (hyperechoic centrally with hypoechoic halo on the transverse sonogram at right angle to the long axis of the tendon). Complete PTT rupture appears as an empty tibia groove at the level of medial malleolus on the transverse sonogram and a wavy fibril pattern over distal end of longitudinal sonogram.

A retrospective study evaluated US by comparing the preoperative sonograms in 17 patients with their intraoperative findings. Surgical findings confirmed the sonograms: 3 with inflammation, 4 with partial tears, and 10 with complete rupture. Another series documented the efficacy of US in 9 patients with surgical confirmation after US assessment. Compared to surgical findings and results of MRI, there were no false positive or false negative findings of tenosynovitis or complete rupture of tendon. It appears that US is a reliable

means of visualizing the extent of symptomatic PTT pathology and may have a role in planning the surgical intervention.

Another diagnostic tool is the MRI in PTT pathology. One study documented the superiority of MRI in defining the tendon substance and soft-tissue structures (73%) as compared to the computed tomography scan (59%) based on intraoperative observations.

One study compared the prognostic value of MRI imaging-based grading versus intraoperative grading in 20 patients who underwent reconstruction of the PTT. Intraoperative grading did not correlate with the outcome following reconstruction of the tendons, although in contrast, MRI grading was predictive of the outcome. One theory is that the superior sensitivity of MRI allows detection of intramural degeneration that was not observed at the time of surgery.

One recent study correlated the secondary MRI changes in diagnosing PTT dysfunction. Twenty-three patients with complete PTT tears and 34 control patients were evaluated by MRI to document the appearance of completely torn versus normal PTT. First, classic MRI "diagnostic" findings of PTT tear (ie, increased tendon girth and internally increased signal intensity) were found frequently in normal tendons and were not specific, reliable indicators of PTT pathology. In contrast, secondary signs such as talonavicular abnormality (failure of long axis of talus to bisect the navicular), the presence of medial tubercle hypertrophy, and the presence of an accessory navicular bone, were useful diagnostic signs of complete PTT tear.

There appears to be great reliance today on special imaging studies, such as MRI, when evaluating tendon dysfunction. It is evident the diagnosis should instead be based on a thorough history and careful physical examination of the patient.

Despite the ability of MRI in assessing the tendon about the foot, one series challenged this concept. The MRI failed to reveal pathologic changes in 7 of 16 patients with intraoperatively proven PTT pathology. In the 7 negative MRI studies, intraoperative evaluation revealed an attenuation and/or elongation of the tendon in 6 patients. Based on these findings, the authors recommended against routine use of MRI in patients with a suspected PTT dysfunction.

Treatment

The treatment of PTT dysfunction is dependent upon the clinical stage at the time of presentation (Table 1). Although many authors believe that conservative management acts mainly as a temporizing measure prior to surgical intervention, nonsurgical treatment should be attempted first for most symptomatic PTT dysfunction patients. Patients with tenosynovitis/stage I usually respond to nonsurgical measures. Patients with advanced disease may improve with nonsurgical measures but must be informed that there is a risk of disease progression.

The goals of nonsurgical management include elimination of symptoms, stress reduction of the compromised tendon, support of the flattened arch, improvement of the hindfoot alignment, and the prevention of the progressive foot deformity. Initial treatment consists of rest, administration of an NSAID, and immobilization (with either a rigid below-knee cast or boot) to prevent overuse and rupture of the tendon. Immobilization for 6 to 8 weeks can improve the symptoms and allow progression to either a stiff-sole shoe with a medial heel or sole wedge or an orthosis, either a University of California/Berkeley orthosis (UCBL) or an ankle-foot orthosis (AFO) (Figs. 7 and 8). If the symptoms continue, additional immobilization or surgical intervention can be contemplated.

One recent series evaluated 49 patients with PTT dysfunction treated by either a molded AFO (40 feet) or UCBL (13 feet). With a mean follow-up of 20.3 months, 33 patients (67%) had excellent or good results. Most of these patients were older, with relatively low activity demands. Six were able to discontinue the orthosis use; the remaining 26 used the orthosis continually from treatment initiation. Patients with fair or poor results after bracing were usually younger with higher activity demands. Often, long-term bracing was not compatible with their lifestyles. Nonsurgical management using an orthosis (UCBL, AFO) appears useful for elderly patients with sedentary lifestyles or for patients at risk secondary to medical problems.

Patients with tenosynovitis stage I who fail 6 to 8 weeks of conservative management may require tenosynovectomy. Tenosynovitis is seen often in younger patients with a seronegative inflammatory disease, an aggressive condition associated with inflammatory infiltrate into the tendon, which may lead to rupture unless arrested.

Surgical treatment has proven effective in a series of 19 patients who underwent tenosynovectomy and debridement of PTT for stage I dysfunction. Seventeen of 19 patients reported subjective improvement and return of function at 30 months follow-up. The authors theorized that surgical intervention arrested the disease progression.

It is critical to differentiate the young patient with an inflammatory disease process (stage I) who benefits from tenosynovectomy from the nonseronegative patient with a degenerative tendon. In the older nonseronegative patient, the failure of nonsurgical treatment with continued symptoms and tendon degeneration may necessitate a supplemental procedure in addition to the tenosynovectomy.

The surgical treatment of stage II PTT dysfunction remains highly controversial. One previously advocated surgical intervention was the PTT reconstruction with a flexor ten-

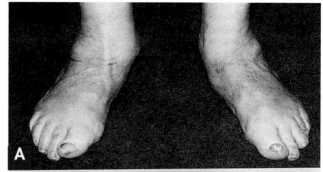
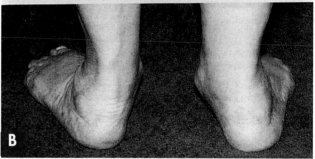

Figure 7

View of patient from the front (**A**) and behind (**B**). Forefoot abduction, heel valgus, and "too-many-toes sign" are seen. (Reproduced with permission from Lin SS, et al: Nonoperative treatment of posterior tibia tendon dysfunction. *Foot Ankle Clin* 1996;1:261.)

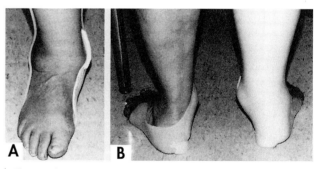

Figure 8

A, Viewed from the front, the right foot is braced with a custom molded ankle–foot orthosis (MAFO). **B,** Viewed from behind, a UCBL shoe insert with medial posting and custom MAFO is used to treat stages II and III PTT dysfunction, respectively. (Reproduced with permission from Lin SS, et al: Nonoperative treatment of posterior tibia tendon dysfunction. *Foot Ankle Clin* 1996;1:261.)

don transfer. Prior to a flexor tendon transfer, several anatomic factors should be considered including hindfoot flexibility, amount of forefoot varus (should be < than 5° of fixed varus), and the activity level of the patient.

Either the FHL or FDL have been used for tendon transfer, although the FDL is most commonly used. FHL dissection is more complicated because of its close proximity to the neurovascular bundle and because its donor site deficit is greater. In contrast, it is not necessary to perform a tenodesis of the FHL to the stump of the newly harvested FDL because multiple interconnections exist between the two. Also, the contiguous proximity of the PTT to the FDL makes the latter a more suitable tendon for PTT reconstruction.

Success with an isolated FDL transfer for advanced stages of PTT dysfunction (stage II or III) has been reported, but results have deteriorated over time secondary to insufficiency of transferred FDL tendon. Although the mechanism for the FDL failure is unclear, one recent case report documented a complete rupture of the FDL tendon 42 months after successful transfer for PTT rupture. These concerns have led to newer techniques for reconstruction of a flexible flatfoot deformity.

One new technique recently proposed is a medial displacement calcaneal osteotomy to correct the valgus heel angulation. This procedure has been advocated in combination with tenosynovectomy in patients with advanced stage I disease or in conjunction with a flexor tendon transfer for stage II. The procedure shifts the os calcis medially and realigns the valgus heel under the mechanical axis of the leg. The end result is reduction of the deforming valgus force of the gastrocnemius-soleus muscle group and potential antagonistic force on the FDL transfer.

Radiographs of 18 patients with PTT dysfunction were reviewed 12 to 26 months after FDL tendon transfer, combined with a medial displacement calcaneal osteotomy. On AP weightbearing radiographs, the mean talus-first metatarsal angle decreased from 21° to 8.5° (mean improvement, 12.5°) and the mean talonavicular coverage angle decreased from 34° to 21° (mean improvement, 13°). On the lateral weightbearing radiographs, the talar-first metatarsal angle decreased from -22° to -9° (mean improvement, 13°) and the distance from the medial cuneiform increased from 9 to 16 mm (mean improvement, 7 mm). While improved radiographic parameters were evident throughout the series, it is still unknown whether these changes will remain stable over time.

Another proposed procedure involves lengthening the lateral column of the foot with interposition tricortical iliac crest bone graft, supplementing the FDL tendon transfer. One author reported improvement in the flatfoot deformity with respect to various radiographic parameters (lateral talocalcaneal angle, lateral talo-first metatarsal angle, AP talometatarsal angle, calcaneal pitch, talonavicular coverage angle) with calcaneal lengthening. In vitro studies have supported this concept because the motion of

the talonavicular joint is maintained to a great extent after a lateral column arthrodesis as well as a minimal amount of the subtalar motion.

Another option for stage II PTT insufficiency is a combination of lateral column lengthening with medial displacement osteotomy of the calcaneus in addition to the FDL tendon transfer and percutaneous heel cord lengthening. The authors believe these extra-articular procedures, when combined, rebalance the mechanical forces but with minimal displacement at each site. Of 17 patients (20 cases) with stage II PTT, most improved dramatically (51.4 versus 82.8; p < 0.01; AOFAS hindfoot scores). Radiographic measurement showed significant correction of the pes planovalgus deformity. With an average follow-up of 17.5 months, correction of the deformity has been maintained in majority of cases. The authors concluded the combination surgical procedure alleviates the symptoms and corrects the deformity associated with PTT stage II; however, the long-term results are unknown.

Another proposed technique involves a subtalar arthrodesis in conjunction with the FDL tendon transfer to correct the collapse of the talocalcaneal angle and the lateral talar subluxation over the calcaneous. Criticism of this technique includes the increased risk of arthritis in the joints contiguous to the subtalar arthrodesis. In addition, minimal arthritis exists in the subtalar joint for many patients with stage II PTT dysfunction.

A rigid valgus deformity (stage III) of the hindfoot or a hindfoot corrected to neutral with a fixed forefoot supination deformity usually will necessitate some form of arthrodesis. Numerous procedures have been advocated for advanced PTT dysfunction, including an isolated talonavicular, double (talonavicular and calcanealcuboid), subtalar, and triple arthrodesis. The choice of joint(s) ideal for arthrodesis depends on the extent and location of the deformity, as well as the degree of arthritis present. Using a cadaveric model, a recent study analyzed an acquired flatfoot deformity to determine the amount of correction obtained with selective hindfoot fusion. Although the talonavicular, double, and triple arthrodesis was able to fully correct the deformity, the subtalar and calcaneocuboid arthrodeses failed to completely correct this. Although triple joints are interconnected, the various hindfoot arthrodeses differ in their ability to correct malalignment.

Although the ideal procedure for stage III PTT dysfunction has not been determined, triple arthrodesis, with its long history of successful treatment for neuromuscular deformities in children, has been described with modifications for adult-acquired PTT flatfoot deformity. A triple arthrodesis is indicated only for patients with a fixed hindfoot deformity and lateral foot pain. A recent series of triple arthrodeses in older patients with flatfoot deformity was associated with a high rate of postoperative complications, including development/progression of arthritis in the contiguous joints (ie, ankle joint). A severe deformity with a rigidly fixed hindfoot allows progression of the talus into a valgus alignment at the tibiotalar articulation (stage IV). The authors cautioned that while triple arthrodesis will eliminate pain secondary to arthritis, this procedure should be used only as a salvage attempt for severe fixed deformities or major arthritic changes in the subtalar and transverse tarsal joints. Stage IV PTT dysfunction or tibiotalar malalignment may necessitate a tibiotalar calcaneal arthrodesis.

Peroneal Tendons

Introduction

The peroneus longus (PL) and peroneus brevis (PB) are the major lateral tendons of the ankle. Working as the major pronators and evertors of the foot, these tendons participate during the push-off phase of gait and supplement the lateral stability of the ankle. The function and unique anatomy of the PB/PL subject them to large physiologic loads that, in various foot positions, can lead to a pathologic condition. Several clinical conditions (PB subluxation/dislocation, PB tendinitis/split tears, and painful os peroneal syndrome) will be described in greater detail.

Anatomy

The lateral compartment consists of the PL and the PB. Both muscles become tendinous prior to their turn at the tip of lateral malleolus. The PL muscle is distinct, with three turns prior to its insertion at the base of the first metatarsal (as well as the insertional slips to the first cuneiform and the base of the second metatarsal). Lying posterolateral to the PB, the PL tendon first turns at the tip of the lateral malleolus, turns next below the trochlear process of the calcaneus, turns finally at the groove of the cuboid, and then crosses the plantar surface of the foot obliquely. The PB tendon is distinct from PL and lies directly behind the posterior lateral malleolus on its pathway to the styloid process of the fifth metatarsal base.

In order to understand the clinical presentation of peroneal tendons, an osteology review is critical (Fig. 9). The tendons lie directly in the retromalleolar sulcus. Although most fibular sulci are concave (with a documented sulcus width of 5.0 to 10.0 mm and a depth up to 3 mm), several anatomic studies documented an 18% to 28% incidence of a flat or convex shape. These anatomic variations of the fibula may predispose the patient to certain pathologic conditions.

One important soft-tissue structure of the lateral foot is the peroneal retinaculum. The PB/PL lie within a synovial sheath that begins approximately 3.5 cm proximal and 4.0 cm distal to the tip of the fibula. This tendon sheath (as well as the peroneal tendons) runs through a fibro-osseous tunnel that facilitates its passage on the lateral side of the foot. Medially,

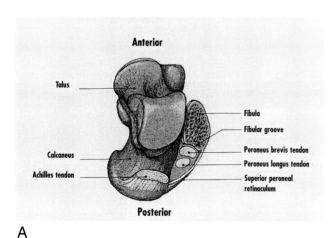

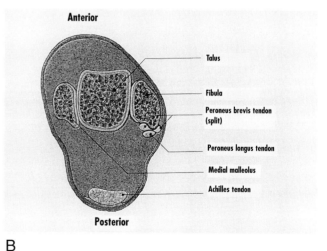

Figure 9

A, Cross-section of peroneus brevis and peroneus longus tendons within the fibular groove, contained by superior peroneal retinaculum. **B,** Cross-section of peroneal tendons at the fibular groove showing the mechanism of injury. The peroneal brevis is compressed by the longus, which lies posterior, into the sharp edge of fibula. This results in splitting of peroneus brevis tendon. The superior peroneal retinaculum is not shown. (Reproduced with permission from Yodlowski ML, Mizel MS: Reconstruction of peroneus brevis pathology. *Oper Tech Orthop* 1994;4:150.)

the tunnel consists of a posterior talofibular and calcane-ofibular ligament. The anterior aspect of the tunnel consists of the retromalleolar sulcus of the fibula. The posterior component consists of a calcaneofibular ligament and the posterior aspect of the retinaculum. The peroneal retinaculum, as well as its insertion into a fibrocartilaginous rim, forms the lateral wall of the fibro-osseous tunnel. Usually greater than 3 to 4 cm in length, the fibrocartilaginous rim increases and enhances the stability of the fibular groove by deepening the retromalleolar sulcus.

The peroneal retinaculum consists of two distinct portions (the superior and inferior aspects). Originating from the lateral aspects of the retromalleolar sulcus in conjunction with the fibrocartilaginous rim, the superior peroneal retinaculum (SPR) overlies the peroneal tendons and inserts into the Achilles tendon and superior aspect of the calcaneus. The importance of the SPR in tendon stability has been shown by a cadaveric study through sequential sectioning of the soft-tissue constraints. Isolated release of the SPR resulted in instability and the potential for dislocation of the peroneal tendons when the foot is in a calcaneovalgus position. In contrast, isolated sectioning of the inferior peroneal retinaculum did not. It is evident that the SPR provides stability by preventing the lateral subluxation of the peroneal tendons.

Many anomalous muscles have been described in relationship to the peroneal tendons. The peroneus quartus (PQ) is one of a group of accessory muscles unique to humans with its origin in the distal leg (frequently the peroneal muscles) and its distal attachment in variable positions. The PQ muscle has been classified based on its insertion: peroneocuboideus (insertion into cuboid), peroneoperoneolongus (insertion into PL tendon), and peroneocalcaneus externum (insertion into calcaneus). Several subtypes of the peroneocalcaneal variant have been described including peroneus accessorius (when the origin is in the tendinous portion of PB and the insertion is into the PL) and peroneus digiti minimi (origin is PB muscle to either proximal phalanx of fifth metatarsal or extensor aponeurosis of the fifth metatarsal). Simplification of this complex terminology has been proposed by an anatomic study under the heading of "variations of the peroneus quartus.

Initially believed to be rare, the PQ was present in 21.7% of the ankles in one study. In 17 legs (63% of the total specimens), the most common form of PQ originated from the muscular portion of PB in the lower aspect of leg and inserted into the peroneal tubercle of calcaneus, with or without connection with the inferior portion of annular ligament. A retrospective review of 136 ankle MRI studies found a 10% (14 of 136) prevalence. In contrast, a majority of accessory tendons inserted into the retrotrochlear eminence of the calcaneus rather than into the peroneal tubercle.

Recognition of the PQ is important because of its association with ankle pain, instability, and peroneal tendon subluxation. The association of PQ with peroneal subluxation is due to an encroachment phenomenon in the fibro-osseous tunnel, often leading to incompetency of the superior peroneal retinaculum. As use of MRI becomes more prevalent, recognition of the PQ may prevent misinterpretation of this finding (Fig. 10). One potential clinical application of PQ is in

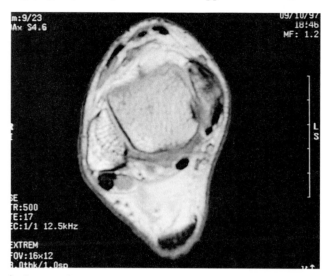

Figure 10
Axial MRI of ankle demonstrating presence of "peroneus quartus."

lateral ankle reconstructive procedures. Its substantial size and avoidance of the donor problems related to the sacrifice of the PB are the main benefits; however, further studies are necessary to confirm its role as a donor tendon.

Peroneus Brevis Tendinitis/Split Tears
PB tendinitis/split tear was believed to be rare; however, recent studies have documented that abnormalities of PB are more prevalent than previously thought. PB tendinitis/split tears should be considered in patients who present with chronic lateral ankle pain, swelling, and instability. In one series, PB tendon attrition was documented in 14 of 124 cadaveric ankles (11.3%). Another cadaveric study found 37 of 57 ankles (21%) with thinning or splitting of the PB tendon. Another series reported PB changes in 14 of 47 patients (30%) undergoing a lateral ankle stabilization procedure.

The degree of tendon attrition varies from peroneal tendinitis to multiple longitudinal splits of PB, to a complete rupture with substantial fraying of the remaining portions. The lesions varied in size between 1.9 cm (range, 1 to 4 cm) to 3.3 cm (range, 2.5 to 5.0 cm). Regardless of the size, the central portion of longitudinal PB split is centered over the distal tip of fibula. Histologic analysis of the tendon split regions revealed characteristic splaying of the collagen bundle with proliferation of the blood vessels and fibrovascular connective tissue. Signs of inflammatory infiltrates were not present and normal cellularity with collagen orientation was present in the regions of tendons not altered. Although a chronic wear and tear defect of the collagen existed, there was sufficient vascularity to mount a healing response.

Several theories have been proposed for the etiology of the PB split tears. One theory proposes a chronic wear and tear phenomenon secondary to maturity. Another theory involves hypovascularity, which occurs in young athletes as well as in mature and elderly patients. An anatomic study found that a sufficient blood supply exists in regard to the peroneal tendons. The current theory for the etiology of PB tendinitis/split tears is a "dynamic mechanical insult" at the fibular groove. Recent cadaveric studies confirmed the role of the SPR as the key restraining force holding the peroneal tendons in their normal anatomic location. Incompetency of the SPR combined with repetitive mechanical compression of PL causes the PB tendon to splay and actually split over the sharp fibrocartilaginous edge of the fibula.

Several anatomic factors contribute to the dynamic mechanical insult theory and the competency of the SPR. Variability in the shape of the fibula and its fibrocartilaginous ridge (normally a concave groove of the fibula is present, but 18% to 26% of specimens had a shallow or convex sulcus) could contribute to the incompetency of the SPR. Other anatomic conditions, such as a sharp fibrocartilaginous ridge as opposed to a round one, may contribute to PB tendon splitting.

One series describes another phenomenon, the encroachment within the fibular sulcus secondary to anomalous muscles. Congenital factors have been implicated in contributing to this overcrowding phenomenon within the peroneal tendon sheathe. These include PL/PB hypertrophy, a low-lying anomalous muscle (ie, PQ), and other congenital abnormalities of the PB tendon. By "overcrowding," the SPR may be partially attenuated/detached from the posterior border of the fibula and allow the peroneal tendons to subluxate laterally over the sharp posterior ridge of the fibula.

In conclusion, PB tendinitis/split tears is a dynamic mechanical lesion caused by a combination of anatomic factors and the incompetency of the SPR. These findings, in conjunction with the PL compression and the sharp posterior lateral edge of the fibula, lead to PB tendinitis/split tear. This theory may explain the wide gamut of patients ranging

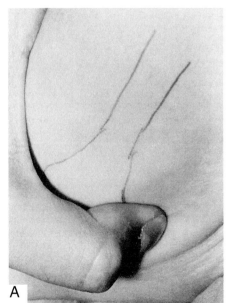
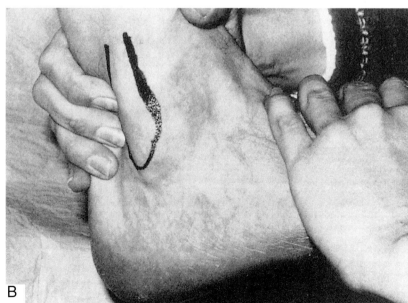

Figure 11

A, Photograph showing the position of the examiner's thumb spanning the posterior ridge of the fibula to the calcaneus and compressing the peroneal tendons and superior peroneal retinaculum as the foot is actually moved from a plantarflexed, inverted position to a dorsiflexed and everted position. **B,** Photograph showing that, alternatively, the examiner may place the index, middle, and long fingertips directed posteriorly over the posterior edge of the fibula while resisting ankle eversion with the opposite hand. (Reproduced with permission from Sobel M, Geppert MJ, Olson EJ, Bohne WH, Arnoczky SP: The dynamics of peroneus brevis tendon splits: a proposed mechanism, technique of diagnosis, and classification of injury. *Foot Ankle* 1992;13:413–422.)

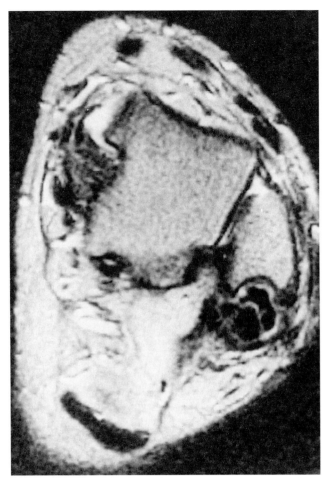

Figure 12

Axial MRI of ankle demonstrating chronic peroneus brevis lesion with multiple longitudinal tears.

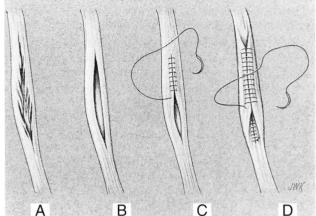

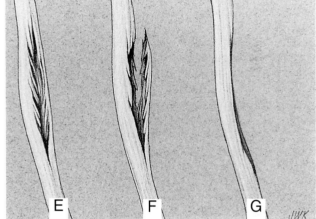

Figure 13

Top, If a major longitudinal tear is identified in the peroneus brevis tendon (**A**), it can be debrided along the frayed edges (**B**), repaired with 6-0 nylon suture (**C**), and the remaining portion of the tendon tubularized over the repair (**D**). **Bottom,** A tear involving the anterior one third of the peroneus brevis tendon (**E**). This may be sharply debrided (**F**) and completely excised (**G**). (Reproduced with permission from Yodlowski ML, Mizel MS: Reconstruction of peroneus brevis pathology. *Oper Tech Orthop* 1994;4:150.)

from young athletes with lateral ankle instability to mature, elderly individuals who present with little or no obvious risk factors.

Physical Examination

Often, it is difficult to ascertain the etiology of chronic lateral ankle discomfort (Fig. 11). The "peroneal tunnel compression test" has been proposed. With the patient seated on the edge of the examination table with the knee bent at 90°, the examiner places his or her thumb over the SPR from the posterior ridge of the fibula down to calcaneus. While the foot is actively moved from a plantarflexed inverted position to dorsiflexed everted position, reproduction of pain is considered a positive sign. One common finding is the "wet leather sign" or squeaking of the involved tendon. Additional findings include triggering or clicking of the peroneal tendon

within the fibular groove, possibly secondary to the anterior half of the PB attempting to subluxate.

Clinical findings can be confirmed by MRI. A recent cadaveric study found that perpendicular axial cuts at the level of the posterior ridge of the fibula by MRI enabled identification of muscle anomalies, such as PQ, as well as longitudinal attrition of the PB tendon (Fig. 12).

The treatment of PB tendinitis/split tears has not been evaluated in any large series. For patients refractory to conservative treatments, exploration of the peroneal sheath is recommended. Usually, findings include an attenuated superior peroneal retinaculum in conjunction with a PB tendinitis/split tear. If a split/tear is present, debridement of the tendon edge and repair of the PB split tear and/or tubularization of the tendon is recommended (Fig. 13). Associated anatomic factors, such as a convex fibular groove, an anomalous low-lying PB muscle or PQ, should also be addressed. Afterward, reefing of the SPR is indicated to improve the stability and prevent the resubluxation of the newly repaired tendon. If there are multiple frayed tears with substantial degeneration, the pathologic section may be excised with the proximal and distal end of PB tenodesed to PL.

Traumatic Peroneal Subluxation/ Dislocation

Traumatic subluxation/dislocation of the peroneal tendons is rare but has been reported after a variety of sports activities. The clinical presentation differs depending on the chronicity of the lesion. With an acute event, the peroneal tendon injury is immediately obvious, often with a snap heard during injury. Frequently, the patient is unable to continue with previous physical activities. While the patient commonly complains of pain in the lateral aspect of the ankle, the diagnosis often is confused with ankle sprain or instability. The spontaneous reduction of the tendon and the hemorrhage/edema of the lateral ankle can obscure and delay the primary diagnosis. In a chronic presentation, the patient experiences episodes of the "giving way" of the ankle, lateral instability, and a painful snap along the lateral ankle with activities.

Although controversy exists regarding ankle position at the time of injury, the basic premise is that a strong peroneal contracture overcomes the anatomic constraints of the fibro-osseous sheath. One theorized mechanism is the position of the ankle in dorsiflexion. In this position, the peroneus tendons tighten and produce an anteriorly directed force upon the fibula. An everted subtalar joint creates a laterally directed force component. Through contractions of the peroneal muscles, the SPR is avulsed off the fibula.

Another theorized mechanism is the position of ankle in inversion, which tightens the calcaneofibular ligament. The tightened calcaneofibular ligament narrows the fibro-osseous tunnel and pushes the peroneal tendon directly against the SPR and its periosteal insertion. Again, a violent muscle contraction is theorized to force the tendon to avulse and strip the SPR along with its periosteal attachments from the fibula. The end result is similar, with the formation of the pseudopouch and peroneal tendon pathology.

Regardless of the specific mechanism(s), a violent muscle contraction of peroneal tendon with an anteriorly and laterally directed force appears to be necessary to overcome the soft-tissue constraints. Other injuries that can occur include lateral ankle instability with lateral ligament disruption/tear; fracture of the lateral process of talus, the base of the fifth metatarsal, or the process of the calcaneus; OCD of talus; and/or rupture of the Achilles tendon.

Analysis of the pseudopouch reveals several interesting findings. The detached retinaculum commonly remains in continuity with the periosteum and forms a pseudopouch in which the subluxated/dislocated peroneal tendons reside. Often, a thin cortical sheet of bone is sheared off the fibula at the time of injury. Unrepaired, this roughened osseous surface can cause the dislocated tendon to become frayed or partially ruptured.

These injury patterns have been classified into three distinct grades based on surgical examination. In grade I, the retinaculum with its periosteum is stripped off the lateral malleolus and the fibrocartilaginous ridge by the dislocating tendons. In grade II, the distal lateral 1 to 2 cm of the dense fibrocartilaginous ridge is elevated along with retinaculum. In grade III, the retinaculum avulses a thin fragment of bone along with the fibrocartilaginous ridge.

Acute Injury: Nonoperative Treatment Four small studies evaluated the results of cast immobilization for acute peroneal tendon subluxation/dislocation. Of the 14 patients in these four studies, only 7 had satisfactory-to-good results. Additional studies have reported limited success with soft compressive dressings. One author reported only 9 of 17 patients had good-to-excellent outcomes with taping, J pads, and crutch ambulation. Another author reported a 73% recurrence rate (ie, failure) in 38 patients treated by compressive bandaging for several weeks. Another series reported only 3 of 10 patients with a good outcome. Four other studies comprising 13 patients reported a 100% failure rate. Although these series lack standardization and have many variables, it is evident the conservative approaches have a limited role with peroneal tendon subluxation/dislocation.

Acute Setting: Surgical Treatment Surgical repair of acute injuries has been advocated by more and more authors due to the suboptimal nonsurgical results, the increased difficulty of treatment with chronic lesions versus acute injury, and the simplicity of the surgery for an acute injury. Several studies have reported excellent results of primary repair with incision, plication, and suturing of the attenuated SPR to the fibrocartilaginous ridge. Variations of the surgical repair include reattachment of the redundant retinaculum via drill holes through the fibula with deepening of the retromalleolar sulcus. One author reported only 3 failures (mainly grade II lesions) in 61 patients. Another series reported success in 9 of 10 patients, with only one early failure secondary to suture rupture. Reoperation was successful and 9 were able to return to their previous sports activities. A similar outcome was noted in another series with only one recurrence in their 16 patients at final follow-up.

Three studies have documented success with grade III (peroneal tendon subluxation/dislocation with a cortical rim avulsion of the fibula) using open reduction and fixation with either a suture, Kirschner wires, and/or screws.

Chronic Setting: Surgical Treatment Chronic subluxation/dislocation of peroneal tendon must be repaired surgically. The numerous reconstructive procedures are: anatomic reconstructive repair, local soft-tissue supplementation, groove-deepening procedure, sliding bone-block technique, and rerouting procedure.

First, an attenuated SPR in continuity with the periosteum allows a direct repair of attenuated SPR. This technique involves scarification of the lateral malleolar surface and either suture or drill holes to hold down the SPR. One series described 6 of 7 patients returning to previous sports activities with good motion, no pain, and no recurrence of dislocation. Another option includes the use of suture anchors. Similar to the Bankart repair for chronic dislocation of the shoulder, the anatomic repair is becoming increasingly popular to correct soft-tissue instability.

Often, the SPR is absent or insufficient and alternative techniques have been advocated. One of the original methods advocated was the use of tendon slip from Achilles tendon swung downward on its calcaneal insertion and implanted into the lateral malleolus. One series reports good long-term results in 15 patients after 6.8 years. Only 1 patient was symptomatic at the final follow-up review. Another author reported an "excellent outcome in 11 patients stabilized with slips of the tendo Achillis." Other soft-tissue options include a plantaris slip, PB, and use of anomalous soft tissues including bifid PB or tendon of the PQ. Other options include a osteoperiosteal flap or the subsequent modification of the Chrisman-Snook procedure utilized as with the lateral ligament reconstruction. Unfortunately, few clinical series report the outcome of these techniques and further confirmation of their application is necessary prior to any definitive recommendation.

Groove-deepening procedures may be accomplished by the sliding bone-block technique or the decancellization of the posterolateral aspect of the fibula and recession of its cortex. The sliding bone-block technique has been created by a displacement of a posterior lateral fibula bone graft, followed by internal fixation. While a few series have reported excellent results using modified techniques, one series did report a 31% (36 cases) postoperative complication rate involving intra-articular screws, fracture of the malleolus, loose foreign body, (eg, as loose screws), and fracture of the bone graft.

Over 42% of the patients complained of painful hardware. The author cautioned that the majority of the complications were due to harvesting too small a bone graft and difficulties with internal fixation. The high complication rate indicates that the operating surgeon must be extremely familiar with this procedure.

The other groove-deepening technique involves raising the periosteal cortical flap with a medial hinge from the posterolateral aspect of the fibula. Decancellization of the posterior fibula deepens the groove approximately 6 to 9 mm, and the cortical periosteal flap is recessed back into its position. The original series reported excellent results in all 9 patients. Another author combined this technique with the primary soft-tissue anatomic reconstruction technique. For patients with a flat or convex fibular sulcus, this option is a viable consideration.

Another technique is a rerouting procedure that substitutes the calcaneofibular ligament for the incompetent superior peroneal retinaculum. The calcaneofibular ligament is used to reconstruct an inframalleolar tunnel, with the calcaneofibular ligament lateral and the calcaneus medial. The author reported excellent results in 10 ankles with a 4.0-year follow-up period. All but 1 patient were able to return to their original sport activities.

It is evident that several treatment options exist for chronic peroneal tendon subluxation/dislocation. The technique chosen should not only be based on the experience of the surgeon with the technique, but also on the specific anatomic pathology of the patient. The anatomic repair is becoming increasingly popular. If the superior peroneal retinaculum is torn or attenuated, direct repair and anatomic reinforcement is usually the treatment of choice. If the superior peroneal retinaculum is absent or insufficient, a soft-tissue reconstruction procedure with local augmentation may be ideal. Other anatomic findings (ie, convex sulcus) often necessitate a groove-deepening procedure in addition to the soft-tissue reconstruction.

Painful Os Peroneum Syndrome

Plantar lateral foot pain consists of a spectrum of clinical and radiographic presentations. Recently, authors coined the term painful os peroneum syndrome (POPS) for the clinical presentation of lateral foot pain associated with an os peroneum.

Anatomy
The os peroneum is an accessory juxta-articular ossicle within the substance of the PL tendon near or plantar to the cuboid bone (Fig. 14). While it has been reported that the "os

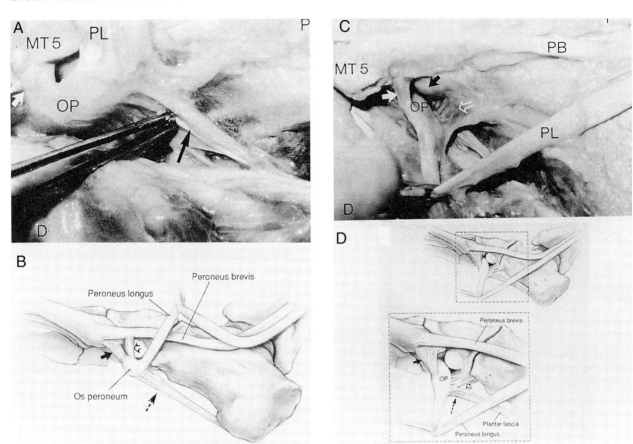

Figure 14

Photograph of cadaveric specimen (**A**) and corresponding illustration (**B**) demonstrating 3 of the 4 soft-tissue attachments of the os peroneum sesamoid complex: (1) the plantar fascial band (black arrow in specimen and dashed black arrow on illustration); (2) the fifth metatarsal band (white arrow in specimen and short solid black arrow on illustration) which extends from the os peroneum (OP) to the base of the fifth metatarsal (MT5); and (3) the band to peroneus brevis tendon (hollow black arrow on illustration). **C,** A photograph of the cadaveric specimen from a different view and corresponding illustration demonstrates the fourth component of the soft-tissue attachments of the os peroneum, sesamoid complex, the cuboid band (hollow white arrow (**C**) and hollow black arrow (**D**), the plantar fascial band (dashed black arrow) (**D**), and the os peroneum articular facet on the cuboid (black arrow) are also identified. PB= peroneus brevis tendon, PL = peroneus longus tendon, OP = os peroneum, MT 5-fifth metatarsal base, P = proximal, D = distal. (Reproduced with permission from Sobel M, Geppert MJ, Olson EJ, Bohne WH, Arnoczky SP: The dynamics of peroneus brevis tendon splits: a proposed mechanism, technique of diagnosis, and classification of injury. *Foot Ankle* 1992;13:413–422.)

peroneum is always present as an unossified cartilaginous or fibro-cartilaginous stage," radiographic studies have documented a 5% to 14% incidence in asymptomatic individuals. A radiographic series documented 143 cases of os peroneum in 1,000 radiographs, of which a bipartite os peroneum was present in 27 cases and only one demonstrated a multipartite os peroneum.

The os peroneum is located either along the lateral border of the calcaneus at the calcaneal-cuboid articulation or beneath the plantar aspect of the cuboid in the cubital tunnel. The os peroneum has 4 strong soft-tissue anchors that connect it to the plantar fascia, fifth metatarsal base, cuboid,

and PB tendon and prevent substantial displacement of the os peroneum. In addition, a moderate- to well-developed groove exists in many of the cuboid specimens that maintains and facilitates the PL excursion. Other anatomic structures that maintain the peroneal tendons are the bony processes in the lateral wall of the calcaneus, the peroneal tubercle (trochlear process of the peroneum), and the anterior calcaneus peroneal facet.

The PL tendon maintains intimate contact with the lateral wall of the calcaneus and is surrounded by a synovial sheath that extends 2.5 to 3.5 cm proximal to the tip of fibula and distal to the region of cuboid tunnel. The anterior calcaneus peroneal facet consists of a well-developed cartilaginous region that facilitates the os peroneum and the PL tendon articulation with the lateral aspect of the cuboid.

Diagnosis

It is apparent that the os peroneum is affected by a spectrum of posttraumatic, attritional, or overuse conditions that may include one or more of the following 5 types of painful os peroneum syndrome. In type I, there is an acute os peroneum fracture or diastasis of a multipartite os peroneum, which may result in discontinuity of the PL tendon. In type II, there is a chronic (healing or healed) os peroneum fracture or diastasis of multpartite os peroneum with callus formation (that may result in a lateral stenosing peroneal tenosynovitis). In type III, there is attrition or partial rupture of the PL tendon proximal or distal to the os peroneum. In type IV, there is frank rupture of the PL with discontinuity proximal or distal to the os peroneum. In type V, a gigantic peroneal tubercle on the lateral aspect of the calcaneus entraps the PL and/or the os peroneus during the tendon excursion.

POPS should be considered in patients with plantar lateral foot pain. Other considerations include the classic differential diagnosis of ankle sprain, PB or extensor tendon rupture/tear, fracture of the base of the fifth metatarsal, fracture of anterior process of the calcaneus, and fracture of the cuboid or the lateral process of talus. Factors reported to be related to POPS include diabetes mellitus, osteomyelitis, and/or varus deformity of the leg.

The development of POPS may be elucidated by the anatomic relationship between the PL tendon, the os peroneum, the lateral wall of calcaneus, and the groove of the cuboid. Several authors believe that the mechanism is a combination of supination and inversion forces. These forces are responsible for the well-developed groove in the lateral wall of calcaneus. These same forces, accentuated by a supination and an inversion force, such as a twist of the ankle or weight-bearing slip off the side of a curb, for example, can cause os peroneum fracture.

POPS is either an acute or chronic presentation. This differentiation is critical in determining treatment. The acute presentation consists of sudden onset of pain associated either with disruption of the PL tendon integrity or an os peroneum fracture or diastasis of multipartite fragments. Although less common than the chronic presentation, the symptoms often are traumatic enough to necessitate a visit to the emergency room. In contrast, the chronic condition may wax and wane over months. Mimicking a sprained ankle or foot, multiple exacerbations after an inversion ankle injury often lead to an orthopaedic consultation. The chronic presentation is consistent with the attrition or partial rupture of the PL tendon and/or diastasis of multipartite os peroneum.

Questioning usually reveals well-localized tenderness and thickening along the distal course of the PL tendon, distal to the fibula to either the peroneal tubercle of the calcaneus or the cubital tunnel. Associated pain may exist along the sural nerve distribution.

The physical examination of POPS confirms the symptoms described by the patient. Usually, there is thickening and tenderness of the PL and PB tendon sheaths. Pain may be elicited with resisted plantarflexion of the first ray, during the heel rise of gait, and when the foot is placed into an inverted supinated position. Some patients may describe weakness or pain with forced eversion. Still, unless a frank rupture exists, strength of the peroneal tendons with plantarflexion and eversion is near normal. Others describe the sensation of stepping on a stone in association with the malalignment of the os peroneum from its normal calcaneocuboid articulation. The distalmost branches of the sural nerves cross over the peroneal tendons and lateral to the calcaneocuboid joint, cubital tunnel, and base of the fifth metatarsal. Sural nerve dysesthesia or the presence of Tinel sign at lateral calcaneus may be elicited.

Radiographic

The os peroneum and its pathology are best identified via plain radiograph with an oblique view of the foot. A symptomatic multipartite os peroneum on the lateral or oblique radiograph is a strong indication of fracture. A radiographic study has confirmed the rarity of multipartite os peroneum in asymptomatic individuals. Diagnosis of an os peroneum fracture is facilitated by obtaining comparison views of the contralateral foot. A Harris (axial) view of the calcaneus or a CT scan can identify the presence of a large calcaneal peroneal tubercle. Radionuclear bone scan may be useful for the patient with a vague history of pain to identify a possible os peroneum fracture, but it is generally ineffective in revealing a proximal or distal tendon rupture. While tendons are best analyzed by MRI, no one study has documented its effectiveness in this clinical entity.

The treatment of POPS differs for acute versus chronic conditions. Seven patients who had less than 1 month of symptoms with various conservative methods (strapping, soft dressings, and casts) had satisfactory to excellent outcomes. In contrast, there are only 2 case reports of the results of surgical intervention after acute presentation. Generally, casting for 4 weeks is advocated for patients who present with less than a 1-month history of symptoms. Local steroid injection should not be used, because 2 case reports described complete rupture of peroneal tendons.

Surgical approach is advocated for patients with symptoms of more than 1 month's duration. Surgical treatment consists of exploration of the PL tendon and either removal of the os peroneum and repair of PL or tenodesis of the PL remnant to the PB tendon. One clinical series reported satisfactory results in 5 of 8 patients using this technique.

Treatment for this type V POPS (presence of a gigantic peroneal tubercle on the lateral aspect of the calcaneus) consists of excision of the peroneal tubercle. Two case reports have demonstrated satisfactory outcome following excision of this pathological tubercle.

Extensor Tendon

The tibialis anterior (TA), extensor hallucis longus (EHL), and extensor digitorum longus (EDL) are the three important extensor tendons of the foot. These tendons and their distal muscle fibers pass under the retinaculum of the distal portion of the tibia. Each tendon is distinct with a fibrous canal surrounded by its own fibro-osseous sheath. Although rupture of the extensor tendons has been reported, the incidence is low. First, the extensor tendons are less subject to wear and tear than are the flexor tendons, because the extensor tendons function primarily during the nonloaded swing phase of gait. Another reason is the reliable blood supply of TA tendon. Anatomic study of 12 cadaveric specimens found an adequate blood supply throughout the course of the TA tendon with no hypovascular region. No relationship was noted between the increasing age and alterations in the blood supply.

Ruptures of the TA can be attributed to four distinct etiologies based on 63 published cases: open direct trauma (laceration), closed indirect trauma (contusion), inner trauma (sudden force upon dorsum of the foot in dorsiflexed position), and spontaneous rupture (associated with steroid or generalized systemic disease, such as diabetes mellitus). Spontaneous rupture of the TA is extremely rare. While acute pain exists in 42% of the cases, the pain resolves rapidly. Often, this leads to a delay in diagnosis (average 2.6 months in one series). Rupture occurs most commonly 0.5 to 3.0 cm proximal to the bony insertion, where the tendon passes under the inferomedial band of the inferior extensor reticulum. These injuries occur mainly in older men sustaining a plantarflexion stress upon the foot; some reports cite a history of corticosteroid injections. Two distinct clinical presentations exist: sedentary elderly patients who typically report a several-month history of insidious, painless foot drop and active elderly patients after an acute traumatic event. The latter group's functional level is very high, often with active sports participation. These patients have a short period of pain that is attributable to an acute event. Physical examination typically reveals a palpable defect between the extensor

retinaculum and the anterior tibial insertion site. Due to the insidious onset, some patients with TA rupture have been mistakenly diagnosed with a neurologic disorder, such as peroneal nerve palsy, herniated nucleus pulposus, or neoplasm.

The optimal treatment for TA rupture continues to be controversial and is dependent on the lifestyle and functional demands of the individual patient. For patients with a traumatic laceration, primary repair has been advocated after appropriate washout. For patients with spontaneous TA rupture and a low functional demand, the optimal treatment may be nonsurgical with bracing or no treatment at all. For active patients who desire an improved functional outcome, surgical repair is usually necessary. It is important to remember that pain is rarely present, and the tendon repair is mainly for increased function. A variety of surgical techniques exist including a direct repair or, if necessary, a turn-down slide or VY lengthening of the ruptured tendon. Published reports of patients with substantial tendon defects describe the use of other extensor tendons (EHL or PB) to reconstruct a deficient TA tendon. Other interposition grafts have been used, such as plantaris tendon. Although primarily repair is generally recommended, there are no random comparative series that evaluate primary repair versus tendon reconstruction. In one series, the patients with spontaneous TA rupture who were treated surgically with a variety of reconstructive techniques had increased strength and functional improvement after surgery.

For patients who present with rupture of EHL secondary to laceration, primary repair is also advocated. Although spontaneous healing of extensor tendons has been documented in children, primary repair continues to be the mainstay of treatment. However, similar to the TA, no controlled comparative series exists assessing the results of primary repair versus tendon transfer.

Annotated Bibliography

Achilles Tendon

Astrom M, Gentz CF, Nilsson P, Rausing A, Sjoberg S, Westlin N: Imaging in chronic Achilles tendinopathy: A comparison of ultrasonography, magnetic resonance imaging, and surgical findings in 27 histologically verified cases. *Skeletal Radiol* 1996; 25:615–620.

A comparison of the information gained by ultrasonography and magnetic resonance imaging in chronic Achilles tendinopathy.

el-Khatib H: Island adipofascial flap for resurfacing of the

Achilles tendon. *Plast Reconstr Surg* 1996;98:1034–1038.

Ten patients were studied and the island adipofascial flap provides a durable and thin coverage for the Achilles tendon after a soft-tissue defect left an exposed tendon.

Mandelbaum BR, Myerson MS, Forster R: Achilles tendon ruptures: A new method of repair, early range of motion, and functional rehabilitation. *Am J Sports Med* 1995;23:392–395.

A prospective study of 29 athletes who had Achilles tendon ruptures treated with early range of motion and the Krackow suture technique.

McGarvey WC, Singh D, Trevino SG: Partial Achilles tendon ruptures associated with fluoroquinolone antibiotics: A case report and literature review. *Foot Ankle Int* 1996;17:496–498.

A case report of a patient with bilateral partial Achilles tendon ruptures associated with ciprofloxacin therapy and review of the current literature on this complication.

Nehrer S, Breitenseher M, Brodner W, et al: Clinical and sonographic evaluation of the risk of rupture in the Achilles tendon. *Arch Orthop Trauma Surg* 1997;116:14–18.

The authors studied the clinical course and sonograms in 36 patients with achillodynia to find a prognostic parameter enabling them to estimate the risk of rupture.

Porter DA, Mannarino FP, Snead D, Gabel SJ, Ostrowski M: Primary repair without augmentation for early neglected Achilles tendon ruptures in the recreational athlete. *Foot Ankle Int* 1997;18:557–564.

A report of the results of primary repair without augmentation for the neglected Achilles tendon rupture with proximal release and imbrication.

Troop RL, Losse GM, Lane JG, Robertson DB, Hastings PS, Howard ME: Early motion after repair of Achilles tendon ruptures. *Foot Ankle Int* 1995;16:705–709.

An evaluation of the clinical outcome of patients treated with limited immobilization and early motion after repair of acute Achilles tendon ruptures.

Wallenbock E, Lang O, Lugner P: Stress in the Achilles tendon during a topple-over movement in the ankle joint. *J Biomech* 1995;28:1091–1101.

A biomechanical study of stress in the Achilles tendon.

Flexor Hallucis Longus

Boruta PM, Beauperthuy GD: Partial tear of the flexor hallucis longus at the knot of Henry: Presentation of three cases. *Foot Ankle Int* 1997;18:243–246.

The purpose of this article is to present 3 cases of partial tear of the FHL and to discuss the pertinent physical findings, imaging studies, and surgical treatment available.

Hamilton WG, Geppert MJ, Thompson FM: Pain in the posterior aspect of the ankle in dancers: Differential diagnosis and operative treatment. *J Bone Joint Surg* 1996;78A:1491–1500.

A retrospective review was performed of the results of surgical treatment of stenosing tenosynovitis of the flexor hallucis longus tendon or posterior impingement syndrome or both in 37 dancers. The results were good or excellent in 28 of 34 ankles in professional dancers, compared with only 2 of 6 in amateur dancers.

Inokuchi S, Usami N: Closed complete rupture of the flexor hallucis longus tendon at the groove of the talus. *Foot Ankle Int* 1997;18:47–49.

A case report of closed complete rupture of flexor hallucis tendon at the groove in the posterior process of the talus and a review of closed complete rupture of FHL.

Kolettis GJ, Micheli LJ, Klein JD: Release of the flexor hallucis longus tendon in ballet dancers. *J Bone Joint Surg* 1996;78A:1386–1390.

Thirteen female ballet dancers underwent surgical release of flexor hallucis longus tendon for isolated stenosing tenosynovitis. The results were reviewed after mean duration of 6 years and 6 months. The authors concluded that surgical release of FHL is effective for the treatment of isolated stenosing tenosynovitis in female ballet dancers.

Posterior Tibial Tendon

Anderson JG, Hansen ST: Fracture-dislocation of the ankle with posterior tibial tendon entrapment within the tibiofibular interosseous space: A case report of a late diagnosis. *Foot Ankle Int* 1996;17:114–118.

A case report of posterior tibial tendon entrapment within the tibiofibular interosseous space following a closed fracture dislocation of the ankle.

Chao W, Wapner KL, Lee TH, Adams J, Hecht PJ: Nonoperative management of posterior tibial tendon dysfunction. *Foot Ankle Int* 1996;17:736–741.

A series of 49 patients with PTT dysfunction were evaluated after treatment with molded AFO (n = 40) and UCBL shoe insert with medial posting (n = 13). Sixty-seven percent of the patients had good-to-excellent results, at an average follow-up period of 14.9 months.

Hintermann B, Gachter A: The first metatarsal rise sign: A simple, sensitive sign of tibialis posterior tendon dysfunction. *Foot Ankle Int* 1996;17:236–241.

The purpose of this prospective study was to validate the "first metatarsal rise sign" by surgical exploration and to compare its sensitivity with other common clinical signs. In a series of 21 consecutive feet with PTT dysfunction, the other clinical signs (too many toes, single heel rise, and double heel rise) were noted to be negative in 20% to 35%. The first metatarsal rise sign was positive in all cases of PTT tendon dysfunction. This simple clinical test may allow recognition of the PTT dysfunction at an early state.

Holmes GB Jr, Mann RA: Possible epidemiological factors associated with rupture of the posterior tibial tendon. *Foot Ankle* 1992;13:70–79.

Rupture of the PTT has been postulated to occur as a result of degenerative changes to the tendon. A review of 67 patients diagnosed with ruptured PTT. Forty-five (60%) had one or more findings in medical history: hypertension, obesity, diabetes mellitus, previous surgery or trauma about the foot, and steroid exposure.

Miller SD, Van Holsbeeck M, Boruta PM, Wu KK, Katcherian DA: Ultrasound in the diagnosis of posterior tibial tendon pathology. Foot Ankle Int 1996;17:555–558.

The effectiveness of US as a diagnostic tool for PTT pathology was evaluated compared to operative findings. In all cases, surgery confirmed the US diagnoses (three inflammation, four partial tears, and ten ruptures). Of interest, two ruptures was undiagnosed by MRI.

Myerson MS: Adult acquired flatfoot deformity: Treatment of dysfunction of the posterior tibial tendon. J Bone Joint Surg 1996;78A:780–792.

An excellent review of the literature for PTT dysfunction discussing the anatomy, pathophysiology, radiographic findings, and treatment options.

Myerson MS, Corrigan J, Thompson F, Schon LC: Tendon transfer combined with calcaneal osteotomy for treatment of posterior tibial tendon insufficiency: A radiological investigation. Foot Ankle Int 1995;16:712–718.

A radiographic analysis was performed of 18 patients with PTT insufficiency after FDL tendon transfer combined with a medial displacement calcaneal osteotomy. Improvement was demonstrated in several radiographic parameters (talar-first metatarsal and talonavicular coverage on AP view and talar-first metatarsal angle and distance from medial cuneiform to the floor). Long-term results are still unknown.

O'Malley MJ, Deland JT, Lee KT: Selective hindfoot arthrodesis for the treatment of adult acquired flatfoot deformity: An in vitro study. Foot Ankle Int 1995;16:411–417.

An acquired flatfoot deformity with significant laxity at the transverse tarsal joint was created experimentally and the amount of correction that was obtained with selective hindfoot fusions was measured radiographically. The authors concluded that talonavicular or double arthrodesis will correct a deformity in a flatfoot with considerable laxity through the transverse tarsal joint but a subtalar fusion will not provide consistent correction.

Ouzounian TJ: Late flexor digitorum longus tendon rupture after transfer for posterior tibial tendon insufficiency: A case report. Foot Ankle Int 1995;16:519–521.

A case presentation of acute failure of a flexor digitorum longus tendon transfer for posterior tibia tendon rupture.

Ouzounian TJ, Myerson MS: Dislocation of the posterior tibial tendon. Foot Ankle 1992;13:215–219.

Seven patients with dislocation or recurrent subluxation of PTT were analyzed. Operative findings included tenosynovitis, shallow or incompetent flexor groove and tearing or absence of flexor retinaculum. At 28 months, all patients were markedly improved and 6 returned to their preinjury level of activity.

Pomeroy GC, Manoli A II: A new operative approach for flatfoot secondary to posterior tibial tendon insufficiency: A preliminary report. Foot Ankle Int 1997;18:206–212.

A combination of surgical procedures (TAL, FDL tendon transfers, lateral column lengthening and medial displacement calcaneal osteotomy) were utilized to treat stage II PTT insufficiency. In 17 patients with 20 cases, the average AOFAS hindfoot score improved from 51.4 to 82.8. Similar improvement of the pes planovalgus deformity was seen in several radiographic parameters. While this combination of procedures did correct the PTT dysfunction, long-term results are still unknown.

Schweitzer ME, Caccese R, Karasick D, Wapner KL, Mitchell DG: Posterior tibial tendon tears: Utility of secondary signs for MR imaging diagnosis. Radiology 1993;188:655–659.

Secondary signs of PTT dysfunction using MRI were evaluated in 23 patients with complete PTT tears and 34 control patients. The presence of secondary signs including talonavicular abnormalities, medial tubercle hypertrophy, and an accessory navicular bone were useful secondary signs of complete PTT dysfunction.

Peroneal

Cheung YY, Rosenberg ZS, Ramsinghani R, Beltran J, Jahss MH: Peroneus quartus muscle: MR imaging features. Radiology 1997;202:745–750.

A retrospective review was performed in 136 consecutive ankle MRI studies. The prevalence of the peroneus quartus muscle was 10% (14 of 136 cases). The site of insertion was variable and included the calcaneus, peroneus longus tendon, peroneus brevis tendon, and cuboid bone. Contrary to previous studies, peroneocalcaneal variant of the PQ muscle appears to insert in the retrotrochlear eminence of the calcaneus rather than the peroneal tubercle.

Extensor Tendon

Forst R, Forst J, Heller KD: Ipsilateral peroneus brevis tendon grafting in a complicated case of traumatic rupture of tibialis anterior tendon. Foot Ankle Int 1995;16:440–444.

A case report of ipsilateral peroneus brevis tendon grafting in complicated tibialis anterior tendon ruptures.

Ouzounian TJ, Anderson R: Anterior tibial tendon rupture. Foot Ankle Int 1995;16:406–410.

This study consists of one of the largest reported series evaluating rupture of anterior tibial tendon. Five patients were treated without surgery and 7 underwent surgical treatment using a variety of individualized reconstructive techniques. The authors recommended surgical reconstruction in appropriate patients.

Classic Bibliography

Conti S, Michelson J, Jahss M: Clinical significance of magnetic resonance imaging in preoperative planning for reconstruction of posterior tibial tendon ruptures. *Foot Ankle* 1992;13: 208–214.

Floyd DW, Heckman JD, Rockwood CA Jr: Tendon lacerations in the foot. *Foot Ankle* 1983;4:8–14.

Frenette JP, Jackson DW: Lacerations of the flexor hallucis longus in the young athlete. *J Bone Joint Surg* 1977;59A:673–676.

Frey C, Shereff M, Greenidge N: Vascularity of the posterior tibial tendon. *J Bone Joint Surg* 1990;72A:884–888.

Funk DA, Cass JR, Johnson KA: Acquired adult flat foot secondary to posterior tibial-tendon pathology. *J Bone Joint Surg* 1986;68A:95–102.

Geppert MJ, Sobel M, Hannafin JA: Microvasculature of the tibialis anterior tendon. *Foot Ankle* 1993;14:261–264.

Johnson KA, Strom DE: Tibialis posterior tendon dysfunction. *Clin Orthop* 1989;239:196–206.

Johnson KA: Tibialis posterior tendon rupture. *Clin Orthop* 1983;177:140–147.

Mann RA, Thompson FM: Rupture of the posterior tibial tendon causing flat foot: Surgical treatment. *J Bone Joint Surg* 1985;67A:556–561.

Myerson M, Solomon G, Shereff M: Posterior tibial tendon dysfunction: Its association with seronegative inflammatory disease. *Foot Ankle* 1989;9:219–225.

Peterson DA, Stinson W: Excision of the fractured os peroneum: A report on five patients and review of the literature. *Foot Ankle* 1992;13:277–281.

Romash MM: Closed rupture of the flexor hallucis longus tendon in a long distance runner: Report of a case and review of the literature. *Foot Ankle Int* 1994;15:433–436.

Rupp S, Tempelhof S, Fritsch E: Ultrasound of the Achilles tendon after surgical repair: Morphology and function. *Br J Radiol* 1995;68:454–458.

Sobel M, Bohne WH, Levy ME: Longitudinal attrition of the peroneus brevis tendon in the fibular groove: An anatomic study. *Foot Ankle* 1990;11:124–128.

Sobel M, DiCarlo EF, Bohne WH, Collins L: Longitudinal splitting of the peroneus brevis tendon: An anatomic and histologic study of cadaveric material. *Foot Ankle* 1991;12:165–170.

Sobel M, Geppert MJ, Olson EJ, Bohne WH, Arnoczky SP: The dynamics of peroneus brevis tendon splits: A proposed mechanism, technique of diagnosis, and classification of injury. *Foot Ankle* 1992;13:413–422.

Sobel M, Levy ME, Bohne WH: Congenital variations of the peroneus quartus muscle: An anatomic study. *Foot Ankle* 1990;11:81–89.

Sobel M, Pavlov H, Geppert MJ, Thompson FM, DiCarlo EF, Davis WH: Painful os peroneum syndrome: A spectrum of conditions responsible for plantar lateral foot pain. *Foot Ankle Int* 1994;15:112–124.

Stuart MJ: Traumatic disruption of the anterior tibial tendon while cross-country skiing: A case report. *Clin Orthop* 1992; 281:193–194.

Thompson FM, Snow SW, Hershon SJ: Spontaneous atraumatic rupture of the flexor hallucis longus tendon under the sustentaculum tali: Case report, review of the literature, and treatment options. *Foot Ankle* 1993;14:414–417.

Wapner KL, Hecht PJ, Shea JR, Allardyce TJ: Anatomy of second muscular layer of the foot: Considerations for tendon selection in transfer for Achilles and posterior tibial tendon reconstruction.

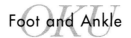
Chapter 21
Arthritis and Deformities of the Hindfoot and Ankle

Introduction

The past several years have seen an evolution in the management of arthritis and deformities of the ankle and hindfoot. Treatment options include a large array of surgical procedures and nonsurgical modalities. Longer-term clinical results and outcomes analysis studies are providing the information needed to individualize the best treatment choices for the patient and physician.

Successful management of these complex problems requires an accurate diagnosis through a detailed history and physical examination, an understanding of the biomechanics of the foot and the appropriate use of imaging studies. Often, well-prescribed pharmacologic and orthotic treatments can provide relief for these disabling conditions. Bracing and shoewear modifications can also result in significant functional improvements and reduction of pain. Should these methods fail, however, surgical treatment may be indicated.

Arthritis

By definition, arthritis is an inflammation of the joint. Unfortunately, this definition gives very little insight as to the etiology of this disabling disease. Osteoarthritis and posttraumatic arthritis are generally similar in that both are mechanical in nature. Typically, they are monarticular, or at least asymmetric. Clinically, the symptoms worsen with activity and may extend well into the night. The cartilage injury leads to increased water content and decreased compliance. There are alterations in the ratio of collagen molecules and an increase in proteoglycan breakdown. The ineffective cartilage then transfers increased load to the underlying subchondral bone, leading to repetitive injury and repair. Radiographs show loss of joint space and subchondral sclerosis, with osteophytes and cysts typically occurring on the same side of the joint in the area of maximum load.

Trauma is the most common cause of ankle and hindfoot arthritis. Posttraumatic arthritis of the tibiotalar joint can occur after ankle fractures, tibial plafond fractures, talus frac-

tures, or combined injuries. Particular care in restoration of fibular rotation and length, as well as stabilization of the syndesmosis, is needed to minimize the incidence of posttraumatic arthrosis when treating ankle fractures. In pilon fractures, the degree of cartilage and soft-tissue injury is often underestimated and carries a large prognostic factor. Talus fractures can cause posttraumatic arthritis in the ankle joint, the subtalar joint, or in both. Additionally, osteonecrosis of the talus can develop secondary to disruption of its blood supply and from the high energy associated with these fractures. The incidence of osteonecrosis is directly related to the degree of displacement of the talus fracture. Fracture healing may not be affected by osteonecrosis, but reconstructive surgical options are limited by its presence. Subtalar arthritis is a frequent complication of both the surgical and nonsurgical treatment of calcaneus fractures.

In contrast to the "bone-forming" sclerosis and osteophytes of osteoarthritis and posttraumatic arthritis, the inflammatory arthropathies, such as rheumatoid arthritis, may show significant osteopenia and erosions, and tend to involve joints in a symmetric fashion. Clinically, the hallmark is inflammation of the synovial-lined joints, tendon sheaths, and bursae with pain and stiffness in the morning. The synovium becomes permeable to infiltrating leukocytes and joint effusions tend to occur. The thick, inflamed lymphoid synovium becomes the pannus that is responsible for the cartilage and subchondral bone destruction. Initially, the pannus invades the exposed area directly adjacent to the articular cartilage. Although forefoot and midfoot arthropathy are more common, ankle involvement can occur, with pronounced valgus deformity of the hindfoot.

Of the seronegative arthropathies that can affect the hindfoot, ankylosing spondylitis, Reiter's syndrome, and psoriatic arthritis are among the most common. Reiter's syndrome has a predilection for the lower extremities. It is the seronegative arthropathy most likely to have the presenting complaint in the foot. The synovial pathology can be indistinguishable from rheumatoid arthritis. Hindfoot pain can be the presenting complaint in these patients, although it is more frequently caused by enthesopathy of the tendoachilles and plantar fascia than by ankle or subtalar arthritis. Radiographically, it appears as a fluffy periosteal reaction at the calcaneal attachment of the plantar fascia and erosions at the tendoachilles insertion. There is typically less ostopenia than in rheumatoid arthritis and, in some patients, there can be increased bone density.

Crystalline arthropathies, of which gout is the prototype, usually involve the great metatarsophalangeal joint or the tarsometatarsal joint, but may also involve the hindfoot. The symptoms are acute, intermittent pain and swelling in a single or few joints. Flares can occur after ingestion of a purine-rich diet, such as red meat or alcohol. The initial radiographic findings are soft-tissue swelling. Later, erosions with a punched out appearance and an overhanging rim of bone appear, while the joint space remains largely preserved. The soft-tissue tophus will usually calcify when larger. Calcium pyrophosphate deposition disease (CPPD) can mimic gout with acute and episodic attacks of arthritis, thus the name pseudogout. It may also present as progressive arthritis with joint space narrowing, osteophytes, and cysts. The radiographic and clinical course for pseudogout is very similar to that of osteoarthritis, with the addition of the characteristic calcific deposits in the joints and surrounding soft tissues. The most common location in the foot is the talonavicular joint, but any of the joints can become involved.

Tumors may lead to hindfoot pain and deformity. Osteoid osteoma may present in the younger patient with these complaints. Symptoms can be worse at night and can respond to salicylates. The diagnosis is suspected with increased uptake on nuclear scans, but usually requires a computed tomography (CT) scan or magnetic resonance imaging (MRI) with thin cuts to detect the nidus. Cystic lesions can be a component of osteoarthritis, an intraosseous ganglion, or associated with pigmented villonodular synovitis. Synovial chondromatosis frequently involves the ankle joint.

Recurrent hemarthroses can cause arthritis and deformity of the ankle and hindfoot. Iatrogenic hemarthrosis of the ankle joint has been attributed to anticoagulation with warfarin. Hemophiliacs can also develop a variety of hindfoot manifestations. Early in the disease, recurrent hemarthroses cause pain and swelling. With time, the bleeding episodes diminish in frequency, but leave a thickened and fibrotic joint capsule. Equinus deformities are common in this group. Also reported are subperiosteal hemorrhages called pseudotumors, which can cause severe destruction of bones such as the calcaneus.

Despite the widespread use of prophylactic antibiotics, both septic arthritis and osteomyelitis continue to produce severe hindfoot arthritis and deformities. Osteomyelitis can be suppurative or nonsuppurative. Suppurative infections tend to be quite fulminant, while the symptoms of nonsuppurative infections are usually indolent in their presentation. Often the correct diagnosis is missed or delayed. Tubercular infections will show a regional osteopenia, and joint space narrowing will occur later than in typical bacterial arthritis. Cartilage destruction occurs initially at the nonweightbearing areas of the joint. Diagnosis is made through skin testing and definitively with a biopsy and culture. Treatment is predominately medical with isoniazid, ethambutol, or rifampin for 12 months or greater and may be combined with casting or bracing.

Neuroarthropathy may involve the ankle and the hindfoot. The most common cause is neuropathy secondary to diabetes, but it can be found in paralytic injuries or peripheral nerve injuries. There are well-described stages of neuropathic arthropathy. Initially, the foot appears hyperemic, edematous, erythematous, and warm, often mimicking infection. Radiographs show fragmentation of the bone and cartilage, capsular distention, and subluxation or collapse. The second stage is early repair with decreased swelling, redness, and warmth. Radiographs show resorption of the fragments and sclerosis of the bone ends. The final stage is one of reconstruction with rounding of the bone ends and loss of the sclerosis. Predominant ankle involvement leads to instability, which can require prolonged bracing or immobilization. Surgical treatment may be required to correct deformity that is unbraceable or to relieve bony prominence. Hindfoot arthritis involving the subtalar, talonavicular, or calcaneocuboid joints is also common, but these are less likely to require surgical intervention.

Deformity

Longstanding lateral ligament instability of the ankle may result in significant tibiotalar arthritis. The resulting tilt can cause an increase in the stress on the medial side of the ankle, with eventual asymmetric joint space narrowing. Weightbearing films are necessary to show the translation or the tilt of the talus.

Adult acquired flatfoot may be related to dysfunction of the posterior tibial tendon. The subsequent loss of the longitudinal arch, and the development of progressive hindfoot valgus and forefoot abduction initially are flexible, but can become rigid. Eventually, a fixed forefoot varus develops to compensate for the hindfoot valgus. Pain can be more pronounced laterally at this stage and may indicate subtalar arthrosis or fibular impingement. For more advanced deformity with arthritis, an isolated subtalar arthrodesis and tendoachilles lengthening can be considered. A triple arthrodesis may be required for significant fixed deformity.

Neuromuscular disease can lead to significant hindfoot deformity. An example is hereditary sensorimotor neuropathy or Charcot-Marie-Tooth disease. Typically, the tibialis anterior, the intrinsics, and the peroneus brevis are affected. The peroneus longus and toe extensors are spared, resulting in the characteristic plantarflexed first ray, claw toes, and hindfoot varus of the cavovarus foot. Treatment is based on hindfoot flexibility, which can be tested with the Coleman block test. A variety of tendon transfers can be performed for flexible hindfoot deformity, including anterior transfer of the posterior tibial tendon through the interosseous membrane, an extensor digitorum longus to peroneus tertius transfer, or peroneus longus to brevis transfer. In those patients with fixed deformity, treatment options usually require bony procedures such as calcaneal and first metatarsal osteotomies or triple arthrodesis.

History and Physical Examination

A thorough history will many times provide the necessary information to begin an accurate differential diagnosis. Questions pertaining to history of trauma, instability, swelling, fever, night pain, or progressive sensory changes of the foot can provide clues to underlying disease processes. Additional questions regarding the onset of symptoms, the duration, and any aggravating factors, as well as rest pain, can be quite helpful. The location of the symptoms can sometimes be difficult for the patient to specify, but it can be the key to arriving at an accurate diagnosis. Pain in the lateral hindfoot or sinus tarsi points toward the subtalar joint, while pain in the anterior ankle or dorsum of the foot is typical of ankle joint involvement. Pain while walking on uneven ground is characteristic of subtalar arthrosis. If the cause was not traumatic, questions regarding other joint involvement should be pursued. Psoriatic arthritis and osteoarthritis often involve the distal interphalangeal (DIP) joints of the hands. Rheumatoid arthritis usually involves the metacarpophalangeal joint, while Reiter's syndrome seldom involves the hand. Crystalline arthropathies, pigmented vilonodular synovitis and tumors tend to be monoarticular or at least asymmetric. Details regarding shoewear and previous shoe inserts or orthotic devices are important. Response to previous forms of treatment can provide valuable information as to the proper diagnosis and subsequent treatment alternatives. Current medical problems and medications can be helpful to evaluate for the presence of such conditions as diabetes, stroke, or neuropathy. Family history can be important when working up a neuromuscular deformity. Cigarette smoking needs to be discussed, particularly when considering a surgical procedure, such as arthrodesis. A recent study revealed a significant increase in the rate of nonunion for ankle fusions in cigarette smokers versus nonsmokers.

Physical examination begins with inspection of each joint in the ankle and hindfoot, including an assessment of range of motion, strength, and painful motion, localization of tenderness and swelling, stability, and alignment. A complete physical examination includes evaluation while the patient is standing and walking. Deformity can be underestimated if the patient is examined only in the nonweightbearing or sitting position. It is helpful to have the patient in shorts to view the knees. Noting the alignment of the hindfoot from behind during midstance can reveal asymmetry or significant deformity. Heel walking will test the muscle strength of the dorsiflexors, as well as eliciting heel pain. The ability to perform a single limb heel rise with restoration of the longitudinal arch and inversion of the heel requires a functioning tibialis posterior tendon. Heel cord tightness should be tested with the transverse tarsal joints reduced and the forefoot supinated to avoid dorsiflexion through the midfoot, producing false dorsiflexion in hindfoot valgus. The appearance of the skin may reveal signs of vascular insufficiency or signs of venous stasis. Callosities in the mid- or forefoot can be a sign of hindfoot, ankle, or midfoot deformity. Vibration sense and monofilament testing at times can reveal a previously undiagnosed peripheral neuropathy. Range of motion of the ankle, subtalar, and midfoot joints should be documented and assessed for pain.

Selective injections of local anesthesia into specific joints can help to localize the most painful joints. This can be an invaluable technique in the preoperative planning process and may help to identify the most symptomatic joint.

Gait Analysis

Gait analysis has allowed us to objectively test parameters of the gait cycle in patient populations with ankle arthritis before and after ankle arthrodesis and total ankle arthroplasty. Ankle arthritis leads to decreases in velocity, stride length, and cadence. More time is spent in double limb stance, with decreased single limb stance on the affected side. Force-plate analysis reveals that there is decreased vertical ground reaction force in ankles with arthritis compared with controls. There is decreased plantar and dorsiflexion strength in ankles with arthritis compared to normal ankles.

To be successful, treatment needs to improve on these parameters and alleviate pain. Comparing ankle arthrodesis with total ankle arthroplasty using the above parameters provides some interesting insight. Patients with total ankle arthroplasty continue to have decreased ankle strength, and marked decrease in velocity, stride length, and cadence. Force-plate analysis also reveals decreased vertical ground reaction force in the arthroplasty group. These findings are similar to those for preoperative ankle arthritis. In contrast, patients with ankle fusions had near normal walking velocity and cadence, with visual analysis being normal in two thirds of those patients, despite a shortened stride length. Both ankle fusions and total ankle arthroplasties have decreased time in single limb stance.

Imaging

Quality radiographs are essential for accurate diagnosis of ankle and hindfoot disorders. Radiographic evaluation begins with weightbearing anteroposterior and lateral views of both ankles as well as weightbearing anteroposterior views of the feet. The degree of deformity or joint space collapse can be underestimated if the views are not weightbearing. Mortise views of the ankles and medial oblique views of the feet can also be helpful. Broden's view provides visualization of the subtalar joint, while Harris views reveal axial alignment of the calcaneus. The weightbearing hindfoot alignment view provides reproducible radiographs of the coronal plane of the hindfoot, which are quite useful in preoperative planning of hindfoot arthrodesis and osteotomy procedures (Fig. 1).

Technetium bone scans are helpful in the diagnosis of occult arthritis or fractures, as well as stress reactions. Three-phase bone scans are also used to determine the presence or absence of other painful conditions, such as reflex sympathetic dystrophy or sympathetically mediated pain syndrome. Resolution

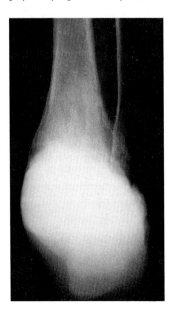

Figure 1

The hindfoot alignment view described by Saltzman and El-Khoury. The moment arm of the hindfoot in the coronal plane is determined by measuring the distance from a line drawn through the weightbearing axis of the tibia to the inferior most point of the calcaneus. Positive values are for hindfoot valgus.

for bone scans has improved, and they can be diagnostic for activity in specific joints of the hindfoot complex.

Tomograms are especially useful in the evaluation of arthrodesis procedures with hardware, but they require a skilled technologist and can be cumbersome to evaluate. Recent advances in trispiral CT have enhanced its utility for similar purposes and have dramatically reduced the time needed to generate quality images. CT scanning remains the standard for evaluation of complex injuries such as fractures of the talus and the calcaneus.

Much attention has been given to the use of MRI in the diagnosis of foot disorders. Always known for its detail of the soft tissues, recent software advances have allowed the MRI to distinguish between subtle bone features such as a contusion, edema, or infection. Tumors and extent of their involvement can be detailed as well. Gadolinium, which enhances tissues with viable circulation, can assist in detecting otherwise indistinguishable tissue differences.

Nonsurgical Treatment

Nonsteroidal anti-inflammatory drugs (NSAIDs), which block the cyclo-oxygenase pathway in the production of prostaglandins, can provide significant relief to patients with hindfoot arthritis. Recent formulations have been developed for single daily dosing, which increases patient convenience and therefore compliance. Precautions should always be given regarding epigastric symptoms and potential gastrointestinal side effects. Periodic chemistry profiles are recommended to assess renal and hepatic function.

A variety of shoe inserts and modifications, as well as braces, can be effective in the treatment of hindfoot arthritis and deformity. Soft plastizote shoe inserts are available both as custom and over-the-counter orthoses to reduce friction and provide shock absorption. They can have a medial post or just longitudinal arch support. Patients who have tarsal or hindfoot pain and a flexible deformity can be treated with a UCBL insert to maintain hindfoot neutral position. Adding a solid ankle, cushion heel (SACH) or rocker bottom to the patient's shoe can improve gait and comfort. An ankle-foot orthosis (AFO) can provide predictable pain relief for ankle or hindfoot arthritis by immobilizing the affected joints. Modifications to offload the ankle joint can be made by adding a patellar tendon bearing component. An alternative to the standard AFO is an ankle gauntlet AFO with a custom inner boot. By restricting inversion/eversion and allowing minimal ankle plantarflexion and dorsiflexion, this brace may benefit those patients with primarily hindfoot arthrosis. It consists of a molded rigid liner to support the hindfoot and

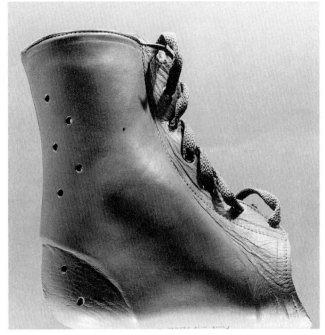

Figure 2
The leather ankle gauntlet ankle-foot orthosis with custom inner boot to control hindfoot inversion and eversion. Note that it also limits ankle dorsi- and plantarflexion.

is encased in a leather sleeve to provide a snug fit and maintain a low profile. It can be worn inside an athletic or a standard lace-up shoe and in some patients is better tolerated than the more rigid orthoses (Fig. 2).

Ambulatory aids, such as a cane used in the contralateral hand, have been shown to benefit patients with ankle or hindfoot arthritis by offloading the affected limb. Intra-articular corticosteroid injections can provide temporary pain relief.

Surgical Treatment

Synovectomy
Synovectomy of the ankle joint may be indicated for chronic inflammatory synovitis that has been refractory to aggressive medical management for 6 months or longer. Rheumatoid arthritis, hemophilia, pigmented villonodular synovitis, synovial chondromatosis and septic arthritis have all been treated with synovectomy by dif-

ferent authors. Both open and arthroscopic synovectomy have been advocated. Results have varied, and questions remain concerning the efficacy of this procedure, due in part to the lack of controlled studies and to the natural history of these inflammatory arthropathies.

Cheilectomy
Ankle cheilectomy is indicated in selected patients with symptomatic anterior ankle osteophytes. These osteophytes usually form on the distal tibia, but may also develop on the dorsal talus, resulting in bony abutment between the talus and the anterior distal tibia. Patients may notice restricted dorsiflexion or anterior ankle pain when climbing stairs. The resulting equinus compensation can result in a back-kneed gait or an externally rotated foot progression angle. Tenderness over the anterior joint line can usually be elicited on examination and the osteophytes may be palpable. Care is taken to correlate the radiographs with the physical examination, as osteophytes are common in this region and may not be the source of pain. If NSAIDs fail to provide adequate relief, surgical cheilectomy may be indicated (Fig. 3). A cheilectomy can be performed arthroscopically or easily via an arthrotomy. Results of arthroscopic and open cheilectomy are similar.

Osteotomy
Fibular osteotomy for fracture malunion can be an effective treatment for early posttraumatic ankle or hindfoot arthritis.

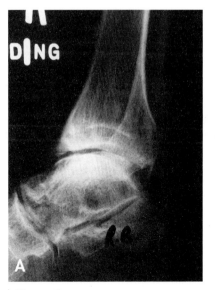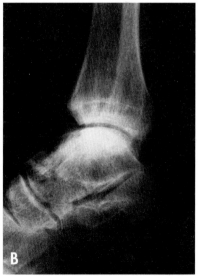

Figure 3
A, Preoperative lateral ankle radiograph demonstrates anterior osteophytes on distal tibia. **B,** Postoperative lateral view confirms a satisfactory decompression following cheilectomy.

Fibular fracture malunions are most frequently shortened and externally rotated, which results in subluxation of the talus within the mortise. Lengthening the fibula with iliac crest bone graft and correction of the rotation with internal fixation may help to restore the ankle mortise and the talocrural angle. This procedure may slow the progression of posttraumatic arthritis and provide symptomatic improvement.

Indications for realignment and fibular osteotomy include distortion of the normal tibiofibular-talar alignment associated with pain. Plain weightbearing ankle radiographs can reveal alterations in the normal bony architecture about the mortise, including disruption of "Shenton's line," an increased medial clear space, or talar tilt. CT scans with axial cuts across the tibiofibular interval and ankle mortise can accurately determine the amount of talar shift and the position of the fibula relative to the tibia when compared to the normal ankle. Contraindications for this procedure include advanced degenerative changes within the ankle joint, impaired vascularity, or inadequate soft tissues. Additionally, realignment should not be attempted in any patient with abnormal sensation such as an early Charcot joint.

Ankle Arthrodesis

Ankle arthrodesis remains the standard reconstructive technique for treatment of disabling ankle arthritis. A solid fusion provides predictable pain relief and a stable, plantigrade foot. The primary indication for ankle arthrodesis remains symptomatic arthritis from any cause unresponsive to conservative measures. Posttraumatic arthritis remains the most common preoperative diagnosis for ankle fusion. Other indications for arthrodesis are rheumatoid arthritis, degenerative or osteoarthritis, osteonecrosis of the talus, neuromuscular conditions, and failed previous surgeries, such as total ankle arthroplasty. Additional indications for ankle arthrodesis include severe deformities that are not braceable or result in skin breakdown. These may be seen in those patients with neuropathic arthropathy, but in these patients the rate of complication and failure is relatively high.

Numerous surgical techniques have been described in the literature with new variations on each ankle arthrodesis method and, in general, each author reporting satisfactory results. Standard fusion principles include apposition of bleeding, cancellous bone surfaces, use of fresh, autologous graft (when needed), compression across the fusion site, and rigid fixation. A trend toward internal fixation with compression screws has coincided with a decrease in the reported rates for nonunion. Surgical approaches, screw types, and screw placement vary, with most authors recommending at least two screws for fixation and some advocating local or

fibular onlay grafting.

Successful salvage of complex ankle problems, such as nonunion, infected nonunion, large bony defects, neuropathic joints, ongoing sepsis, severe osteopenia, and combined ankle and hindfoot arthrosis, can be challenging and may require the use of a number of techniques for arthrodesis, including intramedullary fixation and external fixation.

Regardless of the specific technique, final position of the foot is critical. The preferred alignment is neutral plantarflexion-dorsiflexion, with hindfoot valgus of 5° to 10°, external rotation of 5° to 10°, and neutral mediolateral and slight posterior translation of the talus with respect to the tibia. This posterior translation minimizes the lever arm of the foot, which results in decreased vaulting during gait and decreased load through the midfoot joints.

For an arthrodesis with minimal or no deformity, arthroscopic or mini-open procedures have been described, which simply remove the remaining articular cartilage and dense subchondral bone. These procedures offer the advantage of less soft-tissue dissection with less periosteal stripping, minimal postoperative pain, and a decreased time to union in some reports. However, the arthroscopic procedure is especially technically demanding and has a steep learning curve. As a result, the miniarthrotomy technique has gained recent favor in those patients without deformity. For patients with ankle deformity, an open procedure is required.

Many procedures have been described through a variety of approaches, including anteromedial, anterolateral, posterior, or combined medial and lateral transmalleolar. The anteromedial incision is longitudinal and is positioned medial to the anterior tibial tendon. The anterolateral approach is lateral to the extensor digitorum longus and peroneus tertius tendons and is centered over the ankle joint. The posterior approach is through a curvilinear incision along the medial aspect of the achilles tendon, and full-thickness skin and subcutaneous flaps are created to minimize skin slough. The achilles tendon may be retracted or divided and repaired to facilitate exposure.

The combined medial and lateral transmalleolar approach consists of curvilinear incisions over the medial malleolus and anterior margin of the distal fibula, paralleling the tendons respectively. Care must be taken to protect the superficial peroneal nerve laterally and the saphenous nerve medially as dissection is carried to bone. The malleoli are exposed and the fibula is transected proximal to the ankle joint line. It can be split longitudinally and used as morcelized or onlay graft. The dissection can then be extended around the anterior or posterior margins as needed for resection and realignment.

Preparation of the fusion site may include osteotomies through the distal tibia and talar dome perpendicular to the longitudinal axis of the leg, producing parallel, flat surfaces. Shortening can be minimized by judicious bony resection, and care is taken to prevent thermal injury to the bone when performing osteotomies with power saws. A chevron-type osteotomy has also been described to maximize surface area, bony contact, and stability. Bone loss may necessitate the use of local or iliac crest bone graft, with large defects requiring tricortical intercalary grafts to minimize limb shortening.

Fixation options are many, including use of internal compression screws, cannulated screws, plates and screws or staples, percutaneous or longitudinal pins, and external fixators. The use of 3 large cancellous screws has been shown to be superior to 2 screws in biomechanical laboratory testing (Fig. 4). Intraoperative use of fluoroscopy or plain radiographs helps to prevent intrusion into the subtalar joint and to assess satisfactory hardware placement and bony apposition. Supplemental fibular onlay grafting has been shown to add stability to the screw fixation. Anterior distal tibial sliding bone graft techniques (Blair) have been successful in those patients with ankle arthrosis and talar osteonecrosis without subtalar involvement.

Clinical results of ankle arthrodesis have been satisfactory in over 80% of patients at long-term follow-up. Radiographic union has usually occurred by 4 months, and maximum clinical benefit is obtained by 6 to 12 months postoperatively. Thirty to forty percent of normal tibiopedal motion persists following ankle fusion via the transverse tarsal and tarsometatarsal joints. Subtalar motion following ankle arthrodesis is usually decreased, but this limited motion may have been present prior to surgery in many patients with ankle arthrosis. Longer-term studies on ankle arthrodesis have demonstrated progressive degenerative changes at the transverse tarsal and tarsometatarsal joints. These radiographic changes were usually asymptomatic.

Complications with ankle fusions are frequent in the literature, including delayed union, nonunion, malunion, wound infection and slough, limb-length discrepancy, subtalar pain and stiffness, and neurovascular injury, to name a few.

Subtalar Joint Arthrodesis

Isolated subtalar arthrodesis is indicated for symptomatic subtalar arthrosis unresponsive to conservative treatment. The etiology of subtalar arthritis can be posttraumatic, osteoarthritis, inflammatory, or deformity due to neuromuscular disease or posterior tibial tendon insufficiency. Subtalar joint arthritis is relatively common following intra-articular calcaneus and talus fractures, and it can also be the end result of subtalar instability. Subtalar arthrodesis has also been useful in the treatment of acquired adult flatfoot deformity secondary to tibialis posterior tendon dysfunction or rupture and talocalcaneal coalition.

Signs of subtalar arthrosis include lateral ankle and hindfoot pain, difficulty walking on uneven terrain or sides of hills, painful and restricted hindfoot motion, and tenderness over the sinus tarsi. Distinguishing between subtalar pain and pain from subfibular (calcaneofibular) impingement, peroneal tendinitis, or sural neuroma can be difficult.

NSAIDs may provide significant relief, especially in the early stages of subtalar arthritis. Hindfoot orthoses and braces that limit inversion and eversion and yet allow ankle plantar and dorsiflexion can greatly enhance ambulation. Intra-articular corticosteroid injections can provide temporary relief, but if symptoms persist, subtalar arthrodesis may be indicated.

In patients with limited deformity, the

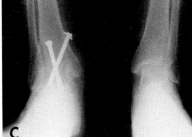
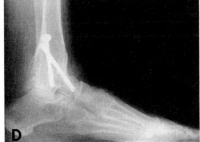

Figure 4

A, Standing anteroposterior ankle radiographs reveal advanced degenerative arthrosis on the right. **B,** Standing lateral ankle view confirms joint space collapse with anterior osteophytes. **C,** Postoperative AP view taken at 1 year shows bony union with 2 crossed screws. **D,** Weightbearing postoperative lateral radiograph at 1 year reveals a solid arthrodesis in satisfactory position.

subtalar arthrodesis can be performed by resecting the remaining articular cartilage and dense subchondral bone through an oblique lateral hindfoot incision, opposing the two bony surfaces with or without bone graft, and applying rigid fixation, such as a compression screw. The moldable bone graft technique can correct significant hindfoot varus or valgus by using bony resection to correct deformity and then packing the subtalar fusion site with morcelized iliac crest bone graft, allowing the surgeon to then place the hindfoot into a plantigrade position prior to fixation (Fig. 5). A large, smooth Steinmann pin generally provides satisfactory fixation with a high rate of union, although compression screws are also frequently used. A tendoachilles lengthening is frequently needed to allow adequate reduction when severe deformity exists preoperatively. Nonunions are rare due to the large surface area and large bed of cancellous bone graft. Varus alignment should be avoided, as it locks the transtarsal joints, producing stiffness and overload of the lateral midfoot and forefoot.

Intra-articular calcaneus fractures can result in significant hindfoot arthrosis and malalignment, with increased heel width, loss of heel height, lateral wall impingement, peroneal tendon subluxation and impingement, calcaneofibular impingement, and anterior ankle impingement due to loss of normal talar declination angle. Appropriate decompression, hindfoot realignment and subtalar joint tricortical distraction bone block arthrodesis can provide significant improvement for these patients.

Talonavicular Joint Arthrodesis

Isolated talonavicular arthrodesis is indicated for arthritis confined to the talonavicular joint. Posttraumatic and rheumatoid arthritis are the most frequent causes. Symptoms usually include pain with weightbearing and difficulty with

uneven surfaces, similar to those for patients with subtalar arthrosis. However, tenderness is localized over the talonavicular joint, usually dorsally, and can many times be confused with anterior ankle symptoms. Hindfoot motion is usually restricted or painful, thus distinguishing it from ankle joint involvement. Selective injections of local anesthetic can be helpful in defining the painful joint. NSAIDs, corticosteroid injections, and immobilization with a hindfoot orthosis or an AFO may provide satisfactory relief.

Surgical arthrodesis may be an option for those patients with refractory talonavicular arthritis. Previous studies have recommended combining talonavicular with calcaneocuboid arthrodesis, citing issues of stability. Most reports, however, support isolated talonavicular arthrodesis with favorable long-term results. Either a medial or dorsal approach, centered over the talonavicular joint, can be used. After incising the capsule, the joint surface is removed. Bone graft may then be placed, if indicated, followed by rigid internal fixation. Compression screws, pins, and staples have all been advocated.

Although successful fusion will alleviate talonavicular pain, up to 37% of patients will go on to develop adjacent joint arthrosis in the subtalar, calcaneocuboid, or naviculocuneiform joints at long-term follow-up. Additionally, fusion of the talonavicular joint will effectively eliminate subtalar and calcaneocuboid motion. Postoperative gait analysis reveals gait patterns very similar to those of patients with subtalar arthrodesis. Some authors have advocated this procedure to halt progression of hindfoot valgus malalignment in those patients with rheumatoid arthritis. Others have proposed isolated talonavicular arthrodesis for correction of the flatfoot deformity associated with tibialis posterior tendon dysfunction by restoring the longitudinal arch.

Calcaneocuboid Joint Arthrodesis

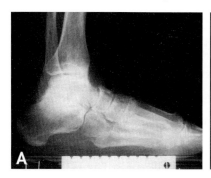 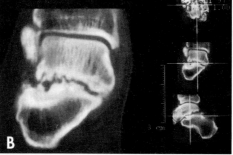 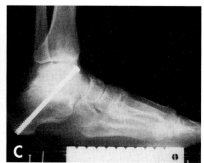

Figure 5

A, Standing lateral radiograph post subtalar arthrodesis elsewhere is suspicious for nonunion. **B,** Subtalar nonunion is confirmed on this spiral CT with coronal reconstruction. **C,** Standing lateral radiograph taken at 10 weeks postrevision subtalar arthrodesis with autologous bone grafting and insertion of a compression screw reveals satisfactory early consolidation across the fusion site. The patient is full weightbearing without pain.

Isolated calcaneocuboid arthritis is rare. When it occurs, an isolated calcaneocuboid arthrodesis can be performed through a longitudinal incision centered over the joint. The extensor digitorum brevis is sharply elevated from the anterior calcaneus, with a distally based flap, to expose the joint. As in isolated talonavicular fusion, the joint surfaces are denuded and bone graft is placed, when indicated. Fixation can be with compression screws, pins, or staples. Cadaveric studies have demonstrated that this single joint fusion preserves 50% to 80% of hindfoot inversion and eversion when compared to a triple arthrodesis. As a result, this procedure has been combined with a lateral column lengthening and various medial soft-tissue procedures to substitute for the dysfunctional tibialis posterior tendon in flexible acquired adult flatfoot deformity. Restoration of the arch is achieved by lengthening the lateral column with a tricortical iliac crest bone graft placed across the calcaneocuboid joint. The disadvantage of this procedure is the lengthy recovery period, a higher incidence of complications, and the need for the graft.

Double Arthrodesis

Motion analysis studies have demonstrated that the subtalar and transverse tarsal (Chopart's) joints are closely interrelated. Consequently, an isolated fusion of one joint restricts motion through the other two, while a fusion of two of the hindfoot joints severely restricts motion through the remaining third joint. However, some authors have advocated that, because talonavicular fusion essentially eliminates subtalar motion, the addition of the calcaneocuboid joint (double arthrodesis) does not further restrict hindfoot motion. A double arthrodesis may provide a more stable fusion construct. Some correction of deformity such as abduction and valgus is possible, to a limited extent, by selective osteotomy to remove bone medially and plantarward. Others routinely favor triple arthrodesis in those patients where more than one joint is involved. Significant deformity may require triple arthrodesis for satisfactory correction.

Triple Arthrodesis

Triple arthrodesis fuses each of the three hindfoot joints, talonavicular, calcaneocuboid, and talocalcaneal (subtalar), and may be considered when significant arthrosis develops in these joints. A triple arthrodesis may also be considered as a salvage procedure for severe deformity, pain, and instability as in patients with acquired adult flatfoot deformity in which there is rigid hindfoot valgus and fixed forefoot varus. Triple arthrodesis may also be indicated in those patients with severe foot deformities associated with neuromuscular disease.

Standard fusion principles are particularly important when performing a triple arthrodesis. Obtaining a satisfactory

reduction while maintaining bony apposition and placement of rigid fixation can at times be challenging. The use of bone graft and judicious bony resection can facilitate a successful fusion with a well-aligned, plantigrade foot (Fig. 6). Recovery can be prolonged and may take up to 1 year. Nonunion is reported in up to 25% of cases, with the talonavicular joint being the most common site. Ankle range of motion can be reduced up to 33%, especially in plantarflexion, and there is near complete loss of inversion and eversion. Results are not as good for those patients with neurologic imbalances, such as Charcot-Marie-Tooth disease, with a potential for recur-

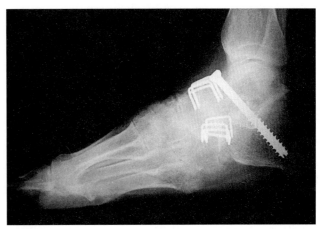

Figure 6
Standing lateral radiograph of a healed triple arthrodesis performed for psoriatic arthritis.

rence of deformity and late ankle arthrosis. Complications following triple arthrodesis are more frequent in those patients with sensorimotor peripheral neuropathy.

Tibiotalocalcaneal Arthrodesis

Tibiotalocalcaneal arthrodesis (TTCA) is indicated as a salvage procedure for painful ankle and subtalar arthrosis unresponsive to NSAIDs, injections, and bracing. Ankle arthrodesis alone may not be appropriate in those patients where there is a high likelihood of residual hindfoot pain. Selective intra-articular injections of local anesthetic are essential to determine if the fusion should be extended across the hindfoot. This procedure is particularly useful in patients with failed total ankle arthroplasty, posttraumatic osteonecrosis of the talus, failed ankle arthrodesis, rheumatoid arthritis with severe osteopenia, unbraceable deformity secondary to neuromuscular disease or neuroarthropathy, and posttraumatic arthrosis. Contraindications are similar to those for ankle arthrodesis and include impaired circulation or a history of indolent or active infection. These challenging problems are often found in patients with multiple prior procedure, and coexisting medical conditions, as well as osteopenic bone. As a result, the postoperative complication rate can be increased.

Preoperative evaluation includes history and physical examination to determine the etiology, degree of deformity,

skin condition, and vascular and sensory status of the extremity. Weightbearing plain radiographs of the foot and ankle are usually sufficient to determine the extent of hindfoot involvement. Coronal CT images through the hindfoot and technetium bone scans can be helpful when evaluating the talocalcaneal articulation. Occasionally, magnetic reso-

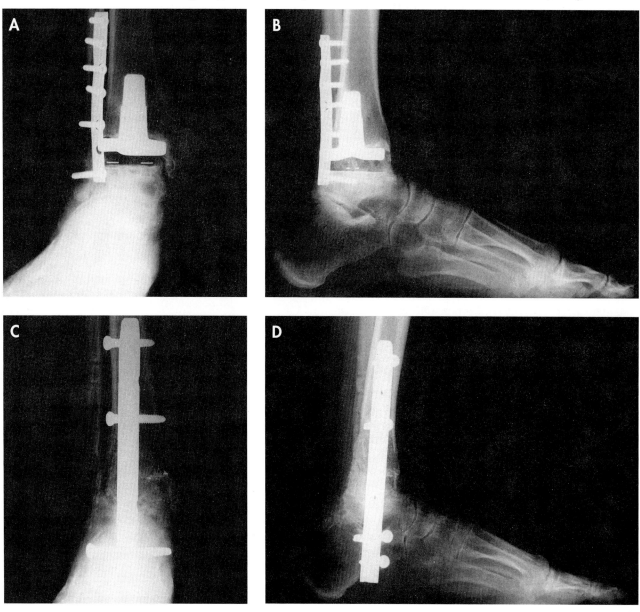

Figure 7

A, A mortise ankle radiograph of a painful total ankle arthroplasty. Subsidence of the tibial component is accompanied by osteolysis, as well as cystic changes in the medial malleolus. **B,** Weightbearing lateral radiograph of the same patient with a failed total ankle arthroplasty. **C,** Standing anteroposterior ankle radiograph of the same patient after implant and hardware removal and tibiotalocalcaneal arthrodesis using a locked, intramedullary nail and iliac crest bone graft. D, Standing lateral radiograph of the same patient showing a healed arthrodesis using an intra- and extra-articular posterior bone graft.

nance imaging may be needed to demonstrate the extent of avascular bone within the talus in cases of posttraumatic talar osteonecrosis.

TTCA, when performed through the posterior approach, avoids prior incisions or traumatized skin and provides maximum exposure for preparation of the intra-articular and extra-articular recipient bone graft sites. The procedure allows for a large correction of deformity and accurate repositioning of the foot in a plantigrade position. These arthrodeses generally require large amounts of bone graft and rigid internal fixation to be successful. Recently, an intramedullary nail has been developed for this procedure to provide more rigid fixation and decrease the complications associated with external fixation (Fig. 7).

Both a posterior and a combined medial/lateral approach have been described. The posterior approach is performed with the patient prone. A curvilinear incision is made along the medial border of the tendoachilles. Full-thickness flaps are made and the tendinous portion of the Achilles is divided in the coronal plane. Dissection is carried through the deep fascia in the midline and the flexor hallucis muscle is detached from the posterior tibia and intraosseous membrane and is retracted medially to protect the neurovascular bundle. The ankle and subtalar joints are then exposed and prepared. Massive autogenous bone graft is used, both intra- and extra-articularly. Fixation can then be provided with a locked intramedullary nail. Other methods of fixation include multiple screws, plate and screws, blade plate, or external fixation. Regardless of the choice of fixation, accurate positioning of the foot with respect to the leg is paramount. Although some tibiopedal motion through the transverse tarsal and tarsometatarsal joints can occur, transverse plane motion is essentially nonexistent. Due to the limited ability of adjacent joints to compensate, even small degrees of varus/valgus malalignment are not well tolerated. Neurovascular structures at risk with nail insertion include the lateral plantar nerve and artery.

As a salvage procedure, the results of TTCA have proved satisfactory in 87% of 30 patients at short-term follow-up and in 75% of 21 patients with follow-up ranging from 2.5 to 7 years. Many of these patients had undergone two or more previous surgical procedures and were considering below-the-knee amputation.

Tibiocalcaneal Arthrodesis
Tibiocalcaneal arthrodesis refers to a fusion of the distal tibia directly to the calcaneus. In those cases where the talar body

is absent or not salvageable, the remaining fragments of the talar body are excised and the tibia is rigidly fixed to the calcaneus with internal or external fixation. Alignment is crucial, as with all ankle and hindfoot fusions. Despite reported acceptable clinical results, considerable shortening of the extremity is a disadvantage. Resection of the malleoli may prevent shoewear impingement.

Pantalar Arthodesis
Pantalar arthrodesis is reserved for those rare cases in which ankle and subtalar arthritis is associated with hindfoot arthritis. Patients with severe rheumatoid arthritis may present with this constellation of symptoms. Also, some patients who have previously undergone triple arthrodesis may go on to develop subsequent ankle arthrosis, requiring extension of the fusion across the ankle joint. The operation can more easily be performed in two stages, but may be accomplished in a single setting when indicated. Special attention toward alignment in the forefoot should be made to avoid varus or valgus, resulting in medial or lateral pressure.

Total Ankle Arthroplasty
Implant arthroplasty of the ankle joint was developed as an alternative to arthrodesis or joint debridement for those patients with isolated inflammatory or osteoarthritis. Indications for total ankle arthroplasty include elderly patients with more sedentary lifestyles. Numerous implant designs have been evaluated over the last 3 decades, with mixed results. While short-term studies have provided encouraging data, longer-term analyses have demonstrated deterioration of clinical results, with migration of components and eventual failure. Salvage of these failed total ankle patients has proved challenging because of the significant bone loss and tenuous skin flaps.

Previous implant designs could not withstand the unusually large compressive, shear, and rotatory forces across a relatively small surface area at the level of the ankle joint. The design of implants continues to evolve, however, and it is hoped that the combination of newer designs and superior materials, as well as improvements in surgical technique, will result in improved long-term results. Although total ankle arthroplasty clinical research continues to generate encouraging results at short- to medium-term follow-up, these results have not yet stood the test of time.

Annotated Bibliography

Carr JB, Hansen ST, Benirschke SK: Subtalar distraction bone block fusion for late complications of os calcis fractures. *Foot Ankle* 1988;9:81–86.

Late complications of calcaneus fractures including subtalar arthrosis, loss of calcaneal height, and decreased lateral talocalcaneal angle may be addressed by subtalar arthrodesis with distraction, insertion of a bone block, and rigid internal screw fixation. Satisfactory results were obtained in 13 of 16 feet with minimum follow-up of 19 months. Restoration of hindfoot height was achieved.

Clain MR, Baxter DE: Simultaneous calcaneocuboid and talonavicular fusion: Long-term follow-up study. *J Bone Joint Surg* 1994;76B:133–136.

A retrospective review of 16 double arthrodesis procedures followed for an average of 83 months. Twelve of 16 were rated excellent or good. All healed except one asymptomatic talonavicular joint. Progressive ankle arthritis was seen in 6 ankles and 7 naviculocuneiform joints.

Cobb TK, Gabrielsen TA, Campbell DC II, Wallrichs SL, Ilstrup DM: Cigarette smoking and nonunion after ankle arthrodesis. *Foot Ankle Int* 1994;15:64–67.

A case control-matched study of primary ankle nonunions with healed primary arthrodeses. In the absence of other risk factors for nonunion, the relative risk of ankle nonunion for a smoker was 16 times higher than for a nonsmoker.

Glick JM, Morgan CD, Myerson MS, Sampson TG, Mann JA: Ankle arthrodesis using an arthroscopic method: Long-term follow-up of 34 cases. *Arthroscopy* 1996;12:428–434.

A multicenter retrospective review of 34 arthroscopic ankle arthrodesis procedures is presented. 33 of 34 successfully fused at an average of 9 weeks. 86% had excellent or good clinical score at 7.7-years average follow up. Disadvantages discussed are the inability to correct deformity, and technical difficulty of arthroscopic burring.

Greene WB: Synovectomy of the ankle for hemophilic arthropathy. *J Bone Joint Surg* 1994;76A:812–819.

Five patients were evaluated at an average follow-up of five years for synovectomy of the ankle due to hemophilia and recurrent hemarthroses. Recovery was easier than for synovectomy of the knee and elbow. Ranges of motion increased and episodes of hemarthrosis were significantly decreased.

Jensen NC, Kroner K: Total ankle joint replacement: A clinical follow up. *Orthopedics* 1992;15:236–239.

Results of total ankle replacement in 30 ankles of 25 patients were presented. Follow-up was available in 23 of the 30 ankles and averaged 57 months (3-year minimum). Clinical results indicated improvement in pain and function, but the authors expressed disappointment in comparison with the outcome of the ankle arthrodesis.

Kile TA, Donnelly RE, Gehrke JC, Werner ME, Johnson KA: Tibiotalocalcaneal arthrodesis with an intramedullary device. *Foot Ankle Int* 1994;15:669–673.

The authors report their experience with a salvage technique in the initial 30 patients in whom both the ankle and the subtalar joints were fused utilizing an intramedullary nail. Trauma was the most common preoperative diagnosis. Satisfactory results were reported in 87% of patients at relatively short-term follow-up, many of whom had been offered below knee amputation.

Kitaoka HB, Romness DW: Arthrodesis for failed ankle arthroplasty. *J Arthroplasty* 1992;7:277–284.

Results were reported for 38 ankles of 36 patients with mean follow-up of 8 years. External fixation was used in 36 and bone graft in 32. A union rate of 89% was reported.

Krause JO, Brodsky JW: The natural history of type 1 neuropathic feet. *Foot Ankle Clin* 1997;2:2–21.

Review of a large series of neuropathic feet. Includes classification of the joints involved and their predicted clinical course. Diagnostic as well as treatment algorithms are recommended.

Moeckel BH, Patterson BM, Inglis AE, Sculco TP: Ankle arthrodesis: A comparison of internal and external fixation. *Clin Orthop* 1991;268:78–83.

Results of arthrodesis using internal fixation in 40 and external fixation in 28 ankles were presented. A higher complication rate was noted in the external fixation group. Authors suggested advantages of internal fixation, though this study was nonrandomized.

Ouzounian TJ: Triple arthrodesis. *Foot Ankle Clin* 1996; 1:133–150.

A detailed review of the history, indications, techniques and approaches, as well as the results of triple arthrodesis is provided. The effects on gait and motion of the adjacent joints of the foot are included.

Paremain GD, Miller SD, Myerson MS: Ankle arthrodesis: Results after the miniarthrotomy technique. *Foot Ankle Int* 1996; 17:247–252.

Fifteen consecutive in situ ankle arthrodeses were performed utilizing an open miniarthrotomy technique and were followed for an average of 12 to 19 months. Union occurred in all patients. Seven of 15 had postoperative synovitis lasting 2 to 6 weeks.

Pochatko DJ, Smith JW, Phillips RA, Prince BD, Hedrick MR: Anatomic structures at risk: Combined subtalar and ankle arthrodesis with a retrograde intramedullary rod. *Foot Ankle Int* 1995;16:542–547.

An anatomic study of 6 cadaver feet with an intramedullary rod placed through the plantar calcaneus. Structures at risk are identified and ideal position of the nail at the plantar surface defined as the junction of the sustentaculum and the body.

Russotti GM, Cass JR, Johnson KA: Isolated talocalcaneal arthrodesis: A technique using moldable bone graft. *J Bone Joint Surg* 1988;70A:1472–1478.

Results are presented of a technique using morselized autogenous iliac crest bone graft with pin or screw fixation in 45 feet of 41 adults. Follow-up averaged 57 months. Results were considered excellent in 87%. Union was achieved in 44 of 45 feet and no secondary degenerative changes of associated joints were observed.

Saltzman CL, el-Khoury GY: The hindfoot alignment view. *Foot Ankle Int* 1995;16:572–576.

A standardized method of radiography to measure weightbearing coronal plane tibiocalcaneal alignment is described. It can be useful for radiographic assessment of pre and postoperative hindfoot alignment.

Schon LC, Bell W: Fusions of the transverse tarsal and midtarsal joints. *Foot Ankle Clin* 1996;1:99–102.

A detailed review of the anatomy, motion, indications, and results of arthrodesis procedures of the transtarsal joints; individual, as well as various combinations.

Stuart MJ, Morrey BF: Arthrodesis of the diabetic neuropathic ankle joint. *Clin Orthop* 1990;253:209–211.

Thirteen patients with insulin-dependent diabetes mellitus and a history of trauma underwent ankle arthrodesis. Follow-up averaged 42 months, and union was achieved in 7 of 13. Thirteen complications occurred in 8 patients. Results were satisfactory in 50%.

Thordarson DB, Markolf KL, Cracchiolo A III: Arthrodesis of the ankle with cancellous-bone screws and fibular strut graft: Biomechanical analysis. *J Bone Joint Surg* 1990;72A: 1359–1363.

The authors assessed stability of internal compression arthrodesis fixation technique using 2 cancellous screws in 18 cadaveric feet with and without a fibular onlay graft. The onlay graft added to the stability of the two-screw technique in all modes of testing, particularly in osteopenic bone.

Unger AS, Inglis AE, Mow CS, Figgie HE III: Total ankle arthroplasty in rheumatoid arthritis: A long-term follow-up study. *Foot Ankle* 1988;8:173–179.

The authors report results of 23 ankle replacements with average follow-up of 5 years. Clinical results were excellent in 2, good in 13, fair in 4, and poor in 4. Radiographic analysis indicated migration and settling of the talar component in 14 of 15 and radiolucencies in 14 of 15. Tilting of the tibial component occurred in 12.

Wynn AH, Wilde AH: Long-term follow-up of the Conaxial (Beck-Steffee) total ankle arthroplasty. *Foot Ankle* 1992;13:303–306.

Thirty-six ankle replacements, of which 32 were primary arthroplasties, were performed on 30 patients. Follow-up averaged 10.5 years. The authors reported a complication rate of 60%, including wound dehiscence in 39%, deep infection in 6%, malleolar fracture in 22%, and impingement in 14%. Ninety percent were radiologically loose at 10 years, and in 10 patients, salvage by arthrodesis was attempted. The authors no longer recommend Conaxial ankle replacement.

Yablon IG, Leach RE: Reconstruction of malunited fractures of the lateral malleolus. *J Bone Joint Surg* 1989;71A:521–527.

A retrospective review of fibula malunions treated with fibular osteotomy 5 years after fracture. Shortening and rotation were corrected and the gap filled with local bone graft. Twenty of 26 returned to preinjury level of activity. The authors recommend treatment with osteotomy when malunion is diagnosed in the presence of symptoms.

Classic Bibliography

Abdo RV, Wasilewski SA: Ankle arthrodesis: A long-term study. *Foot Ankle* 1992;13:307–312.

Bennett GL, Graham CE, Mauldin DM: Triple arthrodesis in adults. *Foot Ankle* 1991;12:138–143.

Buck P, Morrey BF, Chao EY: The optimum position of arthrodesis of the ankle: A gait study of the knee and ankle. *J Bone Joint Surg* 1987;69A:1052–1062.

Buechel FF, Pappas MJ, Iorio LJ: New Jersey low contact stress total ankle replacement: Biomechanical rationale and review of 23 cementless cases. *Foot Ankle* 1988;8:279–290.

Cracchiolo A III, Cimino WR, Lian G: Arthrodesis of the ankle in patients who have rheumatoid arthritis. *J Bone Joint Surg* 1992;74A:903–909.

Demottaz JD, Mazur JM, Thomas WH, Sledge CB, Simon SR: Clinical study of total ankle replacement with gait analysis: A preliminary report. *J Bone Joint Surg* 1979;61A:976–988.

Fogel GR, Katoh Y, Rand JA, Chao EY: Talonavicular arthrodesis for isolated arthrosis: 9.5-year results and gait analysis. *Foot Ankle* 1982;3:105–113.

Gellman H, Lenihan M, Halikis N, Botte MJ, Giordani M, Perry J: Selective tarsal arthrodesis: An in vitro analysis of the effect on foot motion. *Foot Ankle* 1987;8:127–133.

Graves SC, Mann RA, Graves KO: Triple arthrodesis in older adults: Results after long-term follow-up. *J Bone Joint Surg* 1993;75A:355–362.

Harrington KD: Degenerative arthritis of the ankle secondary to long-standing lateral ligament instability. *J Bone Joint Surg* 1979;61A:354–361.

Holt ES, Hansen ST, Mayo KA, Sangeorzan BJ: Ankle arthrodesis using internal screw fixation. *Clin Orthop* 1991;268:21–28.

Innis PC, Krackow KA: Weightbearing roentgenograms in arthritis of the ankle: A case report. *Foot Ankle* 1988;9:54–58.

Kitaoka HB, Anderson PJ, Morrey BF: Revision of ankle arthrodesis with external fixation for non-union. *J Bone Joint Surg* 1992;74A:1191–1200.

Kumar R, Madewell JE: Rheumatoid and seronegative arthropathies of the foot. *Radiol Clin North Am* 1987;25: 1263–1288.

Ljung P, Kaij J, Knutson K, Pettersson H, Rydholm U: Talonavicular arthrodesis in the rheumatoid foot. *Foot Ankle* 1992;13:313–316.

Offierski CM, Graham JD, Hall JH, Harris WR, Schatzker JL: Late revision of fibular malunion in ankle fractures. Clin Orthop 1982;171:145–149.

Ogilvie-Harris DJ, Mahomed N, Demaziere A: Anterior impingement of the ankle treated by arthroscopic removal of bony spurs. *J Bone Joint Surg* 1993;75B:437–440.

Papa JA, Myerson MS: Pantalar and tibiotalocalcaneal arthrodesis for post-traumatic osteoarthrosis of the ankle and hindfoot. *J Bone Joint Surg* 1992;74A:1042–1049.

Scranton PE Jr, McDermott JE: Anterior tibiotalar spurs: A comparison of open versus arthroscopic debridement. *Foot Ankle* 1992;13:125–129.

Shih LY, Wu JJ, Lo WH: Changes in gait and maximum ankle torque in patients with ankle arthritis. *Foot Ankle* 1993;14: 97–103.

Thordarson DB, Markolf K, Cracchiolo A III: Stability of an ankle arthrodesis fixed by cancellous-bone screws compared with that fixed by an external fixator: A biomechanical study. *J Bone Joint Surg* 1992;74A:1050–1055.

Ward AJ, Ackroyd CE, Baker AS: Late lengthening of the fibula for malaligned ankle fractures. *J Bone Joint Surg* 1990;72B: 714–717.

Weber BG, Simpson LA: Corrective lengthening osteotomy of the fibula. *Clin Orthop* 1985;199:61–67.

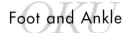

Chapter 22
Arthritis of the Midfoot

Anatomy and Biomechanics

The midfoot is composed of multiple articulations and ligamentous connections between adjacent tarsal bones and metatarsal bases. Three distinct articular compartments are present: medial, containing the first metatarsocuneiform joint; central, containing the second and third metatarsocuneiform joints, and the intercuneiform joints; and lateral, containing the cubometatarsal joints. These compartments form the basis of a columnar division of the foot, into medial, central, and lateral. A complex and variable ligamentous configuration consisting of dorsal, plantar, and interosseous ligaments provides a stout soft-tissue envelope. The three cuneiforms and cuboid form a transverse arch, with the apex at the third metatarsocuneiform articulation.

Midfoot motion has been quantitated in the sagittal plane and in rotation, with approximately 10° occurring in both planes at the cubometatarsal joints, and considerably less (0.6° to 3.5°) at the cuneiform-metatarsal joints. Motion occurs at the naviculocuneiform articulation, but decreases from medial to lateral. The planes of motion and the forces exerted on the foot are responsible for the typical deformity of pronation, dorsiflexion, and abduction seen with midfoot arthrosis.

The second metatarsal base is recessed between the medial and lateral cuneiforms by approximately 8 mm and 4 mm, respectively. The strong, oblique interosseous Lisfranc ligament connects the second metatarsal base with the medial cuneiform. This ligament, approximately 8 to 10 mm in length and 5 to 6 mm thick, is the largest in the tarsometatarsal complex. The second plantar ligament, the strongest plantar ligament, connects the medial cuneiform to the second and third metatarsal bases. The bony and ligamentous structures of the second tarsometatarsal joint provide the primary stabilization of the midfoot. In the cadaver foot, dorsolateral displacement of this joint results in considerable loss of contact area, with a 3-mm displacement causing 38.6% decrease in articular contact. Small degrees of displacement require CT scanning to diagnose, as plain radiography may not provide adequate visualization of the dorsal or dorsolateral subluxation that is typical with tarsometatarsal injuries.

The first metatarsocuneiform joint is stabilized in weight-bearing primarily by its plantar ligament. A clinical study has shown that, in the asymptomatic foot, first metatarso-

cuneiform motion averages 4.37° in the sagittal plane, and thumb hyperflexibility correlated with increased motion. Multiple variables, including intermetatarsal 1-2 angle, sex, age, elbow and knee hyperextension, and distal cuneiform shape, did not correlate with first metatarsocuneiform motion. The morphology of this joint is variable, and descriptions have been based on the medial inclination, lateral radiographic slope, and type of articular facet with the second metatarsal.

A recent cadaver investigation of the tarsometatarsal joints found that as loads on the leg increased, contact forces increased in the medial three joints. However, loads up to twice body weight did not increase contact forces in the lateral two joints, which may help to explain the small incidence of symptomatic arthrosis in the cubometatarsal articulation.

Degenerative Arthrosis

Arthrosis of the tarsometatarsal complex occurs as primary degenerative arthrosis as well as following trauma. In a recent series, patients with primary arthrosis tended to be older (60 versus 40 years), and have a larger extent of disease and greater deformity when compared to those with posttraumatic arthrosis (Fig. 1). Primary arthrosis may, however, affect only 1 joint and be without deformity. Dorsal osteophytes are typically present with severe involvement, but these can also be present in isolated joint involvement, and compression of peroneal nerve branches can cause nerve impingement symptoms. Despite advances in the treatment of injuries to the tarsometatarsal joints, posttraumatic arthrosis remains prevalent and is observed even following presumably subtle injuries, possibly secondary to articular cartilage damage. Factors associated with the development of posttraumatic arthrosis include persistent malalignment, especially with collapse of the medial longitudinal arch, and demonstrable articular injury.

Pain is the most common presenting complaint. Deformity may cause problems with shoewear and bracing because of pressure against bony prominences. The standing examination of both feet is important to determine the degree and location of deformity. The sitting examination of both feet includes determination of the deformity, flexibility, motion

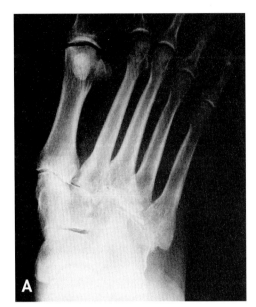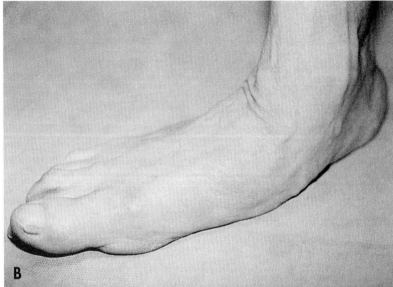

Figure 1

A, Primary degenerative arthritis of the midfoot with involvement of all columns. **B,** Clinical appearance of characteristic flatfoot deformity.

measurements, neurovascular and skin assessment, and careful palpation of each midfoot joint. The midfoot can be stressed with a pronation-abduction maneuver. Transverse plane alignment of the metatarsal heads is also determined while the patient is seated.

The radiographic evaluation of the arthritic midfoot includes standing anteroposterior, lateral, and oblique radiographs. It is useful to image both feet to determine the degree of deformity, which can be assessed by measuring the anteroposterior talus-first metatarsal, talus-second metatarsal, and lateral talus-first metatarsal angles. In cases with deformity, there is often loss of talar head coverage by the navicular.

It is sometimes difficult to determine the extent of arthrosis with the use of plain radiographs and the physical examination. Although controversial, in these cases a bone scan and/or CT scan can be useful on a preoperative basis. These imaging modalities should be carefully interpreted and used in conjunction with the physical examination, which it may be useful to repeat on separate occasions. Some authors have discussed the use of selective injections of local anesthetic, however, this can be difficult to perform accurately, is painful to the patient, and may be misleading because of the synovial compartmentalization of the midfoot joints.

Nonsurgical Treatment
Nonsurgical treatment modalities for midfoot arthrosis include a rocker-bottom sole, with or without stiffening pro-

vided by an extended steel shank or full length carbon fiber insert. An ankle-foot arthrosis with a full-length foot plate will provide additional support for more severe involvement. A custom or off-the-shelf orthotic device may be useful to provide cushioning, support for the longitudinal arch, and metatarsal head relief, but patients with deformity may not tolerate arch support due to a plantar bony prominence. Shoe wear modifications, padding, and skip lacing techniques can help decrease pressure from dorsal osteophytes. The goal of nonsurgical treatment is to decrease motion and forces across the midfoot and to relieve pressure on bony prominences.

Surgical Treatment
Surgical treatment is indicated when nonsurgical modalities are exhausted and the patient is unable to perform daily activities. Osteophyte resection is performed when symptoms are secondary to nerve impingement or skin irritation from the prominence. Arthrodesis of the involved joints is otherwise indicated. Generally agreed upon surgical principles regarding midfoot arthrodesis include the following. Deformity should be realigned, and in patients without deformity an in-situ fusion is performed; all joints with symptomatic arthrosis or part of the deformity should be included; longitudinal incisions are used with protection of the cutaneous nerves; and rigid internal fixation with meticulous joint preparation is necessary. Bone graft is often unnecessary for primary surgery.

The surgical approaches to the midfoot are based on joint involvement. Single joint arthrosis can be approached directly dorsal to the joint, and dorsomedial to the first tarsometatarsal joint. Recommendations regarding the approach to multiple joints vary. An accepted method is to approach the first tarsometatarsal joint dorsomedially, the second and third tarsometatarsal joints through an incision centered between the metatarsals two and three, and the fourth and fifth tarsometatarsal joints between the fourth and fifth metatarsals. The cubometatarsal joints infrequently require arthrodesis, as shown in 2 recent studies; 2 of 32, and 5 of 41 feet required lateral column arthrodesis.

An in-situ arthrodesis is performed in feet without deformity. All articular cartilage is removed from the involved joints, and the subchondral bone is feathered with a small osteotome or drilled with a small caliber bit. Internal fixation is achieved with the use of interfragmentary screws to provide compression. Cannulated 4.0-mm screws allow excellent fixation in the midfoot, however, 3.5-mm to 4.5-mm cortical or partially threaded cancellous screws have also been used. Screw patterns vary, but fixation generally proceeds from proximal to distal, and from medial to lateral if the naviculocuneiform or intercuneiform joints are involved. It is beneficial to retain the cuboid-lateral cuneiform articulation to allow some residual lateral midfoot motion. In patients undergoing naviculomedial cuneiform arthrodesis, the naviculo-middle cuneiform joint may need to be released or included to obtain satisfactory compression. It is important to maintain the metatarsal heads at a symmetric level. In isolated first metatarsocuneiform arthrodesis, when there is shortening of the medial column, it may be necessary to plantarflex the first metatarsal slightly, to maintain its weightbearing role.

Deformity correction often requires bony resection medially, and it occasionally requires lengthening of the lateral soft tissues, particularly the peroneus brevis tendon. The use of a small external fixator on the lateral column can be helpful to assist with the correction. It has been recommended to correct any deformity, particularly if there is greater than 2 mm or 15° of displacement. Bone graft may be necessary to fill any bony defects or gaps. Fixation, as with an in-situ arthrodesis, can be accomplished with interfragmentary screw fixation. The use of medial col-

umn plating is helpful to maintain alignment in deformity cases, and has been reported in a series of 9 patients. All obtained fusion, with good or excellent results in 7, and reliable correction of deformity (Fig. 2).

Two recent studies have provided data on the outcome of midfoot arthrodesis for primary and posttraumatic degenerative arthrosis. In one report, 40 patients followed for an average of 6 years had a 93% satisfaction rate. The union rate was 98%, or 176 of the 179 joints involved. Correction of deformity as measured by both the change in the anteroposterior and lateral talus-first metatarsal angle was approximately 8° in both planes. In the other report, 32 patients with posttraumatic arthrosis had considerable improvement in their clinical foot score, with only one asymptomatic nonunion. The extent or location of the arthrodesis, patient age, need for revision surgery, and work-related status of the original injury were shown to have no significant effect on outcome. The most frequent complications in both series included: neuroma formation; metatarsalgia related to malunion; and wound slough. Malunion occurred in 7 out of the combined total of 72 patients, and involved plantarflexion of the second metatarsal in all and the third or first metatarsal in 4. Of these 7 patients, 2 underwent surgical treatment with a dorsal closing-wedge osteotomy, and 5 were managed successfully with a metatarsal pad or cushioned in-sole.

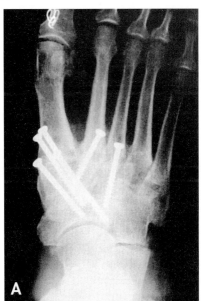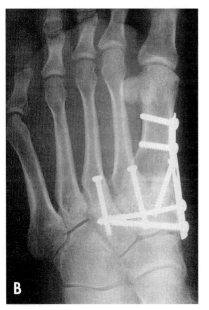

Figure 2

A, Midfoot arthrodesis for posttraumatic arthritis, utilizing interfragmentary screw fixation. The lateral column is left intact and is asymptomatic, despite radiographic degenerative arthritis. **B,** The medial plate technique is useful in cases requiring correction of deformity.

Extended Midfoot Arthrosis

A subset of patients with midfoot arthrosis present with extensive pathology involving a considerable portion of the medial column, from the talonavicular joint to the medial cuneiform or first metatarsal. Often this results from significant trauma, particularly involving the tarsal navicular and surrounding joints. Occasionally, there is collapse of only the lateral portion of the navicular. A variable degree of involvement may be present within the central and lateral columns.

Treatment in these cases is complex due to the extent of disease. In most cases, nonsurgical treatment may be accomplished with a custom ankle-foot orthosis. Surgical treatment alternatives include inlay or interpositional iliac crest bone grafting. The inlay technique involves the creation of a medial or dorsal rectangular slot from the talus to the involved cuneiforms or metatarsal bases. This can be formed with a burr, and a tricortical graft is inlaid with distraction of the foot. The involved joints are not prepared separately, but are spanned by the graft. Fixation may be achieved with screws through the graft into the midfoot and hindfoot, or with the use of long mini or small fragment implants. In patients with osteopenic bone, supplementary external fixation may be useful in the early phases of graft incorporation.

The interpositional technique includes resection of the affected bone segment and replacement with tricortical iliac crest graft. The use of 2 grafts to fill the segment, with the superior side of the crest positioned dorsally, has been advocated. Fixation can be achieved with screws or with a plate spanning the defect. With either technique, postoperative care requires immobilization and nonweightbearing for a minimum of 2 to 3 months. Often graft incorporation requires up to 6 months, and premature weightbearing may lead to loss of fixation and nonunion.

Midfoot Neuroarthropathy

Neuroarthropathy, defined as a progressive degenerative and destructive arthropathy occurring secondary to loss of joint sensory innervation, causes significant disability in the foot. Disorders associated with neuropathic arthropathy include diabetes, syphilis, syringomyelia, pernicious anemia, leprosy, spina bifida, congenital insensitivity to pain, Charcot-Marie-Tooth disease, and idiopathic and other etiologies of peripheral neuropathy. Diabetes is currently the most common cause in this country, and neuroarthropathy occurs in approximately 0.15% to 2.5% of diabetics. The midfoot is the most common location of involvement, representing 60% to 70% of cases in the foot and ankle.

The neuroarthropathic midfoot typically collapses into a rocker bottom deformity with a plantar prominence. A plantarmedial deformity with forefoot abduction results with medial and central column involvement. If there is lateral column involvement, a complete rocker deformity will result, with dorsal subluxation of the entire forefoot. In one recent study, 58% of feet undergoing midfoot surgical reconstruction also had hindfoot deformity consisting of dorsilateral peritalar subluxation.

The vast majority of midfoot neuroarthropathic feet are stable and can be managed with long-term bracing or, in patients with minimal deformity, custom plastizote orthotic devices in extra-depth or custom shoewear. Treatment is based on relieving pressure on bony prominences, minimizing shear forces, and providing stability. Patient education in this process is critical, with the primary goal being avoidance of skin breakdown and ulceration.

The surgical indications in the neuroarthropathic midfoot include recurrent ulceration despite adequate nonsurgical care, and unbraceable deformity. The goal of treatment is to obtain an ambulatory, ulcer-free, and shoeable plantigrade foot, thus avoiding the need for amputation. A stable deformity with a plantar bony prominence associated with recurrent or chronic ulceration is managed with an exostectomy of the offending bone. Arthrodesis is indicated in patients with severe or unstable deformity.

Arthrodesis must be considered with caution because there is potential for significant complications. Only compliant patients, who have adequate vascular supply, without active infection, should be considered. Contraindications include active neuroarthropathy with bony resorption or fragmentation, ongoing infection, gangrene, and vascular insufficiency. Surgical reconstruction includes preoperative planning, careful attention to surgical technique, meticulous soft-tissue handling, and strict postoperative management. Longitudinal incisions are used to expose the deformity, which is realigned by taking down the involved joints, and with osteotomies if fixed deformity is present. Internal fixation must be rigid and may be achieved with plates and/or interfragmentary screw fixation. Percutaneous Achilles tendon lengthening is frequently necessary.

In a series of 21 feet undergoing arthrodesis in the midfoot and hindfoot, limb salvage was obtained in 18. Seventy percent of ulcers healed at an average time of 6 weeks, with no midfoot ulcer recurrence. Fusion in successful cases was achieved in approximately 5 months. Two cases developed a nonunion, with hardware failure, and 2 underwent a below-knee amputation for postoperative osteomyelitis. Other complications included wound dehiscence, recurrent deformity, forefoot ulceration, and death. Overall, complications related to surgery occurred in 38% of cases. Of the salvaged feet, 87% were able to wear extra-depth, wide-toe box, off-the-shelf shoes with inserts.

Recent trends regarding the rocker-bottom diabetic foot deformity have included the development of a new classification system based on location and severity of the deformity. Cadaveric and clinical study of surgical management with plantar closing-wedge osteotomies and plantar plate fixation has demonstrated early satisfactory results.

Inflammatory Arthritis

Rheumatoid arthritis is the most common inflammatory arthritic disorder affecting the foot. The midfoot typically does not present with the significant involvement that is seen in the forefoot and hindfoot. Synovitis may be present with or without associated radiographic changes. Joint ankylosis may occur, but is usually not of functional significance. Involvement of the medial column, particularly the first metatarsocuneiform joint, may lead to a flatfoot deformity and contribute to the development of a hallux valgus deformity. Nonsurgical management includes corrective orthosis for flexible deformities or an accommodative device if the deformity is rigid. Surgical treatment includes arthrodesis of the involved joints with correction of deformity.

The seronegative spondyloarthropathies, a group of inflammatory disorders similar to rheumatoid arthritis, include ankylosing spondylitis, psoriatic arthritis, and Reiter's syndrome. They are characterized by a nonspecific inflammatory process involving synovial joints, tendon sheaths, joint capsules, tendon and ligament bony attachments (entheses), and fibrocartilaginous structures. The process is typically of low intensity, chronic, and associated with fibrosis and ossification, which differentiates it from rheumatoid arthritis. Although the foot is often affected, the midfoot is rarely involved in these conditions. Enthesopathy is common, with a frequent site of involvement being the plantar fascia origin, with resulting heel pain. Whereas the rheumatoid foot demonstrates generalized osteopenia, loss of joint space, and bony destruction, the seronegative disorders demonstrate periarticular calcifications, periostitis, bony erosions, joint ankylosis, subchondral sclerosis, and calcification of the entheses.

Ankylosing spondylitis primarily involves the axial skeleton. Calcaneal entheses are most commonly affected in the foot. Approximately 90% of caucasians with this disorder are HLA-B27 positive. Reiter's syndrome, also commonly HLA-B27 positive, and psoriatic arthritis are similar both clinically and radiographically. Both may present with a more acute course than ankylosing spondylitis. Reiter's syndrome commonly affects the foot, but in an asymmetric pattern, whereas psoriasis tends to be symmetric and also affects the hands. Reiter's syndrome can affect the hindfoot and midfoot, with the development of bony ankylosis. The classic Reiter's triad of urethritis, conjunctivitis, and arthritis is infrequently seen, with most patients exhibiting only certain components of the triad. The arthritic process in psoriasis usually follows the cutaneous manifestations, but is present prior to skin involvement in 10% to 20% of patients. The treatment of these disorders is focused on the medical management of the inflammatory process. Cushioned insoles or heel inserts are useful in the management of associated heel pain.

The juvenile with seronegative spondyloarthropathy often presents with lower extremity involvement. Midfoot involvement was observed clinically in 15 of 40 patients, with an average age of 11.2 years in 1 study. Spontaneous fusion of joints in the midfoot may occur, and bracing or orthoses may be helpful to maintain a plantigrade foot during the active stage of the disease.

Arthritis of the Forefoot

Anatomy and Biomechanics

The cam-shaped first metatarsophalangeal joint is characterized by a convex metatarsal head and concave proximal phalangeal base. Stability is provided by stout medial and lateral collateral ligaments, metatarsosesamoid suspensory ligaments, and a thick plantar plate. The musculotendinous structures that power the hallux include the extensor hallucis brevis and longus, flexor hallucis brevis and longus, abductor hallucis, and adductor hallucis. A recent cadaver study reported that injury to the metatarsophalangeal joint complex resulting from a dorsiflexion force can occur in variable patterns and may involve the medial capsule or plantar plate, with plantar disruption occurring distal or proximal to the sesamoids. This helps to explain the various injury patterns observed at this joint.

Motion of the first metatarsophalangeal joint is approximately 84° in dorsiflexion and 23° in plantarflexion. Normal barefoot gait uses approximately 60° of dorsiflexion, and this decreases to 30° in stiff sole shoes. The joint moves with a sliding action and changing instant centers of motion within the metatarsal head.

Two boat-shaped sesamoids lie in articular sulci beneath the first metatarsal head, with nearly flat, upper articular surfaces and concave lower portions that are embedded within the 2 tendon slips of the flexor hallucis brevis. The larger medial sesamoid has an incidence of bipartism of approximately 7% to 11%; the incidence in the lateral sesamoid is less than 1%. Bilateral bipartite sesamoids occur with an incidence of approximately 25%. The motion of the sesamoids averages approximately 72°, and is restricted by strong ligamentous attachments. The sesamoids serve to protect the metatarsal head and flexor hallucis longus tendon, distribute load transmission to the medial forefoot, and, via a pulley effect, increase the flexor strength to the hallux. Recent cadaver studies have demonstrated that the effective tendon moment arm of the flexor hallucis brevis is significantly decreased by excision of both sesamoids, while that of the flexor hallucis longus is also decreased by isolated sesamoid resection. These studies have shown that the flexor hallucis longus is the principal flexor of the first metatarsophalangeal joint.

Hallux Rigidus

Degenerative arthrosis of the first metatarsophalangeal joint, or hallux rigidus, is characterized by painful limitation of motion, primarily dorsiflexion, typically with the formation of dorsal osteophytes. The incidence in the adult population aged 60 years and older is 1 in 45. Juveniles are affected with a similar process, with an incidence of 1 in 4,500.

The precise etiology remains unknown, but multiple anatomic factors, trauma, and other causes have been proposed. A recent report found no significant differences with respect to metatarsus primus elevatus, first metatarsal declination, lateral one-two intermetatarsal angle in adults, with and without hallux rigidus. The condition generally begins with synovitis and articular degeneration of the dorsal metatarsal head, with subsequent dorsal osteophyte formation. Bone formation tends to be on the dorsal and lateral aspects of the metatarsal head, often without significant medial involvement. Patient complaints usually relate to activity and shoewear. Examination demonstrates a painful dorsal prominence, which, in the early phases of the process, presents as a small ridge. Pain is reproduced with metatarsophalangeal joint dorsiflexion, occasionally lateral deviation due to dorsolateral osteophytes, and plantarflexion due to capsular and extensor tendon stretching over the dorsal osteophytes. Metatarsophalangeal motion is restricted secondary to mechanical impingement from the dorsal osteophytes as well as the general arthritic condition of the joint.

Nonsurgical treatment includes the use of an adequate toe box to accommodate the enlarged joint. Stiffening of the sole, with or without a rocker bottom, is also beneficial, and can be achieved with a steel shank or a full length thin carbon fiber or plastic insert, which can be interchangeable between most shoes. Nonsteroidal anti-inflammatory medication is useful, particularly in the early phases of the process.

Current surgical recommendations for most cases include joint debridement (cheilectomy) or arthrodesis. Debridement is indicated for mild to moderate arthrosis with dorsal impingement. The procedure includes synovectomy, release of plantar capsular adhesions, and resection of the dorsal 25% to 33% of the metatarsal head, relieving impingement and providing an increase of passive dorsiflexion. The medial eminence is generally retained; however, it is important to resect lateral osteophytes. A dorsal approach is usually advocated, but satisfactory results have also been reported with a medial approach. Cheilectomy typically increases postoperative metatarsophalangeal motion by approximately 20°, and patient satisfaction rates have been reported between 70% and 90%. Arthrosis may progress in the joint following cheilectomy, and recurrence of dorsal spurring has been reported in up to 30% of cases. Unsatisfactory results are associated with inadequate or excessive bone resection, or when performed in the presence of severe arthrosis (Fig. 3).

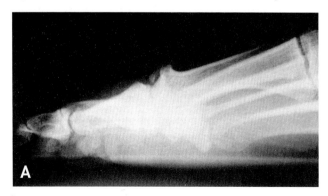 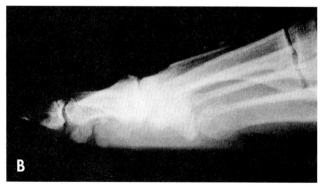

Figure 3

A, Hallux rigidus, characterized by dorsal impinging osteophytes. **B,** Postoperative radiograph following cheilectomy.

A cheilectomy may be combined with a proximal phalangeal osteotomy (Moberg procedure) to increase the dorsiflexion arc of motion and, theoretically, to decompress the joint. An osteotomy may be performed as an isolated procedure in patients who lack dorsiflexion but do not have dorsal impingement. A concern with the combination procedure is that the cheilectomy relies on early motion, which could lead to healing difficulties with an osteotomy. An osteotomy in a patient who lacks plantarflexion may lead to an unacceptable dorsiflexed posture of the hallux.

Arthrodesis is indicated for severe arthrosis; hallux valgus with degenerative arthrosis or severe deformity; salvage procedure following cheilectomy, joint arthroplasty, hallux valgus surgery, or infection; and for neuromuscular deformity or instability. This procedure generally relieves pain at the expense of motion (Fig. 4). The preferred position of arthrodesis is approximately 10° to 15° dorsiflexion from the sole of the foot, 15° to 20° valgus, and neutral rotation. Clinically, this positions the hallux slightly inclined from the sole, and next to, but not encroaching on, the second toe. Many fusion techniques and methods of fixation have been reported, with an average union and success rate of 90%. A biomechanical study has shown that preparation of the joint with conical reamers, and fixation with interfragmentary screws, is more stable than other commonly used techniques, however, clinical union rates are high with most current techniques. The most common complications of arthrodesis include nonunion, malunion, and interphalangeal arthrosis. Excessive dorsiflexion, the most common positioning error, results in shoe impingement and loss of hallucal weightbearing. The clinical significance of interphalangeal arthrosis is variable, with many patients asymptomatic, but its presence is associated with metatarsophalangeal malunion in some studies. Adequate valgus positioning appears to minimize interphalangeal joint arthrosis, and in the rheumatoid patient a valgus position of 20° to 30° may be appropriate, however, this degree of valgus may cause pressure against the second toe, especially in the nonrheumatoid patient.

Arthrodesis with an interpositional bone graft is an effective salvage technique for the failed Keller resection arthroplasty or implant arthroplasty with significant first ray shortening. This technique is more demanding, and may require a longer time to union. A two-stage approach can be used for patients with septic arthritis, with an initial debridement and placement of an antibiotic containing methylmethacrylate spacer. Tricortical iliac crest graft is interchanged with the cement spacer as the second stage. Good results have been reported in 4 of 5 patients using this technique, with resolution of the infection in all. Nonunion of the proximal fusion site was the most common complication.

Arthritis of the Hallucal Sesamoids

Arthritic conditions affect the metatarsosesamoid articulation in much the same way they affect other joints. Degenerative arthrosis can be associated with hallux rigidus, posttraumatic, or secondary to sesamoidal chondromalacia. Inflammatory conditions, such as rheumatoid arthritis and seronegative spondyloarthropathies, can also involve the sesamoids. Typically, the rheumatoid patient has a concomitant hallux valgus deformity. Cystic changes, bony erosion, sclerosis, and calcifications may be seen with the crystalline arthropathies. Patients typically present with tenderness over the affected sesamoid, synovitis, and frequently decreased metatarsophalangeal motion. Nonsurgical treatment modalities, aimed at decreasing stresses on the sesamoid complex and metatarsophalangeal joint, include stiff-sole shoes; metatarsal pad placed just proximal to the sesamoids; and the judicial use of nonsteroidal anti-inflammatory medication or a local steroid preparation injection. One study reported successful treatment of sesamoid-related pain in the athlete with the use of custom-fitted orthotic devices. If nonsurgical care is unsuccessful and pathology is isolated to one sesamoid, the surgical treatment is excision of the involved bone (Fig. 5). When both sesamoids are affected, double excision is contraindicated due to weakening of pushoff, and the potential for hallucal clawing. Treatment is controversial in these rare cases, and metatarsophalangeal joint arthrodesis with or without sesamoid excision has been advocated.

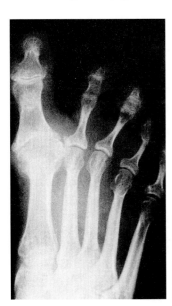

Figure 4

Severe degenerative arthritis of the first metatarsophalangeal joint. The surgical management of this degree of arthritis generally is arthrodesis.

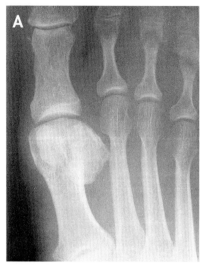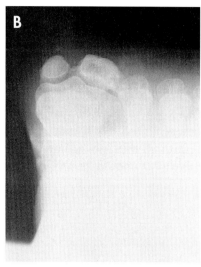

Figure 5

A and **B,** Posttraumatic arthritis of the lateral sesamoid. Management included resection via a dorsal approach.

Rheumatoid Arthritis

Foot and ankle involvement is frequent in patients with rheumatoid arthritis. A review of 99 outpatients from university rheumatology clinics found that 93 had foot or ankle symptoms. The duration of disease correlated with the prevalence of foot symptoms. Ankle symptoms were present in 79, forefoot in 71, and midfoot in 27. Of the 93, 42% rated ankle symptoms worse than forefoot, and 28% rated the forefoot most symptomatic. A moderate or severe hallux valgus deformity was present in approximately one third, and lesser toe deformity was present in 42%. Hallucal deformity is associated with lesser metatarsophalangeal dislocation, with the most common forefoot complaint being metatarsalgia. Despite the frequent occurrence of foot problems, very few patients had received any treatment.

Rheumatoid arthritis tends to be progressive, with intermittent and variable remissions. The lesser metatarsophalangeal joints progress from synovitis to plantar plate destruction, with subsequent dorsal dislocation and hammering of the toes. Nonsurgical treatment includes soft orthotic devices, with unloading of the forefoot by metatarsal pads, and padding to relieve lesser toe discomfort. Extra-depth or custom shoewear is often necessary, and custom orthotic devices may be beneficial.

Surgical treatment should be delayed until comprehensive conservative measures have failed to provide satisfactory pain relief. Currently, most authors advocate surgical reconstruction of the rheumatoid forefoot with first metatarsophalangeal joint arthrodesis and resection of the lesser metatarsal heads. Recurrence of deformity and deterioration of results over time have been problems associated with resection or implant arthroplasty of the hallux.

Surgical forefoot reconstruction uses longitudinal incisions: dorsal to the first metatarsophalangeal joint; between the second and third metatarsals; and between the fourth and fifth metatarsals. The metatarsal heads 2 through 5 are resected in a smooth cascade from medial to lateral, and beveled from dorsal-distal to plantar-proximal. Fixation of the metatarsophalangeal region with the long extensor tendon interposed is done with K-wires. It is important to create a smooth resection pattern with adequate arthroplasty space. The preservation of the proximal phalangeal bases tends to result in improved cosmesis and preserves toe stability through soft-tissue attachments to the proximal phalanx. Lesser toe deformities can usually be managed with a closed osteoclasis. The hallucal arthrodesis is performed so that the tip of the hallux and second toe are at the same level. In a series of 20 patients, 19 were satisfied with the result at 3.7 years. No patient required custom shoes or orthoses, and all but one achieved fusion of the first metatarsophalangeal joint. Ten percent had postoperative painful plantar callosities, whereas earlier studies without first ray arthrodesis have reported incidences of 30% to 60%. An arthrodesis will result in earlier lift-off of the forefoot during gait, which results in decreased lesser metatarsophalangeal joint dorsiflexion forces, thus protecting them from recurrent deformity. Short-term results of forefoot reconstruction tend to be better when the hallux is managed with an arthrodesis, however, long term follow-up studies are lacking, and results with other techniques have tended to show deterioration 4 to 5 years postoperatively.

Occasionally, a patient will present for surgery with uninvolved rays or no hallucal deformity. As a general rule, forefoot arthroplasty should include all lesser metatarsophalangeal joints, even if 1 or 2 are not appreciably affected, because there is a high likelihood of symptoms and disease progression in these rays. The hallux should typically be included even with mild involvement, however, in patients with a normal hallux, it may be preserved if the patient has been forewarned that later surgery may be necessary. In a large series of rheumatoid forefoot reconstructions, 4 feet had preservation of the hallux; 3 of whom 3 to 10 years later required arthrodesis for progressive deformity.

Other surgical reconstructive procedures have been reported for the rheumatoid forefoot. A recent review of 75 feet reported satisfactory results in 83% at 6 years following metatarsal 2 through 5 shortening oblique osteotomy and metatarsophalangeal joint synovectomy, with hallux valgus reconstruction using an implant arthroplasty or osteotomy. Thirty percent had recurrence of lesser ray deformity, and 12% had recurrent plantar callosities. Joint sparing procedures may be indicated for the younger, more active patient with early joint involvement, however, the rheumatoid forefoot tends to have an unpredictable nature which may be a factor in the failure of certain procedures.

Plantar forefoot pressures have been studied pre- and post-operatively in the rheumatoid patient undergoing resection arthroplasty of metatarophalangeal joints 1 through 5. Peak pressures are similar or increased following surgery, but there tend to be fewer regions of abnormally high pressure. It is likely that surgery creates a foot better able to tolerate weightbearing. Elevated forefoot pressures have been measured in patients with a hindfoot valgus posture, and this deformity, especially when greater than 10°, should be addressed prior to forefoot reconstruction with either non-surgical or surgical means.

Lesser Metatarsophalangeal Joint Arthrosis

Arthrosis involving the lesser metatarsophalangeal joints typically results from the sequelae of Freiberg's infraction of the second metatarsal head. This disease, an osteochondrosis of the metatarsal head, usually occurs in adolescence and is felt to be secondary to osteonecrosis following repetitive micro-trauma. Occasionally, patients develop significant degenerative changes characterized by hypertrophy of the joint, bony fragmentation, and dorsal osteopyhtes. Nonsurgical treatment measures are similar to those for hallux rigidus, and also include the judicial use of an intra-articular corticosteroid injection. Surgical treatment includes synovectomy and joint debridement with resection of osteophytes and loose bodies. In more severe cases, a metatarsophalangeal joint arthroplasty may be necessary. This includes joint debridement and resculpturing of the metatarsal head. A K-wire is placed across the joint for approximately 2 weeks, after which motion exercises are initiated. Approximately 50% of normal motion is obtained with this procedure. If the plantar articular surface of the metatarsal head is intact, a dorsal closing wedge osteotomy may be performed in the metatarsal head to preserve the remaining joint surface.

Occasionally, metatarsophalangeal joint arthrosis is post-traumatic in nature. These patients often present with joint incongruity or destruction, with a variable degree of motion loss. The treatment principles discussed above for Freiberg's infraction tend to apply to this population as well.

Seronegative Spondyloarthropathy

These disorders have also been discussed in the midfoot arthritis section.

With respect to the forefoot, ankylosing spondylitis causes deformities similar to those seen in rheumatoid arthritis, with involvement of the metatarsophalangeal joints. The inflammatory process, however, is typically less severe than in rheumatoid arthritis. Joint ankylosis may occur secondary to intra-articular or capsular ossification. Clinical management follows the same principles as in the rheumatoid patient.

Psoriatic arthritis typically affects the distal interphalangeal joints of the toes, and may also cause erosion of the proximal phalanges, with the formation of "pencil in cup" appearance to the joints. This may result in arthritis mutilans, with severe erosive destruction of multiple joints. Distal phalanx tuft erosion and pathologic changes in the nails are also present. The metatarsophalangeal joints may or may not be involved. Reiter's syndrome is similar clinically to psoriasis, but it tends to be less symmetric and to have less interphalangeal joint involvement. Both disorders can cause "sausage digits", caused by generalized soft-tissue swelling of a toe secondary to tenosynovitis.

Crystal-Induced Arthritis

Gout and pseudogout are crystalline deposition disorders that may present with foot involvement. Gout is characterized by the intra-articular presence of monosodium urate crystals, which are needle-shaped and negatively birefringent under a polarizing microscope. It results from a disorder of purine metabolism, but also may occur in certain diseases, and from medications that elevate the serum uric acid. Gout is more frequent in men than women, and typically presents with an acute arthritis or periarticular inflammatory reaction of the first metatarsophalangeal joint. This joint is involved in 50% to 75% of initial attacks, and 90% of patients will have involvement of this joint at some time. An acute attack, manifested by severe pain, swelling, erythema, and warmth about the involved joint, typically lasts for several days and then subsides. The postoperative period is a frequent time of attacks. Diagnosis can often be made on a clinical basis, and crystal analysis of joint fluid will confirm the diagnosis. Serum uric acid level may be normal, and radiographs are typically normal with an initial attack but may later demonstrate periarticular erosions or lesions on both sides of the joint. Joint destruction may occur in chronic cases.

The acute gouty episode of the hallux is treated with rest, elevation, and use of a wooden sole, open toe postoperative shoe. Medical management involves the use of nonsteroidal anti-inflammatory medication (typically indomethacin) or colchicine. Chronic tophaceous gout remains rare, and management includes local debridement of symptomatic or draining deposits. Arthrodesis may be indicated in the presence of significant joint destruction.

Pseudogout results from calcium pyrophosphate dihydrate (CPPD) crystal deposition in joints or periarticular tissue, causing an inflammatory reaction. Crystals are of variable shape and have weak positive birefringence under the polarizing microscope. Radiographs may demonstrate fine intra-articular calcifications, but joint destruction is uncommon. The metatarsophalangeal joints are most commonly affected in the foot, and treatment is symptomatic, with medical management of acute synovitis. If severe joint involvement occurs, the process may be similar to degenerative arthritis or neuroarthropathy with bony fragmentation.

Annotated Bibliography

Midfoot Arthritis

de Palma L, Santucci A, Sabetta SP, Rapali S: Anatomy of the Lisfranc joint complex. *Foot Ankle Int* 1997;18:356–364.

Anatomic dissections demonstrated the synovial compartmentalization of the midfoot into medial, central, and lateral components. Stability is provided by numerous ligaments that are quite variable. The Lisfranc ligament and the second plantar ligament are the most powerful ligaments in the midfoot.

Early JS, Hansen ST: Surgical reconstruction of the diabetic foot: A salvage approach for midfoot collapse. *Foot Ankle Int* 1996; 17:325–330.

The diabetic neuroarthropathic midfoot was reconstructed in 21 feet. Limb salvage was obtained in 18, with a 28-month follow-up. Forty-seven percent were free of complications, and 70% of presenting ulcers healed. There were no recurrent midfoot ulcers.

Ebraheim NA, Yang H, Lu J, Biyani A: Computer evaluation of second tarsometatarsal joint dislocation. *Foot Ankle Int* 1996;17:685–689.

Articular contact area was shown to decrease as articular displacement increases in a cadaver model. Dorsolateral displacement caused the greatest decrease in contact area, with 3 mm causing 38.6% reduction in the contact area.

Horton GA, Olney BW: Deformity correction and arthrodesis of the midfoot with a medial plate. *Foot Ankle* 1993;14:493–499.

Nine feet with midfoot arthritis were treated with arthrodesis using a medial plate, with average follow-up of 27 months. Deformity was present and corrected in 6, all 9 achieved union, and 7 had a good or excellent result.

Komenda GA, Myerson MS, Biddinger KR: Results of arthrodesis of the tarsometatarsal joints after traumatic injury. *J Bone Joint Surg* 1996;78A:1665–1676.

Thirty-two patients with midfoot posttraumatic arthritis were retrospectively evaluated at an average of 50 months after arthrodesis. Twenty-four required correction of deformity, and complications occurred in 11. The authors provide a detailed analysis of their operative technique and results.

Mann RA, Prieskorn D, Sobel M: Mid-tarsal and tarsometatarsal arthrodesis for primary degenerative osteoarthrosis or osteoarthrosis after trauma. *J Bone Joint Surg* 1996;78A: 1376–1385.

The authors report on 41 midfoot arthrodeses for feet with posttraumatic, primary degenerative, and inflammatory arthritis. Average follow-up was 6 years, and 93% were satisfied, with a 98% union rate. This study provides a comparison between patients with primary and posttraumatic arthritis; both had similar clinical results, however, the primary arthritis group was older, with more extensive arthritic involvement.

Myerson MS, Henderson MR, Saxby T, Short KW: Management of midfoot diabetic neuroarthropathy. *Foot Ankle Int* 1994;15:233–241.

The authors detail a treatment protocol for the diabetic midfoot neuroarthropathy based on neuroarthropathic stage, foot stability, ulceration, infection, and ischemia. Their protocol was successful in 82 of 85 feet, and total contact casting was effective in 75% of cases. Nonsurgical treatments were typically successful, but various surgical procedures were performed on 37 feet.

Sangeorzan BJ, Veith RG, Hansen ST Jr: Salvage of Lisfranc's tarsometatarsal joint by arthrodesis. *Foot Ankle* 1990;10: 193–200.

This study provides a retrospective review of 16 patients with posttraumatic midfoot arthritis treated with arthrodesis. Twelve patients had deformity which was realigned, and 45 of 49 joints fused achieved union. Overall there were 69% good and excellent results.

Forefoot Arthritis

Aper RL, Saltzman CL, Brown TD: The effect of hallux sesamoid excision on the flexor hallucis longus moment arm. *Clin Orthop* 1996;325:209–217.

This cadaver study provides evidence that the flexor hallucis longus is the prime flexor of the first metatarsophalangeal joint. Isolated sesamoid resection, as well as total resection caused a significant decrease in the flexor hallucis longus effective tendon moment arm.

Beaman DN, Saltzman CL: Disorders of the hallucal sesamoids, in Adelaar RS (ed): *Disorders of the Great Toe.* Rosemont, IL, American Academy of Orthopaedic Surgeons, 1997, pp 33–42.

This review provides a comprehensive summary of sesamoid anatomy, biomechanics, and the evaluation and management of patients with various hallucal sesamoid disorders. The multitude of arthritic conditions which may affect the sesamoids are presented.

Coughlin MJ, Mann RA: Arthrodesis of the first metatarsophalangeal joint as salvage for the failed Keller procedure. *J Bone Joint Surg* 1987;69A:68–75.

Sixteen feet with failed Keller resection arthroplasties were retrospectively studied following first metatarsophalangeal joint arthrodesis. Excessive shortening was treated with interpositional bone graft in four cases. All feet achieved union with good resolution of preoperative transfer metatarsalgia.

Dereymaeker G, Mulier T, Stuer P, Peeraer L, Fabry G: Pedodynographic measurements after forefoot reconstruction in rheumatoid arthritis patients. *Foot Ankle Int* 1997;18:270–276.

A review of 38 patients at 35-month follow-up found a 93% subjective satisfaction rate with a joint-ablation surgical approach to the rheumatoid forefoot. Fifty-one percent had persistent plantar callosities, and hallucal deformity recurred in 22%. The clinical course correlated with pedodynographic findings in 79% of the patients.

Hanyu T, Yamazaki H, Murasawa A, Tohyama C: Arthroplasty for rheumatoid forefoot deformities by a shortening oblique osteotomy. *Clin Orthop* 1997;338:131–138.

A retrospective review of 47 patients followed an average of 6 years found an 83% satisfaction rate with this joint-sparing surgical approach to the rheumatoid forefoot. Deformities recurred in 30% of the lesser toes and 15% of the great toes. Plantar callosities recurred in 12%.

Hattrup SJ, Johnson KA: Subjective results of hallux rigidus following treatment with cheilectomy. *Clin Orthop* 1988; 226:182–191.

A retrospective review of 58 cases of cheilectomy was presented with complete satisfaction in 53% of cases. The procedure was less successful in cases with more advanced degenerative changes, however, results did not deteriorate with time.

Mann RA, Clanton TO: Hallux rigidus: Treatment by cheilectomy. *J Bone Joint Surg* 1988;70A:400–406.

A retrospective review of 31 cases of cheilectomy was presented with complete pain relief in 71%. Range of motion increased by 20°, and no patient required further surgery. The procedure relieves symptoms by alleviating dorsal joint impingement, and provided a satisfactory result even with significant degenerative changes.

Mann RA, Schakel ME II: Surgical correction of rheumatoid forefoot deformities. *Foot Ankle Int* 1995;16:1–6.

Nineteen of 20 patients undergoing forefoot reconstruction with first metatarsophalangeal joint arthrodesis and lesser metatarsal head resection were satisfied at a follow-up of 3.7 years. Ninety percent had significant pain relief, with 2 patients having residual painful plantar callosities. This procedure provides a successful midterm result, with diminished stress across the lesser toes provided by the hallucal arthrodesis and subsequent earlier forefoot lift-off in gait.

Classic Bibliography

Coughlin MJ: Arthrodesis of the first metatarsophalangeal joint. *Orthop Rev* 1990;19:177–186.

Curtis MJ, Myerson M, Jinnah RH, Cox QG, Alexander I: Arthrodesis of the first metatarsophalangeal joint: A biomechanical study of internal fixation techniques. *Foot Ankle* 1993;14:395–399.

Fritz GR, Prieskorn D: First metatarsocuneiform motion: A radiographic and statistical analysis. *Foot Ankle Int* 1995; 16:117–123.

Guerra J, Resnick D: Arthritides affecting the foot: Radiographic-pathological correlation. *Foot Ankle Int* 1982;2:325–331.

Hasselo LG, Willkens RF, Toomey HE, Karges DE, Hansen ST: Forefoot surgery in rheumatoid arthritis: Subjective assessment of outcome. *Foot Ankle* 1987;8:148–151.

Levi S, Ansell BM, Klenerman L: Tarsometatarsal involvement in juvenile spondyloarthropathy. *Foot Ankle* 1990;11:90–92.

Mann RA, Oates JC: Arthrodesis of the first metatarsophalangeal joint. *Foot Ankle* 1980;1:159–166.

Michelson J, Easley M, Wigley FM, Hellmann D: Foot and ankle problems in rheumatoid arthritis. *Foot Ankle Int* 1994;15: 608–613.

Myerson MS, Miller SD, Henderson MR, Saxby T: Staged arthrodesis for salvage of the septic hallux metatarsophalangeal joint. *Clin Orthop* 1994;307:174–181.

Ouzounian TJ, Shereff MJ: In vitro determination of midfoot motion. *Foot Ankle* 1989;10:140–146.

Prieskorn D, Graves S, Yen M, Ray J Jr, Schultz R: Integrity of the first metatarsophalangeal joint: A biomechanical analysis. *Foot Ankle Int* 1995;16:357–362.

Chapter 23
Amputations Below the Knee

The indications for amputation of an extremity include peripheral vascular disease, infection, trauma, tumor, or congenital anomaly. For successful amputation surgery, it is essential to consider the entire patient, including function, psychological issues, and quality of life, when creating a treatment plan for these difficult problems. Advances in medical and surgical management have helped improve limb salvage; however, in certain situations these attempts can lead to excessive morbidity and possibly death. When considering amputation of all or part of an extremity, the patient should be counseled regarding the surgical, prosthetic, and rehabilitative processes. When considering an amputation and subsequent use of a prosthesis, the clinician should consider the cognitive capacities of the patient. Patients must exhibit the following abilities in order to use a prosthesis effectively: (1) memory, (2) attention, (3) concentration, and (4) organization.

The concept of a team approach is important in amputation surgery. The input of a vascular surgeon and appropriate preoperative testing can help determine a level of amputation that has the capacity to heal in patients with peripheral vascular disease. Additional assistance from nurses, prosthetists, orthotists, pedorthists, and amputee support groups provide invaluable services, allowing patients to return to an improved quality of life.

Preoperative Evaluation

Vascular Disease and Diabetes

The most common indication for amputation in Western society is peripheral vascular disease, with associated infection or gangrene. Approximately half of these patients have diabetes. A Swedish study has noted a decreasing incidence of major amputations and an increasing percentage of amputations performed below the ankle in patients who have been managed by a multidisciplinary footcare team approach. Unfortunately, many failures of conservative management and revascularization procedures still occur. A thorough examination of these patients should include evaluation of skin, perfusion, and immunocompetence. Other medical specialists can help optimize patients' blood glucose levels, as well as renal and cardiac function.

Although palpation of pulses in the foot and ankle is helpful in evaluating large-vessel perfusion, other studies may be necessary. Doppler ultrasound provides objective measurement of blood flow. For healing diabetic foot ulcers, results of studies evaluating the predictive value of systolic ankle and toe blood pressure have been conflicting. An ankle/brachial index > 0.45 has been shown to correlate with successful wound healing. However, vessel walls, which are often calcified, can be noncompliant, and this can lead to a falsely elevated test, indicating more blood flow than is actually present. Measurement of transcutaneous oxygen pressure ($TcpO_2$) and carbon dioxide pressure ($TcpCO_2$) are other noninvasive tests, and appear to be more accurate predictors of wound healing. One study, which factored out variables of tissue nutrition and immunocompetence, found that in 92% of patients with $TcpO_2$ greater than 30 mm Hg at the midfoot and ankle the amputation wound healed. Other modalities in the diagnostic armamentarium include arteriography, which is invasive and may still provide false results, and evaluation of cutaneous temperature with venous occlusion plethysmography.

The nutritional status and immune system function should always be considered in this patient population. These two factors have been shown to correlate directly with wound healing in amputation. Serum albumin levels of greater than 3.0 g/dl and total lymphocyte count of greater than 1,500 cells/mm³ have been shown to be significantly correlated to wound healing capabilities. Patients who demonstrate values below these levels may require nutritional supplementation prior to surgical intervention. If nutrition cannot be optimized prior to surgery, a higher-level amputation may need to be considered. Another important variable is the influence of smoking on complications of amputations. High concentrations of nicotine have been shown to compromise cutaneous blood-flow velocity and to increase the risk of formation of micro-thrombi.

The overall medical condition, activity level, and ambulatory status should also be considered. Finding the most distal level that can be safely healed is the goal in ambulatory patients, with subsequent prosthetic fitting and rehabilitation. Studies have shown that gait velocity and the energy cost of walking are directly related to the level of amputation. The goals in patients who may be bedridden include adequate wound healing, with minimal complications, and the ability to sit, transfer, and tend to personal hygiene.

Infection and Gangrene

Cases of local ischemia and infection must be treated in an expeditious manner. It is often necessary to control the infection prior to definitive amputation procedures. This control is accomplished with incision and drainage of the infected region, leaving the majority of the wound open or using drains where appropriate. The debridement must be done aggressively down to normal-appearing tissue, removing all necrotic tissue. Bed rest, elevation, and compression are instituted, as well as starting broad-spectrum antibiotics once adequate intraoperative cultures are taken. These measures should be maintained until the infectious organisms are identified and more specific antibiotics can be instituted. In severe infections, it may be necessary to return to the operating room for redebridement after approximately 48 hours in order to be certain that all necrotic tissue has been removed.

Once the cellulitis and infection are under control, a more definitive amputation may be necessary. It is again essential that the patient's medical status be optimized from the standpoint of blood supply, nutrition, and immune status. The level of the amputation is determined by the location of the infection, the status of circulation, and the age and activity level of the patient.

Three types of gas-forming gangrene may present as lower extremity infections. Patients with clostridial myonecrosis may be acutely ill, with sepsis, pain, and disorientation. A brownish discharge may be noted, and there may be crepitus of the soft tissues. Open amputation above the level of infection is required, and intravenous penicillin should be started and consideration given to hyperbaric oxygen therapy.

Streptococcal myonecrosis is usually a slower process, and patients are generally less septic than in clostridial infections. Surgical debridement of the involved compartments and penicillin are necessary. In diabetic patients, infections are often polymicrobial and include anaerobic infections caused by gram-negative organisms. These infections also require debridement and appropriate parenteral antibiotics, with consideration for open amputation if systemic sepsis is evident.

Trauma

With the advances made in the technical aspects of reconstruction of bone, blood vessels, nerves, and other soft tissues, heroic efforts to salvage severely injured lower extremities are sometimes attempted. However, the extremity may remain functionless after multiple reconstructive procedures, which can be costly, time-consuming, and stressful to the patient, as well as those responsible for the

patient's care. One recent study compared limb salvage versus early below-knee amputation for the treatment of severe open tibial fractures with soft-tissue loss (Gustillo-Anderson grades IIIB and IIIC). The authors concluded that complications and osseous union were difficult problems, and that limb salvage often led to less satisfactory functional, occupational, recreational, and quality-of-life outcomes than were seen following early amputation. The amputation population also demonstrated quicker recovery time and reduced long-term disability, and they more frequently returned to preinjury job status and incurred lower hospital costs than the limb salvage group.

The absolute indication for amputation in trauma situations is an ischemic limb with a nonreconstructable vascular injury. In many cases, however, the decision to perform early amputation can be difficult for both patient and clinician. The Mangled Extremity Severity Score (MESS) was developed to assist in evaluation of these injuries. The 4 variables assessed include skeletal and soft-tissue injury, limb ischemia, shock, and age of the patient (Table 1). A score of 7 or more was a positive predictor of amputation. The limb ischemia score is doubled if the time of restoring perfusion to a dysvascular extremity exceeds 6 hours. Although these scores are not absolute, they can act as a guide in aiding the clinician to make realistic predictions of outcome and salvage. The goals of limb salvage must also be considered. In the lower extremity, these goals are a painless, functional platform on which to bear weight, one that is durable and has some protective sensation.

Tumors

The primary goal in musculoskeletal tumor procedures is to provide disease-free surgical margins and maintain long-term patient survival. Patients who present with tumors of the foot and ankle present several difficult challenges, including achieving adequate margins, providing soft-tissue coverage, and a lack of distinct anatomic compartments. Although they account for approximately 1% to 5% of all bony and soft-tissue tumors, they are rarely malignant. However, those that are malignant have traditionally been treated with a below-knee amputation. More recent surgical salvage techniques, neoadjuvant chemotherapy, and radiation therapy have been beneficial in managing these tumors. Even with these modalities many patients eventually require amputation. Several recent studies have described various limb-sparing techniques for these difficult neoplasms. This can sometimes be achieved by wide excision versus a midfoot or hindfoot amputation including transmetatarsal, Chopart, Pirogoff, or Syme techniques. If none of these are feasible, a below-knee amputation may be appropriate.

Table 1
Mangled extremity severity score (MESS) variables

Skeletal/soft-tissue injury

Low energy	1
Medium energy	2
High energy	3
Very high energy	4

Limb ischemia

Pulse reduced or absent, normal perfusion	1*
Pulseless; paresthesias; poor perfusion	2*
Cool, paralyzed, insensate, numb	3*

Shock

Systolic blood pressure above 90 mm Hg	0
Transiently hypotensive	1
Persistent hypotension	2

Age (years)

< 30	0
30-50	1
> 50	2

*Score doubled for ischemia > 6 hours
(Reproduced with permission from Johansen K, Daines M, Howey T, et al: Objective criteria accurately predict amputation following lower extremity trauma. *J Trauma* 1990;30:568-573.

Pediatric Amputations
Amputations in the pediatric population may be indicated in cases of congenital limb deficiencies, trauma, and tumors. The treatment concepts for trauma and tumors previously described for adults should be applied in a similar fashion to children. Congenital deficiencies are either longitudinal or transverse, and intercalary deficits are possible as well. A preaxial deficiency in the lower limb is the tibial side, whereas postaxial refers to the fibular side. Indications for lower extremity amputation in this group of patients may include proximal femoral focal deficiency, as well as tibial or fibular hemimelia. In these cases, early amputation may produce a more functional residual limb and improve prosthetic replacement. Several authors have recommended through-knee amputation and early prosthetic fitting for type 1A tibial hemimelia in which there is a complete absence of the tibia or tibial anlage.

Two important concepts to consider in pediatric amputations are residual limb length and terminal overgrowth. All attempts should be made to avoid removal of the distal epiphysis and its growth center. What appears to be a very long diaphyseal amputation may result in a short resultant limb once skeletal maturity is complete. In addition, a diaphyseal amputation can lead to terminal overgrowth via appositional bone growth at the bone end. Therefore, disarticulation procedures are preferred. These techniques help prevent not only loss of residual limb length, but also terminal overgrowth, which can occur in 8% to 12% of acquired pediatric amputations. If terminal overgrowth does occur, it may be salvaged by stump revision with adequate bony resection or autogenous osteochondral stump capping as described by Marquardt.

In a study comparing several types of partial foot amputations with Syme amputations, the authors made several conclusions. Metatarsal ray, transmetatarsal, Lisfranc, midtarsal, and Chopart amputations without equinus contractures had better overall function than did Syme amputation. Those with Chopart amputation, equinus contracture, and inadequate length of the forefoot had poorer overall function than Syme's procedures. Prosthetic fitting of the lower extremity should begin once the child is crawling or pulling to stand at 8 to 12 months of age. It is generally not necessary to force gait training too early, as children are very adaptable to their prostheses, and will develop an efficient gait pattern as their motor coordination improves.

Technical Considerations
Careful and meticulous handling of the soft tissues is important for wound healing and future functional outcome in amputation surgery. These tissues often have impaired circulation or may be traumatized, which increases the risk of wound failure. Skin flaps must be kept thick, avoiding significant soft-tissue dissection between the skin, subcutaneous, fascial, and muscle planes. These soft-tissue flaps should be carefully planned so that adequate coverage is available after bony resection and little tension is present upon closure of the wound. The flaps should be tested prior to closure to determine if further bony resection is necessary.

The classic teaching has been against the use of a tourniquet during amputation surgery. However, a prospective randomized study using patients with diabetes and/or peripheral vascular disease demonstrated no difference in amputation healing for patients with or without a tourniquet. There was also no significant difference between healing rates when comparing Esmarch bandage tourniquets versus pneumatic thigh cuff tourniquets.

The peripheral nerves should be carefully resected, with adequate coverage by muscle to prevent painful neuroma formation. The nerve should be resected with a fresh scalpel and should not be crushed with a clamp prior to transection. Other techniques such as ligation, cauterization, capping, perineural closures, and end-loop anastomoses have not been shown to be more effective than sharp transection and adequate soft-tissue coverage in preventing painful neuromas, phantom pain, or reflex sympathetic dystrophy.

In adults, the periosteum should not be stripped above the level of the bony resection to prevent overgrowth, whereas in children excision of 0.5 cm of the periosteum proximal to the amputation level may prevent bony overgrowth. In all cases, the bone edges should be smooth and rounded.

Stabilizing the underlying muscle after bony resection can improve residual function and prevent atrophy and deformity, as well as provide padding over the end of the bone. Myodesis involves suturing the muscles or tendon to bone, whereas myoplasty involves suturing muscles to periosteum or distally to each other. The goal is to prevent a mobile muscle sling, which can lead to painful bursa formation. Split-thickness skin grafts are generally not recommended in amputation surgery unless a resilient muscle mass is present between the graft and the underlying bone.

When preparing for wound closure, nylon or other nonreactive material should be used, and skin flaps should be tested to be certain there is no tension on the wound edges. If this is questionable, further bone resection may be indicated. It is more optimal to leave the wound open and allow healing by granulation than to leave too much tension on the wound, with possible subsequent flap necrosis. It is also important to palpate the bone ends through the skin to check for sharp or prominent edges that could produce pressure ulceration of the stump. Suction drainage is often used to prevent postoperative hematoma formation and to lessen tension on the wound. In cases of infection, an irrigation system may be used with an inflow catheter of normal saline or Ringer's lactate. The fluid can run through the wound and out the suture line with a loose closure, removing the irrigation catheter after 12 to 24 hours.

Amputation Levels

Terminal Syme's
Indications for this amputation include onychomycosis, severe nail deformity, and recurrent infection. It is most common in the great toe, but it can also be done in the lesser toes.

After removing the nail plate, the entire nail bed and matrix are excised down to the underlying distal phalanx. An oscillating saw can then be used to resect at least 1.0 cm of the distal aspect of the phalanx to allow for closure without significant tissue tension on the wound. This results in a shortened toe; however, it is generally curative, and careful closure can avoid wound problems or a bulbous stump. Complications can include nail regrowth due to some remaining nail matrix.

Great Toe
Maintaining some of the length of the great toe will allow for better function and fewer complications than a disarticulation through the metatarsophalangeal (MP) joint. If at least 1.0 cm of proximal phalanx can be saved, the first ray will receive greater weightbearing, which will lessen the risk of transfer lesions to the lesser metatarsal heads (Fig. 1). This will help reduce the risk of subsequent ulceration beneath these heads. Push-off is also helped because of the preservation of the sesamoids, flexor hallucis brevis, and plantar fascia insertion. It is usually not necessary to repair the tendons at this level of amputation.

Lesser Toes
The lesser toes can be amputated through the MP joints, through the interphalangeal joints, or through the phalanges. There is little difference in function between these techniques, although there will be some loss of stance-phase stability. Saving the base of the proximal phalanx of the toe is recommended to help prevent migration of the adjacent toes, which may fill the dead space. This is most important for complete amputation of the second toe, which can lead to subsequent hallux valgus. The skin flaps for partial toe amputations can be either side-to-side or dorsal-plantar. If the procedure is done through the MP joint, a racquet-shaped incision can be used.

Ray Resection
Amputation of a toe and all or part of the corresponding metatarsal is termed a ray resection. Removal of 2 or 3 rays is termed a partial forefoot amputation. These procedures are very durable and provide a more functional alternative to the transmetatarsal amputation. To maintain forefoot stability, it is generally recommended that no more than 2 rays be removed. The border rays (first or fifth) are the easiest to resect, using a medial or lateral incision with a racquet-type of incision around the base of the toe. The central ray resections can have problems, including prolonged wound healing and toe migration. If more than 1 central ray is to be removed, midfoot amputation should be considered as an

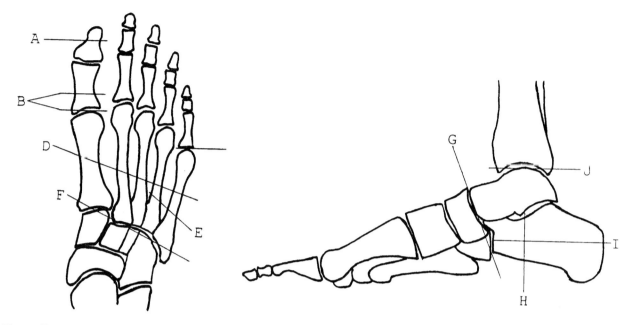

Figure 1

Levels of forefoot, midfoot, and hindfoot amputations. **A,** Terminal Syme's. **B,** Great toe (at base of proximal phalanx preserves some function, or at metatarsophalangeal (MTP) joint). **C,** Lesser toe at MTP joint. **D,** Transmetatarsal. **E,** Ray(s). **F,** Lisfranc. **G,** Chopart. **H,** Pirigoff (includes talectomy, 90° rotation and fixation to distal tibia). **I,** Boyd. **J,** Syme's.

alternative. The bases of the metatarsals should be preserved during ray resections, if possible, in order to prevent instability of the Lisfranc joint complex.

Transmetatarsal

Amputation at the transmetatarsal or Lisfranc joint level is generally very durable and functional. Longer plantar flaps provide the best coverage, but equal dorsal and plantar flaps can be used if necessary. The dorsal incision should be curved proximally from medial to lateral to mimic the level of bony resection. For the transmetatarsal level, the bone should be resected using a beveled cut with an oscillating saw from dorsal distal to plantar proximal. This can help prevent plantar ulcerations from prominent bone surfaces. Each metatarsal should be resected approximately 2.0 to 3.0 mm shorter than the one medial to it in order to create a cascade of length. The fifth metatarsal should also be beveled in a second plane from medial distal to lateral proximal to prevent a lateral prominence.

Muscle balance should be evaluated preoperatively to assess tightness of the heel cord, as well as strength of the anterior and posterior tibialis and peroneals. Because the lever arm is shortened, it is often necessary to lengthen the Achilles tendon. If the insertions of the tibialis or peroneal muscles are released, they should be reattached to prevent future defor-

mity. One may also consider reattachment of the extensor tendons or tibialis anterior tendons to the lateral cuneiform to help prevent equinus and varus deformity. Although amputations through the Lisfranc joint are technically easier from a standpoint of bony resection, they require more soft-tissue balancing and produce a shorter foot than transmetatarsal amputations.

Hindfoot and Syme's

At the level of the transverse tarsal joints, a Chopart amputation has had a reputation for less optimal functional results due to equinovarus deformity. Leaving only the talus and the calcaneus creates a soft-tissue balancing problem, which must be addressed by careful reconstruction. A percutaneous lengthening of the Achilles tendon should be considered to prevent equinus, and the anterior tibial tendon may be reattached to the neck of the talus. These patients may lack push-off at the terminal stance of gait.

Some authors recommend Pirogoff or Boyd amputations for children, to preserve length and growth centers. These can also help prevent heel pad migration and improve socket suspension. The Boyd hindfoot amputation consists of a talectomy with a calcaneal-tibial arthrodesis. The Pirogoff amputation is similar to the Boyd; however, the distal end of the calcaneus is excised and is then turned up and fused to the tibia. In children, some studies have demonstrated improved function with these hindfoot amputations versus the Syme's amputation.

An important option for acute and chronic osteomyelitis of the calcaneus in the diabetic patient is partial or total calcanectomy. This can be done through a plantar longitudinal incision, which can also incorporate elliptical resection of the underlying ulcer on the heel. All necrotic and infected tissue must be adequately debrided, and a drain is recommended in all of these amputations. If the infection is localized and the distal Achilles tendon is free of infection, it may be possible to maintain plantarflexion by repairing the tendon to the non-infected plantar fascia. These wounds may require an extended period of time for complete healing, and postoperative care often requires use of total contact casting. Once healed, an ankle/foot orthosis with a Plastazote and foam insert can be used to fill the defect created. One recent study has shown that this procedure creates a cosmetically acceptable deformity with a good functional outcome. Syme's amputation is a disarticulation of the ankle with removal of the talus and calcaneus, while carefully preserving the plantar skin and heel pad to cover the distal tibia. The malleoli should also be removed to help narrow the stump, which helps with pros-

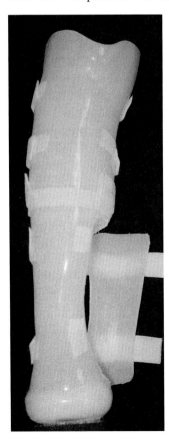

Figure 2

Temporary prosthesis for Syme's amputation. Note distal opening to accommodate bulbous stump.

thetic fitting. In the past, it was recommended that this amputation be done in two stages, delaying the removal of the malleoli by approximately 6 weeks. However, a recent prospective randomized study demonstrated similar wound-healing results in a one-stage versus two-stage procedure in diabetic patients with peripheral vascular disease. The selection criteria for this study included patients who demonstrated no ulcers of the heel pad, no gross pus at the amputation site, no ascending lymphangitis, adequate blood flow, and adequate wound-healing potential. Syme's amputation provides a durable end-stump that allows direct load transfer and provides stable gait pattern, rarely requiring gait training (Fig. 2). One important technical tip is to secure the heel pad to the tibia through drill holes anteriorly or posteriorly. Postoperatively, a cast is recommended once the initial compressive dressing has been removed and the wound has been inspected.

Below-Knee

Amputations performed below the knee are the most common major amputations. A long posteromedial myocutaneous flap is preferable to sagittal flaps (Fig. 3). If possible, this soft-tissue envelope should cover no less than 12 to 15 cm of tibia below the knee joint; however, the residual tibia should be no longer than the junction of the middle and distal thirds. Adhering to the previously mentioned principles of amputation surgery, the distal end of the tibia should be beveled, and myodesis or myoplasty will help secure the soft tissues to prevent shearing of the stump. If there is concern for an insensate stump, in cases such as L4 lumbar myelomeningocele, an option is to implement a long posteromedial myocutaneous flap versus an above-knee amputation. Postoperatively, rigid dressings are often used, and weightbearing can begin within 5 to 21 days of the amputation if the residual limb is capable of transferring the load.

Complications

Pain

Pain following amputation surgery can occur in as many as 85% of patients undergoing these procedures. Most often, this presents as phantom sensation in which the patient can perceive pressure, warmth, cold, wetness, itching, or pain in the portion of the limb that was removed. Studies have reported the incidence of phantom pain to range from 5% to 85%. All of these sensations, including pain, usually resolve over the course of several months to years. Various treatment modalities that have been shown to help in some cases include massage, intermittent compression, increased pros-

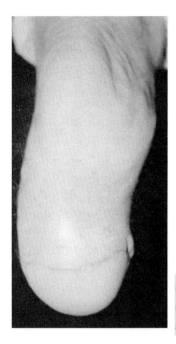

Figure 3

Patient with below-knee amputation using long posterior myocutaneous flap.

thetic use, or transcutaneous electrical stimulation. Some recent studies have demonstrated a diminished rate of postoperative phantom pain with the use of preoperative lumbar epidural blockade, as well as the use of continuous postoperative regional analgesia by nerve sheath block.

Reflex sympathetic dystrophy (RSD) in the residual limb has also been reported following various types of lower extremity amputations. This pain may present as burning, throbbing, tearing, or piercing. Other associated findings in RSD include hyperemia, hyperthermia, edema, and hyperhidrosis. The skin may appear pale or cyanotic and may be mottled and cool. Early diagnosis, with prompt institution of therapy, including desensitization, contrast baths, range of motion, splinting, pneumatic intermittent compression, and transcutaneous nerve stimulation may help reduce the signs and symptoms of this difficult problem.

It is important to rule out other potential causes of pain in the residual limb following amputation. These causes include: a poorly fitting prosthesis, neuromas, exostoses from osteotomy sites, fracture or hematoma following trauma to the stump, and osteomyelitis or abscess formation. These problems may require adaptation of the prosthesis, or may require further surgery to remove the inciting cause. Additional causes of pain may include ischemia, disk herniation, proximal arthritis, or visceral etiologies.

Edema

Postoperative limb edema following lower extremity amputation is a common complication. It may lead to pain, as well as potential wound-healing problems. Early use of a rigid dressing may help reduce this problem, but soft compression dressings may also be used. Care should be taken to avoid a dressing that may be too tight proximally and produce a bulbous stump that is difficult to fit with a prosthesis. If late residual swelling occurs in below-knee amputation, it may lead to a proximal constriction of the socket, causing congestion in the residual limb. This may produce verrucous hyperplasia, a wart-like overgrowth of skin, which can develop fissuring and oozing and lead to secondary infection. The cellulitis may be treated with broad-spectrum antibiotics and avoidance of socket wear. The skin changes may be managed with soaking of the hard keratin layer and using salicylic acid paste. The socket may then be altered to create a total contact fit.

Joint Contractures

Joint contractures generally occur during the time between amputation and prosthetic fitting. If there is evidence of preoperative joint contracture, the condition should be addressed with releases at the time of surgery. The equinus contractures that may occur after Lisfranc and hindfoot amputations may be prevented with adequate soft-tissue balancing at the time of surgery. Those that do occur postoperatively should be treated with early aggressive physical therapy. For below-knee amputations, the use of a long-leg rigid dressing, early postoperative prosthetic fitting, quadriceps strengthening exercises, and hamstring stretching may prevent this complication. Hip flexion contractures can also occur as a result of diminished activity.

Wound Failure

In the diabetic population and in those with ischemic limbs, wound failure as a complication is not uncommon. If the wound is small, it may be managed with local care, including wet-to-dry dressing changes or other similar management. In larger wounds, total contact casting or other rigid dressings may help in management, and may allow continued weightbearing. If the wound is extremely large, or if bone is exposed, the limb can be revised with further bone resection or a more proximal level of amputation.

Dermatologic Problems

Most of the skin problems associated with amputations can be avoided with good hygiene, including maintaining a clean and dry residual limb and prosthesis. The majority of these problems occur with stumps that are weightbearing and result from the shear and pressure stresses on the overlying skin. Epidermoid cysts may occur at the socket brim of below-knee amputations, and may require modification of

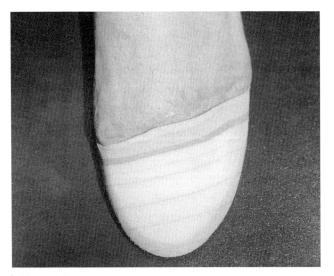

Figure 4

Patient with trans-metatarsophalangeal disarticulations following trauma to the toes. Note shoe insert with toe filler. Carbon fiber base adds rigidity for improved push-off.

the socket to relieve local areas of pressure. Contact dermatitis may be confused with infection and can be caused by acids, bases, and caustic substances that come from detergents and soaps. The stump sock may need to be replaced, and patients should be encouraged to use a mild soap and rinse the sock well. Other causes of dermatitis may be nickel and chrome in the metal, antioxidants in rubber, carbon in neoprene, salts used in leather, and epoxy and polyester resins in sockets. In addition to removing the irritant, treatment can include soaking the limb, application of topical steroid creams, and compression with elastic wraps or shrinkers.

Superficial skin infections may also occur. These include cellulitis and folliculitis, which presents with pustules in hair areas. Antibiotics may be used when appropriate, and the socket may require modification to relieve pressure areas. Candidiasis may lead to scaly, itching skin and can be treated with topical antifungal creams.

Prosthetics

The appropriate use of prosthetics and orthotics for amputations of the foot and lower leg is essential to maintain a functional, long-lasting residual limb. In the foot, many amputations can be managed with custom orthoses that have fillers for the portion of the foot or toe that is missing. (Fig. 4). Once the wound is completely healed, use of the postoperative shoe may be discontinued and a custom orthosis with the appropriate filler may be used for a terminal Syme's, great toe, lesser toe, and ray amputations. For those undergoing trans-

metatarsal or Lisfranc amputations, a stiff-soled shoe may also be necessary, or possibly a lace-up high-top shoe or a polypropylene ankle/foot orthosis to help stabilize the ankle. Chopart amputations are too short to be maintained in a standard shoe and require an ankle/foot orthosis. Syme's amputations require a prosthesis that is large enough to accommodate the bulbous end of the residual limb.

A large variety of prosthetic options are available for the below-knee amputee. Various socket designs may incorporate a liner to improve comfort and accommodate changes in residual limb volume. Patellar tendon bearing sockets that are flexible are most commonly used today, although the majority of weight is borne on the medial tibial flare (Fig. 5). The type of suspension used varies according to patient and prosthetist preference. Different types of suspension include a

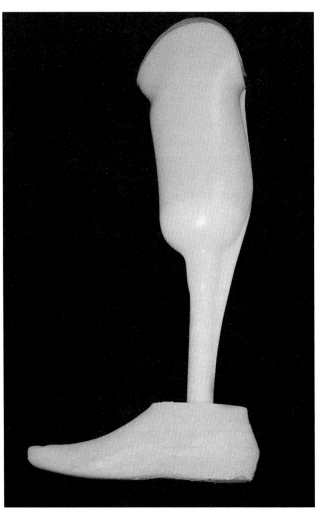

Figure 5

Endoskeleton of below-knee prosthesis.

suprapatellar strap, a waist belt and fork strap for short below-knee amputations, and thigh corsets for those with poor soft tissue or intrinsic knee pain. Suspension sleeves made of latex or neoprene may be combined with a silicon-based liner to create an intimate friction fit. A metal post on the distal end of the liner then locks into the socket to assist the suspension. A variety of prosthetic feet are available, depending on the needs and demands of each individual amputee. Older, sedentary patients may only require a solid-ankle cushion heel (SACH), whereas active patients and competitive athletes may benefit from the newest technology available in energy-storing and elastic-response feet (Fig. 6). These newer feet can be very expensive and require more frequent replacement.

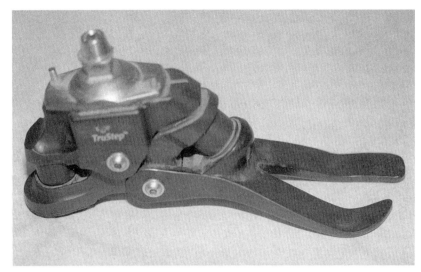

Figure 6

Carbon fiber dynamic response foot which provides inversion and eversion as well as more powerful plantarflexion.

Annotated Bibliography

General Considerations

Brodsky JW: Amputations of the forefoot, in Myerson M (ed): *Current Therapy in Foot and Ankle Surgery.* St. Louis, MO, Mosby-Year Book, 1993, pp 210–216.

The author presents a detailed discussion of amputations of the forefoot. The specific techniques of each procedure are reviewed, as well as the principles of amputation closures and healing, and the problems that can occur with each amputation level.

Choudhury SN, Kitaoka HB: Amputations of the foot and ankle: Review of techniques and results. *Orthopedics* 1997; 20:446–457.

The authors outline the indications and contraindications for various amputations of the foot and ankle. Surgical techniques are also discussed, and an algorithm for decision-making is also provided as a guide. An excellent review of amputation procedures in the congenital, traumatic, and dysvascular patient is discussed.

Myerson M: Amputations of the midfoot and hindfoot, in Myerson M (ed): *Current Therapy in Foot and Ankle Surgery.* St Louis, MO, Mosby-Year Book, 1993, pp 217–224.

This chapter provides a detailed description of techniques for amputations of the midfoot and hindfoot. Emphasis is made on the preoperative evaluation, including evaluation of the vascular and nutritional status of the patient, as well as the management of infection.

Diabetes and Ischemia

Larsson J, Apelqvist J, Agardh CD, Stenstrom A: Decreasing incidence of major amputation in diabetic patients: A consequence of a multidisciplinary foot care team approach? *Diabet Med* 1995;12:770–776.

The authors performed a retrospective review of 294 diabetic patients who underwent 387 amputations of the lower extremity. Following the implementation of a multidisciplinary program for the prevention and treatment of diabetic foot ulcers, the incidence of major amputations decreased 78%, the proportion of amputations below the ankle increased from 28 to 53%, and reamputation decreased from 36 to 22%.

Pinzur MS, Sage R, Stuck R, Osterman H: Amputations in the diabetic foot and ankle. *Clin Orthop* 1993;296:64–67.

This review article provides a less detailed, but overall discussion of the basic concepts of foot and ankle amputation in the diabetic population.

Pinzur MS, Smith D, Osterman H: Syme ankle disarticulation in peripheral vascular disease and diabetic foot infection: The one-stage versus two-stage procedure. *Foot Ankle Int* 1995; 16:124–127.

This study compared a Syme ankle disarticulation using a 1-stage versus 2-stage procedure in a prospective randomized fashion. Randomization was stopped during the study period; however, it was demonstrated that this procedure may be performed safely in a 1-stage procedure in properly selected patients.

Trauma, Pediatrics, Tumors

Chou LB, Malawer MM: Analysis of surgical treatment of 33 foot and ankle tumors. *Foot Ankle Int* 1994;15:175–181.

The authors performed a retrospective review of 33 patients who were treated for benign and malignant tumors of the foot and ankle using limb-sparing techniques. At an average follow-up of 7.2 years, there were no recurrences, and 82% had good or excellent functional results.

Georgiadis GM, Behrens FF, Joyce MJ, Earle AS, Simmons AL: Open tibial fractures with severe soft-tissue loss. *J Bone Joint Surg* 1993;75A:1431–1441.

The authors reviewed the long-term outcomes and quality of life in patients with type IIIB and IIIC open tibia fractures treated with limb salvage versus early below-knee amputation. Those undergoing limb salvage had more complications, more surgical procedures, longer hospital stays, required more time to become fully weightbearing, were less willing or able to work, had higher hospital charges, more frequently considered themselves disabled, and had more problems with occupational and recreational activities than those undergoing early amputation.

Greene WB, Cary JM: Partial foot amputations in children: A comparison of the several types with the Syme amputation. *J Bone Joint Surg* 1982;64A:438–443.

A retrospective comparison was made between several types of partial foot amputations with the Syme amputation in 14 children. Patients with a ray or transmetatarsal amputation were reported to have better function and range of motion than those with a Syme amputation. Patients with a Lisfranc, midtarsal, or Chopart amputation had better overall function, but required more adjustments for gait than those with Syme amputation. Syme amputations did have better results than those patients with Chopart amputation who had an equinus contracture and inadequate forefoot length.

Johansen K, Daines M, Howey T, Helfet D, Hansen ST Jr: Objective criteria accurately predict amputation following lower extremity trauma. *J Trauma* 1990;30:568–572.

In both a retrospective and prospective review, the authors found that a Mangled Extremity Severity Score (MESS) value ≥ 7 predicted amputation with 100% accuracy. This score is based on skeletal/soft-tissue damage, limb ischemia, shock, and age.

Complications

Larsson J, Apelqvist J, Castenfors J, Agardh CD, Stenstrom A: Distal blood pressure as a predictor for the level of amputation in diabetic patients with foot ulcer. *Foot Ankle* 1993; 14:247–253.

The authors prospectively evaluated 161 consecutive diabetic patients with foot ulcers. An ankle pressure below 50 mm Hg was found to never be sufficient for wound healing. A toe pressure below 15 mm Hg was found to seldom be sufficient for wound healing, and these indices gave no further information.

Lind J, Kramhoft M, Bodtker S: The Influence of smoking on complications after primary amputations of the lower extremity. *Clin Orthop* 1991;267:211–217.

A retrospective review of 302 patients who underwent above- or below-knee amputations was performed. In cigarette smokers, the risk of infection and reamputation was 2.5 times greater than in the nonsmoking or cheroot smoking group.

Melzack R: Phantom limbs. *Sci Am* 1992;266:120–126.

This author presents an excellent discussion on the subject of phantom pain and phantom sensation. He discusses the historic and new theories of these phenomena, and the current treatment approaches.

Wyss CR, Harrington RM, Burgess EM, Matsen FA III: Transcutaneous oxygen tension as a predictor of success after an amputation. *J Bone Joint Surg* 1988;70A:203–207.

The authors measured transcutaneous oxygen tension at the foot and proximal and distal to the knee in 162 patients who underwent 206 amputations. They concluded that preoperative values were a more consistent predictor of success or failure of healing a foot or below-knee amputation than were measurements of systolic blood pressure at the ankle.

Classic Bibliography

Brodsky JW, Chambers RB: Effect of tourniquet use on amputation healing in diabetic and dysvascular patients. *Perspec Orthop Surg* 1991;2:71–76.

Larsson U, Andersson GB: Partial amputation of the foot for diabetic or arteriosclerotic gangrene: Results and factors of prognostic value. *J Bone Joint Surg* 1978;60B:126–130.

Smith DG, Stuck RM, Ketner L, Sage RM, Pinzur MS: Partial calcanectomy for the treatment of large ulcerations of the heel and calcaneal osteomyelitis: An amputation of the back of the foot. *J Bone Joint Surg* 1992;74A:571–576.

Wagner FW Jr: The Dysvascular foot: A system for diagnosis and treatment. *Foot Ankle* 1981;2:64–122.

Chapter 24
Current Trends in
Foot and Ankle Imaging

As modern technologies have advanced, so has the ability to image and diagnose diseases of the foot and ankle that previously were diagnosed or suspected purely on clinical grounds. A clinical diagnosis cannot only be confirmed but occult pathologies can also be discovered. However, in order to use these technologies, their potential and limitations must be made known. This chapter will review some of the recent advances in imaging of the foot and ankle and how they may help physicians in their daily clinical practice.

Radiography

Routine radiographs are the first imaging modality of choice because they are a cost-effective way to evaluate many problems of the ankle and foot. The main limitation of radiographs is their insensitivity to soft-tissue abnormalities. Evaluation of osseous structures can also be limited by the complex osseous anatomy of the ankle and foot. For example, the subtalar joint is difficult to visualize even with adequately positioned radiographs. In the trauma patient, adequate radiographs may be difficult to obtain. Certain osseous pathologies, such as stress fractures, can also be occult on radiographs. Despite their limitations, radiographs often can establish a diagnosis or actually help in the interpretation of more advanced imaging studies.

Various stress techniques have been used with radiographs to help indirectly evaluate the soft tissues. In particular, stress radiography has been used to evaluate the ligamentous integrity of the ankle. There is still controversy about the effectiveness of this technique in assessing the lateral collateral ligaments (LCLs) of the ankle. Various apparatuses have been devised in order to make the measurements more consistent, but a large normal range remains. A diagnosis of instability is often made based on comparison with the contralateral ankle, if normal.

Nuclear Medicine

There are 2 nuclear medicine studies important to the ankle and foot: the bone scan and the labeled white cell scan. The bone scan takes advantage of the ability of the radiolabeled substrate methylene diphosphate (MDP) to be incorporated into bone. The isotope used is technetium 99m. The primary determinants of whether the bone will be labeled are blood flow to the area and activity of the osteoblasts. Low blood flow states can lead to diminished labeling; conversely, high blood flow states can lead to increased labeling. Thus, hyperemia (such as that caused by a cellulitis) can cause an apparent increase in uptake in the osseous structures. The 3-phase technique exploits this increased uptake. In this technique, the first set of images are obtained immediately following the intravenous administration of the radioisotope, allowing assessment of the blood flow to the area. The second set of images is obtained shortly after the first set (usually within minutes) and is used to assess soft-tissue activity, which gives a measurement of the degree of hyperemia. Thus, synovitis, cellulitis, and other soft-tissue inflammation will show increased activity on the second phase. The third set of images is obtained several hours after the injection in order to allow for clearance of excess isotope from the soft tissues and lessen background noise. The distribution of activity within the bones is studied during this third phase. In the ideal case, the 3 phases allow distinction of inflammatory responses that primarily involve soft tissue versus those that involve the underlying bone.

Any state in which the osteoblasts are active will cause increased labeling of the bone as well. Therefore, tumors, trauma, and infection can all lead to increased activity in the bone, which becomes a problem particularly when evaluating the diabetic foot for osteomyelitis. Underlying neuropathic changes can lead to increases in both osseous activity and soft-tissue activity. A superimposed cellulitis can also confound the soft-tissue findings as well as lead to even more hyperemia and hence increased labeling of the osseous structures. Thus, 3-phase bone scanning, especially in the diabetic foot, can have a low specificity.

A labeled white cell scan can improve the specificity of bone scanning for infection. This involves withdrawing some of the patient's blood, separating the white cells and labeling them with an isotope (usually indium-111), and reinjecting them into the patient. Subsequent imaging ascertains if the labeled white cells aggregate at the suspected site of infection. The indium-111 white cell scan suffers from the following limitations: poor spatial resolution, often making it difficult to determine exactly where the white cells are localizing, and it may be falsely negative in partially treated infections, chronic osteomyelitis, and in some types of abscesses.

Other uses of bone scanning include: excluding stress fractures, evaluation of tumors (especially metastases), and evaluating reflex sympathetic dystrophy (RSD). The specifics of each of these will be discussed later.

Computed Tomography

Computed tomography (CT) has proved to be an especially useful tool in the evaluation of trauma. Scanning can be performed in either of 2 planes: coronal or axial. Most machines now allow 2-dimensional and 3-dimensional reconstruction. Reconstruction allows assessment of various articulations that may not have been optimally positioned because of various constraints. For example, a casted foot is difficult to position for coronal sections, but with reconstruction, sagittal and coronal images can be obtained to assess the subtalar joint. With the advent of spiral scanning, thin sections can be obtained fairly rapidly and can be readily reconstructed. When spiral scanning is used, I obtain 2- to 3-mm sections at a minimum. The 2-mm sections are particularly useful for reconstruction because they allow 1-mm resolution on reconstruction. In general, the coronal plane is preferred for evaluation of the subtalar joint and the axial plane for evaluation of the midfoot.

Other indications for CT include: calcaneus fracture evaluation; evaluation of fracture healing; determining the presence of stress fractures, especially in the navicular; talus fractures, especially of the lateral process; evaluation of osteochondral defects of the talar dome; and assessment of coalitions. The examination yields the most useful information when it is tailored to the particular problem.

Ultrasound

Ultrasound has been used primarily to assess tendon integrity. It has found its greatest use in evaluation of the Achilles tendon. Evaluation of other tendons is limited because many of them pass through fibro-osseous tunnels, which makes ultrasound difficult. Ultrasound is technically demanding because the examiner must minimize artifacts that can mimic pathology. The examination requires a high-frequency transducer, in the range of 7.5 to 10 MHz. One of its main advantages is its relatively low cost (compared with magnetic resonance imaging [MRI] or CT). Ultrasound is probably most useful in assessing Achilles tendon tears and determining the presence of xanthomas in the Achilles tendon in familial hypercholesterolemia. One disadvantage of ultrasound is that it is difficult to include landmarks on the images that may later be useful to the surgeon.

Magnetic Resonance Imaging

MRI offers the best delineation of the soft tissues of any imaging method. It is also excellent for evaluating pathologic processes involving the marrow. In addition, MRI is a multiplanar technique, allowing imaging of structures lying in various oblique planes. However, it is limited in its ability to image cortical bone. Recent advances in hardware and software technology have increased both the spatial resolution and the speed of MRI. These advances allow better visualization of the small soft-tissue and ligamentous structures of the ankle and foot. Dedicated coils are required for high resolution.

One of the newer techniques is fast spin-echo (FSE) imaging, which allows rapid acquisition of data and hence reduces imaging time. This is particularly advantageous in lengthy sequences such as T2 and inversion-recovery (IR) sequences. One disadvantage of FSE imaging is that the marrow fat continues to have relatively high signal ("bright"), which can obscure marrow pathology.

Several pulse sequences have been developed recently for the evaluation of cartilage. The 2 primary pulse sequences are spoiled gradient echo (SPGR) and FSE proton density, both with fat saturation. The primary advantage of the former is that data can be acquired as a volume; hence, both thin sections and reconstruction in any plane can be obtained. Additionally, the SPGR data can be reconstructed to give "maps" of the cartilage. These sequences are valuable in the ankle for the evaluation of bone bars in the physis of children.

MRI can be used to assess the integrity of ligamentous structures and tendons, tumors, various inflammatory conditions, osteochondral defects, stress fractures, and a host of other pathologies. Because of the complex anatomy of the ankle and foot, the highest diagnostic yield is obtained when MRI is used to address a specific clinical question, such as, is there a tear of the posterior tibial tendon? Although it may often reveal other unsuspected pathology, MRI is probably not best used as a screening tool. Thus, a good clinical history is an essential prerequisite to an MRI examination.

A new technique that has been recently used is magnetic resonance arthrography, which involves the injection of either saline or saline with gadolinium into the tibial-talar joint. This technique is used primarily to evaluate the LCLs and for assessing the stability of osteochondral fragments. Although the technique appears to be more sensitive in determining the integrity of the lateral ligaments, its main disadvantage is that its use turns a noninvasive procedure into an invasive one. It has yet to be determined if this procedure will become cost effective.

Posterior Ankle Pain

Achilles Tendon

One of the more common causes of posterior ankle pain is injury of the Achilles tendon. The spectrum of injury can range from chronic mucinous degeneration of the tendon to acute tearing. Although the Achilles tendon can be visualized on radiographs, this imaging modality is relatively insensitive. The 2 best imaging modalities are MRI and ultrasound. A frank tear can often be adequately assessed on clinical grounds, but if it is clinically difficult to palpate the ends of the tendon, then either MRI or ultrasound can be used to locate the ends of the tendon and to ascertain if the tear is complete. Imaging can be performed with the foot in plantarflexion to determine if the ends of the tendon can be opposed.

With MRI, the best planes for visualizing the tendon are axial and sagittal. The Achilles tendon is normally of low signal on all pulse sequences, has an anterior concavity, and measures no more than 7 mm at a level 2 cm above the bursal projection of the calcaneus. With a complete tear there is total loss of the low signal of the tendon and instead there is usually an amorphous region containing areas of high and intermediate signal on the T2-weighted sequences (Fig. 1). With degeneration of the tendon, there is loss of the normal anterior concavity, thickening of the tendon, and signal within the tendon that is often best appreciated on T1 or proton density-weighted sequences and on IR sequences. The degenerative signal may not be that apparent on T2-weighted signal. These changes are usually seen approximately 2 to 6 cm proximal to the calcaneus.

Os Trigonum Syndrome

A large os trigonum can also be associated with posterior ankle pain. Multiple etiologies are responsible for this syndrome. The os trigonum is a relatively common ossicle occurring adjacent to the trigonal process of the talus. Because this ossicle is so common, it is easy to mistake a trigonal process fracture, either acute or secondary to chronic stress, for os trigonum syndrome. A large os trigonum can cause impingement against the talar plafond in extremes of

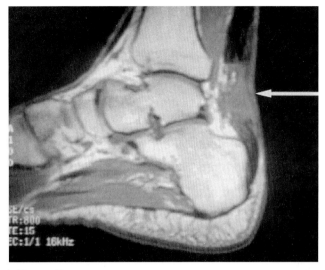

Figure 1

Complete tear of the Achilles tendon. Sagittal T1-weighted magnetic resonance image. The normal tendon should be dark. The arrow points to the area of intermediate signal representing the tear. Also note the thickening of the tendon superior to the tear.

plantarflexion, or it can cause direct mechanical irritation of the nearby flexor hallucis longus (FHL) tendon. Additionally, the synchondrosis between os trigonum and the lateral talar tubercle can become inflamed because of repetitive microtrauma.

Radiographically, the os trigonum is a well-corticated ossicle that projects posterior to the talus. On axial CT or MRI views the ossicle is identified posterior to the lateral tubercle on the posterior aspect of the talus. A prominent lateral process, without the ossicle, is known as the trigonal or Stieda's process. Immediately lateral to the lateral process is the tendon of the FHL. The inferior surface can articulate with the calcaneus and the posterior aspect can serve as an attachment site for the posterior talofibular and posterior talocalcaneal ligaments. A cartilaginous synchondrosis attaches the os trigonum to the talus.

CT can be useful to determine if in fact the "ossicle" seen on a radiograph is a true os trigonum or a fracture of the trigonal process. The ossicle would be expected to have well-corticated margins whereas the fracture should have poorly defined adjacent margins. Difficulty arises in distinguishing an os trigonum from an old/subacute fracture or repetitive trauma. Chronic disruption of the synchondrosis can demonstrate sclerotic and cystic changes on both sides of the synchondrosis. Radionuclide imaging or MRI may be of benefit in the latter case. On the bone scan, increased activity over the ossicle would imply that it is actually a fracture or that the cartilaginous attachment of the os trigonum has been disrupted. MRI could show low signal (dark) in the marrow of the ossicle and the adjacent talus with corresponding high signal (bright) on the T2 or inversion recovery. Increased signal on T2-weighted sequences between the ossicle and the talus implies disruption of the synchondrosis. The additional advantage of MRI is that it allows assessment of the adjacent soft tissues, particularly the FHL. Furthermore, sagittal images performed with the foot in plantarflexion can determine if the os trigonum impinges on the posterior aspect of the plafond.

If a selective injection of the synchondrosis with 1 ml of either lidocaine or a mixture of corticosteroids and local anesthetic relieves the patient's symptoms, then the os trigonum is likely the etiology of the patient's symptoms.

Accessory Soleus

The accessory soleus is an anomalous muscle that has a variable origin and insertion. The muscle can arise from the fibula, the tibia, the flexor digitorum longus, or the normal soleus. The tendon can insert on the Achilles tendon or on the superior or medial surfaces of the calcaneus. The muscle can present as an apparent soft-tissue mass or there may be pain after exercise, possibly because of ischemia within the muscle or a compartment-like syndrome. The diagnosis can be made with radiographs (Fig. 2), CT, or MRI. With MRI,

the "mass" has signal characteristics of muscle (Fig. 3) and its origin and insertion sites can be identified.

Medial Ankle Pain

General Considerations

A 3-part MRI grading scheme is used in the assessment of tendon pathology. Grade 1 tendon injuries are characterized by a thickened tendon with splitting of the fibers; grade 2 injuries demonstrate focal thinning; and grade 3 injuries show complete disruption. Tendinosis is a loss of normal striation and discoloration as seen at surgery. MRI findings include thickening of the tendon with or without internal signal and high T2 signal surrounding the tendon. A grade 1 tear usually demonstrates linear signal as opposed to the more heterogeneous signal seen in tendinosis. There is, obviously, a spectrum of findings because a tendinosis may predispose to a tear. A paratenonitis on MRI scan is characterized by increased signal on T2-weighted sequences surrounding the tendon, which is otherwise of normal thickness and signal intensity.

Posterior Tibial Tendon

The most commonly injured flexor tendon is the posterior

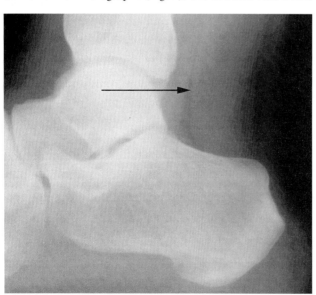

Figure 2

Lateral radiograph of the ankle. The normal pre-Achilles fat (Kager's triangle) is obliterated by a soft-tissue mass (arrow) representing an accessory soleus.

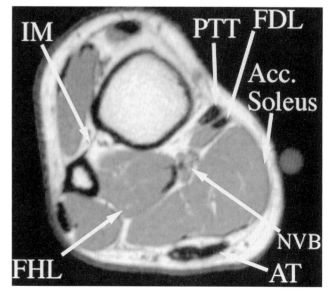

Figure 3

Axial T1-weighted magnetic resonance image demonstrating an accessory soleus. The round area of intermediate signal on the skin adjacent to the accessory soleus is a vitamin E capsule placed where the patient felt a "lump" after exercising. (PTT = posterior tibial tendon, FDL = flexor digitorum longus, NVB = neurovascular bundle, AT = Achilles tendon, FHL = flexor hallucis longus, IM = interosseous membrane.)

tibial tendon (PTT). The PTT helps maintain the arch of the foot. Its primary insertion site is on the medial aspect of the navicular, although it also sends additional tendon slips to the cuneiforms. The normal tendon on MRI passes under the medial malleolus. The tendon is usually of uniform low signal on all pulse sequences and is the largest of the flexor tendons, being roughly 1.5 to 2 times the diameter of the other flexors. PTT tears commonly occur behind the medial malleolus, at the navicular, or 2 to 3 cm proximal to the navicular (Fig. 4).

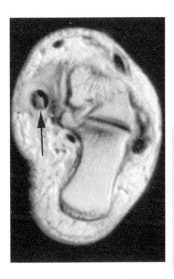

Figure 4

Type 2 tear of the posterior tibial tendon (PTT). Oblique coronal fast spin-echo proton density-weighted image. The arrow points to a markedly thickened PTT with abnormal linear signal extending through the tendon. The intermediate signal surrounding the tendon indicates an associated tenosynovitis.

The 2 main modalities for imaging the PTT are CT and MRI. Although CT can demonstrate changes in the size of the tendon as well as show fluid in the tendon sheath, it does not demonstrate the internal structural changes of a degenerating tendon as well as MRI can. Although MRI has been shown to have a relatively weak correlation with surgical findings, it has been shown to have a better correlation with patient outcome than surgical findings. This may be because of the ability of MRI to demonstrate internal structural changes within the tendon that cannot be visualized by external inspection. In addition, several studies have demonstrated MRI to be highly specific and sensitive. For this reason, I prefer MRI for evaluation of the PTT and for the other ankle tendons as well.

Because of the complex course of the PTT (as well as the other tendons of the ankle), MRI is best performed in several oblique planes. The preferred imaging planes include sagittal, oblique coronal, and oblique axial planes. A potential source of error occurs as the tendon passes at 55° to the main magnetic field. At this point there may be increased signal within the tendon on T1- and proton density-weighted images, which is an artifact termed the "magic angle" effect. The "magic-angle" effect is a physical phenomenon that pro-

duces increased signal in structures with normally low signal with highly ordered collagen fibrils, for example, tendons. This signal becomes less intense on T2-weighted sequences. A technique that can be used to reduce "magic angle" effects is to image the foot in varying degrees of flexion and thus change the area in which the effects occur.

Several findings seen on imaging have been associated with PTT tears and degeneration of the tendon. One of these is the presence of osteophytes along the posteromedial aspect of the medial malleolus. These can be identified with radiography, CT, or MRI. These osteophytes are thought to arise from a reactive periostitis secondary to PTT pathology. However, large osteophytes probably contribute to further attrition within the PTT. Thickening of the flexor retinaculum as well as degeneration or loss of the spring ligament can also be seen with PTT pathology. One relatively common finding with PTT pathology is the presence of an accessory navicular. The type 2 and type 3 accessory naviculars are most commonly associated with tears of the PTT, and will be discussed later in the chapter. An abnormal articulation between the talus and navicular can also be seen.

Flexor Hallicus Longus

Although not as common, changes similar to those seen in the PTT can be seen in the FHL (Fig. 5). The FHL passes through the tarsal tunnel beneath the sustentaculum tali. Tendon tears are noted in ballerinas and in other sports involving toeing off from the great toe. As noted previously, a large os trigonum can impinge on the FHL, contributing to attrition. A similar grading scheme as used for PTT tendon tears can be applied to the FHL. One caveat is that relatively large amounts of fluid (as manifested by high signal on T2-weighted MRI scans) in the FHL tendon sheath can

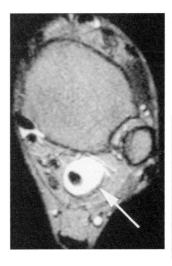

Figure 5

Tenosynovitis of the flexor hallucis longus (FHL). Axial fast spin-echo T2-weighted magnetic resonance image. The arrow points to a marked amount of high signal surrounding a thickened FHL tendon, indicating fluid in the tendon sheath. No abnormal signal is seen within the FHL tendon.

be a normal finding. Therefore, diagnosis of a paratenonitis is somewhat more difficult in the FHL. One important consequence, however, of large amounts of fluid in the FHL is that it may cause a tarsal tunnel syndrome.

Tarsal Tunnel Syndrome

On the medial aspect of the ankle the posterior tibial nerve passes through a confined fibro-osseous space known as the tarsal tunnel; the nerve and its branches are subject to compression by space-occupying lesions. The posterior tibial nerve gives rise to medial calcaneal sensory branches and the medial and lateral plantar branches. Hence, depending on the level of compression, burning pain and paresthesias can be felt in the toes, sole of the foot, or the medial heel. Approximately 50% of the cases of tarsal tunnel are idiopathic, with an identifiable mechanical cause in the other 50%. Mechanical causes include ganglion cysts, nerve sheath tumors, varicosities, tenosynovitis, abductor hallucis hypertrophy, hindfoot valgus, and posttraumatic fibrosis. Surgical decompression is often performed, but can have variable results depending on the series. Identifying a mechanical cause of compression preoperatively can obviously aid in planning surgery. MRI is the best technique for evaluating and identifying the structures of the tarsal tunnel.

A tenosynovitis of the flexor tendons appears as high signal surrounding the tendons on T2-weighted sequences. A ganglion cyst typically is a lobulated discrete structure that is of uniformly high signal on T2-weighted sequences. Neural tumors can have variable signal characteristics, but are usually recognized by their anatomic distribution along the course of the nerve. They can appear elliptical with tapered ends. Venous varicosities are usually of high signal on T2 and IR sequences. Morphologically they are tubular and serpiginous. Scar tissue in the tarsal tunnel (Fig. 6) is of low to intermediate signal on both T1- and T2-weighted sequences. The presence of scar tissue can make it difficult to distinguish the individual structures within the tarsal tunnel because of the loss of fat and the architectural distortion. The flexor retinaculum can also appear thickened.

Medial Collateral Ligament

Diagnosis of a medial collateral (deltoid) ligament tear is usually made on the basis of physical findings and radiographs. However, the structures of the deltoid ligament can be readily visualized on MRI scan and often with CT. There are several components of the deltoid ligament, and the full description of these structures is beyond the scope of this chapter. The posterior tibiotalar and the tibiocalcaneal ligaments are the most readily visualized. The posterior tibiotalar ligament is uniformly thick and often has heterogeneous signal on MRI scan. The tibiocalcaneal ligament is of variable thickness and is usually of low signal intensity. Injuries of these ligaments appear as absence of the structure or discontinuity. With MRI scan, high T2 signal can be seen around the expected location of the ligaments. Because 60% to 67% of posterior tibiotalar ligament injuries are by avulsion, and because this is one of the more commonly injured components of the deltoid, it is not unusual to see an osseous fragment with an otherwise intact ligament.

Accessory Navicular

The accessory navicular bone has been associated with medial foot/ankle pain. It is present in 4% to 21% of the population and is more common in females. Certain types of accessory navicular have also been associated with PTT injuries. The accessory navicular has been classified into 3 types. Type 1 represents a true sesamoid bone within the posterior tibial tendon and has also been termed the os tibiale externum. It is typically asymptomatic. Type 2 is the most common accessory navicular and is an ossification along the medial aspect of the navicular that is attached to the navicular by a cartilaginous synchondrosis. Type 3 can be thought of as a fusion of a type II accessory navicular to the navicular leading to a prominent medial process of the navicular. This type of navicular has also been termed the cornuate navicular.

The type 2 accessory navicular can be symptomatic in 1 of 2 ways. As noted above, it may be indirectly symptomatic because of its association with PTT tears. However, repetitive trauma can lead to inflammation in the synchondrosis, making the type 2 accessory navicular the source of direct pain. There are 2 imaging methods that can be used to confirm the diagnosis of a symptomatic type 2 accessory navicular: MRI and radionuclide bone scan. The latter technique will demonstrate increased activity over the region of the medial navicular. With MRI, edema in the adjacent bone as well as in

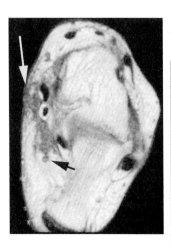

Figure 6

Tarsal tunnel syndrome. Oblique coronal proton density-weighted magnetic resonance image. Diffuse low signal (white arrow) is seen in place of the normal flexor retinaculum. Low signal was also seen on the T2-weighted images consistent with scar tissue. The anterior neurovascular structures (medial plantar nerve, black arrow) are effaced by the scar. Patient had had a prior retinacular release with recurrent symptoms.

suppressed

the synchondrosis can be seen. One advantage of MRI is that it allows assessment of the PTT.

Lateral Pain

Lateral Collateral Ligament

Ankle sprains are a very common injury and inversion is the most common mechanism, representing roughly 90% of all ankle sprains. It is therefore not surprising that injuries to the LCL complex are quite common. Poor initial healing or repetitive injuries can lead to chronic injury to the LCL and ankle instability. The LCL is composed of three ligaments: the anterior talofibular (ATF), calcaneofibular (CF), and the posterior talofibular (PTF). Assessment of the integrity of these structures has relied on physical examination, plain radiography, stress radiography, arthrograms, and surgical exploration. Currently the application of MRI both with and without intra-articular contrast has shown great promise in the assessment of the LCL.

Radiographs are often unremarkable with ankle sprains. Occasionally small ossific avulsion fragments can be identified. Soft-tissue swelling may be evident in the acute phase. Stress radiographs have been used as a more dynamic evaluation of the LCL. One of the great difficulties in performing stress radiographs is applying consistent pressure in the appropriate planes on the ankle. Various mechanical devices have been used to mitigate this problem. Two parameters are measured on stress radiographs: the talar tilt and the anterior draw (anterior displacement of the talus relative to the tibia). To assess talar tilt, the ankle is placed into medial deviation and the angle formed between lines drawn parallel to the talar dome and tibial plafond is measured. The normal range is 0 to 13°. Often the contralateral "normal" ankle is obtained for comparison. A tilt of > 10° probably indicates instability and a difference of > 5° between sides is considered indicative of instability. An anterior translation of the talus of > 6 mm or a difference of > 3 mm between sides is also considered to indicate instability.

Two major problems with stress radiography are that (1) there is a wide "normal" range, and (2) it is assumed that the contralateral ankle is normal. It may well be that there are individuals who are predisposed to ankle injuries and instability because of inherently lax ligaments. With these individuals a wide range of "normal" would be expected and side-to-side comparison would have less meaning. The usefulness of stress radiography, especially in the acute setting, is also questionable in light of findings that suggest that there is a nearly equal distribution of functional instability in patients with mechanical stability (as assessed by stress radiographs) as with those having mechanical instability.

In the acute setting, the integrity of the CF ligament can be evaluated with ankle arthrography. The CF ligament is extrinsic to the capsule and attached to the peroneal tendon sheath. Thus, extravasation of contrast into the peroneal tendon sheath during ankle arthrography indicates a torn CF ligament. This technique becomes less useful in the subacute setting because subsequent scar formation can prevent contrast leakage.

MRI has shown promise in the evaluation of the LCL. Some distinct advantages of MRI are that through the use of oblique imaging planes, it allows direct visualization of the component ligaments, and it allows simultaneous evaluation of the peroneal tendons. Attrition in the peroneus brevis tendon is not uncommon with chronic ankle instabilities, and knowledge of this may aid in surgical planning. Some disadvantages of MRI are that it is not a dynamic study and, like arthrography, scar formation can obscure injury.

When evaluating the ligaments with MRI, 3 questions can be asked: (1) Is the ligament visible and if so is it contiguous? (2) Is there high signal on T2-weighted images extending through the ligament (a variation on the first question) or surrounding the ligament? (3) Is there redundancy or buckling of the ligament? The ATF and CF ligaments are typically of low signal and the PTF has intermediate signal. The ATF ligament is usually best identified on oblique axial images at the level of the malleolar fossa (Fig. 7). The CF ligament is found deep to the peroneal tendons and follows an oblique course from the fibula to the lateral aspect of the calcaneus. It is best identified on oblique coronal images. The PTF ligament can be identified on axial and coronal images as a thick band extending from the posterior fibula to the posterior talus (Fig. 8).

The ATF ligament is the most commonly injured component of the LCL and the CF ligament is the second. The PTF

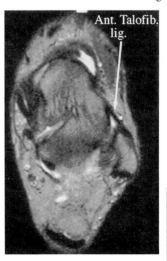

Figure 7

Normal anterior talofibular ligament. Oblique coronal fast spin-echo T2-weighted magnetic resonance image.

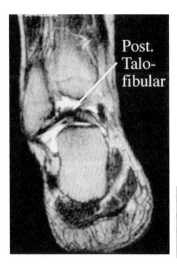

Figure 8

Normal posterior talofibular ligament. Coronal fast spin-echo T2-weighted magnetic resonance image.

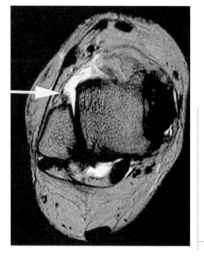

Figure 9

Acute tear of the anterior talofibular ligament (ATF). Oblique axial fast spin-echo T2-weighted magnetic resonance image. High signal is seen extending through the expected location of the ATF ligament. A small stump (arrow) of the ATF ligament is seen attached to the fibula.

is injured only rarely. On oblique axial images, a torn ATF often demonstrates high T2 signal extending through the ligament (Fig. 9). A small remnant of the ligament can sometimes be identified on the fibula. In the chronic setting, ATF tears may be masked by the formation of scar tissue and secondary signs of injury, such as redundancy and buckling of the ligament, may be the only indication of ATF injury. The CF ligament is not as reliably identified as the ATF ligament, perhaps owing to the oblique course of the ligament. However, because the CF ligament is very rarely injured with an intact ATF ligament, an intact ATF ligament is a good indicator of an intact CF ligament.

Recent use of magnetic resonance arthrography has shown it to be more sensitive and specific for LCL tears. For ATF ligament tears the sensitivity and specificity have been reported to be as high as 100%. For the CF ligament, the technique is less sensitive (90%) and specific (83%), but still better than routine MRI. However, it is likely that the pretest probability was high, helping to account for the high specificity. In a routine clinical practice, there might normally be a high pretest probability because presumably only those patients with a high clinical suspicion for ligamentous injury would be selected to undergo magnetic resonance arthrography. There is still debate about whether the added diagnostic information warrants the invasive procedure.

Peroneal Tendon Injuries

Although tendon ruptures and tenosynovitis are not as common in the peroneal tendons as in the other tendons of the ankle, they are associated with chronic LCL tears and can mimic them. In addition to ruptures and tenosynovitis, other disorders that can affect the peroneal tendons include splitting of the tendons, stenosing tenosynovitis, and acute and chronic subluxation. Each of the imaging characteristics of these

disorders will be considered in turn. As with the other ankle tendons, MRI is the best imaging modality for evaluating the tendons and associated structures. Isolated tenography for the actual evaluation of the tendon is only rarely performed today; the procedure is usually performed for the injection of anesthetic (bupivacaine) into the tendon sheath. Relief of symptoms confirms the tendon as the source of pain. A small amount of contrast is often injected first, not only to confirm the location of the needle prior to injection, but also to ensure that there will be no leakage of anesthetic into the ankle or subtalar joint. The contrast also confirms that the whole tendon sheath is filled, which might not happen in a stenosing tenosynovitis. Leakage of anesthetic or incomplete filling of the tendon sheath could produce misleading results.

Several anatomic factors are important in the development of peroneal tendon pathology. The major stabilizer of the peroneal tendons is the superior peroneal retinaculum. The origin of this retinaculum is from the lateral aspect of the fibula, it passes superficial to the tendons and then inserts on the lateral aspect of the calcaneus and Achilles tendon. At the origin of the retinaculum on the fibula a small triangular piece of meniscal-like tissue can occur. The fibula normally has a shallow concave groove at its tip through which the peroneal tendons run. Distally, the tendons pass around the peroneal tubercle of the calcaneus with the peroneus longus tendon passing inferiorly and the peroneus brevis passing superiorly to the tubercle. A normal variant that is frequently encountered is the peroneus quartus muscle. The tendon of this muscle passes medial to the peroneus brevis tendon and should not be mistaken for a tear of the peroneus brevis. Key to identifying a peroneus quartus tendon is the identification of a separate muscle belly.

Fortunately, rupture of the peroneal tendons is rare. The peroneus longus tendon is most commonly injured and an acute tear usually occurs during physical activity. The acute tear typically occurs at the level of the calcaneocuboid joint just distal to the os peroneum. Radiographs may demonstrate proximal retraction of the os peroneum or even fracturing of the os peroneum. MRI will demonstrate the discontinuity of the tendon and, in the acute setting, edema in the surrounding soft tissues. The end of the tendon can also be identified and the amount of proximal retraction assessed. Acute injuries of the peroneus brevis almost always involve an osseous avulsion from the base of the fifth metatarsal. Plain radiographs suffice in this instance.

Chronic tears of the peroneal tendons are manifested as longitudinal splits within the substance of the tendons. Splitting of the peroneus longus tendon occurs distal to the lateral malleolus. Splitting of the peroneus brevis tendon occurs at the level of the lateral malleolus and can propagate distally and proximally. There are several predisposing factors and associated findings with peroneus tendon splitting, including: tears of the LCL and superior retinaculum, osseous spurs on the fibula, "abnormal" muscles such as the peroneus quartus and a low-lying muscle belly of the peroneus brevis, a flat or convex tip of the lateral malleolus, subluxation of the peroneal tendons, and a hypertrophied peroneal tubercle. Most of these other findings probably contribute to peroneal splitting because of increased mechanical stress placed on the peroneus tendons. This is particularly true for the peroneus brevis tendon, which is sandwiched between the peroneus longus tendon and the fibula.

MRI findings with peroneus tendon splits show some overlap with chronic tears of other tendons, but also some unique features. The tendon can appear thickened or attenuated with areas of abnormal signal extending through its substance (Fig. 10). Splitting of the peroneus brevis tendon can alter the morphology of the tendon, often giving it a C-shape that can partly cover the peroneus longus tendon. There may be no signal changes within the tendon but only an irregular contour with clefts. Increased T2 signal, presumably representing fluid, is commonly found in the tendon sheath and in the surrounding soft tissues. Sometimes areas of low signal on all pulse sequences are seen in the surrounding soft tissues and these presumably represent scar tissue. It is important during MRI examination for peroneus tendon tears to look for the associated findings mentioned previously because these abnormalities may need to be addressed during surgery in order for repair to be successful.

As mentioned previously, subluxation of the peroneal tendons can predispose to tendon tears. Subluxation or dislocation of the tendon can be symptomatic as an isolated finding. Associated findings include tears or redundancy of the superior peroneal retinaculum and flattening of the retromalleo-

lar groove, which are similar to tendon tears. With acute dislocations of the peroneal tendons, a small avulsion fragment from the posterolateral lateral malleolus (representing avulsion of the superior peroneal retinaculum) can sometimes be seen on radiographs, MRI, and CT. Because acute peroneal dislocations are often misdiagnosed as lateral ankle sprains (which may also be present) the recognition of the fragment is an important finding in leading to the correct diagnosis. With cross sectional imaging techniques, the actual subluxation of the tendons may not be apparent because the tendons are often displaced only in certain foot positions.

Anterolateral Impingement Syndrome

This syndrome is produced by the entrapment of abnormal soft tissue in the anterolateral gutter of the ankle. The origin of this tissue in most cases is probably posttraumatic, with previous hemorrhage leading to the formation of scar tissue, hypertrophied synovium, and often a meniscus-like tissue. An accessory fascicle of the anteroinferior tibiofibular ligament has also been associated with this syndrome. Anterolat-

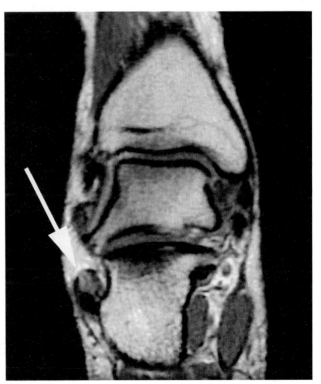

Figure 10

Severe splitting of the peroneus brevis tendon. Oblique coronal proton density-weighted magnetic resonance image. The normal peroneus brevis tendon has low signal. The arrow points to a split peroneus brevis tendon with high signal. The normal peroneus longus tendon is seen just inferior (plantar) to the abnormal tendon.

eral impingement syndrome is often confused with multiple other causes of lateral ankle pain. MRI has recently been used to diagnose this syndrome in patients with a confusing clinical presentation or in those in whom conservative therapy has failed.

The anterolateral gutter is usually best seen on axial images. It is defined by the ATF ligament anteriorly, the lateral malleolus laterally, and the talus medially. It normally contains fibrofatty tissue that follows fat signal on all pulse sequences. The most accurate diagnosis occurs when fluid fills the gutter outlining a discrete soft-tissue mass distinct from the ATF ligament. Fat-suppression images are useful to distinguish fat from soft-tissue masses. Care must be taken not to confuse a torn ATF with a soft-tissue mass.

Sinus Tarsi Syndrome

Abnormality in the sinus tarsi as a cause of ankle pain remains a somewhat controversial subject. It is thought that proliferative synovial tissue, inflammation, and scar tissue in the region of the sinus tarsi can cause ankle pain as well as a feeling of hindfoot instability. The reason for this is not immediately clear because the ligaments of the sinus tarsi do not appear to be primary stabilizers of the hindfoot, but there is an association with LCL injury. Local injection of anesthetic into the lateral aspect of the sinus tarsi can bring relief. The primary mechanism is an inversion injury, although an inflammatory process such as rheumatoid arthritis or gout has also been associated with the syndrome. MRI is the major imaging modality for evaluating the presence of a sinus tarsi syndrome.

Fat within the sinus tarsi provides good contrast for MRI. Any process that replaces the fat is readily recognizable. Two good pulse sequences for evaluating the sinus tarsi are sagittal T1 and IR sequences. On T1-weighted sequences the fat within the canal is normally of high signal (bright) and on IR sequences the fat is normally dark. A T2-weighted sequence in either the sagittal or coronal plane is also useful. Three basic patterns of the sinus tarsi syndrome have been described: (1) low signal on both T1- and T2-weighted sequences suggesting fibrosis; (2) low signal on T1-weighted sequences with diffuse high signal on T2-weighted sequences suggesting either a synovitis or inflammatory changes (Fig. 11); and (3) lobulated areas of low

signal on T1-weighted sequences that have high signal on T2-weighted sequences, suggesting synovial cysts. Other findings associated with the sinus tarsi syndrome are tears of the LCL and PTT. One caveat is that ankles imaged in the acute or subacute phase of injury can demonstrate edema within the sinus tarsi without necessarily developing the syndrome. This edema is most likely related to the trauma. Thus, an accurate clinical history is essential in evaluating the sinus tarsi.

Plantar Fasciitis

The diagnosis of plantar fasciitis is usually based on clinical factors. Patients are usually only referred for imaging studies if they have failed conservative therapy or have an atypical presentation. Arthritides such as rheumatoid arthritis and the seronegative spondyloarthropathies can also cause inflammation in the plantar fascia. The 3 primary imaging tests for evaluating the plantar fascia are radiographs, nuclear medicine 3-phase bone scan, and MRI.

Radiographs are useful for evaluating the osseous structures. There may be a plantar enthesophyte though its significance is often unclear. However, an enthesophyte with poorly defined or whiskery cortical margins can suggest a seronegative arthritis. The presence of erosions suggests rheumatoid arthritis. Thin, linear calcifications can also occasionally be seen within the fascia with calcium pyrophosphate dihydrate deposition.

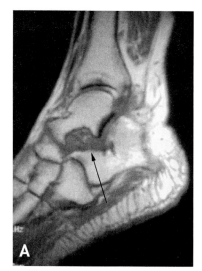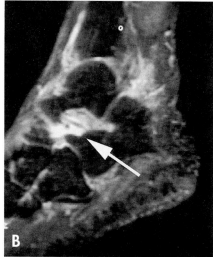

Figure 11

Sinus tarsi syndrome. **A,** Sagittal T1-weighted magnetic resonance image. The arrow points to the sinus tarsi, which normally contains the high signal of fat, but in this case the fat has been replaced. **B,** Sagittal inversion recovery magnetic resonance image. Diffuse high signal (arrow) is seen within the sinus tarsi. Similar changes were seen on T2-weighted sequences. Findings suggest diffuse inflammation/edema in the sinus tarsi.

The 3-phase bone scan usually reveals increased activity over the plantar aspect of the foot near the insertion of the plantar fascia on the second (soft-tissue) phase. On the third phase there may be some increased activity that localizes in the adjacent calcaneus. Markedly increased activity on the third phase would suggest a more inflammatory process and radiographs should be scrutinized for the presence of erosions or a whiskery plantar enthesophyte, which might indicate the presence of an arthropathy.

MRI allows direct imaging of the plantar fascia. The normal plantar fascia is a thin linear area of low signal on all pulse sequences. It normally measures about 3 mm in thickness. With plantar fasciitis, the fascia is thickened, usually > 5 mm, and there may be increased signal on T2 sequences both within the fascia and around it in the adjacent soft tissues. Often, signal increases in the adjacent bone marrow of the calcaneus on IR or fat-suppressed sequences (Fig. 12).

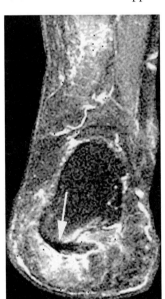

Figure 12

Plantar fasciitis. Coronal fast spin-echo T2-weighted sequence with chemical fat saturation. Diffuse thickening of the plantar fascia (arrow) is seen with marked edema in the plantar soft tissues and in the adjacent calcaneus.

Osseous and Joint Abnormalities

Calcaneus Fractures

The 2 primary methods for evaluating calcaneus fractures are radiography and CT. Radiography is important for the initial assessment and for subsequent follow-up. CT, however, allows a precise and accurate evaluation of the subtalar joint as well as the degree of comminution of the calcaneus. Another advantage of CT is that it allows evaluation of the flexor and peroneal tendons to determine if they are potentially entrapped within the fracture fragments. Follow-up CT scanning can evaluate the degree of subtalar arthrosis as

well as intra-articular fragments, bone spurs impinging on the tarsal tunnel or peroneal tendons, entrapment of tendons, and the location of screws.

The advent of spiral CT scanning has facilitated the rapid acquisition of data and has also allowed high-quality 2-dimensional and 3-dimensional reformations. Because the patient's foot is usually splinted or casted, it is often difficult to place the foot in multiple positions. In general, I try to have the patient place the foot flat on the table and obtain spiral 2-mm acquisitions through the hindfoot up to and through the calcaneocuboid joint. Thin 1-mm, 2-dimensional reformations can then be performed in the sagittal and axial planes. Alternatively, if the hindfoot can only be imaged in the axial plane, then a coronal reconstruction can be performed. Although not a standard practice, I perform 3-dimensional reconstruction for particularly complex fractures where it is difficult to visualize the spatial orientation of the fracture fragments.

The coronal plane is ideal for assessing the posterior facet of the subtalar joint. The degree of displacement and depression of the articular surface can be evaluated. Involvement of the middle facet, although not common, is also best seen in this plane. The flexor tendons and peroneal tendons are also best evaluated in this plane for potential entrapment. An axial reconstruction allows evaluation of the calcaneocuboid joint. The sagittal reconstruction allows assessment of the degree of depression along Böhler's angle.

Stress Fractures

Stress fractures can occur in virtually any bone of the foot and ankle, but are most common in the calcaneus, navicular, and metatarsals. Stress fractures are often occult on radiographs and are usually suspected on clinical grounds. When radiographic changes are present, they are often subtle, with changes that include trabecular sclerosis, periostitis, cortical thickening, or cortical defects. If further imaging is necessary because of confusing clinical findings or other reasons, then either bone scanning, CT, or MRI can be performed.

Bone scanning demonstrates focal increased osseous activity in the location of a stress fracture. One advantage of bone scanning is that it allows assessment of other osseous structures. It is not unusual to find other clinically occult areas of abnormal uptake. These probably represent areas of stress that either have not yet become apparent or are masked by the more advanced stress injury. Disadvantages of bone scanning include the radiation exposure as well as its low specificity.

CT scan is helpful in the evaluation of midfoot tarsal fractures. These fractures are often sagittally oriented and are best demonstrated with coronal imaging. CT can also be used to assess healing. Findings indicating a stress fracture on CT include cortical defects, increased attenuation within the marrow, sclerosis and thickening of trabeculae, and in the long bones of the metatarsals, focal endosteal thickening of the cortex and periosteal new bone.

With MRI, the primary finding of a stress reaction or fracture is marrow edema. Marrow edema is manifested as low signal on T1-weighted sequences and high signal on T2-weighted or IR sequences. At times a linear area of low signal on all sequences is seen and is one of the more reliable signs indicating a stress fracture (Fig. 13). Periosteal edema can also be seen as can endosteal cortical thickening, although the latter is usually better seen on CT. MRI does suffer from a lack of specificity because of the many causes of marrow edema. However, in the appropriate clinical setting, for example, screening an athlete for a stress fracture, a limited evaluation to exclude the presence of a stress fracture/reaction can be performed rapidly and usually at a reduced cost. A T1-weighted sequence and IR sequence can be used effectively and quickly to evaluate for a stress fracture.

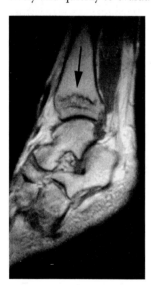

Figure 13

Stress fracture of the distal tibia. Sagittal T1-weighted MR image. A linear area of low signal is seen in the tibial metaphysis (arrow). Note that this area is just superior to the normal physeal scar, which is also of low signal. Inversion recovery sequences demonstrated high signal in the adjacent medullary space.

Osteochondritis Dissecans

This osseous lesion most commonly affects the talus. The primary questions to ask in the imaging assessment of the lesion are: (1) Is the overlying cartilage intact? and (2) Is the fragment displaced or loose? The 2 primary techniques that can be used to answer these questions are CT and MRI both with and without intra-articular contrast. The presence of contrast material in the joint facilitates both the evaluation of the overlying cartilage and the stability of the fragment. The main disadvantage of intra-articular contrast is that it is invasive.

Osteochondritis dissecans of the talus is best imaged in the coronal plane for both CT and MRI. With CT, the fragment

can be seen as a sclerotic or marrow-containing fragment of bone in a subarticular location. If the fragment has become detached, then a frank defect in the talus is seen and a search must be made for an intra-articular body. If intra-articular contrast is used, then imbibition of contrast through the cartilaginous surface is evidence of fissuring of the cartilage, and if contrast extends around the fragment then this is evidence that the fragment is loose in the bed.

Some advantages of MRI compared to CT are its greater sensitivity to fluid in the joint and the ability to use sequences that accentuate cartilage. The presence of fluid in the joint, whether natural or introduced, greatly facilitates the evaluation of osteochondritis dissecans. Fluid extending into the cartilage is the best evidence of a cartilage defect, and a smooth rim of high signal extending around the fragment indicates the fragment is no longer attached to the bed (Fig. 14). The fragment itself can be of uniformly low signal, most likely indicating sclerosis, or may contain marrow signal.

Growth Plate Injuries

MRI can be used to evaluate injuries to the growth plate of the distal tibia as well as the sequelae of such injuries. In particular, MRI can be used to determine if a bony bar is present and to determine its location. Several different pulse sequences make the cartilage of the physis appear bright. Against this bright background the bone bar appears black (Fig. 15). Certain sequences also allow the creation of a 2-dimensional map of the growth plate by using reconstruction techniques developed for magnetic resonance angiography. These maps, along with the multiplanar abilities of MRI, allow precise localization of the bone bar.

Tarsal Coalitions

The 2 most common coalitions are calcaneonavicular and talocalcaneal. In general, coalitions can be fibrous, cartilaginous, or osseous. However, some admixture of these types of coalitions can be found (that is, fibrocartilaginous). Plain radiography can sometimes depict these coalitions, but often is inconclusive. With radiography, it is difficult to distinguishing between the types of coalitions. Bone scans can show abnormal uptake in the regions of coalitions, but the lack of specificity and poor anatomic resolution limits the usefulness of this study. The 2 best studies for depiction of coalitions, especially subtalar coalitions, are CT and MRI.

CT is usually performed in the coronal plane for subtalar coalitions and in the axial plane for calcaneonavicular coalitions. Osseous coalitions are fairly obvious on CT with the bridging bone readily identified. Fibrous or cartilaginous coalitions can be more subtle and often indirect signs are used to make the diagnosis. One of these signs is an altered morphol-

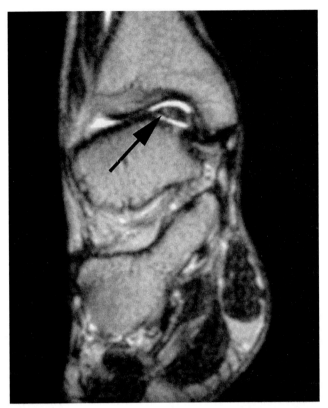

Figure 14

Osteochondritis dissecans of the medial talar dome. Coronal fast spin-echo T2-weighted magnetic resonance image. High signal (arrow) is seen surrounding an osteochondral dissecans fragment, which indicates joint fluid surrounding the fragment, and hence, a loose fragment.

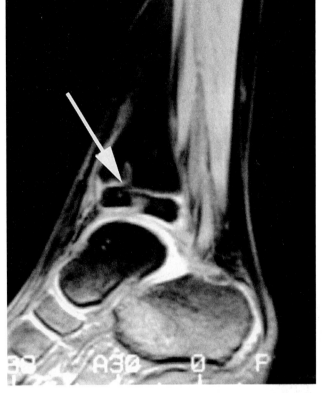

Figure 15

Bone bar through the tibial physis. Sagittal spoiled gradient-echo sequence with chemical fat saturation. The small linear area of low signal (arrow) seen extending through the bright physeal cartilage represents a bony bar. Also note the high signal in the epiphyseal ossification center, which is a sequalae of the child's previous Salter-Harris type 4 fracture.

ogy of the sustentaculum tali. Normally the medial margin of the sustentaculum tali is placed more cephalad than the lateral margin. With a coalition the medial margin is often displaced caudad giving the sustentaculum tali a medial plantar slope. A second sign is hypertrophy of the middle facet. The normally sclerotic subarticular margins of the middle facet also are lost with a fibrous or cartilaginous coalition. The articular surface can appear irregular with cystic changes within the bone.

Similar morphologic changes are seen with MRI. The diagnosis of an osseous coalition is made by marrow extending across the joint space. A cartilaginous coalition is present when there is loss of joint space and cartilage-like signal extending across the joint space. A fibrous coalition is defined by loss of joint space and low to intermediate signal extending across the joint (Fig. 16). A recent study noted that MRI was better than CT in depicting fibrous coalitions. One false positive was found with MRI because of the presence of pannus in the articulation, which mimicked fibrous tissue.

Lisfranc Joint Injuries

Injury of the tarsometatarsal joint (TMT) can range from subtle joint disruption to frank fracture-dislocation. The initial evaluation includes radiographs, which usually reveal disruption of the TMT joint as well as any fractures that may be present. However, disruption of the TMT joint can be subtle and care must be taken to ensure that all metatarsals are properly aligned with the appropriate tarsal bones. Stress views may be needed to assess the TMT joint, but these often have to be performed with the patient under sedation or with an anesthetic.

Recently, MRI has been used to assess the TMT joint. In addition to allowing evaluation of joint alignment, MRI can also allow visualization of the Lisfranc ligament, a vital stabilizer of the TMT joint. The Lisfranc ligament extends from the lateral aspect of the medial cuneiform to the medial aspect of the proximal second metatarsal. This ligament is seen as a hypointense band on oblique axial images obtained

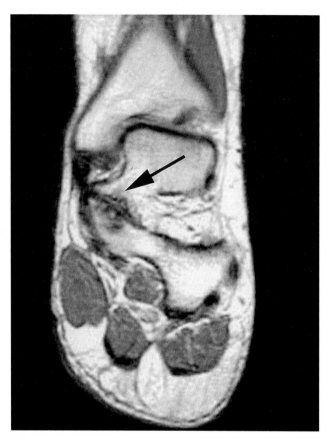

Figure 16

Fibrous coalition of the middle facet of the subtalar joint. Coronal proton density-weighted magnetic resonance image. A hypertrophied middle facet is seen with low and intermediate signal extending across the joint (arrow). Cystic changes are seen on both sides of the coalition.

parallel to the dorsum of the foot. Frank disruptions of the ligament can be identified as well as avulsions from the attachment sites. The tomographic nature of MRI also allows evaluation of alignment of the TMT. In the future, MRI may prove useful for the evaluation of equivocal cases.

Selective Joint Injections

Although this section does not discuss a specific disease process, it has been included here because it deals with several joint abnormalities such as osteoarthrosis and congenital deformities. Specifically this is a technique employed to help determine if the joint in question is in fact causing the patient's symptoms. This technique has been used to predict the outcome of and help select the joint for arthrodesis. The technique involves using fluoroscopic guidance to place a needle into the joint in question and then inject anesthetic, sometimes with steroid. The position of the needle is confirmed with a small injection of contrast. Immediately following the

injection the patient is then questioned regarding subjective pain relief and then evaluated by the orthopaedic surgeon.

In 1 study, there was a high correlation between pain relief after injection and subsequent pain relief following arthrodesis. In some instances, the surgical plan was altered based on the results of the injection. The authors also found poor correlation between the outcome of the injections and the results of previous radiographs, CT, or bone scans. The results of this study suggest that in patients with multiple degenerative joints, not all the joints need to be fused for a successful outcome and the correct joint for fusion can be reliably selected using selective anesthetic injections.

Infection

The best way to image and diagnose infection in general, and osteomyelitis in particular, is controversial. A radiograph should be obtained first. If characteristic changes of osteomyelitis are present, then little further imaging needs to be done in uncomplicated cases. Unfortunately, radiographs are frequently negative, especially in the early stages of the disease, or are complicated by the presence of neuropathic changes (a problem that can be encountered in the diabetic foot). Both nuclear medicine studies and MRI are excellent for excluding an osteomyelitis when the findings are normal (negative predictive value of MRI is 96%). Proponents of nuclear medicine studies point out the high cost of MRI. However, the specificity and sensitivity of nuclear medicine studies is comparable to MRI only when both a bone scan and indium-111 white cell scan are performed. The reported sensitivity of a combined bone scan and white cell scan in the diabetic foot ranges from 73% to 100% and the specificity from 55% to 91% for osteomyelitis. A recent report found the sensitivity and specificity of MRI for osteomyelitis in the diabetic foot to be 82% and 80%, respectively. The cost of 2 nuclear medicine studies combined may reach the cost of one MRI. Proponents of MRI point out that the spatial resolution of MRI exceeds that of nuclear medicine studies, making it possible to accurately plan biopsies and limited surgical resections. Ultimately, the type of examination obtained depends on the particular skills of the interpreting physician as well as the cost in a particular health-care setting.

As already described in the nuclear medicine section, a 3-phase bone scan is performed for the evaluation of osteomyelitis. The classic findings of osteomyelitis are increased blood flow on the arterial phase; increased activity in the surrounding soft tissues on the second phase; and focal increased activity within the bone on the third phase. Unfortunately, similar findings can be seen in the neuropathic foot.

Poor blood supply can also limit the delivery of the radioiso-tope. The indium-111 white cell scan shows activity over the infected area. One problem with the white cell scan is the poor spatial resolution, making it difficult to distinguish an adjacent cellulitis from an osteomyelitis. Digital superimpo-sition of the bone scan with the white scan can sometimes aid in localizing the infection.

The hallmark of osteomyelitis on MRI is the presence of marrow edema. Unfortunately, this is a nonspecific finding, as many processes cause edema. Other findings aid in distin-guishing an osteomyelitis from reactive marrow edema. Some of these findings include evidence of breaching of the cortical bone near an area of soft-tissue inflammation with extension of abnormal signal into the marrow. Confluent areas of high signal on T2-weighted images that have a signal intensity similar to the adjacent soft-tissue infection is anoth-er indirect sign. There is controversy regarding the utility of contrast in the MRI evaluation of osteomyelitis. There are proponents who claim that contrast increases the sensitivity and specificity and others who claim that contrast has no utility. The proponents believe that enhancement within the marrow space that is of the same degree as an adjacent cel-lulitis is a strong indication of osteomyelitis. A large prospec-tive study is probably needed to settle the issue. Contrast can be useful in evaluating soft-tissue or osseous abscesses. A well-demarcated region of high signal on a T2-weighted image with rim enhancement after administration of con-trast suggests the presence of an abscess.

Reflex Sympathetic Dystrophy

Reflex Sympathetic Dystrophy (RSD) is a pain syndrome with associated autonomic dysfunction. It has been reported to occur after even minor trauma or surgery. The best imag-ing method is a 3-phase bone scan. Sensitivity has been reported to be as high as 100% for bone scanning, with a specificity at approximately 66%.

The characteristic findings on radiographs are marked or persistent osteopenia and sometimes soft-tissue swelling. The finding of a persistent osteopenia after a patient has returned to weightbearing status after trauma, along with the appropriate clinical findings, is suggestive of the diagno-sis. On a 3-phase radionuclide bone scan there may be evi-dence of increased blood flow to the foot as well as activity in the soft tissues on the second phase. The third phase is the most characteristic, with diffuse increased isotope uptake throughout the foot and more focal uptake in a juxta-artic-ular distribution. Often there is poor definition of the bones on the third phase.

Recently an attempt has been made to define the MRI char-acteristics of RSD. In acute RSD, skin thickening, soft-tissue edema, and soft-tissue contrast enhancement were found. In the subacute stage, the results were more variable with both skin thickening and thinning, infrequent contrast enhance-ment, and no evidence of edema. With more chronic disease, again there were variable skin changes, but muscle atrophy was noted. Most of these findings are nonspecific and it seems unlikely that MRI would be used as a primary imag-ing modality in RSD. These findings are useful because they may be associated with RSD and could be potentially seen in a patient referred for MRI for foot pain who in fact had unrecognized RSD.

Other Conditions

Morton's Neuroma

Morton's neuroma is not a true neuroma but is in fact per-ineural fibrosis and nerve degeneration around the plantar digital nerve. A Morton's neuroma typically occurs as a painful mass-like lesion between the third and fourth metatarsal heads but can also occur between the second and third metatarsal heads. Both CT and MRI have been used to image Morton's neuromas. Most recent work has concentrat-ed on the use of MRI and this work will be discussed here.

MRI has a reported sensitivity of 87% and a specificity of 100%. However, a recent study suggests that asymptomatic Morton's neuromas may occur. This study indicated that neuromas over 5 mm in diameter were more likely to be symptomatic. Morton's neuromas tend to be isointense on T1- and T2-weighted pulse sequences, making them diffi-cult to visualize. Coronal (that is, the plane transverse to the long axis of the foot) images with T1-weighting have been reported to be the best for visualizing Morton's neuromas. Other pulse sequences reported as useful include fat-sup-pressed postcontrast sequences and IR sequences. On T1-weighted sequences, Morton's neuromas typically appear as intermediate signal intensity masses located between the metatarsal heads. The neuromas are of relatively low signal on T2-weighted sequences and this characteristic allows them to be distinguished from ganglion cysts, true neuro-mas, and intermetatarsal bursal fluid collections. Morton's neuromas typically demonstrate contrast enhancement.

Aggressive Fibromatosis

Plantar fibromatosis is a member of the group of diseases known as the fibromatoses. This tumor is considered benign, but has highly aggressive characteristics and may recur after resection. Because of the aggressive nature of the tumor, it

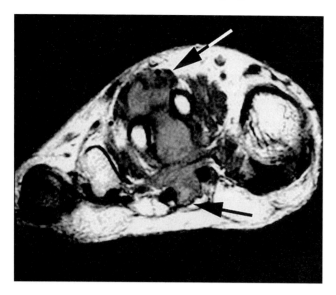

Figure 17

Aggressive fibromatosis. Coronal proton density-weighted magnetic resonance image. Lobulated areas of slightly high to intermediate signal (arrows) are seen extending between the second and third metatarsals and the flexor tendons. The patient had a previous resection of a plantar fibroma with recurrence of the tumor now evident.

infiltrates the surrounding tissues and causes compression of adjacent normal soft tissues.

MRI can clearly display the extent of the lesion, which is vital for surgical planning so that adequate margins can be obtained. The tumor has a characteristic location and signal characteristics. The tumor is isointense to muscle on T1- and T2-weighted images, shows variable contrast enhancement, and usually is hyperintense on IR sequences (Fig. 17). Deeper portions of the tumor sometimes demonstrate areas of increased signal intensity on T2-weighted sequences. The plantar border of the lesion tends to be well circumscribed, whereas the dorsal aspect often shows poorly defined borders and infiltration into the soft tissues. Clear-cell sarcoma is another malignancy that has shown MR signal characteristics similar to plantar fibromatosis.

Annotated Bibliography

Ligamentous Injuries

Chandnani VP, Harper MT, Ficke JR, et al: Chronic ankle instability: Evaluation with MR arthrography, MR imaging, and stress radiography. *Radiology* 1994;192:189–194.

The authors compare stress radiography with standard magentic resonance imaging (MRI) and magnetic resonance arthrography (MRA) in the assessment of lateral collateral ligament injuries. They conclude that MRA is the more sensitive and accurate test for evaluation of the anterior talofibular ligament and that both routine MRI and MRA are useful in the detection of associated injuries.

Tendon Injuries

Khoury NJ, el-Khoury GY, Saltzman CL, Brandser EA: MR imaging of posterior tibial tendon dysfunction. *Am J Roentgenol* 1996; 167:675–682.

This study evaluates the magnetic resonance imaging findings of posterior tibial tendon tears. The authors note that a severe tendinosis and a partial tear may have similar imaging features.

Rosenberg ZS, Beltran J, Cheung YY, Colon E, Herraiz F: MR features of longitudinal tears of the peroneus brevis tendon. *Am J Roentgenol* 1997;168:141–147.

An analysis of the magnetic resonance imaging features of longitudinal tears of the peroneus brevis tendon was performed as well as an analysis of other pathologic and normal conditions associated with these tears.

Tjin A Ton ER, Schweitzer ME, Karasick D: MR imaging of peroneal tendon disorders. *Am J Roentgenol* 1997;168:135–140.

Magnetic resonance imaging features of longitudinal tears of the peroneus brevis are described. Morphologic changes in the tendon as well as associated pathologic changes in the fibula are described.

Os Trigonum Syndrome

Wakeley CJ, Johnson DP, Watt I: The value of MR imaging in the diagnosis of the os trigonum syndrome. *Skeletal Radiol* 1996;25:133–136.

This article presents 3 patients with posterior ankle pain in whom magnetic resonance imaging was able to demonstrate that the pain was related to the os trigonum. The authors describe the imaging features and note that flexion and extension magnetic resonance imaging can be useful in evaluating the os trigonum.

Infections

Morrison WB, Schweitzer ME, Wapner KL, Hecht PJ, Gannon FH, Behm WR: Osteomyelitis in feet of diabetics: Clinical accuracy, surgical utility, and cost-effectiveness of MR imaging. *Radiology* 1995;196:557–564.

The authors compare the cost-effectiveness of magnetic resonance imaging (MRI) with combined skeletal scintigraphy and indium-111 white cell scanning. They find MRI to be comparable to the nuclear medicine studies in cost-effectiveness, but the authors believed that MRI was superior to the nuclear medicine studies in planning limited foot-sparing resections.

Tumors

Morrison WB, Schweitzer ME, Wapner KL, Lackman RD: Plantar fibromatosis: A benign aggressive neoplasm with a characteristic appearance on MR images. *Radiology* 1994;193:841–845.

This article describes the magnetic resonance imaging characteristics of plantar fibromatosis. The authors describe variable signal characteristics and enhancement, but a characteristic morphology of the tumors is studied.

Zanetti M, Ledermann T, Zollinger H, Hodler J: Efficacy of MR imaging in patients suspected of having Morton's neuroma. *Am J Roentgenol* 1997;168:529–532.

The authors tested various pulse sequences and concluded that T1-weighted sequences were best for localizing a Morton's neuroma. The authors also found magnetic resonance imaging to be useful for accurate localization of the lesion.

Selective Joint Injections

Khoury NJ, el-Khoury GY, Saltzman CL, Brandser EA: Intraarticular foot and ankle injections to identify source of pain before arthrodesis. *Am J Roentgenol* 1996;167:669–673.

The authors retrospectively analyzed the results of 20 (22 joints) patients who underwent arthrodesis on the basis of pain relief after selective joint injection with anesthetic. Out of the 20 patients, 17 had significant pain relief after injection and arthrodesis. The authors found that imaging studies were less useful in predicting outcome.

Tarsometatarsal Joint

Preidler KW, Brossmann J, Daenen B, Goodin D, Schweitzer M, Resnick D: MR imaging of the tarsometatarsal joint: Analysis of injuries in 11 patients. *Am J Roentgenol* 1996;167:1217–1222.

This study describes the magnetic resonance imaging (MRI) findings in injuries at the tarsometatarsal joint. MRI was able to detect joint malalignment in all patients studied as well as frequent injuries to Lisfranc's ligament. Intact Lisfranc's ligaments were associated with avulsion fractures.

Classic Bibliography

Cardone BW, Erickson SJ, Den Hartog BD, Carrera GF: MRI of injury to the lateral collateral ligamentous complex of the ankle. *J Comput Assist Tomogr* 1993;17:102–107.

Conti S, Michelson J, Jahss M: Clinical significance of magnetic resonance imaging in preoperative planning for reconstruction of posterior tibial tendon ruptures. *Foot Ankle* 1992;13:208–214.

Craig JG, Amin MB, Wu K, et al: Osteomyelitis of the diabetic foot: MR imaging. Pathologic correlation. *Radiology* 1997;203:849–855.

Erickson SJ, Quinn SF, Kneeland JB, et al: MR imaging of the tarsal tunnel and related spaces: normal and abnormal findings with anatomic correlation. *Am J Roentgenol* 1990;155:323–328.

Karasick D, Schweitzer ME: The os trigonum syndrome: Imaging features. *Am J Roentgenol* 1996;166:125–129.

Khoury NJ, el-Khoury GY, Saltzman CL, Kathol MH: Peroneus longus and brevis tendon tears: MR imaging evaluation. *Radiology* 1996;200:833–841.

Klein MA: MR imaging of the ankle: Normal and abnormal findings in the medial collateral ligament. *Am J Roentgenol* 1994;162:377–383.

Klein MA, Spreitzer AM: MR imaging of the tarsal sinus and canal: Normal anatomy, pathologic findings, and features of the sinus tarsi syndrome. *Radiology* 1993;186:233–240.

Logan PM, Janzen DL, O'Connell JX, Munk PL, Connell DG: Magnetic resonance imaging and histopathologic appearances of benign soft-tissue masses of the foot. *Can Assoc Radiol J* 1996;47:36–43.

Marcus CD, Ladam-Marcus VJ, Leone J, Malgrange D, Bonnet-Gausserand FM, Menanteau BP: MR imaging of osteomyelitis and neuropathic osteoarthropathy in the feet of diabetics. *Radiographics* 1996;16:1337–1348.

Miller TT, Staron RB, Feldman F, Parisien M, Glucksman WJ, Gandolfo LH: The symptomatic accessory tarsal navicular bone: Assessment with MR imaging. *Radiology* 1995;195:849–853.

Mitchell MJ, Bielecki D, Bergman AG, Kursunoglu-Brahme S, Sartoris DJ, Resnick D: Localization of specific joint causing hindfoot pain: Value of injecting local anesthetics into individual joints during arthrography. *Am J Roentgenol* 1995;164:1473–1476.

Mizel MS, Michelson JD, Newberg A: Peroneal tendon bupivacaine injection: Utility of concomitant injection of contrast material. *Foot Ankle Int* 1996;17:566–568.

Schweitzer ME, Caccese R, Karasick D, Wapner KL, Mitchell DG: Posterior tibial tendon tears: Utility of secondary signs for MR imaging diagnosis. *Radiology* 1993;188:655–659.

Schweitzer ME, Eid ME, Deely D, Wapner K, Hecht P: Using MR imaging to differentiate peroneal splits from other peroneal disorders. *Am J Roentgenol* 1997;168:129–133.

Schweitzer ME, Mandel S, Schwartzman RJ, Knobler RL, Tahmoush AJ: Reflex sympathetic dystrophy revisited: MR imaging findings before and after infusion of contrast material. *Radiology* 1995;195:211–214.

Terk MR, Kwong PK, Suthar M, Horvath BC, Colletti PM: Morton neuroma: Evaluation with MR imaging performed with contrast enhancement and fat suppression. *Radiology* 1993; 189:239–241.

Zanetti M, Strehle JK, Zollinger H, Hodler J: Morton neuroma and fluid in the intermetatarsal bursae on MR images of 70 asymptomatic volunteers. *Radiology* 1997;203:516–520.

Index